CLINICAL NEUROSURGERY

CONGRESS OF NEUROLOGICAL SURGEONS

1951

ERUDITIO OBSERVANTIA SOCIETAS

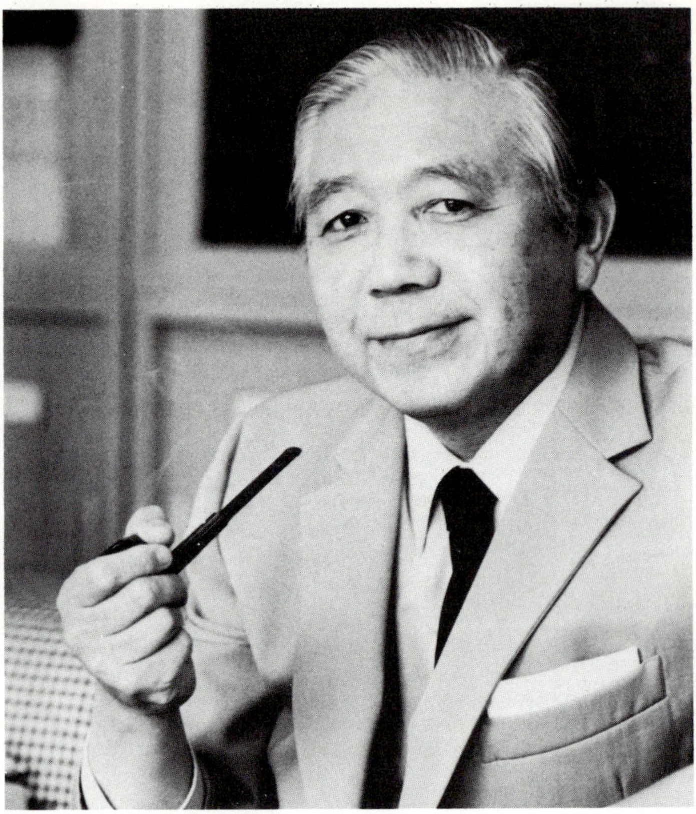

KEIJI SANO, M.D., D.M.SC., F.A.C.S. (HON.)

CLINICAL NEUROSURGERY

Proceedings

OF THE

CONGRESS OF NEUROLOGICAL SURGEONS

Toronto, Ontario, Canada

1982

SANS TACHE

WILLIAMS & WILKINS
Baltimore/London

Made in the United States of America

Library of Congress Cataloging in Publication Data

The Library of Congress cataloged this title as serial:

Congress of Neurological Surgeons.
Clinical neurosurgery. Proceedings. v. 1–1953–00
Baltimore, Williams & Wilkins
v. illus. 24 cm. annual.

1. Nervous system—Surgery. I. Title.

RD593.A1C63 617.48 54-12666 rev

Library of Congress [r57f1]

ISBN 0-683-02025-0

COMPOSED AND PRINTED IN THE
UNITED STATES OF AMERICA

Preface

The Thirtieth Volume of *Clinical Neurosurgery* is dedicated to Keiji Sano, Honored Guest and Principal Speaker at the Thirty-Second Annual Meeting of the Congress of Neurological Surgeons held in Toronto, Ontario, Canada, October 3–8, 1982.

Dr. Sano's presentation embraced his long-standing interests in perturbations of cerebral blood flow and metabolism following subarachnoid hemorrhage and varied manifestations of primary intracranial neoplasms. His insights into mechanistic phenomena underlying the observation of cerebral vasospasms following subarachnoid hemorrhage provide a substrate for development of protocols designed to ameliorate this major source of postsubarachnoid hemorrhage morbidity. Professor Sano's extensive experience in the management of pineal region neoplasms enables a thorough assessment of considerations relevant to masses found within the region of the pineal; his development of an integrated approach to the management of primary glial neoplasms reflects not only his vast experience with the management of such problems but also his superb capacity to synthesize a reasoned management protocol embracing the many disciplines which come to bear upon such efforts.

A biographical sketch defining the role that Professor Sano has played in the evolution of neurosurgery as a discipline in Japan, as well as his outstanding influence on international neurosurgery, is provided by Kenichi Uemura.

The themes of the meeting, "Pediatric Neurosurgery" and "Spinal Surgery," were selected by Dr. Donald H. Stewart, Jr., President, Congress of Neurological Surgeons. Dr. Stewart enjoys a long and distinguished role as a vigorous participant in many Congress activities. He has been a dynamic force in the activities of the Joint Socio-Economic Committee, in which he has occupied a position of distinguished leadership for many years. In his presidential address, Dr. Stewart emphasized the role that our traditional concern for quality has played in the evolution of neurosurgery as a distinguished discipline. Dr. Stewart calls for a renewed and reinforced emphasis on concerns for quality at every level of neurosurgical activity, embracing the process of resident selection, training of our residents and, perhaps most importantly, a continued effort at maintaining the highest standards of quality in all of its ramifications in our neurosurgical practice. A final appeal to the role that we as community leaders must play in humanitarian considerations influencing society at large brought this heartwarming presidential address to its close in a manner undoubtedly leaving all of us privileged to hear this address with a heightened sense of moral and social responsibility.

Volume 30 is divided into three sections. The first of these embraces the Presidential Address, presentations of our Honored Guests, the superb presentation by our Resident Award Winner, Dr. Mervin P. Kril, and selected material from our special courses. Section II focuses on the arena of pediatric neurosurgery, with particular emphasis on problems related to pediatric brain tumors and dysraphic states. An extensive consideration of the arena embracing spinal surgery, including assessment of chemonucleolysis, constitutes Section III.

Dr. Christoper Shields once again demonstrated his indefatigable efforts in his role as the Annual Meeting Chairman; Dr. Donald O. Quest, our distinguished Treasurer, was the Scientific Program Chairman. We are all indeed grateful for their efforts in securing distinguished speakers of international stature and expertise whose presentations constitute the basis from which the text derives.

At this point, the Editor would like to re-emphasize the Peer Review process underlying the genesis of *Clinical Neurosurgery*. The initial, and perhaps most important, phase of this screening process begins with the selection of the scientific program participants. This selection involves an intense review of contributions made by numerous distinguished contributors to selected academic disciplines; the final choice of a given participant represents a consensus of the Scientific Program Committee defining the expertise of the participant. Manuscripts are then solicited by the Editorial Board of *Clinical Neurosurgery* from selected scholars; these manuscripts are then critically reviewed by the Editorial Board of *Clinical Neurosurgery*. Eventually, those manuscripts deemed to represent the highest level of scientific endeavor and merit with respect to a focused discipline are selected to constitute the body of this book.

The Editor gratefully acknowledges the outstanding effort of each Associate Editor in his role in the genesis of this monograph. Sincere appreciation is expressed for the outstanding counsel of Alice Reid of Williams & Wilkins, and grateful appreciation is expressed to Mrs. Nancy Blackard for her continued efforts on behalf of *Clinical Neurosurgery*. The editor would like to express particular appreciation to Shokei Yamada, M.D., Ph.D., for his translation of Dr. Sano's bibliography.

Finally, continued appreciation is extended to President Stewart and members of the Publication Committee of the Congress of Neurological Surgeons for their confidence and support for this Editorial Board.

MARTIN H. WEISS, M.D.
Editor-in-Chief
Associate Editors:
J. LOBO ANTUNES, M.D.
MICHAEL L. J. APUZZO, M.D.
PAUL COOPER, M.D.
MICHAEL EDWARDS, M.D.
RONALD IGNELZI, M.D.
JOHN LITTLE, M.D.
ARTHUR MARLIN, M.D.
LAWRENCE PITTS, M.D.
MICHAEL SALCMAN, M.D.
ROBERT SPETZLER, M.D.
H. RICHARD WINN, M.D.

Honored Guests

1952—Professor Herbert Olivecrona, Stockholm, Sweden
1953—Sir Geoffrey Jefferson, Manchester, England
1954—Dr. Kenneth G. McKenzie, Toronto, Canada
1955—Dr. Carl W. Rand, Los Angeles, California
1956—Dr. Wilder G. Penfield, Montreal, Canada
1957—Dr. Francis C. Grant, Philadelphia, Pennsylvania
1958—Dr. A. Earl Walker, Baltimore, Maryland
1959—Dr. William J. German, New Haven, Connecticut
1960—Dr. Paul C. Bucy, Chicago, Illinois
1961—Professor Eduard A. V. Busch, Copenhagen, Denmark
1962—Dr. Bronson S. Ray, New York, New York
1963—Dr. James L. Poppen, Boston, Massachusetts
1964—Dr. Edgar A. Kahn, Ann Arbor, Michigan
1965—Dr. James C. White, Boston, Massachusetts
1966—Dr. Hugo A. Krayenbühl, Zurich, Switzerland
1967—Dr. W. James Gardner, Cleveland, Ohio
1968—Professor Norman M. Dott, Edinburgh, Scotland
1969—Dr. Wallace B. Hamby, Cleveland, Ohio
1970—Dr. Barnes Woodhall, Durham, North Carolina
1971—Dr. Elisha S. Gurdjian, Detroit, Michigan
1972—Dr. Francis Murphey, Memphis, Tennessee
1973—Dr. Henry G. Schwartz, St. Louis, Missouri
1974—Dr. Guy L. Odom, Durham, North Carolina
1975—Dr. William H. Sweet, Boston, Massachusetts
1976—Dr. Lyle A. French, Minneapolis, Minnesota
1977—Dr. Richard C. Schneider, Ann Arbor, Michigan
1978—Dr. Charles G. Drake, London, Ontario, Canada
1979—Dr. Frank H. Mayfield, Cincinnati, Ohio
1980—Dr. Eben Alexander, Jr., Winston-Salem, North Carolina
1981—Dr. J. Garber Galbraith, Birmingham, Alabama
1982—Dr. Sano Keiji, Toyko, Japan

Officers of the Congress of Neurological Surgeons 1982

DONALD H. STEWART, JR., M.D.
President

JOHN M. TEW, JR., M.D.
President-Elect

EDWARD F. DOWNING, M.D.
Vice President

JOSEPH C. MAROON, M.D.
Secretary

DONALD O. QUEST, M.D.
Treasurer

EXECUTIVE COMMITTEE
J. Fletcher Lee, M.D.

HAL L. HANKINSON, M.D.
ROBERT RATCHESON, M.D.
J. CHARLES RICH, JR., M.D.
MICHAEL SALCMAN, M.D.
CHRISTOPHER B. SHIELDS, M.D.

GEORGE SYBERT, M.D.
ROBERT M. CROWELL, M.D.
JULIAN T. HOFF, M.D.
DAVID L. KELLY, JR., M.D.
EDWARD R. LAWS, JR., M.D.
DAVID STORRS, M.D.

CHRISTOPHER B. SHIELDS, M.D., *Chairman, Annual Meeting Committee*
DONALD O. QUEST, M.D., *Chairman, Scientific Program Committee*

Contributors

A. LELAND ALBRIGHT, M.D., Assistant Professor, Department of Neurosurgery, University of Pittsburgh, Pittsburgh, Pennsylvania (Chapter 15)

MICHAEL L. J. APUZZO, M.D., Professor of Neurological Surgery, University of Southern California, School of Medicine, Los Angeles, California (Chapter 5)

VALLO BENJAMIN, M.D., Professor, Department of Neurological Surgery, New York University, New York, New York (Chapter 30)

DEREK A. BRUCE, M.B., CH.B., Children's Hospital of Philadelphia and University of Pennsylvania School of Medicine, Philadelphia, Pennsylvania (Chapter 25)

PETER W. CARMEL, M.D., Associate Professor of Neurosurgery, Columbia University, College of Physicians & Surgeons, New York, New York (Chapter 20)

NORRIS CARROLL, M.D., Associate Professor of Orthopaedic Surgery, University of Toronto, Toronto, Ontario, Canada (Chapter 22)

MAURICE CHOUX, M.D., Professor, Department of Pediatric Neurosurgery, Hôpital des Enfants de la Timone, Marseilles, France (Chapter 14)

THOMAS B. DUCKER, M.D., Professor and Chairman, Division Neurological Surgery, University of Maryland School of Medicine, Baltimore, Maryland (Chapter 27)

QUENTIN J. DURWARD, M.B., CH.B., Division of Neurosurgery, Department of Clinical Neurological Sciences, Faculty of Medicine, University of Western Ontario, University Hospital, London, Ontario, Canada (Chapter 29)

MICHAEL S. B. EDWARDS, M.D., Assistant Professor of Neurological Surgery, Department of Neurosurgery, University of California, San Francisco, California (Chapter 12)

FRED EPSTEIN, M.D., Associate Professor of Neurosurgery, New York University Medical Center, New York, New York (Chapter 19)

CHARLES R. FITZ, M.D., Associate Professor, University of Toronto; Head, Division of Special Procedures, Department of Radiology, The Hospital for Sick Children, Toronto, Ontario, Canada (Chapter 10)

BARRY N. FRENCH, M.D., F.R.C.S.(C), F.A.C.S., Associate Clinical Professor, Department of Neurological Surgery, University of California, Davis, California (Chapter 17)

MOKHTAR GADO, M.D., Professor, Mallinckrodt Institute of Radiology, Section of Neuroradiology, Washington University School of Medicine, St. Louis, Missouri (Chapter 34)

FLOYD H. GILLES, M.D., Professor of Neuropathology, Childrens' Hospital Medical Center, Boston, Massachusetts (Chapter 9)

DEREK C. HARWOOD-NASH, M.D., Department of Radiology, University of Toronto and The Hospital for Sick Children, Toronto, Ontario, Canada (Chapter 18)

JACQUES HASSOUN, M.D., Neuropathology, Hôpital de la Timone, Marseilles, France (Chapter 14)

E. BRUCE HENDRICK, M.D., F.R.C.S.(C), Professor of Surgery, University of Toronto and The Hospital for Sick Children, Toronto, Ontario, Canada (Chapters 13, 23, and 24)

FRED J. HODGES III, M.D., Mallinckrodt Institute of Radiology, Section of Neuroradiology, Washington University School of Medicine, St. Louis, Missouri (Chapter 34)

JULIAN HOFF, M.D., Professor and Chief of Neurosurgery, University of Michigan Medical Center, Ann Arbor, Michigan (Chapter 31)

HAROLD J. HOFFMAN, M.D., F.R.C.S.(C), Professor of Neurosurgery, University of Toronto and The Hospital for Sick Children, Toronto, Ontario, Canada (Chapters 13, 23, and 24)

ROBIN P. HUMPHREYS, M.D., F.R.C.S.(C), Associate Professor of Surgery, Division of Neurosurgery, Department of Surgery, University of Toronto and The Hospital for Sick Children, Toronto, Ontario, Canada (Chapters 13, 23, and 24)

ALASDAIR G. W. HUNTER, M.SC., M.D. C.M., F.R.C.P.(C), Associate Professor, Department of Pediatrics, University of Ottawa, Ottawa, Ontario, Canada (Chapter 6)

DEREK JENKIN, M.B., Professor of Radiology, University of Toronto, Ontario, Canada (Chapter 11)

MERVIN P. KRIL, M.D., Department of Neurological Surgery, University of Southern California, Los Angeles, California (Chapter 5)

RONALD J. LEMIRE, M.D., Professor of Pediatrics, University of Washington, School of Medicine, Seattle, Washington (Chapter 8)

GABRIEL LENA, M.D., Department of Pediatric Neurosurgery, Neurochirurgein, Hopital des Enfantes de la Timone, Marseilles, France (Chapter 14)

VICTOR A. LEVIN, M.D., Department of Neurological Surgery, School of Medicine, University of California, San Francisco, California (Chapter 12)

JOHN T. LUCAS, Department of Neurosurgery, University of Maryland Hospital, Baltimore, Maryland (Chapter 27)

ROBERT L. MCLAURIN, M.D., Professor and Chairman, Division of Neurosurgery, University of Cincinnati, Cincinnati, Ohio (Chapter 16)

DAVID G. MCLONE, M.D., Ph.D., Division of Pediatric Neurosurgery, Department of Surgery, The Childrens' Memorial Hospital, Northwestern University Medical School, Chicago, Illinois (Chapters 18 and 21)

ARNOLD H. MENEZES, M.D., Associate Professor, Division of Neurosurgery, University of Iowa Hospitals, Iowa City, Iowa (Chapter 28)

THOMAS P. NAIDICH, M.D., Associate Professor of Radiology, Children's Memorial Hospital, Northwestern University Medical School, Chicago, Illinois (Chapter 18)

JASH PATEL, M.D., Mallinckrodt Institute of Radiology, Section of Neuroradiology, Washington University School of Medicine, St. Louis, Missouri (Chapter 34)

S. J. PEERLESS, M.D., F.R.C.S.(C), Division of Neurosurgery, Department of Clinical Neurological Sciences, Faculty of Medicine, University of Western Ontario, University Hospital, London, Ontario, Canada (Chapter 29)

JEROME B. POSNER, M.D., Professor, Department of Neurology, Cornell University Medical College, New York, New York (Chapter 36)

UROS ROESSMANN, M.D., Professor of Neuropathology, Case Western Reserve University, Cleveland, Ohio (Chapter 7)

KEIJI SANO, M.D., D.M.SC., F.A.C.S. (Hon.), Emeritus Professor of Neurosurgery, Faculty of Medicine, Teikyo University, Tokyo, Japan. Honored Guest of the Congress of Neurological Surgeons, 1982. (Chapters 2, 3, and 4)

LUIS SCHUT, M.D., Professor of Neurosurgery, University of Pennsylvania, Children's Hospital of Philadelphia, Philadelphia, Pennsylvania (Chapter 25)

EDWARD L. SELJESKOG, M.D., PH.D., Professor, Department of Neurological Surgery, University of Minnesota Hospitals, Minneapolis, Minnesota (Chapter 32)

NEAL SLATKIN, M.D., Department of Neurology, Cornell University Medical College, New York, New York (Chapter 36)

BENNETT M. STEIN, M.D., Byron Stookey Professor, Chairman, Department of Neurological Surgery, Columbia University, College of Physicians & Surgeons, New York, New York (Chapter 37)

DONALD H. STEWART, JR., M.D., Clinical Assistant Professor, Department of Neurosurgery, Upstate Medical Center, Syracuse, New York, President of the Congress of Neurological Surgeons (Chapter 1)

LESLIE N. SUTTON, M.D., Children's Hospital of Philadelphia and University of Pennsylvania School of Medicine, Philadelphia, Pennsylvania (Chapter 25)

CHARLES H. TATOR, M.D., PH.D., F.R.C.S.(C), Professor of Surgery

(Neurosurgery), University of Toronto, Toronto, Ontario, Canada (Chapter 26)

JOHN C. VANGILDER, M.D., Professor and Chairman, Division of Neurosurgery, University of Iowa Hospitals, Iowa City, Iowa (Chapter 28)

CONSTANCE A. WALLECK, Instructor, School of Nursing, University of Maryland Hospital, Baltimore, Maryland (Chapter 27)

DAVID WATERS, M.D., Section of Neurosurgery, University of Michigan Medical Center, Ann Arbor, Michigan (Chapter 31)

CLARK WATTS, M.D., Professor and Chief, Division of Neurosurgery, University of Missouri-Columbia, Health Sciences Center, Columbia, Missouri (Chapter 33)

PHILIP R. WEINSTEIN, M.D., Professor and Chairman, Division of Neurological Surgery, University of Arizona, Health Science Center, Tucson, Arizona (Chapter 35)

CHARLES B. WILSON, M.D., Department of Neurological Surgery, School of Medicine, University of California, San Francisco, California (Chapter 12)

Biography of Keiji Sano, M.D., D.M.Sc., F.A.C.S. (Hon.)

Dr. Keiji Sano was born on June 30, 1920, in the quiet and scenic town of Fujinomiya in Shizuoka Prefecture which lies at the foot of Mt. Fuji, about 100 kilometers to the west of Tokyo. He was the first son of Dr. and Mrs. Takeo Sano. His father was a well-known surgeon. After Dr. Sano graduated from high school there, he entered the University of Tokyo Faculty of Medicine, from which he graduated with his M.D. degree in 1945.

Because there was no internship in Japan, he joined the First Surgical Department of the University of Tokyo to receive postgraduate training in general surgery from Professor Ohtsuki. Neurosurgery in Japan originated from this department of surgery through the efforts of Kentaro Shimizu (1903–). Dr. Shimizu first joined the Department of Psychiatry after graduating from the University of Tokyo in 1929, but when two of his patients died from misdiagnosed brain tumors, he changed his mind and became a neurosurgeon. In 1932, he joined the First Surgical Department. When Dr. Sano joined the Department, Dr. Shimizu was actively practicing neurosurgery as an Associate Professor of Surgery.

In 1948, Dr. Shimizu became the Professor and Chairman of the First Surgical Department and, thereafter, Dr. Sano specialized in neurosurgery. In 1948 he published several papers on the techniques of percutaneous cerebral angiography. In 1951, he was awarded a degree of Doctor of Medical Science (D.M.Sc.), which corresponds to a Ph.D. in medicine. Dr. Sano obtained a fellowship from the Ministry of Education of Japan to study neurosurgery with Drs. Naffziger and Boldrey at the University of California at San Francisco and neuropathology with Dr. Nathan Malmud from 1951 to 1952.

Dr. Sano was promoted to Lecturer and Chief of the Outpatient Clinic of Neurosurgery in 1965 and then to Associate Professor of Neurosurgery at the Institute of Brain Research, University of Tokyo Faculty of Medicine, in 1957. In the same year he was married to his wife, Sumako. In 1962 the Japanese Government first approved and opened an independent Department of Neurosurgery at the University of Tokyo and appointed Dr. Sano as the first Professor and Chairman of the department. Later in the same year, another Department of Neurosurgery was approved at Niigata University where Dr. Komei Ueki was appointed as the Professor and Chairman. Dr. Sano and Dr. Ueki, pioneering neurosurgeons, worked continuously for almost half a century until neurosurgery was officially recognized as a definite independent discipline of clinical medicine. An additional 10 years were necessary until the Japanese Government decided to open a Department of Neurosurgery in every national university hospital.

In 1948, the first meeting on neurosurgical research was held at Niigata, and after 7 meetings, the Japan Neurosurgical Society was organized in 1952. In 1965, Dr. Sano was elected the President of the Japan Neurosurgical Society. In addition to being the secretary for the society for 20 years of his professorship, he devoted his entire professional life not only to his own neurosurgical research at the University of Tokyo but also to the development of neurosurgery throughout Japan by establishing a standardized postgraduate training curriculum for neurosurgery.

The Japanese Board of Neurosurgery was organized in 1966 with regulations on training curriculum and training institutes; Dr. Sano was the Chairman of the Board from 1967 to 1973 and again from 1979 to 1980. He was also the President of the Japanese Association for Research in Stereo-Encephalotomy in 1966, President of the Asian and Australasian Society of Neurological Surgeons from 1967 to 1971, President of the World Federation of Neurosurgical Societies from 1969 to 1973, Chairman of the 3rd Conference on Surgery of Apoplexy in 1974, President of the Japanese Society of CNS Computed Tomography since 1978, General Chairman of the Workshop on Pituitary Tumors since 1978, Chairman of the 3rd Wilder Penfield Memorial Conference in 1980, President of the 4th Conference on Neurotraumatology in 1981, and President of the Japanese Congress of Neurological Surgeons in 1981.

His contribution to neurosurgical research has been outstanding. Between 1948 and 1981, he published 629 papers (153 in English and 2 in German), including 162 on intracranial and spinal tumors, 119 on cerebrovascular diseases, 80 on head injuries, 48 on stereotactic and functional neurosurgery, 43 on EEG, 32 on other diagnostic methods, 24 on congenital anomalies and pediatric neurosurgery, 20 on operative techniques and paraoperative care, and 16 on epilepsy.

Obviously, the scope of his research has been too wide to review here. I would like to make special mention, though, of his works on thalamotomy for pain, posteromedial hypothalamotomy for pain and behavior disorders, BUdR-antimetabolite-radiation therapy and boron-neutron capture therapy for glioblastoma, and artificial embolization for large AVMs, and his research on the mechanism of vasopasm and of head injuries.

It is with the great pride of all Japanese neurosurgeons that Dr. Keiji Sano, the real establisher of Japanese neurosurgery, was invited to be the Honored Guest of the 32nd Annual Meeting of the Congress of Neurological Surgeons.

KENICHI UEMURA

Bibliography of Keiji Sano, M.D., D.M.Sc., F.A.C.S. (Hon.)

1. Shimizu, K., Sano, K. Pulseless disease. Rinsho Geka (Clin. Surg.), *3:* 377–396, 1948.
2. Shimizu, K., and Sano, K. Intradural pneumography. Shujutsu (Operation), *3:* 1–5, 1949.
3. Sano, K. Chronic localized meningitis: Case report. No to Shinkei (Brain and Nerve), *1:* 125–129, 1949.
4. Sano, K. The method for vertebral artery injection. No to Shinkei (Brain and Nerve), *2:* 28–37, 1950.
5. Sano, K. Transfrontal minicraniotomy. No to Shinkei (Brain and Nerve), *2:* 227–229, 1950.
6. Sano, K. Cerebral angiography. Saishin Igaku (Modern Med.), *5:* 588–598, 1950.
7. Sano, K. Surgical approach to the patient with impaired consciousness. In: *Symposium of Recent Advance in Emergency Treatment*, pp. 38–45. Kinbara-Shoten, Tokyo, 1950.
8. Sano, K. Thalamolaminotomy: Case report. No to Shinkei (Brain and Nerve), *2:* 360–361, 1950.
9. Sano, K. Activation of the brain waves, especially action of trans-π-oxocamphor. Rinsho (Clinic), *4:* 636–642, 1951.
10. Shimizu, K., and Sano, K. Pulseless disease. J. Neuropathol. Clin. Neurol., *1:* 37–47, 1951.
11. Sano, K., and Hayashi, S. Operative method and operative consideration of cavum septi pellucidi and cavum vergae. No to Shinkei (Brain and Nerve), *3:* 221–224, 1951.
12. Sano, K., and Malamud, N. Clinical significance of sclerosis of the cornu Ammonis. Ictal "psychic phenomena." Arch. Neurol. Psychiatry, *70:* 40–53, 1953.
13. Sano, K., and Takeuchi, K. Synergetic movement of the occulomotor nerve and trigeminal nerve-etiology and treatment. Rinsho Ganka (Clin. Ophthalmol.), *8:* 315–320, 1954.
14. Shimizu, K., and Sano, K. Head trauma. In: *Shinryo Iten (Therapeutic Reference Book)*, Vol. 2, pp. 118–154. edited by Y. Miami and T. Fukada, 1954.
15. Sano, K. Cingulectomy in treatment of agitated mental defectives. No to Shinkei (Brain and Nerve), *6:* 146–156, 1954.
16. Sano, K., and Kitamura, K. Foci of psychomotor attacks. No to Shinkei (Brain and Nerve), *6:* 247–272, 1954.
17. Sano, K. Brain tumor and electroencephalogram. Sogo Rinshio

(Gen. Clin. Med.), *3:* 1758–1767, 1954.

18. Sano, K., and Takeuchi, K. Syndrome of crocodile tears. Seishin Shinkei-geka (Psychosurg. Neurosurg.), *57:* 42, 1955.
19. Sano, K., Takeuchi, I., and Nakamura, N. Marin Amat Syndrome and syndrome of crocodile tears. Seishin Shinkei-geku (Psychosurg. Neurosurg.), *56:* 566–567, 1955.
20. Takeuchi, I., and Sano, K. Therapeutic inhalation of carbon dioxide and oxygen. No to Shinkei (Brain and Nerve), *7:* 9–18, 1955.
21. Sano, K., and Takeuchi, I. Marcus Gunn Phenomenon. Rinsho Ganka (Clin. Ophthalmol.), *9:* 614–623, 1955.
22. Sano, K. Cerebral localization by electroencephalography. In: *Physiology of the Central Nervous System*, pp. 35–45. edited by K. Motokawa. Iwanami Shoten, Tokyo, 1955.
23. Sano, K. Surgical treatment in head trauma. Rinsho Geka (Clin. Surg.), *10:* 795–803, 1955.
24. Sano, K. Electroencephalographic diagnosis of diseases of the nervous system. Shinkei-Kenkyu no Shinpo (Adv. Neurol. Res.), *1:* 21–52, 1956.
25. Sano, K. Cerebral angiography. Shinkei-Kenkyu no Shinpo (I Adv. Neurol. Res.), *1:* 40–49, 1956; (II Adv. Neurol. Res.), *1:* 109–139, 1956.
26. Sano, K. Cerebral angiography. Igaku no Ayumi (Adv. Med.), *22:* 307–322, 1956.
27. Sano, K. *Operative Procedures in Head Trauma-Complications and Their Treatment*, pp. 237–253. Igaku-Shoin, Tokyo, 1956.
28. Sano, K. Early diagnosis of brain tumors. Gan no Rinsho (Clin. Practice Cancer), *3:* 121–133, 1957.
29. Sano, K. Surgical treatment of psychomotor attacks. Nihon Geka-Gakkai Zasshi (J. Japanese Soc. Surg.), *58:* 762–766, 1957.
30. Sano, K. *Postoperative Treatment in Neurosurgery*, pp. 40–48. edited by A. Ichikawa, T. Fukuda, and N. Kuji. Kinbara-Shuppon, Tokyo, 1957.
31. Sano, K. Temporal lobe and psychomotor attacks. Shinkei-Kenkyu no Shinpo (Adv. Neurol. Res.), *2:* 65–74, 1957.
32. Sano, K. Cerebral localization by electroencephalography. Igaku no Doko *(Trends in Medicine)*, 10: 85–107, 1957.
33. Sano, K. Roentogenological diagnosis of brain tumors. Saishin Igaku (Modern Med.), *12:* 2222–2234, 1957.
34. Sano, K. Role of electroencephalography in diagnosis of brain tumors. Shinkei-Kenkyu no Shinpo (Adv. Neurol. Res.), *2:* 267–282, 1957.

35. SANO, K. Testing of brain function. Shinkei-Kenkyu no Shinpo (Adv. in Neurol. Res.), *2:* 337–369, 1957.
36. SANO, K., and SATO, F. Advances in electroencephalography. Rinsho Byori (Clin. Pathol.), *Special Issue 6:* 158–168, 1957.
37. SANO, K., and SATO, F. Electroencephalography. Naika (Medicine), *1:* 151–161, 1958.
38. SANO K. Clinical application of electroencephalography. In: *Handbook of Pathological Physiology*, Vol. 8, pp. 29–65. Nakayama-Shoten, 1958.
39. HAYASHI, S., WATANABE, J., and SANO, K. Carotid sinus reflex. Geka no Ryoiki (Fields Surg.), *6:* 97–108, 1958.
40. SANO, K. Neurosurgical consideration on temporal lobe function. Seishin-Shinkei-Gaku Zasshi (J. Psychiatry Neurol.), *60:* 1031–1055, 1958.
41. SANO, K., and YODONAWA, T. Studies on ictal EEG changes (I). EEG. J. (Suppl. 12): 22–25, 1958.
42. SANO, K. Neurosurgical consideration of the orbito-temporo-limbic system. EEG. J. (Suppl 12): 142–147, 1958.
43. SANO, K. Trigemino-oculomotor synkineses. Neurol. Med.-Chirurg., *1:* 29–51, 1959.
44. SANO, K. Tests for neurological function. Nihon Rinsho (Japanese Clin. Med.), *17:* 314–326, 1959.
45. SANO, K., and SATO, F. Electroencephalography. In: *Clinical Laboratory Tests in Pediatric Diseases*, edited by Takatsu and Momiki, pp. 649–680. Igaku-Shoin, Tokyo, 1959.
46. SANO, K. Occlusive diseases of the carotid artery. In: *Medicine in Japan, 1959*, 15th General Meeting of Japanese Society of Medicine, Proceedings of the Scientific Papers, Vol. 4 pp. 474–482, 1959.
47. SANO, K. Electroencephalography in the neurosurgical field. In: *Medicine in Japan, 1959*, 15th General Meeting of Japanese Society of Medicine, Proceedings of the Scientific Papers, Vol. 5, pp. 682–692, 1959.
48. SANO, K., MIWA, T., and CHIGASAKI, H. Cerebellar tumor. Shinkei-Kenkyu no Shinpo (Adv. Neurol. Res.) *3:* 611–621, 1959.
49. SANO, K. Encephalographic findings and diagnostic analysis of brain tumors. In: *Standard Clinical Encephalography*, edited by Japanese Society of Electroencephalography, pp. 75–78, 1959.
50. SANO, K. Surgical indication in brain tumors. Shindan to Chiryo (Diagn. Treatment), *47:* 1062–1067, 1959.
51. SANO, K., and YODONAWA, T. Studies on ictal EEG changes (II). EEG. J. (Suppl. 18): 56–57, 1959.

52. SANO, K. A simple stereotaxic apparatus. Neurol. Med.-Chir., *1:* 253–256, 1959.
53. SANO, K. Cerebellar herniation in vertebral arteriogram—Foraminal sign. Neurol. Med.-Chir., *1:* 180–188, 1959.
54. SANO, K. Introduction to clinical electroencephalography. Rinsho Naika Shonika (Clin. Internal Med. Pediatr.), *14:* 1341–1354, 1959.
55. SANO, K. Diagnostic importance of cerebral angiography. Naika Saishin no Shinpo (Recent Adv. Internal Med.), *4:* 379–408, 1960.
56. SANO, K. Various diagnostic studies for brain tumors and their analysis. Rinsho no Nihon (Clin. Med. Japan), *6:* 259–273, 1960.
57. SANO, K. Pulseless disease: Review of our 6 cases. Shindan to Chiryo (Diagn. Treatment), *48:* 1089–1097, 1960.
58. SANO, K. General review of neurological surgery. Nihon Ishikai Zasshi (J. Japanese Soc. Med.), *44:* 431–444, 1960.
59. SANO, K., and CHIGASAKI, H. Correlation analysis of EEG in neurosurgery I. Autocorrelation analysis of EEG in brain tumors. Proc. IX. Jap. EEG. XIII EMG. Soc. pp. 28–32, 1960.
60. SANO, K. Upper mesencephalic reticulotomy in epilepsy and behavior disorders. Neurol. Med.-Chir., *2:* 138–146, 1960.
61. SANO, K. Olfactory-alarming reflex and olfactory-lacrimatory reflex. No to Shinkei (Brain and Nerve), *13:* 826–827, 1961.
62. SANO, K., and YASAKU, Y. Transfusion in neurosurgical practice. Geka Shinryo (Surg. Pract.), *3:* 27–31, 1961.
63. SANO, K. Pulseless disease and aortic arch syndrome. Naika (Internal Med.), *7:* 456–458, 1961.
64. SANO, K., and TERAO, H. Ossifying fibroma of the skull. No to Shinkei (Brain and Nerve), *13:* 539–547, 1961.
65. SANO, K., CHIGASAKI, H., and OHYA, T. Power electroencephalography. Proc. X. Jap. EEG Soc., pp. 94–97, 1961.
66. SANO, K. Occlusive diseases of the carotid artery based on arteritis. Igaku no Ayumi (Adv. Med.), *37:* 236–246, 1961.
67. SANO, K. Cerebral potential studies-diagnostic analysis. Sogo Rinsho (Gen. Clin. Pract.), *10:* 883–894, 1961.
68. SANO, K. A statistical observation of intracranial tumors. Neurol. Med.-Chir., *3:* 192–200, 1961.
69. SANO, K., and KUWABARA, T. Intra-operative complications during neurosurgical procedures and their management. Geka Chiryo (Surg. Ther.), *5:* 171–180, 1961.
70. SANO, K., and CHIGASAKI, H. Diagnostic evaluation of cerebellar signs. Nihon Rinsho (Japanese Clin. Pract.), *19:* 2007–2014, 1961.
71. SANO, K. Surgical treatment of epilepsy. Geka (Surgery), *23:* 1263–1266, 1961.

72. SANO, K., and NAKAMURA, N. Traumatic intracranial hematoma. Shinkei Kenkyu no Shinpo (Adv. Neurol. Res.), *30:* 11–14, 1962.
73. SANO, K. Brain tumors. In: *Current Therapeutic Guide*, pp. 333–334. Igaku-Shoin, Tokyo, 1961. Pulseless disease. In: *Current Therapeutic Guide*, pp. 141–142. Igaku-Shoin, Tokyo, 1961.
74. SANO, K. Radiation therapy in neurosurgery. Kagaku Ryoho (Chemotherapy), *30:* 11–14, 1962.
75. SANO, K., KITAMURA, K., KUWABARA, T., NAKAMURA, N., SATO, F., and CHIGASAKI, H. Hydrocephalus in children—Pathogenesis and treatment. Shonika Rinsho (Pediatr. Treatment), *25:* 826–834, 1962.
76. SANO, K. Temporal lobe seizures and psychomotor attacks. Igaku no Ayumi (Adv. Med.), *40:* 610–611, 1962.
77. SANO, K. Current review on treatment of hydrocephalus. Med. Culture, *4:* 324–328, 1962.
78. SANO, K. Experiences of reticulotomy in epilepsy. No to Shinkei (Brain and Nerve), *14:* 275–280, 1962.
79. SANO, K. Congenital neurological diseases and treatment. Geka Chiryo (Surg. Treatment), *6:* 649–669, 1962.
80. SANO, K., TERAO, H., NAGASHIMA, C., and KUWABARA, T. Brain tumors in infancy. Shinkei Kenkyu no Shinpo (Adv. Neurol. Res.), *6:* 365–378, 1962.
81. SANO, K. Brain tumors and statistical observations. No to Shinkei (Brain and Nerve), *14:* 751–758, 1962.
82. SANO, K., and KUWABARA, T. Indications for craniotomy in acute head trauma. Geka Chiryo (Surg. Treatment), *4:* 1504–1511, 1962.
83. SANO, K., and KUWABARA, T. *Impaired Consciousness, Medical Symposium, Vol. 1: Current Treatment in Acute Emergency*, pp. 34–47. Shindan to Chiryo-sha (Diagnosis and Therapy, Publisher), Tokyo, 1962.
84. SANO, K. Brain diseases and sleep. Seishin Igaku (Psychiatr. Med.), *4:* 847–860, 1962.
85. SANO, K. Sedative neurosurgery with special reference for posteromedial hypothalamotomy. Neurol. Med.-Chir., *4:* 112–142, 1962.
86. SANO, K., SATO, F., and CHIGASAKI, H. Tissue culture of glioma. Morphol. Neuroglia (J. Nakai ed.) Igaku Shoin, Tokyo, 1963, pp. 133–150.
87. SANO, K., and KUWABARA, T. Osteoma in the optic canal. No to Shinkei (Brain and Nerve), *15:* 441–447, 1963.
88. SANO, K. Neurosurgical procedure for aggressive behavior. Shinkei Kenkyu no Shinpo (Adv. Neurol. Res.), *7:* 615–636, 1963.
89. HATANAKA, H., KITAMURA, K., KAMANO, H., MASUZAWA, H., SANO, K. Steroids and cerebral edema. No to Shinkei (Brain and

Nerve), *15:* 624–633, 1963.

90. SANO, K. Vertebral angiogram for diagnosis of posterior fossa tumors. No to Shinkei (Brain and Nerve), *15:* 821–832, 1963.
91. NAKAMURA, N., KITAMURA, K., KUWABARA, F., SATO, F., CHIGASAKI, Y., and SANO, K. Roentgenological diagnosis of the thalamic tumors. No to Shinkei (Brain and Nerve), *15:* 841–849, 1963.
92. SANO, K., and CHIGASAKI, H. Neurosurgery of infancy. Shonika Rinsho (Clin. Pediatr.), *16:* 907–910, 1963.
93. SANO, K., and TSUTSUMI, H. Cerebral angiography and ultrasonography as diagnostic studies in head trauma. Rinsho to Kenkyu (Clin. Med. Res.), *40:* 1376–1385, 1963.
94. SANO, K., and HATANAKA, H. Steroid treatment for cerebral edema. Saishin Igaku (Modern Med.), *18:* 2478–2492, 1963.
95. SANO, K., HATANAKA, H., KAMANO, S., and MASUZAWA, H. Steroids and the blood-brain barrier with special reference to treatment of brain edema. Neurol. Med.-Chir., *5:* 21–43, 1963.
96. SANO, K., KUWABARA, T., CHIGASAKI, H., and MIYAKE H. Steady potential encephalography (SPEG). Proc. XII Ann. Meet. Jap. EEG Soc., pp. 85–89, 1963.
97. SANO, K., and CHIGASAKI, H. 6 and 14 c/s positive spikes in organic brain diseases. Proc. XII Ann. Meet. Jap. EEG Soc. pp. 16–24, 1963.
98. SANO, K. Present and future of neurological surgery. Geka (Surgery), *26:* 86–89, 1964.
99. HATANAKA, H., KITAMURA, K., NAKAMURA, N., and SANO, K. Hydroencephalodysplasia. Shonika Shinryo (Pediatr. Treatment), *27:* 138–152, 1964.
100. SANO, K. Blood brain barrier. Med. Culture, *6:* 74–81, 1964.
101. SANO, K. Traumatic intracranial hematoma. Nihon Geka-gakkai Zasshi (J. Jap. Soc. Surg.), *65:* 930–938, 1964.
102. SANO, K., and KUWABARA, T. Controversy in neurosurgical technique for treatment of head injury. Geka Shinryo (Surg. Treatment), *6:* 428–433, 1964.
103. SANO, K., TSUTSUMI, H., and AIBA, T. Surgical treatment of cerebrovascular lesions. Rinsho Geka (Clin. Surg.), *19:* 431–442, 1964.
104. SANO, K. "Special Issue" Advances in diagnosis and treatment in neurological surgery. Nihon Iji Shinpo (Jpn. Med. News) (Special Issue), *2085:* 3–10, 1964.
105. HAYAKAWA, I., and SATO, O. Fractional intracarotid infusion of chemotherapeutic agents for treatment of brain tumors. Saishin Igaku (Modern Med.), *19:* 1224–1237, 1964.

106. SANO, K., and SATO, F. Electroencephalography. In: *Electronics for Physicians: Clinical Application*, edited by M. Oshima, pp. 283–326. Nanzando, Tokyo, 1964.

107. SANO, K., and CHIGASAKI, H. Hydrocephalus and Arnold-Chiari malformation. Shinkei Kenkyu no Shinpo (Adv. Neurol. Res.), *8:* 241–262, 1964.

108. SANO, K., and NAWADA, H. Basilar impression and anomalies of the foramen magnum and its vicinity. Shinkei Kenkyu no Shinpo (Adv. Neurol. Res.), *8:* 263–287, 1964.

109. SANO, K., YOSHIOKA, M., and CHIGASAKI, H. 4-14 Cycle positive spikes observed in the organic brain diseases. Rinsho Noha (Clin. Electroencephalogr.), *6:* 19–25, 1964.

110. TSUTSUMI, Y., SANO, K., KUWABARA, K., TAKAKURA, K., HAYAKAWA, I., SUZUKI, T., and KATANUMA, M. A new portable echoencephalograph, using ultrasonic transducers and its clinical application. Med. Electron. Eng., *2:* 21–29, 1964.

111. SANO, K., and NAKAMURA, N. Rehabilitation following head injury. Shinryo (Med. Pract.), *17:* 105–192, 1964.

112. SANO, K., and KUWABARA, T. Indication for neurosurgical operations. Rinsho Igaku (Gen. Clin. Med.), *13:* 1476–1487, 1964.

113. SANO, K., and KITAMURA, K. Headaches—surgical standpoint. In: *My Way of Diagnosis and Treatment*, pp. 285–291. Chugai-Igaku Publisher, Tokyo, 1964.

114. SANO, K. What makes man intelligent? Based on physiological anatomy of the brain. Izumi, September 1964, pp. 26–33.

115. SANO, K., and HATANAKA, H. Blood brain barrier and steroids. Myakkan-gaku (Vasculology), *4:* 72–80, 1964.

116. SANO, K., and HATANAKA, H. Pulmonary edema. Kyobu Shikkan (Chest Dis.), *8:* 1239–1246, 1964.

117. SANO, K., and KUWABARA, T. Early care of the patients with head trauma caused by traffic accident. Saigai Igaku (Trauma Med.), *7:* 539–547, 1964.

118. SANO, K. Head trauma and indication of emergency operations. Nihon Ishikai Zasshi (J. Jpn. Soc. Med.), *52:* 768–776, 1964.

119. SANO, K. Neurosurgical consideration of the subthalamic region in regard to psychomotor function. No to Shinkei (Brain and Nerve), *16:* 815–824, 1964.

120. SANO, K. Controlled pneumoencephalography. Naika (Medicine), *14:* 909–920, 1964.

121. SANO, K., YOSHIOKA, M., and MASUZAWA, A. H. Spontaneous intracerebellar hematoma. Rinsho Shinkei-Gaku (Clin. Neurol.), *4:* 511–512, 1964.

122. SANO, K. *Pulseless disease—Diseases peculiar to Japan*, pp. 153–163. Gendai-Shobo, Tokyo, 1964.

123. SANO, K., and KUWABARA, T. Thalamic tumors. Shinkei Kenkyu no Shinpo (Adv. Neurol. Res.), *8:* 799–820, 1964.

124. SANO, K., YOSHIOKA, N., KOKASHI, M., and ISHIJIMA, T. Surgical treatment of intractable pain-thalamolaminotomy. Shinkei Kenkyu no Shinpo (Adv. Neurol. Res.), *8:* 855–866, 1964.

125. SANO, K. Trauma and intracranial hemorrhage. Shindan to Chiryo (Diagn. Treatment), *52:* 1817–1819, 1964.

126. SANO, K., and KUWABARA, T. National survey of brain tumors and surgical consideration. Rinsho Hoshasen (Clin. Radiation Ther.), *9:* 767–780, 1964.

127. SANO, K. Surgical approach to the extrapyramidal system and diencephalon. Nihon Ishikai Zasshi (J. Jpn. Soc. Med.), *52:* 1217–1238, 1964.

128. SANO, K. Hydrocephalus and its various subtypes. Neurol. Med.-Chir., *6:* 12–17, 1964.

129. SANO, K. Intracranial arterio-venous malformation with special reference to its treatment. Neurol. Med.-Chir., *6:* 28–34, 1964.

130. SANO, K., TERAO, H., HAYAKAWA, I., KAMANO, S., and SAITO, I. Experimental transplantation of the head—two headed dog. Neurol. Med.-Chir., *6:* 35–38, 1964.

131. SANO, K. Intracranial hemorrhage related to head trauma. Geka (Surgery), *26:* 1395–1407, 1964.

132. SANO, K., and KUWABARA, T. Advances in diagnosis and treatment: Neurological surgery. Nihon Iji Shinpo (Jpn. Med. News), *2128:* 67–84, 1965.

133. SANO, K., and AIBA, T. Pulseless disease and similar disorder—Based on aortitis. Kokyu to Junkan (Respiration Circ.), *13:* 168–181, 1965.

134. SANO, K. Hydrocephalus and its various subtypes. No to Shinkei (Brain and Nerve), *17:* 351–353, 1965.

135. SANO, K. Intracranial arteriovenous malformation with special reference to its treatment. No to Shinkei (Brain and Nerve), *17:* 360–364, 1965.

136. SANO, K., NAKAMURA, N., YAMADA, H., and HIRAKAWA, K. Grading system for diagnosis in acute head injury—differential diagnosis between intracranial hematoma, cerebral contusion and cerebral edema. Nihon Iji-Shinpo (Jpn. Med. News), *2143:* 3–8, 1965.

137. SANO, K., YOSHIOKA, M., and KOKASHI, M. Stimulation and ablation of the human posterior subthalamic region. Saishin Igaku (Modern Med.), *20:* 1508–1519, 1965.

138. SANO, K., NAKAMURA, N., YAMADA, H., and HIRAKAWA K. Differential diagnoses in acute head trauma—Statistical analysis for diagnosis. Rinsho Geka (Clin. Surg.), *20:* 701–712, 1965.

139. SANO, K., and AIBA, T. Pulseless disease. Shindan to Chiryo (Diagn. Treatment), *53:* 1154–1165, 1965.

140. SANO, K., and TSUTSUMI, Y. Ultrasonic diagnosis in the central nervous system. Shindan to Chiryo (Diagn. Treatment) (Special Issue: Medical Electronics), 90–93, 1965.

141. SANO, K., KUWABARA, T., SEKINO, K., and MAYANAGI, K. Analysis of five-year survival cases with brain tumor. Rinsho Geka (Clin. Surg.), *20:* 1007–1017, 1965.

142. SANO, K. Diagnostic importance of cerebral angiography in the distribution of carotid artery. Rinsho Shinkei-Gaku (Clin. Neurol.), *5:* 458–460, 1965.

143. SANO, K. Telangiectasia of the basal portion of the cerebral hemisphere—my view. No to Shinkei (Brain and Nerve) *17:* 748–750, 1965.

144. SANO, K., and AIBA, T. Pathological changes of the subclavian artery and subclavian steal syndrome in pulseless disease. Myakkan-Gaku (Vasculology), *5:* 232–233, 1965.

145. SANO, K. Criteria for abnormal brain waves. Rinsho Noha (Clin. Electroencephalogr.) (Special Issue: What do we learn from electroencephalograms?): 90–95, 1965.

146. SANO, K., NAKAMURA, N., YAMADA, H., and HIRAKAWA, K. Diagnosis of the intracranial hematomas without special ancillary studies—Stochastic diagnosis. Geka Chiryo (Surg. Treatment), *13:* 432–446, 1965.

147. SANO, K., YOSHIOKA, M., KASHI, M., ISHIJIMA, T., and OHYE, C. Stereotactic surgery of posterior thalamic lamina. No to Shinkei (Brain and Nerve), *17:* 945–957, 1965.

148. NAKAMURA, N., HIRAKAWA, K., SHIBO, M., SANO, K., and MUKAI, N. Traumatic coma vigil—The first issue, clinical observation, electroencephalography and prognosis. No to Shinkei (Brain and Nerve), *17:* 989-998, 1965.

149. SANO, K., and AIBA, T. Discussion on reoperation in surgical cerebral vascular diseases. Geka-Shinryo (Surg. Treatment), *7:* 1173–1181, 1965.

150. CHIGASAKI, H., TAKAKURA, K., SANO, K., and SHIMAZONO, N. The role of lactic acid, dehydrogenase, isozyme in diagnosis of brain tumors. Shinkei Kenkyu no Shinpo (Adv. Neurol. Res.), *9:* 568–575, 1965.

151. SANO, K. Medical practice for 20 years after World War II: neuro-

logical surgery, particularly for the treatment of brain tumors. Saishin Igaku (Modern Med. (Special Issue), 20: 126–127, 1965.

152. NAKAMURA, N., HIRAKAWA, K., SHINBO, M., SANO, K., and MUKAI, N. Traumatic coma vigil. II. Pathological and anatomical basis. No to Shinkei (Brain and Nerve), *17:* 1121–1134, 1965.

153. SANO, K. Surgery of epilepsy. In: *Nihon Geka Shujutsu Zensho (Japanese Handbook of Operative Procedure)*, Vol. 1, edited by M. Tsuzuki and T. Fukuda, pp. 173–194. Nihon Geka Shujutsu Zensho Kankokai, Tokyo, 1965.

154. SANO, K., and KITAMURA, K. Cerebral hemispherectomy. In: *Nihon Geka Shujutsu Zensho (Japanese Handbook of Operative Procedure)*, edited by M. Tsuzuki and T. Fukuda, pp. 195–202. Nihon Geka Shujutsu Zensho, Kankokai, Tokyo, 1965.

155. SANO, K., and KUWABARA, T. Early diagnosis of the brain and spinal cord tumors in early diagnosis of cancer, pp. 75–87. Ishiyaku Shuppan, Tokyo, 1965.

156. SANO, K., AIBA, T., and JIMBO, M. Surgical treatment of cerebral aneurysms and arteriovenous malformations with special reference to artificial embolization. Neurol. Med.-Chir., *7:* 128–131, 1965.

157. SANO, K., MIYAKE, H., and MAYANAGI, Y. Steady potentials of the brain and its relations to brain metabolism, pp. 30–32. Proc. XIV. Jap. EEG Soc., 1965.

158. SANO, K., SATO, F., HOSHINO, T., and NAGAI, M. Experimental and clinical studies of radiosensitizers in brain tumors, with special reference to BUdR-antimetabolite continuous regional infusion-radiation therapy (BAR therapy). Neurol. Med.-Chir., *7:* 51–72, 1965.

159. SANO, K., AIBA, T., and SHINPO, M. New operative procedure for cerebral arteriovenous malformation-artificial embolization. Nihon Iji Shinpo (Jpn. Med. News), *2123:* 37–40, 1965.

160. SANO, K., SATO, O., and HIYAKAWA, E. I. Adjunctive therapy of brain tumors. Rinsho Geka (Clin. Surg.), *21:* 37–46, 1966.

161. SANO, K. Review of National Congress—3rd Annual meeting of Japanese neurosurgical society. No to Shinkei (Brain and Nerve), *18:* 6–7, 1966.

162. SANO, K. Head trauma, particularly emergency care. Kango-Gaku Zasshi (J. Nursing Sci.), *30:* 32–38; *30:* 40–48, 1966.

163. SANO, K. Symposium on recurrent brain tumors—Introductory speech, Prolegomena. No to Shinkei (Brain and Nerve), *18:* 108–109, 1966.

164. SANO, K., and KUWABARA, T. Advances in diagnosis and treat-

ment—Neurological surgery. Nihon Iji Shinpo (Jpn. Medical News) (Special Issue), *2187:* 10–20, 1966.

165. SANO, K., NAKAMURA, N., YAMADA, H., and HIRAKAWA, K. Statistical estimation for differential diagnosis between acute intracranial hematoma, cerebral contusion and cerebral edema. Saigai Igaku (Trauma Med.), *9:* 1–12, 1966.

166. SANO, K., and AIBA, T. Pulseless disease—Summary of our 62 cases. Jap. Circ. J. *30:* 63–67, 1966.

167. SANO, K., and AIBA, T. Surgery for intracranial aneurysms and arteriovenous malformations, particularly for arteriovenous malformations. No to Shinkei (Brain and Nerve), *18:* 488–497, 1966.

168. SANO, K., and KUWABARA, T. Indications for neurosurgical procedures and pre- and post-operative management. Rinsho to Kenkyu (Clin. Practice Res.), *43:* 616–628, 1966.

169. SANO, K. Management of head trauma for general practice—differential diagnosis between hematoma and cerebral edema. Medicina, *3:* 967–969, 1966.

170. SANO, K. Emergency care—especially differential diagnosis of intracranial hematomas. Kowa Iho (Kowa Med. J.), *66(3):* 6–12, 1966.

171. SANO, K., and HATANAKA, H. Head trauma. In: *Biochemical Approach to Diseases, Vol. 8, Nervous System, No. 1, Diseases of the Nervous System,* edited by J. Shimazono, T. Hayashi, K. Yamada, Y. Yamamura, and K. Yoshinori, pp. 212–269, Nakayama-Shoten, Tokyo, 1966.

172. KITAMURA, K., HATANAKA, H., KAMANO, H., and SANO, K. Steroid treatment for cerebral edema. In: *Pre- and Post-operative Management in Neurosurgical Patients,* edited by D. Jinnai, pp. 127–137. Igaku-Shoin, Tokyo, 1966.

173. SANO, K., and CHIGASAKI, H. Brain tumors. In: *Biochemical Approach to Diseases, Vol. 8, Nervous System, No. 1, Diseases of the Nervous System,* edited by I. Shimazono, T. Hayashi, K. Yamada, Y. Yamamura, and K. Yoshinori, pp. 182–210. Nakayama-Shoten, Tokyo, 1966.

175. SANO, K. Head trauma and its neurological sequelae. In: *Rushidoriru Sosho 1,* 1966.

176. SANO, K. Head trauma. Karada no Kagaku (Science of Human Body), *10:* 16–21, 1966.

177. SANO, K. Head trauma—differential diagnosis in acute stage. Sogo Rinsho (Gen. Clin. Med.), *5:* 1367–1374, 1966.

178. SANO, K. Diagnosis and treatment of intracranial hematomas. Chiryo to Hoken (Treatment and Welfare), *8:* 323–327, 1966.

179. SANO, K. Organization of emergency care system. Toshi Mondai (Problems of City Organization), *57(10):* 28–40, 1966.

180. SANO, K. Relationship between neurosurgery and internal medicine. Saishin Igaku (Mod. Med.), *21:* 2140–2142, 1966.

181. SANO, K., AIBA, T., JIMBO, M., and NAGAI, T. Analysis of circulatory peculiarity in the cerebral arteriovenous malformations. Myakkan-Gaku (Vasculology), *6:* 64–65, 1966.

182. SANO, K. Ultrasonic diagnosis in head trauma. In: *Ultrasonics in Medicine*, pp. 251–257. Igaku-Shoin, Tokyo, 1966.

183. SANO, K. Ultrasonic plethysmo-encephalography. In: *Ultrasonics in Medicine*, pp. 263–267. Igaku-Shoin, Tokyo, 1966.

184. SANO, K. Head trauma. Insatsu-kyoku Iho (Med. News-Dept. Printing), *12(2):* 17–40, 1966.

185. SANO, K. Tumors and mass producing diseases. In: *Clinical Neurology*, edited by T. Tsubaki, K. Sano, and Y. Isojima, pp. 505–567. Igaku-Shoin, Tokyo, 1966.

186. SANO, K. Hereditary and developmental anomalies. In: *Clinical Neurology*, edited by T. Tsubaki, K. Sano, and Y. Isojima, pp. 645–676. Igaku-Shoin, Tokyo, 1966.

187. SANO, K., and KUWABARA, T. Early diagnosis of brain and spinal cord tumors. Naika (Int. Med.), *18:* 1204–1212, 1966.

188. SANO, K. Analysis of neurological sequelae following head trauma. Ijin-Yakujin (Physicians and Pharmaceuticals), *15(11):* 5–7, 1966.

189. SANO, K., and NAKAMURA, N. Clinical analysis of factors influencing the prognosis of head trauma. Shindan to Chiryo (Diagnosis and Treatment), *54:* 2163–2170, 1966.

190. SANO, K. Evoked potentials in response to thalamic stimulation and its application to stereotactic surgery in humans, especially in thalamolaminotomy as a treatment of intractable pain. Shinkei-kenkyu no Shinpo (Adv. Neurol. Res.), *10:* 521–524, 1966.

191. SANO, K., JIMBO, M., and SAITO, I. Aneurysms of vertebral-basilar artery, especially transpharyngeal approach. No to Shinkei (Brain and Nerve), *18:* 1197–1203, 1966.

192. SANO, K., YOSHIOKA, M., OGASHIWA, M., ISHIJIMA, B., and OHYE, C. Thalamolaminotomy—A new operation for relief of intractable pain. In: *Advances in Stereoencephalotomy*, Part II, edited by E. A. Spiegel and H. T. Wycis, pp. 63–66. Karger, Basel, 1966.

193. SANO, K., YOSHIOKA, M., OGASHIWA, M., ISHIJIMA, B., and OHYE, C. Postero-medial hypothalamotomy in the treatment of aggressive behaviors. In: *Advances in Stereoencephalotomy*, Part II, edited by E. A. Spiegel and H. T. Wycis, pp. 164–167. Karger, Basel, 1966.

194. SANO, K., MIYAKE, H., and MAYANAGI, K. Measurement of D.C.

potentials in the brain and its clinical application. In: *Analysis of Electrical Activities in the Brain and Its Application*, edited by B. Fujimori, et al., pp. 251–270. Igaku-Shoin, Tokyo, 1966.

195. SANO, K. Peculiarity in trauma—Head trauma. Nihon Geka-Gakkai Zasshi (J. Jpn. Soc. Surg.), *67:* 2062–2068, 1966.

196. SANO, K., YOSHIOKA, M., ARAI, N., and YOSHIMASU, M. Cavum septi pellucidi and cavum vegae. Rinshon Shinkei-gaku (Clin. Neurol.) *6:* 726–733, 1966.

197. SANO, K. Survey of the organization of services for the treatment of acute head injury in Japan. Proceeding of the IIIrd International Congress of Neurological Surgery, Copenhagen, 23–28 August 1965, pp. 39–45. Excerpta Medica, Amsterdam, 1966.

198. SANO, K., CHIGASAKI, H., and TAKAKURA, K. Diagnostic value of LDH isozyme studies in intracranial tumour. Proceeding of the IIIrd International Congress of Neurological Surgery, Copenhagen, 23–28 August 1965, pp. 575–579. Excerpta Medica, Amsterdam, 1966.

199. SANO, K., HOSHINO, T., and NAGAI, M. Studies on incorporation of a radiosensitizer (5-bromo-2-deoxyuridine) into brain tumor cells and their clinical application. Nippon Acta Neuroradiol. *7:* 4–11, 1966.

200. SANO, K. Review on head trauma. Tama Igakukai-shi (Tama Med. J.), *1:* 5–16, 1966.

201. SANO, K., NAGAI, M., TSUCHIDA, T., and HOSHINO, T. New diagnostic method of brain tumors by cell culture of the cerebrospinal fluid. Millipore filter-cell culture method (preliminary report). Neurol. Med. Chir. *8:* 17–27, 1966.

202. SANO, K., and SAITO, I. Immunological studies of pulseless disease. Neurol. Med. Chir. *8:* 28–39, 1966.

203. SANO, K., HOSHINO, T., NAGAI, M., TSUCHIDA, T., and SATO, F. Studies on a radiosensitizer (5-bromo-2′-deoxyuridine) in the treatment of malignant brain tumors. Neurol. Med. Chir. *8:* 227–231, 1966.

204. SANO, K., JIMBO, M., SAITO, I., TERAO, H., and HIRAKAWA, K. Artificial emobolization with liquid plastic. Neurol. Med. Chir. *8:* 198–201, 1966.

205. SANO, K. Diagnostic value of stationary potentials in the brain. Shindan to Chiryo (Diagnosis and Treatment), *55:* 146–148, 1967.

206. SANO, K., and MAYANAGI, K. Tumors in the pinneal region. Geka Chiryo (Surg. Treatment), *16:* 232–237, 1967.

207. SANO, K., and NAKAMURA, N. Head trauma in children. Nihon Ishikai Zasshi (J. Jpn. Soc. Med.), *57:* 477–487, 1967.

208. SANO, K., and HOSHINO, T. Research on treatment of brain tumors

with radiation-sensitizing substances. Nihon Gan-chiryo Gakkai-Shi (J. Jpn. Soc. Cancer Treatment), *2:* 23–32, 1967.

209. SANO, K., and SATO, O. Chemotherapy of malignant brain tumors. Nihon Gan-chiryo Gakkai-Shi (J. Jpn. Soc. Cancer Treatment), *2:* 33–42, 1967.

210. SANO, K., and HATANAKA, H. Blood brain barrier. In *General Physiology, Physiology of the Brain*, edited by T. Tokizane, pp. 817–838. Igaku-Shoin, Tokyo, 1967.

211. SANO, K., HOSHINO, T., NAGAI, M., TSUCHIDA, T., and SATO, F. Radiation-sensitising substances in treatment of brain tumors—Research in radiation therapy. No to Shinkei (Brain and Nerve), *19:* 339–344, 1967.

212. SANO, K., and NAKAMURA, N. Advances in diagnosis and treatment—Neurological surgery. Nihon Iji-Shinpo (Jpn. Med. News) (Special Issue), *2243:* 3–13, 1967.

213. SANO, K., and HATANAKA, H. *Blood Brain Barrier—Peripheral Circulation and Pathophysiology*, edited by Massho Junkan Kenkyukai (Research Group of Peripheral Circulation), pp. 336–345. University of Tokyo Press, Tokyo, 1967.

214. SANO, K., YOSHIOKA, M., KOKASHI, M., ISHIJIMA, T., OHYE, C., SEKINO, H., and MAYANAGI, K. Regulatory mechanism in the human brain stem. No to Shinkei (Brain and Nerve), *19:* 439–446, 1967.

215. SANO, K. Emergency care of children in head trauma. Shonika Rinsho (Clin. Pediatr), *20:* 416–420, 1967.

216. SANO, K., SHINBO, M., and SAITO, I. Aneurysms of middle cerebral artery. No to Shinkei (Brain and Nerve), *19:* 581–588, 1967.

217. SANO, K. Traumatic intracranial hematomas—extradural, intradural and intracerebral hematomas. In: *Kyo no Chiryo Shishin (Today's Therapeutic Guide)*, pp. 229–232. Igaku-Shoin, Tokyo, 1967.

218. SANO, K., KUWABARA, T., SAITO, O., NAGAI, M., TAKIZAWA, and ANCHO. Hemangioblastoma in the brain. No to Shinkei (Brain and Nerve), *19:* 643–653, 1967.

219. HIRAKAWA, K., NAKAMURA, N., and SANO, K. Spontaneous cure of chronic subdural hematoma: Resolving subdural hematoma (Vol. I, Symptomatology and x-ray findings). No to Shinkei (Brain and Nerve), *19:* 661–670, 1967.

220. SANO, K. Metastatic brain tumor and treatment. Nihon Gan-Chiryo Gaku-Shi (J. Jpn. Soc. Cancer Treatment), *2:* 121–122, 1967.

221. SANO, K.,, and KUWABARA, T. Surgery of the nervous system. In: *Handbook of Modern Pediatrics*, Vol. 16A, edited by M. Arakawa,

T. Nakayama, N. Yamada, and M. Katsusai, pp. 77–179. Nakayama-Shoten, Tokyo, 1967.

222. SANO, K., MIYAKE, H., and MAYANAGI, Y. Steady potentials in various stress conditions in man. Electroencephalography and clinical neurophysiology, Suppl. 25. In: *Recent Advances in Clinical Neurophysiology*, edited by L. Widén, pp. 264–275. Elsevier, Amsterdam/London/New York, 1967.

223. SANO, K. Emergency surgery of head trauma—operative procedures and indication. Rinsho Kagaku (Clin. Sci), *3:* 900–910, 1967.

224. SANO, K. Brain tumors. In: *Kyo no Shindan-Shishin (Today's Diagnostic Guide)*, pp. 318–319. Igaku-Shoin, Tokyo, 1967.

225. SANO, K. Neurological sequelae of head trauma. Chiryo to Hoken (Treatment and Welfare), *9:* 1173–1177, 1967.

226. SANO, K.,, and TERAO, H. Transpharyngeal approach to the lesions located anterior to the brain stem. Rinsho Geka (Clin. Surg.), *22:* 1267–1272, 1967.

227. SANO, K., HIRAKAWA, K., and NAKAMURA, N. Head trauma and ophthalmological complications, particularly traumatic optic nerve lesion. Saigai Igaku (Trauma Med.), *10:* 595–606, 1967.

228. SATO, O., SANO, K., and HORIGUCHI, M. Measurement of fatty acid; fatty acid composition in the normal human white matter and gray matter and cerebrospinal fluid. No to Shinkei (Brain and Nerve), *19:* 773–777, 1967.

229. SANO, K. Brain tumors. Karada no Kagaku (Sci. Human Body), *17:* 61–66, 1967.

230. SANO, K. Surgical approach to personality change—Psychosurgery for aggressiveness. Kagaku Ryoho (Chemotherapy), *52:* 1–6, 1967.

231. SANO, K., KUWABARA, T., JIMBO, M., and SAITO, I. Pathophysiological analysis of cerebral juxta-basal telangiectasia. In: *Intracranial Diseases with Anomalous Vascular Network*, edited by T. Kudo, pp. 77–83. Igaku-Shoin, Tokyo, 1967.

232. SANO, K.,, and ISHIJIMA, T. Central mechanism of pain. In: *Handbook of Physiology, Vol. 6, Physiology of the Sensory Function*, edited by Y. Katsuki, pp. 588–613. Igaku-Shoin, Tokyo, 1967.

233. SANO, K. Traumatic visual impairment. Nihon Ganka-Gakkai Zasshi (J. Jpn. Soc. Ophthalmol.), *71:* 1939–1949, 1967.

234. SANO, K., JIMBO, M., and SAITO, I. Immunological analysis of pulseless disease. Myakkan-Gaku (Vasculology), *7:* 100–101, 1967.

235. SANO, K. Diagnosis and surgical treatment of subarachnoid hemorrhage. Tochigi-ken Igakkai Kaishi (J. Tochigi Prefecture Soc. Med.), *6:* 107–116, 1967.

236. SANO, K. Embolization of cerebral arteriovenous malformations—

Clinical use of liquid silicone. Current medicine by pictorial explanation. In *New Treatment*, pp. 57–59. Igaku-Shoin, Tokyo, 1967.

237. SANO, K. Stereotactic encephalotomy (II) psychosurgery. Current medicine by pictorial explanation. In: *New Treatment*, pp. 73–74. Igaku-Shoin, Tokyo, 1967.

238. NAGAI, M., HOSHINO, T., TSUCHIDA, T., SATO F., and SANO, K. Atlas of tissue culture of brain tumors, Part 1. No to Shinkei (Brain and Nerve), *19:* 954–961, 1967.

239. NAGAI, M., HOSHINO, T., TSUCHIDA, T., SATO, F., and SANO K. Atlas of tissue culture of brain tumors, Part 2. No to Shinkei (Brain and Nerve), *19:* 1055–1062, 1967.

240. SANO, K. Central mechanism of pain, based on stereotactic thalamotomy. Proceedings of the 17th General Meeting of Japanese Society of Medicine. In: *Medicine in Japan, 1967*, Vol. 3, pp. 952–956, 1967.

241. NAGAI, T., JIMBO, M., and SANO, K. Cerebro-pulmonary scan using macroaggregated albumin as a quantitation of intracerebral arterio-venous shunting. J. Nuclear Med., *8:* 709–722, 1967.

242. NAGAI, M., HOSHINO, T., TSUCHIDA, T., SATO, F., and SANO, K. Atlas of tissue culture of brain tumors, Part 3. No to Shinkei (Brain and Nerve), *19:* 1175–1184, 1967.

243. SATO, O., and SANO, K. Research on composition of fatty acids in cultured brain tumors. No to Shinkei (Brain and Nerve), *19:* 1193–1197, 1967.

244. NAKAMURA, N., HIRAKAWA, K., and SANO, K. Natural healing of chronic subdural hematoma—Resolving subdural hematoma (in Part 2, Pathological process and its analysis). No to Shinkei (Brain and Nerve), *19:* 1209–1219, 1967.

245. TERAO, H., TSUKAMATO, Y., and SANO, K. Von Rechlinghausen's disease and brain tumors. No to Shinkei (Brain and Nerve), *19:* 1235–1245, 1967.

246. SANO, K. Surgery of accoustic neurinomas. Geka Shinryo (Surg. Treatment), *9:* 1293–1294, 1967.

247. SANO, K., YOSHIOKA, M., OGASHIWA, M., ISHIJIMA, B., OHYE, C., SEKINO, H., and MAYANAGI, Y. Central mechanisms of neck movements in the human brain stem. The 3rd International Symposium on Stereoencephalotomy, Madrid, 1967. Confin. Neurol., *29:* 107–111, 1967.

248. SANO, K., YOSHIOKA, M., OGASHIWA, M., ISHIJIMA, B., OHYE, C., SEKINO, H., and MAYANAGI, Y. Autonomic, somatomotor and electroencephalographic responses upon stimulation of the hy-

pothalamus and the rostral brain stem in man. The 3rd International Symposium on Stereoencephalotomy, Madrid, 1967. Confin. Neurol., *29:* 257–261, 1967.

249. Sano, K., Nakamura, N., Hirakawa, K., Masuzawa, M., Hashizume, K., Hayashi, T., and Fujii, S. Mechanism of dynamics of closed head injuries (preliminary report). Neurol. Med. Chir., *9:* 21–33, 1967.

250. Sano, K., Ogashiwa, M., Sekino, H., Mayanagi, Y., and Yoshimasu, N. Follow-up studies on the hypothalamotomy. Neurol. Med. Chir., *9:* 288–290, 1967.

251. Sano, K. The role of the internal medullary lamina in pain. Anales del XII Congreso Latinoamericano de Neurocirugia, Lima, Oct. 1967, pp. 937–952.

252. Sano, K. Stimulation and destruction of the postero-medial hypothalamus by means of stereotaxis in man. Anales del XII Congreso Latinoamericano de Neurocirugia, Lima, Oct. 1967, pp. 981–990.

253. Nagai, M., Tsuchida, T., Hoshino, T., and Sano, K. Millipore filter-cell culture method from the cerebrospinal fluid as new diagnostic study. Shinkei Kenkyu no Shinpo (Adv. Neurol. Res.), *11:* 811–817, 1967.

254. Sano, K. Statistical method for diagnosis in head trauma. Sogo Rinsho (Gen. Clin. Pract.), *17:* 26–33, 1968.

255. Sano, K., Jimbo, M., Saito, I., and Kitamura, T. Embolization of the vascular tumors with liquid plastic. Rinsho Geka (Clin. Surg.), *23:* 67–75, 1968.

256. Sano, K. Challenge to cancer-brain tumor. Jikken Chiryo (Exp. Treatment), No. 429, 1968.

257. Ueda, H., Ishikawa, K., Okabayashi, A., Kirisawa, N., Kusunoki, T., Takahashi, N., Sano, K., Sunada, T., Nasu, T., Yamaoka, K., and Yoshitoshi, K. Clinical and pathological analysis of aortitis syndrome. Shaishin Igaku (Mod. Med.), *23:* 181–188, 1968.

258. Sano, K., Jimbo, M., and Saito, I. Subarachnoid hemorrhage. Sogo Rinsho (Gen. Clin. Practice), *17:* 231–239, 1968.

259. Sano, K., and Nakamura, N. Advances in diagnosis and treatment—Neurological surgery. Nihon Iji Shinpo (Jpn. Med. News) (Special Issue), *2291:* 3–12, 1968.

260. Shiraki, H., Sano, K., and Tsubaki, T. Protection of the brain. Iwanami-Shinsho, *675:* 224, 1968.

261. Sano, K. Brain and spinal cord abscess. In: *Today's Therapeutic Guide*, p. 229. Igaku-Shoin, Tokyo, 1968.

262. Sano, K., Hoshino, T., and Nagai, M. Radiosensitization of brain

tumor cells with a thymidine analogue (bromouridine). J. Neurosurg., *28:* 530–538, 1968.

263. SANO, K. What to gain from studying abroad? Medicina, *5:* 685–687, 1968.

264. SANO, K. Analysis of emergency care in head trauma—Summary and my view. Chiryo (Treatment), *50:* 1576–1579, 1968.

265. AKASHI, K., NAGAI, M., CHIGASAKI, H., and SANO, K. Cranium bifidum and its special form "cephalocele basalis." No to Shinkei (Brain and Nerve), *20:* 813–823, 1968.

266. SANO, K., MIYAKE, H., and MAYANAGI, Y. Diagnostic value of steady potential recording in man. Proceedings of the Australian Association of Neurologists Reporting the Second Congress of the Asian and Oceanian Association of Neurologists, Melbourne, 1967, Vol. 5, pp. 27–32, 1968.

267. SANO, K., OGASHIWA, M., and SEKINO, H. Clinical and physiological data obtained in stereotaxic surgery of the hypothalamus. Proceedings of the Australian Association of Neurologists Reporting the Second Congress of the Asian and Oceanian Association of Neurologists, Melbourne, 1967, Vol. 5, pp. 267–275, 1968.

268. SANO, K. Surgery of cerebrovascular lesions focused on treatment of aneurysms and areteriovenous malformations. Nihon Ishikai Zasshi (J. Jpn. Soc. Med.), *60:* 639–655, 1968.

269. TERAO, H., YOSHIMASU, M., and SANO, K. Intracranial melanoma—Reports on 6 cases and bibliographic consideration. No to Shinkei (Brain and Nerve), *20:* 991–999, 1968.

270. SANO, K. Advances in clinical encephalography—Correlation analysis, evoked potentials, and D.C. potentials. Shinkei Kenkyu no Shinpo (Adv. Neurol. Res.), *12:* 419–436, 1968.

271. SANO, K. Non-symptomatic diseases and their treatment—Neurological surgery. Shindan to Chiryo (Diagnosis and Treatment), *56:* 113–114, 1968.

272. MASUZAWA, H., HAYAKAWA, I., YAMADA, F., HIRAKAWA, K., and SANO, K. Special form of occulomotor dysfunction secondary to facial trauma—Blow-out fracture. Nihon Saigai-Igaku Kaishi (J. Jpn. Soc. Trauma Med.), *16:* 425–438, 1968.

273. NAKAMURA, N., HIRAKAWA, K., MASAZAWA, H., HASHIZUME, K., SANO, K., HAYASHI, T., FUJII, S., and KOBAYASHI, H. What determines the life and death? Dynamics of head trauma. No to Shinkei (Brain and Nerve), *20:* 1204–1212, 1968.

274. SANO, K. Traffic accident and head trauma. Nihon Kotsu-Igaku-Kai Zasshi (J. Jpn. Soc. Traffic Med.), *22:* 242–248, 1968.

275. SANO, K. Intracranial tumors of infancy and childhood. XII Con-

greso International de Pediatria, Memorias, Mexico, 1968, Vol. II, pp. 278–281.

276. HATANAKA, H., MASUZAWA, T., AMANO, K., and SANO, K. Basic and clinical studies on boron-neutron capture therapy. Nippon Acta Neuroradiol., *9:* 37–40, 1968.
277. SAITO, I., NAGAI, M., TSUCHIDA, T., and SANO, K. Cranial and intracranial chondroma. No to Shinkei (Brain and Nerve), *20:* 1053–1060, 1968.
278. SANO, K. Brain tumors. Gendai no Katei-Igaku (Modern family medicine, 2). In: *Diseases and Treatment, 1*, pp. 293–298. Gakushu Kenkyu-sha, Tokyo, 1969.
279. SANO, K. Head trauma. (Modern family medicine, 2). In: *Diseases and Treatment, 1*, pp. 293–298. Gakushu Kenkyu-sha, Tokyo, 1969.
280. SANO, K. Radiation treatment of brain tumors. Nihon Ishikai Zasshi (J. Jpn. Soc. Med.), *61:* 283–299, 1969.
281. SANO, K. Surgery of cerebrovascular diseases—Focused on aneurysms and arteriovenous malformations. Nihon Geka-Gakkai Zasshi (J. Jpn. Soc. Surg.), *70:* 14–150, 1969.
282. SANO, K., and SATO, F. Artificial skull. In: *Handbook of Modern Surgery (Organ Transplantation, Vol. 25)*, pp. 171–176. Nakayama-Shoten, Tokyo, 1969.
283. SANO, K. Statistical method for diagnosis in head trauma. In: *Statistical Method for Diagnosis*, edited by A. Takahashi, pp. 162–179. Todai Shuppan-kai (University of Tokyo Press), Tokyo, 1969.
284. SANO, K. Atlas of brain tumors (1)—Statistics of brain tumors, especially of gliomas. No to Shinkei (Brain and Nerve), *21:* 462–465, 1969.
285. SANO, K. Atlas of brain tumors (2)—Astrocytoma, astroblastoma. No to Shinkei (Brain and Nerve), *21:* 610–613, 1969.
286. SANO, K. Atlas of brain tumors (3)—Ependymoma. No to Shinkei (Brain and Nerve), *21:* 730–733, 1969.
287. SANO, K. Atlas of brain tumors (4)—Medulloblastoma, pituicytoma. No to Shinkei (Brain and Nerve), *21:* 850–851, 1969.
288. SANO, K. Atlas of brain tumors (5)—Oligodendroglioma, spongioblastoma, and choroid plexus papilloma. No to Shinkei (Brain and Nerve), *21:* 958–961, 1969.
289. SANO, K. Atlas of brain tumors (6)—Meningioma. No to Shinkei (Brain and Nerve), *21:* 1074–1077, 1969.
290. SANO, K. Atlas of brain tumors (7)—Neurinoma. No to Shinkei (Brain and Nerve), *21:* 1211–1213, 1969.

291. SANO, K. Atlas of brain tumors (8)—Pituitary tumor and craniopharyngioma. No to Shinkei (Brain and Nerve), *21:* 1327–1329, 1969.
292. SEKINO, H., TSUCHIDA, T., NAKAMURA, N., SANO, K., MATSUMOTO, M., MIURA, N., and TAKAHASHI, T. Intracranial adenoid cystic carcinoma—Reports on 2 cases. No to Shinkei (Brain and Nerve), *21:* 709–714, 1969.
293. SANO, K. Diagnosis of brain tumors. Sogo Rinsho (Gen. Clin. Practice), *18:* 1281–1296, 1969.
294. TOKIZANE, T., FUJIMORI, B., SHIMAZONO, Y., and SANO, K. *Guide to Modern Electroencephalography*, p. 452. Nanzando, Tokyo, 1969.
295. SANO, K. Head trauma and pharmaceutical treatment of neurological sequelae: general review. Yakubutsu Ryoho (Pharmaceut. Ther.) (Special Issue), *2:* 977–979, 1979.
296. SANO, K. Electroencephalography and other clinical methods to study cerebral electrical activities. Ika-Kikai-Gaku Zasshi (J. Med. Instrumentation), *39:* 628–637, 1969.
297. SAITO, I., and SANO, K. Immunological study of pulseless disease. Igaku no Ayumi (Adv. Med.), *70:* 289–292, 1969.
298. SANO, K. Neutron-capture treatment. Rinsho Kagaku (Clin. Sci.), *9:* 1247–1249, 1969.
299. HIRAKAWA, K., NAKAMURA, N., MASUZAWA, H., HASHIZUME, K., and SANO, K. Analysis of skull fracture and orbital fracture. No to Shinkei (Brain and Nerve), *21:* 963–973, 1969.
300. AKASHI, K., CHIGASAKI, H., SANO, K., and KUWABARA, T. Spina bifida and analysis of the cases. No to Shinkei (Brain and Nerve), *21:* 1147–1154, 1969.
301. SANO, K. Analysis of cerebrovascular impairment—Neurosurgical standpoint. Shinyaku to Chiryo (New Drugs and Treatment), *128:* 19–26, *129:* 19–26, 1969.
302. SANO, K. Five-year follow-up of head trauma—particularly following intracranial hematomas and depressed fractures. Nihon Ishikai Zaisshi (J. Jpn. Soc. Med.), *62:* 431–434, 1969.
303. SANO, K. Cerebral angiography. In *Handbook of Modern Surgery 26A: Brain and Spinal Cord 1*, pp. 130–181. Nakayama-Shoten, Tokyo, 1969.
304. SANO, K. Brain tumors—Clinical testing. Sogo Rinsho (Gen. Clin. Med.) (Special Issue), *18:* 2015–2016, 1969.
305. SANO, K., NAKAMURA, N., HIRAKAWA, R., MASUZAWA, H., HASHIZUME, K., and MIZONOKAMI, T. 5-Year post-operative follow-up for intracranial hematoma and depressed fracture. Nihon Geka-Gakkai Zasshi (J. Jpn. Soc. Surg.), *70:* 1312–1314, 1969.

306. SANO, K. Operative procedure for head. In: *Handbook of Clinical Surgery 1*, pp. 96–119. Kinbara-Shuppan, Tokyo, 1969.

307. HOSHINO, T., and SANO, K. Radiosensitization of malignant brain tumours with bromouridine (thymidine analogue). Acta Radiologica, *8:* 15–26, 1969.

308. SANO, K. Recent trends in head injury. Shinyaku to Chiryo (New Drugs and Treatment), *131:* 3, 1969.

309. SANO, K. *Neurological Surgery* (Pictorial explanation of living 5, Health), p. 166. Shufu no Tomo-sha, Tokyo, 1970.

310. SANO, K., AIBA, T., and SAITO, I. Angiography in pulseless disease. Radiology, *94:* 69–74, 1970.

311. SANO, K., and KUWABARA, T. Recent advances in diagnosis and treatment—Neurological surgery. Nihon Ihi Shinpo (Jpn. Med. News) (Special Issue), *2899:* 9–18, 1970.

312. SANO, K. Stereotactic surgery of subthalamic area and emotional control. Shinkei-kenkyu no Shinpo (Adv. Neurol. Res.), *14:* 157–163, 1970.

313. SANO, K. Present and past in medical treatments. Shindan to Shinryo (Diagnosis and Treatment), *58:* 971–979, 1970.

314. SANO, K. Treatment of brain tumors. Nihon Ishikai Zasshi (J. Jpn. Soc. Med.), *64:* 253–258, 1970.

315. SANO, K. Treatment of brain tumors with atomic energy—Boron-neutron capturing treatment. Igaku no Ayumi (Adv. Med.), *74:* 468–469, 1970.

316. SANO, K. Trauma—Cerebral trauma series 4. Chugai Iho (Chuga Med. News), *23:* 332–343, 1970.

317. SANO, K., SAITO, I., BASUGI, N., ASANO, T., FUKUSHIMA, T., KIRITANI, S., and FUJIMURA, O. A new method of blood flow measurement by means of digitally controlled dynamic radiography. A preliminary report. Ann. Bull. Res. Inst. Logopedics and Phoniatrics of University of Tokyo, *4:* 115–119, 1970.

318. SANO, K. Atlas of brain tumors (9), Tumors of pineal body—pinealoma, teratoma. No to Shinkei (Brain and Nerve), *22:* 6–8, 1970.

319. SANO, K. Atlas of brain tumors (10), Hemangioblastoma. No to Shinkei (Brain and Nerve), *22:* 126–128, 1970.

320. SANO, K. Atlas of brain tumors (11), Metastatic brain tumor, melanoma and sarcoma. No to Shinkei (Brain and Nerve), *22:* 234–236, 1970.

321. SANO, K. Atlas of brain tumors (12), Congenital tumors. No to Shinkei (Brain and Nerve), *22:* 350–352, 1970.

322. SANO, K., MAYANAGI, Y., SEKINO, H., OGASHIWA, M., and ISHIJIMA, B. Results of stimulation and destruction of the posterior

hypothalamus in man. J. Neurosurg., *33:* 689–707, 1970.

323. SANO, K., YOSHIOKA, M., MAYANAGI, Y., SEKINO, H., YOSHIMASU, N., and TSUKAMOTO, Y. Stimulation and destruction of and around the interstitial nucleus of cajal in man. Confin. Neurol., *32:* 118–125, 1970.

324. SANO, K., YOSHIOKA, M., SEKINO, H., MAYANAGI, Y., YOSHIMASU, N., and TSUKAMOTO, Y. Functional organization of the internal medullary lamina in man. Confin. Neurol., *32:* 374–380, 1970.

325. SANO, K. Analysis of injuries caused by traffic accident and their treatment. Gekkan Kotsu (Monthly Traffic), *2(2):* 8–18, 1971.

326. SANO, K. Irradiation and drugs for brain tumor. Shindan to Chiryo (Diagnosis and Treatment), *59:* 107–112, 1971.

327. SANO, K., and KUWABARA, T. Recent advances in diagnosis and treatment—Neurological surgery. Nihon Iji Shinpo (Jpn. Med. News) (Special Issue), *2447:* 26–34, 1971.

328. SANO, K. What are involved in neurological surgery. Kango-gijutsu (Nurs. Pract.), *208:* 112–118, 1971.

329. SANO, K., SATO, O., and SAITO, I. Microneurosurgery—Introduction of surgical microscope in neurosurgery. Nihon Iji Shinpo (Jpn. Med. News), *2437:* 37–40, 1971.

330. SAITO, I., FURUHATA, T., HASHIZUME, K., SATO, O., and SANO, K. Total removal of spinal cord hemangioblastoma. No to Shinkei (Brain and Nerve), *23:* 13–17, 1971.

331. SAITO, O., FURUHATA, T., TSUCHIDA, T., SEKINO, H., NAKAMURA, N., and SANO, K. Arachnoid cyst. No to Shinkei (Brain and Nerve), *23:* 33–39, 1971.

332. SANO, K. Recent review on neurosurgical treatment. Geka Chiryo (Surg. Treatment), *24:* 274–281, 1971.

333. SANO, K. Advances in diagnostic studies of brain tumors—Essentials for diagnosis. Shinryo (Clin. Exam. Treatment), *24:* 273–286, 1971.

334. SAITO, I., and SANO, K. Surgical treatment of aneurysms of the anterior communicating artery. Proceedings of 3rd discussion group meeting on special subjects in neurological surgery, pp. 79–98, 1971.

335. SANO, K. Advances in brain tumors. Nihon Igakukai Sokai Zasshi. Proceedings of the 18th general meeting of Japanese Society of Medicine, pp. 271–277, 1971.

336. SANO, K. Treatment of brain tumors. Asian Med. J., *14:* 303–312, 1971.

337. SANO, K. Advances in chemotherapy of cancer—Combined treatment with special irradiation and chemotherapeutic agents in

brain tumors. Sogo Rinsho (Gen. Med. Pract.) (Special Issue), *20:* 1401–1406, 1971.

338. MANAKA, N., and SANO, K. Diagnostic value of stationary potentials for organic brain diseases—Comparison between the stationary potentials during craniotomy and those in the pre- and post-operative stages. No to Shinkei (Brain and Nerve), *23:* 1131–1142, 1971.
339. SANO, K. Recent advances in cerebrovascular diseases in neurosurgical field. Kowa Iho (Kowa Med. J.), *15(5):* 2–7, 1971.
340. SAITO, I., TSUCHIDA, T., and SANO, K. Pharmaceutical treatment of cerebrovascular occlusive diseases. Kowa Iho (Kowa Med. J.), *15(5):* 48–51, 1971.
341. SANO, K. Advances in treatment of brain tumors. In Special Issue: Advances in treatment of malignant tumors. Naika (Medicine), *28:* 678–684, 1971.
342. SAITO, O., SEKINO, H., MAYANAGI, Y., and SANO, K. Simple method of third ventriculography. Rinsho Geka (Clin. Surg.), *26:* 1615–1619, 1971.
343. SANO, K., NAGAI, M., ARAI, N., and HOSHINO, T. Long-term follow-up of BAR therapy in malignant brain tumors. Nihon Gan-Chiryo Gakkai-Shi (J. Jpn. Soc. Cancer Treatment), *6:* 224–230, 1971.
344. SANO, K. Surgery of intracranial aneurysms. No to Shinkei (Brain and Nerve), *23:* 1252–1264, 1971.
345. SANO, K. My way of treatment—Treatment of pulseless disease No. 2. Rinsho Kagaku (Clin. Sci.), *7:* 1651–1653, 1971.
346. SANO, K. Surgery of the head. In: *New Handbook of Surgical Procedures*, Vol. 1, pp. 421–564. Nanzando, Tokyo, 1971.
347. SANO, K. Operative technique of brain tumors—Video publication. In: *Handbook of Modern Clinical Medicine.* Chikuma-Shobo, Tokyo, 1971.
348. SANO, K. General review of brain tumors. In: *Handbook of Modern Surgery 26B, Brain, Spinal Cord II*, pp. 3–47. Nakayama-Shoten, Tokyo, 1971.
349. SANO, K. Effects of stimulation and destruction of the posterior hypothalamus in cases of behaviour disorders and epilepsy. *Special Topics in Stereotaxis*, edited by W. Umbach, pp. 22–41. Hippokrates-Verlag, Stuttgart, 1971.
350. HIRAKAWA, K., HASHIZUME, K., NAKAMURA, N., and SANO, K. Mechanical study on the traumatic optic nerve injury. Neurol. Med. Chir., *11:* 34–45, 1971.
351. MASUZAWA, H., HIRAKAWA, K., NAKAMURA, N., and SANO, K. Engineering aspects of human skull fracture—Experimental

study and theoretical consideration on brain damage. Neurol. Med. Chir., *11:* 46–65, 1971.

352. SEKINO, H., FUKUSHIMA, T., HORI, T., ISHIJIMA, B., and SANO, K. Neuronal activity of the human pretectal area (preliminary report). Neurol. Med. Chir., *11:* 79–83, 1971.
353. ISHIJIMA, B., and SANO, K. Responses of specific and nonspecific thalamic nuclei to the selective A-δ and C-fiber stimulation, and their interactions in cat's brain. Neurol. Med. Chir., *11:* 84–100, 1971.
354. TAKAKURA, K., and SANO, K. Sites of action of chemotherapeutic drugs on brain tumor metabolism. In: *The Experimental Biology of Brain Tumors*, edited by W. F. Kirsh, E. G. Paoletti, and P. Paoletti, pp. 429–456. Charles C Thomas, Springfield, Ill., 1972.
355. SANO, K. *Brain Tumors—Pathology and Clinical Aspect*, p. 178. Igaku-Shoin, Tokyo, 1972.
356. SATO, O., and SANO, K. Hydrocephalus, Arnold-Chiari malformation, Dandy-Walker syndrome, hydroencephalodysplasia, and cephalocele. Shinkei-Kenkyu no Shinpo (Adv. Neurol. Res.), *16:* 275–280, 1972.
357. SANO, K. Recent advances in treatment of brain tumors. Gan no Rinsho (Clin. Pract. Cancer), *18:* 293–298, 1972.
358. SANO, K., and NAKAMURA, N. Recent advances in diagnosis and treatment—Neurological surgery. Nihon Iji Shinpo (Jpn. Med. News) (Special Issue), *2503:* 14–22, 1972.
359. SANO, K. Head trauma and neurological sequelae—General review. In *Current Therapeutic Practice 1*, edited by K. Oshima, T. Hayashida, and Iji Nippo-sha, pp. 519–521. Osaka, Tokyo, 1972.
360. SANO, K. Brain abscess. In: *Guide to Current Treatment*, pp. 278–279. Igaku-Shoin, Tokyo, 1972.
361. SANO, K. Differential diagnosis in head trauma—Intracerebral hematoma and cerebral edema—Basic knowledge for internists. Medicina, *9:* 419–421, 1972.
362. SANO, K. Brain tumors and management. Mainichi Life, (October issue): 164–166, 1972.
363. SANO, K. Surgical treatment of subarachnoid hemorrhage. Modern Medicine, (August issue): 12–15, 1972.
364. MANAKA, M., and SANO, K. Brain tumors and brain wave. Gendai Chiryo (Curr. Med. Treatment), *4:* 673–679, 1972.
365. SANO, K., NAKAMURA, N., HIRAKAWA, K., and HASHIZUME, K. Correlative studies of dynamics and pathology in whip-lash and head injuries. Scand. J. Rehab. Med., *4:* 47–54, 1972.
366. TAKAKURA, K., MIKI, Y., KUBO, O., OGAWA, N., MATSUTANI, M.,

and SANO, K. Adjuvant immunotherapy for malignant brain tumors. Jap. J. Clin. Oncol., *12:* 109–120, 1972.

367. SANO, K. Head trauma and neurological sequelae—General review. Tokyo, *20:* 3–13, 1972.

368. SANO, K., SEKINO, H., and MAYANAGI, Y. Results of stimulation and destruction of the posterior hypothalamus in cases with violent, aggressive or restless behaviours. In: *Psychosurgery*, edited by E. Hitchcock, L. Laitinen, and K. Vaernet, pp. 57–75. Charles C Thomas, Springfield, Ill., 1972.

369. SATO, O., and SANO, K. Microsurgery in neurosurgical field—Application to surgery of brain tumors. Geka Chiryo (Surg. Treatment), *27:* 275–281, 1972.

370. SAITO, I., and SANO, K. Microsurgery in neurosurgical field: Application to surgery of intracranial aneurysms. Geka Chiryo (Surg. Treatment), *27:* 298–304, 1972.

371. SANO, K. Brain tumors. In special issue: Treatment of cancer. Shindan to Chiryo (Diagnosis and Treatment), *60:* 1916–1921, 1972.

372. SANO, K. Glioma. Gan no Rinsho (Clin. Pract. Cancer), *48:* 3–11, 1972.

373. SANO, K., and SAITO, I. Recent advances in studies of pulseless disease. Rinsho Geka (Clin. Surg.), *27:* 1373–1379, 1972.

374. SANO, K., NAGAI, M., ARAI, T., and HOSHINO, T. Follow-up results of BAR therapy of malignant brain tumors. In: *Present Limits of Neurosurgery*, edited by I. Fusek and Z. Kunc, pp. 71–75 (Proceeding of the 4th European Congress of Neurosurgery, Prague, June 28–July 2, 1971). Avicenum, Czechoslovak Medical Press, Prague, 1972.

375. HATANAKA, H., and SANO, K. A revised boron-neutron capture therapy for malignant brain tumors. *Present Limits of Neurosurgery*, edited by I. Fusek and Z. Kunc, pp. 83–85 (Proceeding of the 4th European Congress of Neurosurgery, Prague, June 28–July 2, 1971). Avicenum, Czechoslovak Medical Press, Prague, 1972.

376. SANO, K., HATANAKA, H. and KAMANO, S. Steroids and the blood-brain barrier with special reference to astrocytic cells. In: *Steroids and Brain Edema*, edited by H. J. Reulen and K. Schürmann, pp. 177–182. Springer-Verlag, Berlin, 1972.

377. MANAKA, N., and SANO, K. Measurement of cerebral stationary potentials—Amplitude of SP in experimental animals and correlation with brain death. No to Shinkei (Brain and Nerve), *24:* 1573–1582, 1972.

378. SANO, K. How to operate on cerebral aneurysms safely? In: *Safe*

Operative Procedures, edited by A. Ichikawa, et al., pp. 75–79. Kinbara-shuppan, Tokyo, 1972.

379. SANO, K. New trends in treatment of malignant tumors—Neurological surgery. Shindan to Chiryo (Diagnosis and Treatment), *60:* 2059–2061, 1972.

380. SANO, K., SEKINO, H., TSUKAMOTO, Y., YOSHIMASU, N., and ISHIJIMA, B. Stimulation and destruction of the region of the interstitial nucleus in cases of torticollis and see-saw nystagmus. Confin. Neurol., *34:* 331–338, 1972.

381. SANO, K. Psychosurgery. In: *Handbook of Modern Surgery 26D*, pp. 215–218. Nakayama-Shoten, 1972.

382. SANO, K., and SAITO, I. Pulseless disease. Summary of our experiences and studies. Schweiz. Arch. Neurol. Neurochir. Psychiatr., *111:* 417–433, 1972.

383. SANO, K. Correlation between dynamics and pathology in head injuries. In: *Neurotraumatologia*, edited by R. Carrea, J. C. Christiensen, and L. Turjanski, pp. 143–172 (Proceedings of the International Conference of Neurotraumatology, August 27–29, 1972). Buenos Aires, Reprografias JMA s. a. 1972.

384. SANO, K., SEKINO, H., and YOSHIMASU, N. The internal medullary lamina in emotive, motor and sensory functions, pp. 162–165. Neurology, India, Proceedings, Suppl. II, 1972.

385. SANO, K., and MANAKA, N. Analysis of ictal waves—Epileptic attacks and D.C. potentials. Rinsho Noha (Clin. Electroencephalogr.), *15:* 1–8, 1973.

386. SANO, K. Subarachnoid hemorrhage in children. No to Hattatsu (Brain and Development), *5:* 7–9, 1973.

387. SANO, K., and SATO, O. Tumors and mass producing diseases. In: *Handbook of Clinical Medicine 1*, Chap. II, pp. 1–65. Kinbara-Shuppan, Tokyo, 1973.

388. SANO, K., and SATO, O. Trauma. In: *Handbook of Clinical Medicine 1, Individual Section*, Chap. II, pp. 67–99. Kinbara-Shuppan, Tokyo, 1973.

389. SANO, K., and SATO, O. Congenital diseases and developmental anomalies. In: *Handbook of Clinical Medicine-Individual Section*, Chap. II, pp. 101–132. Kinbara-Shuppan, Tokyo, 1973.

390. SANO, K. Hereditary and developmental anomalies and hydrocephalus. In: *Handbook of Modern Surgery*, Vol. 26C, *Brain, Spinal Cord III*, pp. 239–275. Nakayama-Shoten, Tokyo, 1973.

391. SATO, O., TAMURA, A., TERAOKA, A., SEKINO, H., and SANO, K. Treatment of pituitary adenomas and analysis of the results. No to Shinkei (Brain and Nerve), *25:* 285–294, 1973.

392. NAGAI, M., TERAOKA, A., NOMURA, K., MATSUTANI, M., and SANO, K. Morphological changes of malignant glioma cells effected by dibutyryl adenosine-3′,5′-cylic monophosphate. No to Shinkei (Brain and Nerve), *25:* 295–306, 1973.

393. MATSUI, T., AMANO, K., KITAMURA, K., SANO, K., and OSHIMA, T. Microstereo-angiography. No to Shinkei (Brain and Nerve), *25:* 307–313, 1973.

394. SANO, K. Treatment in Japan—brain tumor. Shindan to Chiryo (Diagnosis and Treatment), *61:* 518–522, 1973.

395. FUKUSHIMA, T., ISHIJIMA, B., HIRAKAWA, K., NAKAMURA, N., and SANO, K. Ventriculofiberscope: A new technique for endoscopic diagnosis and operation (technical note). J. Neurosurg., *38:* 251–256, 1973.

396. SANO, K. Neurological surgery. In special issue: Review of clinical medicine—Advances in diagnosis and treatment. Nihon Iji Shinpo (Jpn. Med. News), *2552:* 13–24, 1973.

397. SANO, K., and MANAKA, N. Stationary potential encephalograph. Gan no Rinsho (Clin. Pract. Cancer), *19:* 383–385, 1973.

398. SANO, K. Immune reaction of cerebrospinal fluid protein. In special issue: Cerebrospinal fluid, its analysis and clinical significance. Nihon Rinsho (Jpn. Clin. Pract.), *31:* 1025–1028, 1973.

399. SANO, K. Present and past of pulseless disease. Nihon Ishikai Zasshi (J. Jpn. Med. Soc.), *69:* 1281–1286, 1973.

400. SANO, K. Spinal cord tumors. In: *Guide to Current Treatment*, p. 95. Igaku-Shoin, Tokyo, 1973.

401. SANO, K. Spinal cord diseases—Recent trends. Ijin-Yakujin (Physicians and Pharmaceuticals), *22(5):* 3–4, 1973.

402. SANO, K., and MANAKU, N. Stationary potential encephalography. Igaku no Ayumi (Adv. Med.), *86:* 31–35, 1973.

403. SANO, K. Current state of microneurosurgery. No-shinkei Geka (Neurol. Surg.), *1:* 93–102, 1973.

404. MANAKU, N., and SANO, K. Stationary potential encephalogram—characteristics and origin. Rinsho Noha (Clin. Electroencephalogr.), *15:* 494–499, 1973.

405. SATO, O., and SANO, K. Roentgenologic diagnosis—Cerebral blood vessels. Shindan to Chiryo (Diagnosis and Treatment), *61:* 1429–1437, 1973.

406. SANO, K. Operations of vertebrobasilar artery aneurysms. No-Shinkei Geka (Neurol. Surg.), *1:* 193–199, 1973.

407. SANO, K. Cerebral symptomatology. In: *Handbook of Modern Gynecology and Obstetrics*, 6B, *Symptomatology of Gynecology*, II, edited by M. Suzuki, pp. 141–146. Nakayama-Shoten, Tokyo, 1973.

408. MANAKU, N., and SANO, K. Clinical application of cerebral D.C. potentials. Noha to Shindenzu (Electroencephalogr. Electromyography), *2:* 107–109, 1973.

409. HATANAKA, H., and SANO, K. A revised boron-neutron capture therapy for malignant brain tumors. I. Experiences on terminally ill patients after Co-60 radiotherapy. Z. Neurol., *204:* 309–332, 1973.

410. SATO, O., and SANO, K. Transoccipital transtentorial approach to posterior fossa lesions. Shujutsu (Operations), *27:* 979–984, 1973.

411. AMANO, K., and SANO, K. Single cell recording from the central grey of the midbrain. No-Shinkei Geka (Neurol. Surg.), *1:* 319–327, 1973.

412. SATO, O., TAMURA, A., SEKINO, H., and SANO, K. Brain tumors in infants. No to Shinkei (Brain and Nerve), *25:* 1447–1454, 1973.

413. SAITO, I., OCHIAI, Y., SATO, O., SANO, K., YAMADA, H., ORIHATA, T., YASAKU, Y., MITSUI, Y., HAWAKAWA, I., TSUCHIDA, T., YANAGIHASHI, K., ISHIJIMA, B., and FUKUSHIMA, T. Diagnosis and treatment of vascular tumors in the spinal cord. No-Shinkei Geka (Neurol. Surg.), *1:* 491–502, 1973.

414. SANO, K. Chemo-radiotherapie der malignen Hirngeschwülste. Therapiewoche, 23, *50:* 4939–4946, 1973.

415. MANAKA, N., MAYANAGI, Y., and SANO, K. Diagnostic value of stationary potentials during resection of epileptic foci, pp. 109–112. Proceedings of the 6th Meeting of the Discussion Group for Selected Subjects in Neurosurgery, 1973.

416. SANO, K., and SATO, O. Long follow-up for treatment of cancers—Brain tumors. Geka Chiryo (Surg. Treatment), *30:* 23–28, 1974.

417. HATANAKA, H., SANO, K., AMANO, K., MOGAMI, H., HAYAKAWA, T., KEJIO, Y., MISHIMA, Y., MIYAMOTO, M., WATANABE, A., and MINOBE, S. Four-year study of boron-neutron capture therapy of brain tumors in Japan and future project. Nihon Beka-Gakkai Zasshi (J. Jpn. Soc. Surg.), *75:* 1611–1613, 1974.

418. SANO, K. Diagnosis based on statistical analysis. No to Shinkei (Brain and Nerve), *26:* 31–32, 1974.

419. SANO, K., and HANDA, H. *Management of Neurosurgical Operating Rooms*, p. 412. Igaku-Shoin, Tokyo, 1974.

420. SANO, K., and SATO, O. *Preoperative Management of Neurosurgical Patients*, edited by K. Sano and H. Handa, pp. 1–28. Igaku-Shoin, Tokyo, 1974.

421. SANO, K. Review of clinical medicine—Neurological surgery. Nihon Iji Shinpo (Jpn. Med. News) *2605:* 12–23, 1974.

422. SANO, K., and KUWABARA, T. *Pediatric Neurosurgery*, p. 311. Igaku-Shoin, Tokyo, 1974.

423. SANO, K. Head trauma in children. In: *Handbook of Clinical Pediatric Surgery*, Vol. III-I, edited by M. Katsusai, pp. 130–144. Kinbara-Shuppan, Tokyo, 1974.

424. SANO, K. Emergency treatment of head trauma. Sogo Rinsho (Gen. Clin. Practice), *23:* 1098–1109, 1974.

425. HIRAKAWA, K., HASHIZUME, K., MIZONOUE, T., TAKAHASHI, H., MITSUI, Y., UEDA, H., MATSUTANI, M., and SANO, K. Differential diagnoses for chronic subdural hematoma: Statistical observation in 309 adult cases. Nihon Geka-Gakkai Zasshi (J. Jpn. Soc. Surg.), *75:* 1622–1625, 1974.

426. SANO, K., FUKUSHIMA, T., and HIRAKAWA, K. Ventriculofiberscopy in paediatric neurosurgery. In: *Progress in Paediatric Neurosurgery*, edited by K. A. Bushe, O. Spoerri, and J. Shaw, pp. 176–179. Hippokrates-Verlag, Stuttgart, 1974.

427. SANO, K., NAGAI, M., and SATO, O. Chemotherapy of brain tumors in children. In: *Progress in Paediatric Neurosurgery*, edited by K. A. Bushe, O. Spoerri, and J. Shaw, pp. 229–232. Hippokrates-Verlag, Stuttgart, 1974.

428. SANO, K., and SATO, O. Statistics in clinical medicine in Japan—Brain tumors. Nihon Rinsho (Jpn. Clin. Practice), *32:* 2158–2169, 1974.

429. SANO, K. Pulseless disease, present and past. Asian Med. J., *17:* 331–338, 1974.

430. SANO, K., and ISHII, S. *Recent Progress in Neurological Surgery* edited by K. Sano and S. Ishii (International Congress Series No. 320), p. 346. Excerpta Medica, Amsterdam, 1974.

431. SANO, K. Surgery of the hypothalamus (in commemoration of Otfrid Foerster). In: *Recent Progress in Neurological Surgery*, edited by K. Sano and S. Ishii (International Congress Series No. 320), pp. 210–218. Excerpta Medica, Amsterdam, 1974.

432. SANO, K., SEGAWA, H., and SATO, O. Aging and brain tumors—Brain tumors observed in geriatric patients. In: *Lecture Series of the Treatment of Geriatric Diseases*, No. 4, edited by Y. Kuroiwa, pp. 79–84. Kinbara-Shuppan, Tokyo, 1974.

433. MANAKA, S., SANO, K., FUCHINOUE, T., and SEKINO, H. Mechanism of action of CDP-choline in parkinsonism. Experientia, *30:* 179–180, 1974.

434. SANO, K., KUDO, T., and KITAMURA, K. *Treatment of Head Trauma*, p. 323. Kinbara-Shuppan, Tokyo, 1974.

435. SANO, K., and SATO, O. Treatment of head trauma in acute stage. In: *Treatment of Head Trauma*, edited by K. Sano, et al., pp. 1–17. Kinbara-Shuppan, Tokyo, 1974.

436. SANO, K., and SATO, O. Head trauma in children. In: *Treatment of*

Head Trauma, edited by K. Sano, et al., pp. 177–188. Kinbara-Shuppan, Tokyo, 1974.

437. SAITO, I., and SANO, K. Surgical treatment of subarachnoid hemorrhage in acute stage. Geka Chiryo (Surg. Treatment), *16:* 1215–1221, 1974.
438. MANAKA, N., MAYANAGI, Y., and SANO, K. Abnormal cerebral stationary potentials in the epileptic foci and pathophysiological explanation. No to Shinkei (Brain and Nerve), *26:* 889–895, 1974.
439. MANAKA, N., and SANO, K. Experimental studies on intrathecal infusion of CDP-choline. No to Shinkei (Brain and Nerve), *26:* 889–895, 1974.
440. SANO, K. Advances in neurological surgery—Essentials for internists. Medicina, *11:* 1372–1373, 1974.
441. SANO, K., SEKINO, H., and AMANO, K. Pain surgery in neurological surgery. Nihon Rinsho- Geka Igakkai Zasshi (J. Jpn. Soc. Clin. Surg.), *35:* 672–675, 1974.
442. SANO, K. Indications for and results of making central lesions in the brain for epileptic patients. In: *Epilepsy*, edited by P. Harris and C. Mawdsley, pp. 215–221. Churchill Livingstone, Edinburgh, 1974.
443. SANO, K., and MANAKA, S. Stationary potential changes in epilepsy. In: *Epilepsy*, edited by P. Harris and C. Mawdsley, pp. 74–77. Churchill Livingstone, Edinburgh, 1974.
444. FUCHINOUE, T., MANAKA, S., HIRAKAWA, K., and SANO, K. Diagnostic value of stationary potential measurement in head injuries. Neurol. Med. Chir., *14(Part I):* 19–27, 1974.
445. SANO, K., JIMBO, M., SAITO, I., and BASUGI, N. Artificial embolization of inoperable angioma with polymerizing substance. In: *Cerebral Angiomas—Advances in Diagnosis and Therapy*, edited by H. W. Pia, J. R. W. Gleave, E. Grote, and J. Zierski, pp. 222–229. Springer-Verlag, Berlin, 1975.
446. SANO, K., and MANAKA, N. Testing of cerebral stationary potentials—New method for electrophysiology of the brain. Nihon Iji Shinpo (Jpn. Med. News), *2654:* 37–40, 1975.
447. SANO, K. Variety of brain tumors—Mortality has reduced since introduction of the surgical microscope. Mainichi Life (Special Issue for Cancer), February issue: 94–102, 1975.
448. SANO, K., and MANAKA, N. M E in neurosurgical field. Iyo-Denshi to Seitai-Kogaku (Med. Electr. Bioengineering), *13:* 43–48, 1975.
449. SANO, K., SEKINO, H., HASHIMOTO, I., AMANO, K., and SUGIYAMA, H. Posteromedial hypothalamotomy in the treatment of intractable pain. Confin. Neurol., *37:* 285–290, 1975.

450. SANO, K. Immunology of brain tumors in children—Focused on a long-term follow-up. Proceedings of the 2nd Research Meeting of Japanese Pediatric Neurosurgery 1974, pp. 61–63. Neuron-sha, Tokyo, 1975.

451. SANO, K. Operative or conservative treatment: Stroke—surgeon's view. Chiryo (Treatment), *57:* 1587–1590, 1975.

452. SANO, K. Posterior hypothalamic lesions in the treatment of violent behavior. In: *Neural Bases of Violence and Aggression*, edited by W. S. Fields and W. H. Sweet, pp. 401–420. W. H. Green, St. Louis, 1975.

453. MIZONOKAMI, T., and SANO, K. Diagnostic importance of cerebral stationary potentials in head trauma. No to Shinkei (Brain and Nerve), *27:* 945–957, 1975.

454. SAITO, I., and SANO, K. Microsurgery of the angiomas of the spinal cord. In: *Microsurgery*, edited by H. Handa, pp. 137–144. Igaku Shoin, Tokyo, 1975.

455. SATO, O., TAMURA, A., and SANO, K. Brain tumors of early infants. Child's Brain, *1:* 121–125, 1975.

456. SANO, K. Takayasu disease—Pulseless disease—Takayasu arteritis. Shinkei Naika (Neurology), *3:* 15–22, 1975.

457. SANO, K., and MANAKA, N. Electrical activity in the brain (1). Rinsho Noha (Clin. Electroencephalogr.), *17:* 642–648, 1975.

458. SANO, K., and MANAKA, N. Electrical activity in the brain (II). Rinsho Noha (Clin. Electroencephalogr.) *17:* 703–710, 1975.

459. SANO, K., and MANAKA, N. Electrical activity in the brain (III). Rinsho Noho (Clin. Electroencephalogr.), *17:* 761–768, 1975.

460. SANO, K. Advances in diagnostic studies of cerebrovascular diseases. Shinyaku to Chiryo (New Drugs and Treatment), *202:* 3–4, 1975.

461. SANO, K. Indication for surgical treatment of ruptured intracranial aneurysms, timing, and prognosis. In special issue: Stroke—Recent review. Naika (Medicine), *36:* 589–593, 1975.

462. SANO, K. Subarachnoid hemorrhage due to rupture of intracranial aneurysms. In special issue: Surgery of stroke. Rinsho Geka (Clin. Surg.), *30:* 1567–1575, 1975.

463. SANO, K. Surgery of stroke. Rinsho Geka (Clin. Surg.), *30:* 1527–1528, 1975.

464. SANO, K. Advances in treatment of cerebrovascular diseases—Surgery. Nihon Ishikai Zasshi (J. Jpn. Soc. Med.), *74:* 1351–1361, 1975.

465. TSUBAKI, K., SANO, K., and GOSHIMA, Y. *Clinical Neurology*, 2nd Ed., p. 929. Igaku-Shoin, Tokyo, 1976.

466. SANO, K. Tumors and mass forming diseases. In: *Clinical Neurology*,

2nd Ed., edited by T. Tsubaki, K. Sano, and Y. Goshima, pp. 635–695. Igaku-Shoin, Tokyo, 1976.

467. SANO, K. Hereditary and developmental anomalies. In: *Clinical Neurology*, 2nd Ed., edited by T. Tsubaki, K. Sano, and Y. Goshima, pp. 775–804. Igaku-Shoin, Tokyo, 1976.

468. SANO, K., ed. *Atlas of Stereoscopic Neurology*, p. 114. University of Tokyo Press, Tokyo, 1976.

469. SANO, K. Pinealoma in children. Child's Brain, *2:* 67–72, 1976.

470. SANO, K. Surgery of cerebrovascular diseases—Aneurysms, arteriovenous malformations. Nihon Geka-Gakkai Zasshi (J. Jpn. Soc. Surg.), *77:* 458–462, 1976.

471. SANO, K. Advances in neurosurgery—Benign brain tumors. Nihon Rinsho (Jpn. Clin. Med.), *34:* 1008–1011, 1976.

472. SANO, K. A long-term result of pineal tumors in children, pp. 77–78. Proceedings of 3rd Research Meeting of Japanese Pediatric Neurosurgery, 1976.

473. SANO, K. Treatment of congenital hydrocephalus. Shoni no No-Shinkei (Pediatr. Neurol.), *1:* 7–8, 1976.

474. MASUZAWA, H., and SANO, K. Hydrocephalus—Treatment of congenital hydrocephalus. Shoni no No-Shinkei (Pediatr. Neurol.) *1:* 99–105, 1976.

475. KURUMADO, K., MORI, W., MATSUTANI, M., and SANO, K. Virus-like particles in human pinealoma. Acta Neuropathol., *35:* 273–276, 1976.

476. SAITO, O., KANAZAWA, I., KAMIYA, H., YAMASHITA, R., and SANO, K. Contrast enhancement in cranial computed tomography—Analysis of ICI method. No to Shinkei (Brain and Nerve), *28:* 1225–1235, 1976.

477. SANO, K. Diagnosis and treatment of tumours in the pineal region. Acta Neurochir., *34:* 153–157, 1976.

478. SANO, K. Chemistry of brain tumors—Radiation treatment. Shinkei Geka (Neurol. Surg.), *16(Part II):* 379–386, 1976.

479. AMANO, K., KITAMURA, K., SANO, K., and SEKINO, H. Relief of intractable pain from neurosurgical point of view with reference to present limits and clinical indications. A review of 100 consecutive cases. Neurol. Med. Chir., *16(Part II):* 145–153, 1976.

480. SANO, K. New year review of neurological surgery. Doctor Salon, *21:* 39–42, 1976.

481. SATO, O., and SANO, K. Von Hippel-Lindau disease. Shinkei Naika (Neurology), *5:* 515–523, 1976.

482. KONO, T., MATSUYA, M., HOSHINO, T., SANO, K., SHITARA, N., and TAKAKURA, K. Chemotherapy of malignant brain tumors

with combination of adriamycin and BCNU. Shinkei Geka (Neurol. Surg.), *16(Part II):* 545–553, 1976.

483. SATO, O., KOBAYASHI, M., and SANO, K. Simultaneous biplane angioautotomography for the analysis of intracranial aneurysms. *Advances in Neurosurgery,* edited by R. Wüllenweber, et al., pp. 281–286. Springer-Verlag, Berlin, 1977.

484. ASANO, T., and SANO, K. Pathogenetic role of no-reflow phenomenon in experimental subarachnoid hemorrhage in dogs. J. Neurosurg., *46:* 454–466, 1977.

485. SANO, K. Principle of surgical treatment of ruptured intracranial aneurysms. In: *Technical Details in Surgical Treatment,* edited by K. Ishikawa and T. Manabe, pp. 78–79. Kinbara-Shuppan, Tokyo, 1977.

486. SANO, K. Brain tumors. In: *Today's Therapeutic Guide,* pp. 86–87. Igaku-Shoin, Tokyo, 1977.

487. KIM, Z., and SANO, K. Role of platelets and red cells in cerebrovascular insufficiency. Shinkei-Geka (Neurol. Surg.), *17(Part II):* 135–144, 1977.

488. SANO, K. Intralaminar thalamotomy (thalamolaminotomy) and postero-medial hypothalamotomy in the treatment of intractable pain. In: *Progress in Neurological Surgery,* edited by H. Krayenbühl, et al., Karger, Basel, 1977.

489. SAITO, I., TAMURA, A., and SANO, K. A long-term result of ruptured anterior communicating aneurysms after operative procedures in acute stage—Especially the follow-up of morbidity. Shinkei Geka (Neurol. Surg.), *17(Part II):* 233–241, 1977.

490. SANO, K., HANDA, H., and ISHII, S. Pioneers in Japanese neurosurgery. Surg. Neurol., *7:* 321–323, 1977.

491. MASUZAWA, H., KIM, Z., and SANO, K. Chiari type IV anomaly—Surgery of anomalies in the central nervous system, pp. 178–181. Proceedings of the 4th Research Meeting of Japanese Pediatric Neurosurgery, 1977.

492. YASUOKA, M., KIRINO, T., KIM, Z., MASUZAWA, H., and SANO, K. Clinical aspect of spinal bifida cystica—Hydrocephalus as a complication and prognosis of neurological function of the lower extremities, pp. 247–251. Proceedings of the 4th Research Meeting of Japanese Pediatric Neurosurgery, 1977.

493. SANO, K. Long-term prognosis of the 3rd ventricle tumors in children, including the recurrence—Prognosis of pineal tumors. Shoni no Shinkei (Pediatr. Neurol.) (Special Issue), *2:* 125–130, 1977.

494. SANO, K. Functional recovery after trauma of the nervous system—

Especially the coordinating movement of the cranial nerves and other symptoms. Gaisho (Trauma), *7:* 442–532, 1977.

495. SANO, K., MANAKA, N., KITAMURA, K., KAGAWA, M., TAKEUCHI, I., KOKASHI, M., NAKAMURA, N., ISHII, S., HIRAI, H., and TSUBAKI, N. Effects of intrathecal injection of CDP-choline in the patients with impaired consciousness. Shinkei-Kenkyu no Shinpo (Adv. Neurol. Res.), *21:* 835–849, 1977.
496. SANO, K., and SAITO, I. A long-term result of intracranial aneurysms after introduction of the surgical microscope. No to Shinkei (Brain and Nerve), *29:* 977–985, 1977.
497. SAITO, I., UEDA, Y., and SANO, K. Significance of vasospasm in the treatment of ruptured intracranial aneurysms. J. Neurosurg., *47:* 412–429, 1977.
498. SANO, K., MANAKA, N., KITAMURA, K., KAGAWA, M., TAKEUCHI, I., KOKASHI, M., KAMEYAMA, M., TOGI, H., and YAMADA, H. Grading method for statistical analysis of the patients with mild impairment of consciousness—Characteristic symptomatology. Shinkei-Kenkyu no Shinpo (Adv. Neurol. Res.), *21:* 1052–1065, 1977.
499. SANO, K. Trauma due to traffic accident and its treatment—Focused on head trauma. In: *2nd Collection of the Lectures on Combined Symposium in Traffic Science*, pp. 99–115. Kotsu Kagaku Kyogikai (Traffic Science Council), 1977.
500. MANAKA, N., MIZONOKAMI, T., KONDO, T., HORI, T., and SANO, K. Effects of thyrotropin releasing hormone tartrate (TRH-T) on unconsciousness. No to Shinkei (Brain and Nerve), *29:* 1075–1081, 1977.
501. SANO, K. Present status of stereotaxic functional neurosurgery, pp. 246–259. Actas y Trajos del XVI Congreso Latinoamericano de Neurocirugia, Caracas, Oct. 12–17, 1975, 1977.
502. SANO, K. Emotional behaviour and the hypothalamus in the light of stereotaxic surgery, pp. 185–194. Commemoration of Professor Egas Moniz. Egas Moniz Centenary Scientific Reports, Lisbon, 1977.
503. SANO, K. Therapeutic results of brain tumors in children, pp. 46–49. Shoni Gan (Cancer in Children), No. 11 (Recordings from Research Meeting of Pediatric Brain Tumors), 1977.
504. KWAK, S., and SANO, K. Classification of hypertensive intracerebral hemorrhage by CT scan. Saishin Igaku (Mod. Med.), *32:* 2299–2305, 1977.
505. SANO, K. Section of the portio minor of the trigeminal nerve for the treatment of the Marcus Gunn phenomenon. Mod. Probl. Paediat., *18:* 258–262, 1977.

506. SANO, K., UEDA, Y., and SAITO, I. Subarachnoid hemorrhage in children. Child's Brain, *4:* 38–46, 1978.

507. SANO, K. Diagnosis by statistical method—Head trauma. In special issue: Statistical diagnosis. Saishin Igaku (Mod. Med.), *33:* 26–27, 1978.

508. SANO, K. Introduction to subarachnoid hemorrhage—Focused on treatment of ruptured intracranial aneurysm. In Special Issue: Subarachnoid hemorrhage—Neurological surgery—Essentials for internists. Nihon Rinsho (Jpn. Clin. Med.), *36:* 460–466, 1978.

509. ASANO, T., TAMURA, A., MII, K., and SANO, K. The role of humoral agents released by platelet aggregation in the pathogenesis of transient ischemic attacks. Neurol. Med. Chir., *18(Part I):* 59–66, 1978.

510. SANO, K. Future of pediatric neurology from the standpoint of pediatric neurosurgeons. No to Hattatsu (Brain and Development), *10:* 195, 1978.

511. SANO, K. What are brain tumors? Kango Gijutsu (Nursing Technique), *24(3):* 9–17, 1978.

512. MANAKA, N., and SANO, K. Monitoring of the level of consciousness. Sogo Rinsho (Gen. Clin. Med.), *27:* 871–876, 1978.

513. SANO, K. Selection of treatment. Shindan to Chiryo (Diagnosis and Treatment), *66:* 106–110, 1978.

514. TERAMOTO, A., MATSUYA, M., HIRAKAWA, K., SANO, K., NAGAMURA, Y., and WATANABE, K. Immuno-histochemical observation of pituitary adenoma—Enzyme antibody method. Shinkei Geka (Neurol. Surg.), *18(Part II):* 209–214, 1978.

515. SHITARA, N., KAWANO, T., NAGAMUNE, A., TAKAKURA, K., and SANO, K. Basic research on phase-synchronization in brain tumors, II. Variations in cell cycle depending on various anticancer chemotherapeutics and on physical factors. Shinkei Geka (Neurol. Surg.), *18(Part II):* 199–207, 1978.

516. SANO, K., and SAITO, I. Timing and indication of surgery for ruptured intracranial aneurysms with regard to cerebral vasospasm. Acta Neurochir., *41:* 49–60, 1978.

517. MASUZAWA, H., and SANO, K. Metrizamide computer tomography of the cisterna magna and the spinal cord. Shinkei Kenkyu no Shinpo (Adv. Neurol. Res.), *22:* 321–332, 1978.

518. SANO, K. Non-surgical treatment of malignant brain tumors. Shinkei Kenkyu no Shinpo (Adv. Neurol. Res.), *22:* 878–880, 1978.

519. SANO, K. Chemo-radiotherapy of malignant brain tumors. In: *Proceedings of the 6th International Congress of Neurological Surgery, São Paulo, June 19–25, 1977*, edited by R. Carrea and D. L. Vay

Co., pp. 79–87. Excerpta Medica, Amsterdam/Oxford, 1978.

520. Kirino, T., and Sano, K. Physiological anatomy of the facial nerve—Old structure and new function of the facial nerve. Shinkei Naika (Neurol. Med.), *9:* 211–226, 1978.

521. Takakura, T., and Sano, K. Clinical use of chemotherapeutic agents—Combined treatment of malignant brain tumors. In Special Issue: Current immunotherapy of cancers—Practice of immunochemotherapy of cancers. Rinsho Geka (Clin. Surg.), *33:* 1427–1431, 1978.

522. Manaka, S., and Sano, K. Thyrotropin-releasing hormone tartrate (TRH-T) shortens concussion effects following head impact in mice. Neurosci. Lett., *8:* 255–258, 1978.

523. Sano, K., and Saito, I. Microsurgery of ruptured intracranial aneurysms. Relation to cerebral vasospasm, Seara Med. Neurochir., *7:* 175–183, 1978.

524. Mayanagi, Y., Hori, T., and Sano, K. The posteromedial hypothalamus and pain behavior with special reference to endocrinological findings. Applied Neurophysiol., *41:* 223–231, 1978.

525. Kwak, S., Inoh, S., Nagashima, T., and Sano, K. Classification of hypertensive intracerebral hemorrhage by means of computed tomography. Neuroradiology, *16:* 159–161, 1978.

526. Saito, I., and Sano, K. Vasospasm following rupture of cerebral aneurysms. Neurol. Med. Chir., *19:* 103–107, 1979.

527. Kondo, T., Manaka, S., Nagamune, A., Tsujita, Y., Hirakawa, K., and Sano, K. Electrophysiological study on pituitary adenoma cells in tissue culture. In: *Treatment of Pituitary Adenomas*, edited by R. Fahlbusch and K. V. Werder, pp. 179–182. Georg Thieme, Stuttgart, 1978.

528. Sano, K., and Manaka, N. *Clinical Use of the CT Scanner of the Head, CT Scanner-Computer Tomography Equipment*, pp. 214–228. Corona-Sha, Tokyo, 1979.

529. Sano, K. Diagnostic tool for localization of cerebral lesions. ME News-Foundation for Research Development in Medical Therapeutic Technology, *9:* 7–11, 1979.

530. Sano, K. Indications for surgical treatment of ruptured intracranial aneurysms and timing for operations. Shindan to Chiryo (Diagnosis and Treatment), *67:* 119–123, 1979.

531. Sano, K. Brain tumors. Clinical aspect of cancers—Early diagnosis of cancers, Series of early treatment, pp. 89–96. Kyowa Hakko-Kogyo Hakko (Kyowa Fermentation Industry Publication), 1979.

532. Takakura, K., Shitara, N., Kawano, T., Yamamoto, H., and Sano, K. Cell cycle of brain tumors and combined treatment.

Gan to Kagaku-Ryoho (Cancer and Chemotherapy), *5(Suppl.)*: 31–40, 1979.

533. HASHIMOTO, I., MANAKA, S., and SANO, K. The role of extracellular potassium in early epilepsy. Neurol. Res., *1:* 39–49, 1979.

534. WAKAI, S., MATSUTANI, M., MIZUTANI, H., and SANO, K. Tight junctions in choroid plexus papillomas. Acta Neuropathol. *45:* 159–160, 1979.

535. SANO, K., MANAKA, N., and HARI, T. Clinical research on treatment of unconsciousness with TRH tartrate. First report. Preliminary report on control study for dosage determination. Rinsho to Kenkyu (Clin. Res.), *56:* 1950–1960, 1979.

536. SANO, K., KITAMURA, K., TAKEUCHI, K., et al. Clinical research on treatment of unconsciousness with TRH tartrate. Second report. Double blind clinical study. Shinkei Kenkyu on Shinpo (Adv. Neurol. Res.), *23:* 184–210, 1979.

537. TAMURA, A., ASANO, T., SANO, K., TSUMAGARI, T., and NAKAJIMA, A. Protection from cerebral ischemia by a new imidazole derivative (Y-9179) and pentobarbital. A comparative study in chronic middle cerebral artery occlusion in cats. Stroke, *10:* 126–134, 1979.

538. SANO, K. Neurological surgery—Surgery of autonomic nervous system. In: *Handbook of New Clinical Surgery*, Vol. 3, edited by K. Sano, K. Nakayama, and S. Sakakibara, p. 603. Kinbara Shuppan, Tokyo, 1979.

539. SANO, K. Brain tumor neurological surgery–Surgery of autonomic nervous system. In: *Handbook of New Clinical Surgery*, Vol. 3, edited by K. Sano, K. Nakayama, and S. Sakakibara, pp. 73–145. Kinbara Shuppan, Tokyo, 1979.

540. SANO, K. Stereotaxic thalamolaminotomy and posteromedial hypothalamotomy for the relief of intractable pain. In: *Advances in Pain Research and Therapy*, Vol. 2, edited by J. J. Bonica and V. Ventafridda, pp. 475–485. International Symposium on Pain of Advanced Cancer. Raven Press, New York, 1979.

541. SANO, K., and ASANO, K. Treatment—Surgical aspect—Aneurysms, arteriovenous malformations, hypertensive cerebral hemorrhages, idiopathic cerebral hemorrhages, cerebrovascular insufficiency, cerebrovascular occlusive diseases. In: *Stroke—Basic Science and Clinical Practice*, edited by K. Kitamura and M. Kameyama, pp. 280–290. Asakura-Shoten, Tokyo, 1979.

542. MAYANAGI, Y., and SANO, K. Long-term follow-up results of the posteromedial hypothalamotomy. In: *Modern Concepts in Psychiatric Surgery*, edited by E. R. Hitchcock, H. T. Ballantine, Jr.,

and B. A. Meyerson, pp. 197–204. Elsevier/North-Holland Biomedical Press, Amsterdam, 1979.

543. MANAKA, S., and SANO, K. Stationary potential of the brain: Part I. Basic studies. Neurol. Med. Chir., *19:* 643–653, 1979.

544. SANO, K., MANAKA, S., MIYAKE, H., MAYANAGI, Y., and FUCHINOUE, T. Stationary potential of the brain: Part II. Clinical studies. Neurol. Med. Chir. *19:* 655–664, 1979.

545. OCHIAI, C., MASUZAWA, H., MANAKA, S., SANO, K., KITAMURA, K. and KOMATSUZAKI, A. Supine-lateral approach versus sitting operation. Statistical analysis of brainstem, cranial nerve and cerebellar function in 165 acoustic neurinomas. Neurol. Med. Chir., *19:* 629–635, 1979.

546. SHIMIZU, H., MASUZAWA, H., and SANO, K. Bilateral acoustic tumors: its clinical features and surgical treatment. Neurol. Med. Chir., *19:* 623–627, 1979.

547. ASANO, T., and SANO, K. Substances for brain protection. No-Shinkei Geka (Neurol. Surg.), *7:* 549–554, 1979.

548. SHITARA, N., TAKAKURA, K., and SANO, K. Interferon and brain tumors. No-Shinkei Geka (Neurol. Surg.), *7:* 645–652, 1979.

549. AOYANAGI, T., MANAKA, N., and SANO, K. Research on two dimensional montage of brain waves. Rinsho Noha (Clin. Electroencephalogr.), *21:* 482–489, 1979.

550. SANO, K. New treatment of brain tumors in children. In: *Basics of Child Neurology*, edited by Y. Fukuyama, pp. 396–402. Shindan to Chiryo-Sha (Diagnosis and Treatment), Tokyo, 1979.

551. GOTO, O., KIM, Z., and SANO, K. Morphological changes of platelets during impairment of microvascular circulation—Clinical analysis by scanning electron microscopy. No to Shinkei (Brain and Nerve), *31:* 937–943, 1979.

552. TERAMOTO, A., SANO, K., NAGAMURA, Y., and WATANABE, K. Immuno-histochemical observations of the pituitary adenoma by enzyme-antibody method—Regarding residual pituitary tissue and capsule. Shinkei Geka (Neurol. Surg.), *19:* 895–902, 1979.

553. SANO, K. Neoplasms of the brain. In: *Medicine, Individual sections, Vol. 8, Neurological Diseases*, edited by M. Kameyama, pp. 301–344. Nankodo, Tokyo, 1979.

554. EGUCHI, T., MANAKA, N., SANO, K., SUGIYAMA, H., IZUKI, Y., BABA, M., KUMAGAYA, N., and NAWADA, H. A method to determine the operative indication in completed stroke-Hyperbaric treatment. Proceedings of the 8th Surgical Research Meeting on Stroke (Surgery for Ischemic Cerebrovascular Disease), pp. 89–94, 1979.

555. MATSUZAWA, H., SHIMIZU, H., and SANO, K. Advantages of metrizamide myelogram and its side effect. No to Shinkei (Brain and Nerve), *31:* 843–854, 1979.

556. TAMURA, A., and SANO, K. Effects of recirculation in ischemic brain tissue—Correlation between local cerebral blood flow and tissue damage. No to Shinkei (Brain and Nerve), *31:* 1005–1015, 1979.

557. SAITO, I., SHIGENO, T., ARITAKE, K., TANISHIMA, T., and SANO, K. Vasospasm assessed by angiography and computerized tomography. J. Neurosurg. *51:* 466–475, 1979.

558. TAKAKURA, K., and SANO, K. Role of immunopotentiators on brain tumor therapy. In: *Multidisciplinary Aspects of Brain Tumor Therapy*, edited by P. Paoletti, M. D. Walker, G. Butti, and R. Knerich, pp. 223–234. Elsevier/North-Holland Biomedical Press, Amsterdam, 1979.

559. SANO, K., and SAITO, I. Indication and timing of operation and vasospasm. In: *Cerebral Aneurysms—Advances in Diagnosis and Therapy*, edited by H. W. Pia, C. Langmaid, and J. Zierski, pp. 208–216. Springer-Verlag, Berlin/Heidelberg/New York, 1979.

560. SANO, K. Neuroradiological diagnosis. Computer tomography. In: *Cerebral Aneurysms—Advances in Diagnosis and Therapy*, edited by H. W. Pia, C. Langmaid, and J. Zierski, pp. 195–196. Springer-Verlag, Berlin/Heidelberg/New York, 1979.

561. SANO, K. Internal carotid posterior communicating anterior choroidal region aneurysms. Microsurgical treatment. In: *Cerebral Aneurysms—Advances in Diagnosis and Therapy*, edited by H. W. Pia, C. Langmaid, and J. Zierski, pp. 252–259. Springer Verlag, Berlin/Heidelberg/New York, 1979.

562. SANO, K. Basilar artery aneurysms—Transoral transclival approach. In: *Cerebral Aneurysms—Advances in Diagnosis and Therapy*, edited by H. W. Pia, C. Langmaid, and J. Zierski, pp. 326–328. Springer Verlag, Berlin/Heidelberg/New York, 1979.

563. SANO, K. Giant cerebral aneurysms—Management. In *Cerebral Aneurysms—Advances in Diagnosis and Therapy*, edited by H. W. Pia, C. Langmaid, and J. Zierski, pp. 342–344. Springer Verlag, Berlin/Heidelberg/New York, 1979.

564. SANO, K. Special technical problems—Wrapping technique—present place. In: *Cerebral Aneurysms—Advances in Diagnosis and Therapy*, edited by H. W. Pia, C. Langmaid, and J. Zierski, pp. 393–395. Springer Verlag, Berlin/Heidelberg/New York, 1979.

565. SANO, K. Operative treatment of complications—Intracerebral haematomas. In: *Cerebral Aneurysms—Advances in Diagnosis and*

Therapy, edited by H. W. Pia, C. Langmaid, and J. Zierski, pp. 402–407. Springer Verlag, Berlin/Heidelberg/New York, 1979.

566. SANO, K. Prognosis of operative treatment—Personal experiences. In: Cerebral Aneurysms—Advances in Diagnosis and Therapy, edited by H. W. Pia, C. Langmaid, and J. Zierski, pp. 428–432. Springer Verlag, Berlin/Heidelberg/New York, 1979.

567. SANO, K., SHITARA, N., and TAKAKURA, K. Interferon productivity of human lymphocytes with the induction of Poly I:C in cases of malignant glioma. In: *Advances in Neurosurgery*, Chap. 7, edited by F. Marguth, M. Brock, E. Kazner, M. Klinger, and P. Schmiedek, pp. 376–380. Springer Verlag, Berlin/Heidelberg/New York, 1979.

568. WAKAI, S., FUKUSHIMA, T., FURIHATA, F., and SANO, K. Association of cerebral aneurysms with pituitary adenoma. Surg. Neurol. *12:* 503–507, 1979.

569. SANO, K., MANAKA, N., KITAMURA, K., KAGAWA, M., TAKEUCHI, T., KOKASHI, M., KAMEYAMA, M., TOGI, H., and YAMADA, H. Statistical research in grading of patients with mild impairment of consciousness—Follow-up studies and selection of symptoms and signs for grading. Shinkei Kenkyu no Shinpo (Adv. Neurol. Res.), *23:* 1207–1218, 1979.

570. SANO, K., MANAKA, N., KITAMURA, K., KAGAWA, M., TAKEUCHI, K., KOKASHI, M., KAMEYAMA, M., TOGI, H., and YAMADA, H. Statistical research in grading of unconsciousness. Shinkei Gaisho (Trauma of the Nervous System), *2:* 105–112, 1979.

571. SANO, K. Clinical medicine in the 1980's—Treatment of neurosurgical diseases. Mainichi Life, *2:* 41–43, 1980.

572. SANO, K. Introduction to recent advances in neurological surgery. Rinsho Seijin-Byo (Clin. Pract. Adult Dis., *10:* 9–10, 1980.

573. SANO, K. Head trauma. In: *Surgery Mook 11, Head Trauma*, edited by K. Sano, p. 251. Kinbara-Shuppan, Tokyo, 1980.

574. SANO, K. Definition and classification of head trauma. In: *Surgery Mook 11, Head Trauma*, edited by K. Sano, pp. 1–6. Kinbara-Shuppan, Tokyo, 1980.

575. AOYANAGI, T., MASUZAWA, H., SANO, K., NORIHIRA, M., and KOBAYASHI S. Compliance of the brain. No to Shinkei (Brain and Nerve), *32:* 47–56, 1980.

576. TSUCHIDA, T., MIYAJI Y., HAYAKAWA I., HIRAKAWA K., and SANO, K. Brain tumors and cyclic nucleotides (first report)—cAMP and cGMP concentration in various brain tumors. No to Shinkei (Brain and Nerve), *32:* 59–67, 1980.

577. SANO, K. Pulseless disease—Series of circulatory diseases, by pic-

torial explanation. Nihon Ishikai Zasshi (J. Jpn. Soc. Med.), *83(3):* 1980.

578. SASAKI, T., ASANO, T., and SANO, K. Cerebral vasospasms and free radical reaction. Shinkei Geka (Neurol. Surg.), *20:* 145–153, 1980.
579. FUKUSHIMA, T., and SANO, K. New transsphenoidal approach to the pituitary body—Sublabial rhinoseptoplastic technique. No-shinkei Geka (Neurol. Surg.), *8:* 229–235, 1980.
580. SANO, K. Perspective in international neurosurgery: Neurosurgery in Japan. Neurosurgery, *6:* 337–339, 1980.
581. SANO, K. Advances in surgical treatment of brain tumors. Gan to Kagaku-Ryoho (Cancer and Chemotherapy), *7(Suppl. 1):* 264–273, 1980.
582. SANO, K. Emergency Care in Cerebral Vascular Diseases—Essentials for Emergency Care 4. In: *Lecture Series of Continuing Education for Emergency Doctors in 1979,* pp. 1–26. Tokyo Municipal Department of Welfare, Tokyo, 1980.
583. MASUZAWA, H., and SANO, K. Diseases of the spinal cord. Rinsho to Kenkyu (Clin. Pract. Res.), *57:* 1043–1048, 1980.
584. MANAKA, N., and SANO, K. The level of consciousness. Sogo Rinsho (Gen. Clin. Med.), *29:* 1475–1479, 1980.
585. KIRINO, T., and SANO, K. Changes in the contralateral dentate gyrus in Mongolian gerbils subjected to unilateral cerebral ischemia. Acta Neuropathol. *50:* 121–129, 1980.
586. SASAKI, T., MAYANAGI, Y., SHIMAZAKI, H., KUBOTA, M., ASANO, T., and SANO, K. Cerebrovascular spasms and lipid peroxidation reaction. Igaku no Ayumi (Adv. Med.), *113:* 970–972, 1980.
587. MANAKA, N., TERAMOTO, A., TAKAKURA, K., SANO, K., and MASUZAWA, H. Effectiveness of radiation therapy for craniopharyngiomas in children–Analysis of various doses of radiation. Shoni no No-Shinkei (Pediatr. Neurol.), *5:* 113–119, 1980.
588. TAKIZAWA, T., and SANO, K. Laser neurosurgery. In: *Laser Medicine, Basic Science and Clinical Application,* edited by K. Atsumi, et al., pp. 191–197. Nakayama-Shoten, Tokyo, 1980.
589. FUKUSHIMA, T., and SANO, K. Sublabial rhinoseptoplastic technique for transsphenoidal pituitary surgery by a hinged-septum method (technical note). J. Neurosurg., *52:* 867–870, 1980.
590. TAKAMAKURA, K., and SANO, K. Brain Tumors—Incidence in each hemisphere. Shinkei Kenkyu no Shinpo (Adv. Neurol. Res.), *24:* 668–670, 1980.
591. SANO, K. Hypertensive cerebellar hemorrhages—Pathological changes of cerebellar vasculature, pictorial explanation. Nihon Ishi-Kai Zasshi (J. Jpn. Soc. Med.), *84(4):* 1980.

592. SANO, K. Neurological surgery. In: *Introduction of Surgery*, edited by K. Ishikawa, M. Ishida, and T. Tanaka, pp. 431–600. Bunkoko, Tokyo, 1980.

593. TANISHIMA, T., and SANO, K. Research on hemoglobin and cerebrovascular spasms (1st report)—Correlation between hemoglobin and cerebrovascular spasms. Shinkei Gaeka (Neurol. Surg.), *20:* 481–489, 1980.

594. TANISHIMA, T., and SANO, K. Research on hemoglobin and cerebrovascular spasms (2nd report)—Calcium blocker and other antagonists against the cerebrovascular spasms. Shinkei Geka (Neurol. Surg.), *20:* 817–822, 1980.

595. SANO, K. A multipurpose all-angle clip applier for aneurysm surgery (technical note). J. Neurosurg., *53:* 260–261, 1980.

596. FUKUSHIMA, T., and SANO, K. Simple retractor holder for the Mayfield skull clamp. Surg. Neurol., *13:* 320, 1980.

597. MANAKA, S., HORI, T., TAKAHASHI, H., SANO, K., KOSUGI, Y., TAKAHASHI, T., and SEKINE, M. Auditorische EEG-Registrierung. Z. EEG-EMG, *11:* 81–83, 1980.

598. SANO, K., KITAMURA, K., TAKEUCHI, K., and KAMEYAMA, M. Cerebrovascular diseases, head trauma, and brain tumors on geriatric patients—Research on results of treatment on patients with mild impairment of consciousness and determination of the grading (3rd report)—Research articles. Foundation for Therapeutic Research on Metabolic Abnormalities, *7:* 80–92, 1980.

599. WAKAI, S., SEGAWA, H., KITAHARA, S., ASANO, T., SANO, K., OGIHARA, K., and TOMITA, S. Teratoma in the pineal region in two brothers (case reports). J. Neurosurg. *53:* 239–243, 1980.

600. SANO, K. Advances in neurological surgery—Focused on stroke. In Special Issue: Clinical Practice of Stroke Clinician. *27(294):* 2–6, 1980.

601. SANO, K., HANDA, H., and ASANO T. Cell damage secondary to cerebral ischemia—Influence of active oxygen and free radicals, p. 198. Neuron-Sha, Tokyo, 1980.

602. SANO, K., TAKAKURA, K., and FUKUSHIMA, T. Hormone producing pituitary tumor—Pathology and clinical practice, p. 163. Kowa Hakko-Kogyo Hakko (Kowa Fermentation Industry Publication), Tokyo, 1980.

603. YOSHIDA, N., INO, S., ASANO, T., SANO, K., KUBOTA, M., SHIMAZAKI, H., and UEDA, N. Destruction of the lipid membrane in the experimental cerebral ischemia—Tissue damage and peroxidation after recirculation—Cerebral ischemic and tissue damage. In: *Active Oxygen and Free Radicals*, edited by K. Sano, H. Handa, and T. Asano, pp. 30–50. Neuron-Sha, Tokyo, 1980.

604. SASAKI, T., WATANABE, T., WAKAI, S., KIRINO, T., ASANO, T., and SANO, K. Experimental studies on cerebrovascular spasms—Lipid peroxidation. In: *Active Oxygen and Free Radicals*, edited by K. Sano, H. Handa, and T. Asano, pp. 90–97. Neuron-Sha, Tokyo, 1980.

605. YOSHIDA, S., INOH, S., ASANO, T., SANO, K., KUBOTA, M., SHIMAZAKI, H., and UETA N. Effect of transient ischemia on free fatty acids and phospholipids in the gerbil brain. Lipid peroxidation as a possible cause of postischemic injury. J. Neurosurg. *53:* 323–331, 1980.

606. TAMURA, A., ASANO, T., and SANO, K. Correlation between rCBF and histological changes following temporary middle cerebral artery occlusion. Stroke, *11:* 487–493, 1980.

607. SANO, K., and MAYANAGI, Y. Long-term follow-up results of posteromedial hypothalamotomy. In: *Advances in Epileptology (The 10th Epilepsy International Symposium)*, edited by J. A. Wada and J. K. Penry, pp. 257–261. Raven Press, New York, 1980.

608. ASANO, T., TANISHIMA, T., SASAKI, T., and SANO, K. Possible participation of free radical reactions initiated by clot lysis in the pathogenesis of vasospasm after subarachnoid hemorrhage. In: *Cerebral Arterial Spasm*, edited by R. H. Wilkins, Proceedings of the II International Workshop, Amsterdam, 1979, pp. 190–201. Williams & Wilkins, Baltimore/London, 1980.

609. SANO, K., and SAITO, I. Timing of microsurgical treatment of ruptured intracranial aneurysms. In: *Cerebral Arterial Spasm*, edited by R. H. Wilkins, Proceedings of the II International Workshop, Amsterdam, 1979, pp. 447–454. Williams & Wilkins, Baltimore/London, 1980.

610. SANO, K., and SAITO, I. Early operation and washout of blood clots for prevention of cerebral vasospasm. In: *Cerebral Arterial Spasm*, edited by R. H. Wilkins, Proceedings of the II International Workshop, Amsterdam, 1979, pp. 510–513. Williams & Wilkins, Baltimore/London, 1980.

611. SAITO, I., and SANO, K. Vasospasm after aneurysm rupture: incidence, onset, and course. In: *Cerebral Arterial Spasm*, edited by R. H. Wilkins, Proceedings of the II International Workshop, Amsterdam, 1979, pp. 294–301. Williams & Wilkins, Baltimore/London, 1980.

612. IWAZAKI, Y., WAKAI, S., MATSUI, M., TAKAKURA, K., and SANO, K. Brain tumors in children. Shoni no No-Shinkei (Pediatr. Neurol.), *5:* 391–398, 1980.

613. FUKUSHIMA, T., KIRINO, T., MAEBARA, T., TAKAKURA, K., and SANO, K. CT images of the pituitary adenoma: Analysis of our 76

cases. CT Kenkyu (CT Research), *2:* 161–166, 1980.

614. SANO, K., WAKAI, S., SEGAWA, H., ASANO, T., and TAKAKURA K. Regional blood flow in normal pressure hydrocephalus measured by the Xenon enhanced CT scan. In: *Research Reports-1979 for Selected Diseases by the Ministry of Welfare*, edited by Research Group on Idiopathic Ventriculomegaly, pp. 87–90, 1980.
615. TAKAKURA, K., MATSUYA, M., SHITARA, N., and SANO, K. Immunotherapy of malignant tumors in neurosurgical field. In: *Immunotherapy of Cancer—Basic Research and Clinical Application*, edited by K. Iguchi and T. Hattori, p. 151–161. Nanzando, Tokyo, 1980.
616. TAKAKURA, K., and SANO, K. Recent advances of chemo-radiotherapy for brain tumors in children. In: *Recent Advances in Management of Children with Cancer*, pp. 201–210. The Children's Cancer Association of Japan, 1980.
617. SANO, K., and OCHIAI, C. Spontaneous brain stem (pontine) haematomas. In: *Spontaneous Intracerebral Haematomas. Advances in Diagnosis and Therapy*, edited by H. W. Pia, C. Langmaid, and J. Zierski, pp. 156–159. Springer Verlag, Berlin/Heidelberg/New York, 1980.
618. SANO, K., and YOSHIDA, S. Cerebellar haematomas. Indications and prognosis. *Spontaneous Intracerebral Haematomas. Advances in Diagnosis and Therapy*, edited by H. W. Pia, C. Langmaid, and J. Zierski, pp. 348–356. Springer Verlag, Berlin/Heidelberg/New York, 1980.
619. Sano, K., and OCHIAI, C. Brain stem haematomas. Clinical aspects with reference to indications for treatment. In: *Spontaneous Intracerebral Haematomas. Advances in Diagnosis and Therapy*, edited by H. W. Pia, C. Langmaid, and J. Zierski, pp. 366–371. Springer Verlag, Berlin/Heidelberg/New York, 1980.
620. SANO, K. Temporo-polar approach to aneurysms of the basilar artery at and around the distal bifurcation (technical note). Neurol. Res., *2:* 361–367, 1980.
621. SANO, K., ASANO, T., TANISHIMA, T., and SASAKI, T. Lipid peroxidation as a cause of cerebral vasospasm. Neurol. Res., *2:* 253–272, 1980.
622. SANO, K. Anecdotes of Harvey Williams Cushing. No-Shinkei Geka (Neurol. Surg.), *9:* 32–35, 1981.
623. ASANO, T., SASAKI, T., AND SANO, K. Lipid peroxidation and cerebrovascular spasms. No to Shinkei (Brain and Nerve), *33:* 33–46, 1981.
624. SANO, K., WAKAI, S., OCHIAI, C., and TAKAKURA, K. Characteris-

tics of intracranial meningiomas in childhood. Child's Brain, in press.

625. SANO, K., and MATSUTANI, M. Pinealoma (germinoma) treated by direct surgery and postoperative irradiation. A long-term follow-up. Child's Brain, in press.

626. SANO, K. *Brain Tumors—Clinical Aspect and Pathology*, 2nd Ed. p. 216. Igaku-Shoin, Tokyo, 1981.

627. MATSUI, T., TERAMOTO, A., FUKUSHIMA, T., MANAKA, N., and SANO, K. Radiological measurement of normal sella turcica—Statistical analysis of 1000 cases in Japan. No to Shinkei (Brain and Nerve), 33:187–194, 1981.

628. SASAKI, T., WAKAI, S., ASANO, T., WATANABE, T., KIRINO, T., and SANO, K. The effect of a lipid hydroperoxide of arachidonic acid on the canine basilar artery. An experimental study on cerebral vasospasm. J. Neurosurg., *54:* 357–365, 1981.

629. SANO, K. 30-Year progress of neurological surgery in Japan. Mainichi Life, April issue: 46–55, 1981.

Contents

III

POSTERIOR FOSSA TUMORS IN CHILDHOOD

IV

SPINAL DYSRAPHISM

I

CHAPTER

1

Presidential Address: "Quality and Neurosurgery"

DONALD H. STEWART, JR., M.D.

In speaking to you this morning, I would like to address the general topic of quality in neurosurgery. I would like to examine this question from three vantage points: first, from the position of the Congress of Neurological Surgeons; second, from the perspective of postgraduate education; and third, from the perspective of the practice of neurological surgery as it affects the neurosurgeon and the public.

The Congress of Neurological Surgeons has from its inception 32 years ago been dedicated to quality neurosurgery. The succinct constitution and by-laws promulgated by the founders of this organization are well worth your rereading. In reviewing the achievements of the Congress over the past 32 years, it is evident that its purposes have been served well by its leaders and members. Our goals have been accomplished reasonably well in the absence of a rigid organizational structure.

The goal of advancing neurological surgery by the dissemination of scientific knowledge has been achieved by the publication of *Clinical Neurosurgery*, which includes the major papers given at each annual meeting. I am certain this is a reference for you and others interested in neurological surgery in the world. Our monthly publication, *Neurosurgery*, is a great success, and is so because of the spirit and dedication of those of you who have participated in its formation and development. Both are prestigious quality publications and stand as examples of this organization's dedication to the dissemination of knowledge.

The efforts of the Congress to bring younger neurosurgeons into this organization have been remarkable. The development of the Residents Committee, the Residents Membership Committee, and this year the inclusion of residents on all the committees of the Annual Meeting Committee have enhanced the operation of this organization. The development of Special Courses on Monday has been a great success, and the more recent development of the Audiotape Program and the very well-received Videotape Library are activities which serve the interests of our members in the finest way. All are examples of our continuing commitment to quality service and professional growth.

The Congress of Neurological Surgeons was happy to be the first organization of neurosurgeons in the United States to formally donate a sum of $25,000 to the Research Foundation begun by the American Association of Neurological Surgeons. Your Executive Committee feels that the acquisition of knowledge and understanding of the nervous system are of paramount importance. To this end, we felt that our support of this Research Foundation and its goals was of high priority.

We are proud of the newly formed Certification Committee under the leadership of Dr. David Kelly. This effort, directed at those neurosurgeons who seek assistance in preparation for Board examination, is a reaffirmation of our dedication to excellence.

To improve the quality of neurosurgery, both from an internal organizational perspective and to represent neurosurgeons more effectively in dealing with organizations other than our own, the Congress over the last 10 years has been a participant in joint activities with the American Association of Neurological Surgeons. We are pleased with the achievements of the Joint Education Committee, the Joint Committee on Devices and Drugs, and the Joint Socio-Economics Committee. The idea of a Spine Section was initiated by your past president, Dr. Al Rhoton. The Washington Committee, with the effective guidance of our Washington representative, Mr. Charles Plante, and the able chairmanship of Dr. Louis Finney is maturing and is of significant value to organized neurosurgery.

We petitioned for and were awarded one delegate to the AMA House of Delegates, which allows us a true participatory role along with the AANS delegate in that national body.

It has been inferred in the past that there is great difficulty attendant in the creation of joint activities because of the lack of control from the top in such situations and because of the communication difficulties which arise (1).

Perhaps we should here acknowledge that years ago the Congress of Neurological Surgeons decided that the purposes of this society and its members might be better served by delegating the governance of the Congress to a well-balanced Executive Committee, responsive and accountable to its membership but not subject to the cumbersome, slow, and internecine activities of a House of Delegates. Witness the often hesitant and contradictory actions of the American Medical Association, the American Bar Association, and numerous other organizations representing large groups.

The business of representing neurosurgeons is complex, and it *is* tedious to deal with more than a few people. If it is time-consuming for the leadership—so be it. A participatory organization has never been the most efficient, but it is the most effective in the long run.

As we increase our own membership, it might be somewhat more difficult for any umbrella organization to claim that it is the sole representative of the neurosurgeons of the United States unless there is built into that organization a truly representative form of internal government.

Neurosurgeons have, in increasing numbers, become involved as participants in public policy development in matters relating to health care. Some of you are aware of our joint efforts, carried out through the Washington Committee, to create coalitions whose purpose would be to effect changes in the liability tort laws which would result in a more efficient liability system, a reduced cost to society, and a more just method of compensating injured persons. Such a coalition for tort reform has been formed in the State of New York. It would be premature to discuss any acheivements. We have, however, the support of the Business Council of the State of New York, representing all of the large and small businesses of the state. In addition, we have the support of the Blue Cross-Blue Shield organizations, the State Medical Society, the New York State Hospital Association, and the representatives of all the insurance companies which sell liability and casualty insurance in the state. We have begun to put together a legislative package which we hope will ameliorate the liability crisis which we face. Our work has just begun, and no victories can be claimed as yet.

Our coalition contains significant power brokers from business and industry, and we feel organizationally competent to challenge the unholy grip of the powerful trial lawyers association on the legislature and courts of that state.

The cost of the present tort system which compensates parties injured as a result of auto accidents, faulty products, or professional negligence, whether it be medical, architectural, engineering, or legal, is enormous. The public has yet to see that the cost of the system has reached the point of reducing their discretionary income. The return of 20 to 30¢ of the premium dollar to the injured party and the payment of over 50¢ of the premium dollar to the law profession for their self-professed and self-serving role as the protectors of the welfare of our citizens constitutes not only a gross social injustice but is, in fact, a social outrage.

We have not been blessed by a Supreme Court such as that here in Canada, which has decided that in the public interest there shall be by judicial decision a maximum payment of $100,000 for "pain and suffering (3)."

You have read recently that the Manville Corp. has applied for bankruptcy as a result of lawsuits brought against it. It is likely that other such defaults will occur. These destructive effects on industry and subsequently on our own economy have arisen as a result of a litiginous society led by its profiteering advocates, hoping to cash in on their insurance lottery tickets and get more than the system can produce.

I hope each of you will seize the opportunity to develop or participate in a coalition for tort reform in your own state as we strive for the development of quality and soundness in public policy.

It is apparent to me that we have reason to be proud of our efforts directed towards quality education, quality research, and quality public policy. I do not think we can become complacent; rather, we should build on this foundation. In the following few minutes I will propose a number of changes which I hope will receive your careful consideration.

My second point is related to the quality of postgraduate neurosurgical training. I would like to begin by noting that we have provided about 100 training programs in the United States, giving the opportunity to bright young men and women to begin to become familiar with the surgical management of diseases of the nervous system (9). We can be well satisfied with our organizational accomplishments which have provided adequate numbers of well-trained individuals who may serve the public's clinical needs.

A question of importance concerns the pre-entry evaluation of these postgraduate students. In the United States there is a popular sentiment for college aptitude tests, law school aptitude tests, medical school aptitude tests, and graduate record exams. These were designed to allow a more rational and objective selection process for the progression of individuals from one higher level of education to another. I believe that the postgraduate training programs for neurosurgery should be considered of no less importance in view of the fact that they consume more of one's life than any single preceding segment of education. The pre-entry evaluation of individuals wishing to enter neurosurgical training and the subsequent selection process might well be improved by an analogous standardized testing process. Such a screening examination might well help determine the necessary temperament, motivation, and interests, as well as the broad educational achievements so necessary to a group contemplating a narrowing of the educational focus.

Next, I would like to propose that the training of neurosurgeons be done in a more flexible fashion. At present, many graduates of neurosurgical training programs go on to do fellowships in one special area or another prior to their certification or prior to their entrance into practice. They do so because they have felt a need for further experience before launching into a professional career or for the purpose of complimenting the educational experience already received. The present requirements regarding specific durations of time spent in one program are wise, but that requirement should not act as an impediment to a rotation of a resident from one geographical area to another while still in his formal training. With the observed fact that some training programs are heavily weighted with expertise in one specific area and offer minimal exposure in other areas, it would not seem unreasonable to ascertain by a system of rotation that the trainee has had exposure in depth to the areas for which he will be held responsible by the public.

The Special Requirements used by the Residence Review Committee specify certain times to be spent studying areas such as the basic sciences, neurology, neuroradiology, and clinical neurosurgery. It seems unwise to consider these minimum time periods as maximums. It would seem more reasonable to adopt a system which is more flexible and matched to the educational needs of the trainees. Some individuals mature rather rapidly in terms of their acquisition of knowledge and technical skills; some mature more slowly.

In the interest of making training programs run smoothly, not only in neurosurgery but in other subspecialty areas, there is frequently the commitment on the part of a Program Director to an individual prior to the time he or she has even finished medical school. Such a commitment has implications for the Program Director and raises expectations on the part of the trainee. People change; energies and goals become altered; personalities become known and understood. I propose at the minimum a mandatory yearly review of the accomplishments of the trainee and a commitment to proceed further with the educational effort only after a positive evaluation has been accomplished. At present, many Program Directors perform in this mode.

Approximately 30% of the training programs in the United States do not require passage of the written Part One of the American Board of Neurological Surgery for completion of the training program. Certification by the American Board of Neurological Surgery is a voluntary process. The successful completion of Part One of this examination, which does not have to be taken for credit, at least gives some objective indication as to the measure of educational advancement of the trainee. I urge consideration in the interest of quality education of making this a mandatory requirement of all training programs. Indeed, I believe we can take a page from our Canadian colleagues and require complete certification of the trainee in neurosurgery prior to entering the practice of neurosurgery.

The responsibility for the determination of quality and competence cannot be left entirely to the credentialing bodies of the various hospital staffs and hospital Boards of Trustees. The initial responsibility is ours, not theirs.

To achieve these suggested changes in the format of training of the neurosurgeon will require some changes in the Special Requirements of the Residency Review Committee (2). As you know, this is a long, laborious, and politically difficult job but one which I am confident that the Congress is willing to support. To achieve these suggested changes will also require a cooperative, constructive, and unselfish spirit among the Program Directors, as well as an adjustment of the present requirements for certification by the American Board of Neurological Surgery. Certainly, it will require a different set of expectations on the part of the trainee.

The goal of the Congress of Neurological Surgeons, as well as the other neurosurgical organizations, is to serve the interests of the public health and welfare. It is imperative that we act responsibly to ensure that the product of our training institutions is what we wish it to be and what the public expects it to be. Inherent are immediate risks but also inherent may be the greater loss of future public credibility if we fail to assume this responsibility. Through these efforts, I believe that organized neurosurgery can demonstrate its lofty ideals and perhaps more adequately ensure the continuing recognition by society of the quality of the neurosurgical practitioner and ensure to the highest possible degree that we are what we say we are.

My third point relates to the quality of the formal practice of neurosurgery. I would like to address this issue from the perspective of the public we serve and from that of the neurosurgeon. We must develop a coordinated system of manpower production which is responsive not only to the needs of the public but also to the professional needs of the neurosurgeon. Any discussion of manpower, of necessity, must include numbers. Over the last 6 to 8 years there have been increasing cries from various quarters that there are too many neurosurgeons. The issue has been aired in numerous articles in our literature. The President's Graduate Medical Education National Advisory Council, as you know, arrived at figures, with our cooperation, which indicated that 8 years from now there will be an excessive number of neurosurgeons (5).

The practicing neurosurgeons in our country, as well as some of the formal educators who have participated in the deliberations of the Joint Socio-Economics Committee over the last 10 years, have frequently reiterated their concern that there are too many neurosurgeons. This is a particularly frequent complaint in those parts of the United States that are heavily populated urban areas, but the complaint occasionally arises even from the rural community.

Last year at the Congress meeting in Los Angeles, Dr. Frank Padberg presented data retrieved from 339 applications submitted by neurosurgeons for fellowship in the American College of Surgeons between 1977 and 1981 (7). These persons had a median age of 40.9 years and a median time after certification by the American Board of Neurological Surgery of 2.98 years. The median yearly surgical workloads of these individuals constituted 29.1 cranial procedures and 36.2 laminectomies, adding up to 70.62 cranial and spinal operations per year and, with various other procedures, a total of 106 operations per year. These median figures afford some insight into what the public can expect from neurosurgeons who have been certified for almost 3 years and in practice for 5 years, and some insight into the economics of neurosurgery.

The figures presented by Dr. Padberg are of interest because I believe they represent about 2/3 or less of the surgical workload of the neurosurgeon, as determined a few years ago by a survey done by the Congress of Neurological Surgeons.

Those of you present in New Orleans several years ago recall the data presented by Dr. Charles Drake in his Presidential Address to the American Association of Neurological Surgeons (4). In that address, he reviewed figures relating to surgical workloads of neurosurgeons in the United States. That information caused some concern on the part of many neurosurgeons because he pointed out the relatively large number of persons doing a relatively small number of specific neurosurgical procedures. A recent article in the Mayo Clinic Proceedings outlined the number of cerebral aneurysms which are operated on yearly in the United States (10). The figures indicate that, on the average, there are approximately five surgical aneurysm cases per neurosurgeon.

Dr. Robert Petersdorf, in an article in the *Bulletin* of the American College of Surgeons, has perhaps addressed the issue accurately when he states that "Although it has been said that in the health services arena, supply creates its own demand, the demand for the procedure-oriented subspecialist is probably limited." He went on to state that "increased competition has made a sham of the concept of regionalization. The idea of having large urban hospitals, usually associated with medical schools, serve as tertiary care facilities, with smaller hospitals providing secondary and primary care, is sound." However, as he noted, "the idea has not worked out, partly because the tertiary care teaching hospitals that are dependent on referrals have trained their own competition, and the competition is now caring for the difficult patients, who used to be referred to the teaching center, in well-equipped and well-staffed community hospitals in the suburbs and small towns" (8).

One might ask if it is possible to maintain a continuing degree of expertise as well as economic solvency in a practice resulting in 100 median operations per year. The matter should be of profound importance to the public at large, the members of this organization, and the Program Directors, who are in large part independent of significant controls and who essentially control the number of trainees entering practice.

If, in fact, the per-individual caseload is declining, as suggested by these studies, and if the projected surgical workload for the future will be less than it is now, one can ask "When does the practice of neurological surgery become less than desirable from the economic and professional quality point of view?" None of the factors contributing to the costs of running a practice of neurological surgery has ever declined . . . . staff assistants, supplies, rent, energy, transportation, liability insurance, etc. Using simple arithmetic and maximal reasonable reimbursement rates and the figures given above, and making allowance for the income produced by nonsurgical work, it is not unreasonable to suggest that we may be approaching a phase in neurosurgery which will require very careful analysis if the interests of neurosurgeons and the public are to be preserved.

We are at the moment witnessing an interesting assessment by the public of its former commitment to pay for medical services provided for those covered by Medicare and Medicaid. These plans are continually being reassessed by our elected officials and the voters. Any reduction in the amounts that government can expend for these services is going to impact, not only on physicians, but also on the more expensive hospital services being used. As a result, there will again be increased effort on the part of physicians and institutions to shift charges for services rendered to the private sector. The magnitude of the cost-shifting is already felt as a threat, and it is likely that a reverse squeeze on physicians, as well as institutions, will come from the private insurance sector. This will significantly affect the income of physicians in a negative fashion and, I might add, that might not be unreasonable in certain situations.

What is of concern to me when we look at the number of trainees entering the practice of neurological surgery, the figures I have just presented, the surgical workload trends, and the various economic forces that are operative, is the question of how we, as a group, can maintain the very high degree of skill implicit in the trust bestowed upon us by society. Ideally, it would seem that the only measure of importance is that of performance of practice-acquired skills and the judgments attendant to them.

I think we may no longer endure the disconnected and noncoordinated system of manpower production that we now enjoy. I am aware that the very mention of any consideration of efforts directed at these questions raises within our ranks a divisiveness so overwhelming as to nullify any effective action on our part.

The internal turf problems appear insurmountable. The fear of action by the Federal Trade Commission stifles any concerted effort at quality maintenance for the public good.

The process and responsibilities associated with the production of neurosurgeons over the last 30 years are no longer totally appropriate. Different forces exist, and as a result different strategies must be adopted if we are to be responsible to the changing scene in which we live and work. I fear that we are too provincial in our views and suffer from an inability to engage in broader planning efforts, free from our own divisiveness and forces which we perceive as inhibiting.

As a beginning, I therefore propose that we go outside of our own neurosurgical organizations and secure the services of a prestigious body which will examine the data and make recommendations regarding a reasonable public policy for manpower production in neurosurgery. The fear of antitrust activity might be overcome by a report of an independent body such as the Rand Corp. or the Academy of Medicine. The Federal Trade Commission does recognize arguments related to a "rule of reason" which allow an opportunity to explain the public benefit of what appears to be an anticompetitive policy (6).

The guiding principle of any effort, whether as a result of outside study or internal action, is that we wish to continue to improve the quality of neurosurgical expertise available to our patients. To adopt this proposal and go forward with it has some risks. I do not think we can lose in the long run, but to achieve this goal will be uncomfortable to many. It will be more uncomfortable in the long run if we do not arise to the occasion now.

To address these areas of concern may seem to many as an impossible task and one fraught with such risk personally, politically, economically, and legally, that they should not be considered. I suggest that this is not the case; we must deal with them now. I say this because to address these problems is to address the quality of the state of the art of neurological surgery and the quality of the existence of those we treat.

Before concluding these remarks, I would like to share with you one final personal conviction. I believe that of even greater importance than the issues I have just discussed is that of securing peace in this world. Perhaps as physicians, we are knowledgeable of the medical consequences of nuclear war. We are certainly not experts in the process related to the politics of the production of nuclear weapons.

We are, however, placed in the peculiar position of being the ones who would participate in the care of those damaged by the use of these weapons, and we are also, as human beings, as susceptible as anyone to the potential annihilating forces associated with their use.

I believe we have two opportunities: we must become better informed as to the medical consequences of thermonuclear warfare and we must help disseminate this information to our nonmedical colleagues. In addition, we must join actively in the debate surrounding the issue. By doing so, it is my hope that we might help forge an international policy which will result in the termination of the construction of nuclear weapons and the ultimate destruction of nuclear weapons themselves. To engage ourselves in this quest for peace is to act for our own human preservation and that of our children.

REFERENCES

1. Clark, W. K. Structure and function: Organization of a medical specialty for the rest of the 20th century. J. Neurosurg., *57:* 301–308, 1982.
2. Clark, K. Accreditation and approval of residency positions in neurological surgery in the United States: An overview. Neurosurgery, *9:* 601, 1981.
3. Dickson, Mr. Justice Brian—personal communication.
4. Drake, C. G. Considerations for strength and quality. Presidential Address. J. Neurosurg., *49:* 483–501, 1978.
5. Final Report of the Graduate Medical Education Advisory Committee to the Secretary of the Department of Health and Human Resources (7 vols.), Sept. 30, 1980, Publication DHS HRD 81-651. Washington, D.C.
6. James, A. E. Certain aspects of the interrelationship of law and medicine. Duke University Medical Center. Perspectives, *2:* 10–16, 1982.
7. Patterson, R. H., Jr. The neurosurgeon: What he really does. Neurosurgery, *11:* 100–101, 1982.
8. Petersdorf, R. G. The doctor's dilemmas. Bull. Am. Coll. Surg., *66:* 15–20, 1981.
9. Residency Programs in Neurological Surgery, United States and Canada. Neurosurgery, *11:* 100–211, 1982.
10. Whisnant, J. P., Sundt, T. M. and Phillips, L. H. Aneurysmal subarachnoid hemorrhage. Mayo Clin. Proc., *57:* 471–475, 1982.

CHAPTER

2

Cerebral Vasospasm and Aneurysm Surgery

KEIJI SANO, M.D., D.M.SC., F.A.C.S.(HON.)

Venienti occurite morbo—Confront disease at its onset
Aulus Persius Flaccus (A.D. 34–62)
Satires iii:64

But on Occasion's forelock watchful wait.
John Milton (1608–1674)
Paradise Regained
Book III, 1: 173

Rupture of intracranial saccular aneurysms is the most frequent cause of subarachnoid hemorrhage (SAH). When conservatively treated, about 70% of the cases with ruptured aneurysms eventually die (32). The two greatest causes of death in SAH patients are bleeding, or rebleeding, of aneurysms and cerebral vasospasm, or cerebral arterial spasm, which may lead to cerebral infarction (2).

The following case is an example of cerebral vasospasm. A 65-year-old woman had a sudden attack of severe headache and was diagnosed by lumbar puncture as having SAH. On admission on Day 2 after SAH, her consciousness was considerably disturbed, but there was no motor weakness. Her status was diagnosed as Grade III of Hunt (22). Figures 2.1*A* and *B* are her computed tomography (CT) scans on Day 2. High density can be noted in the suprasellar, interhemispheric, ambient, and Sylvian cisterns. Figures 2.1*C* and 1*D* are her angiograms taken on Day 4, which show an anterior communicating aneurysm and narrowing of the anterior cerebral and middle cerebral arteries on the right side. Because of her age and her general condition, surgery was postponed. On Day 9, her consciousness disturbance deteriorated to a semicomatose state and left-sided motor weakness was noted. CT showed a light degree of low density in the right hemisphere as seen in Figure 2.1*E*. On Day 10 she exhibited left hemiplegia, and CT revealed a marked low density in the right hemisphere (Fig. 2.1*F*), which suggested right middle cerebral infarction. Her general condition became worse and worse to the degree of Grade V of Hunt. She died on Day 16 after SAH despite administration of various kinds of drugs.

Therefore, the most important purpose of surgery of ruptured intra-

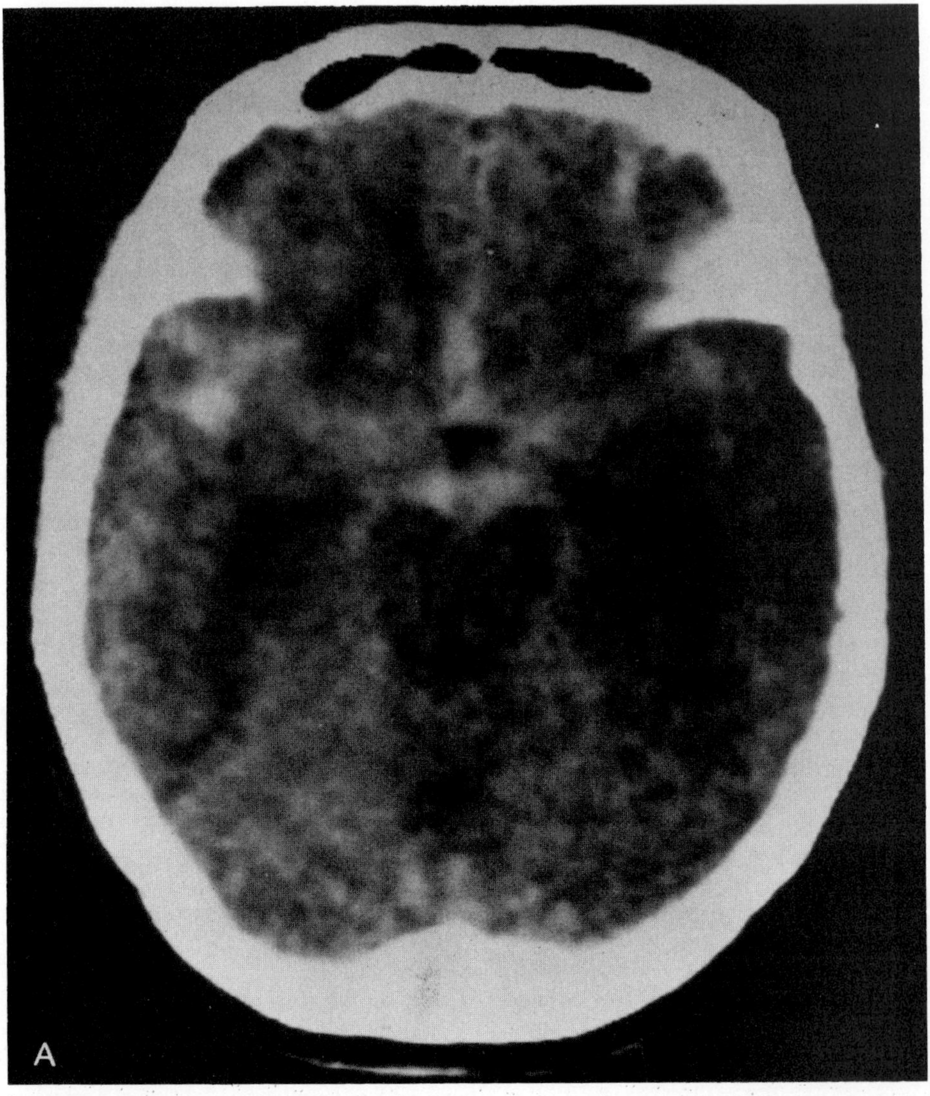

FIG. 2.1. (*A*) CT on Day 2 of SAH in a 65-year-old woman in Grade III. High density in the suprasellar, interhemispheric, and ambient cisterns. (*B*) The same case. High density in the interhemispheric, Sylvian, and insular cisterns.

cranial aneurysms is (a) to prevent rebleeding of aneurysms and, (b) if at all possible, to prevent development of cerebral arterial spasm by early surgery and removal of subarachnoid blood clots which may later be degraded to produce vasoactive substances (6, 46).

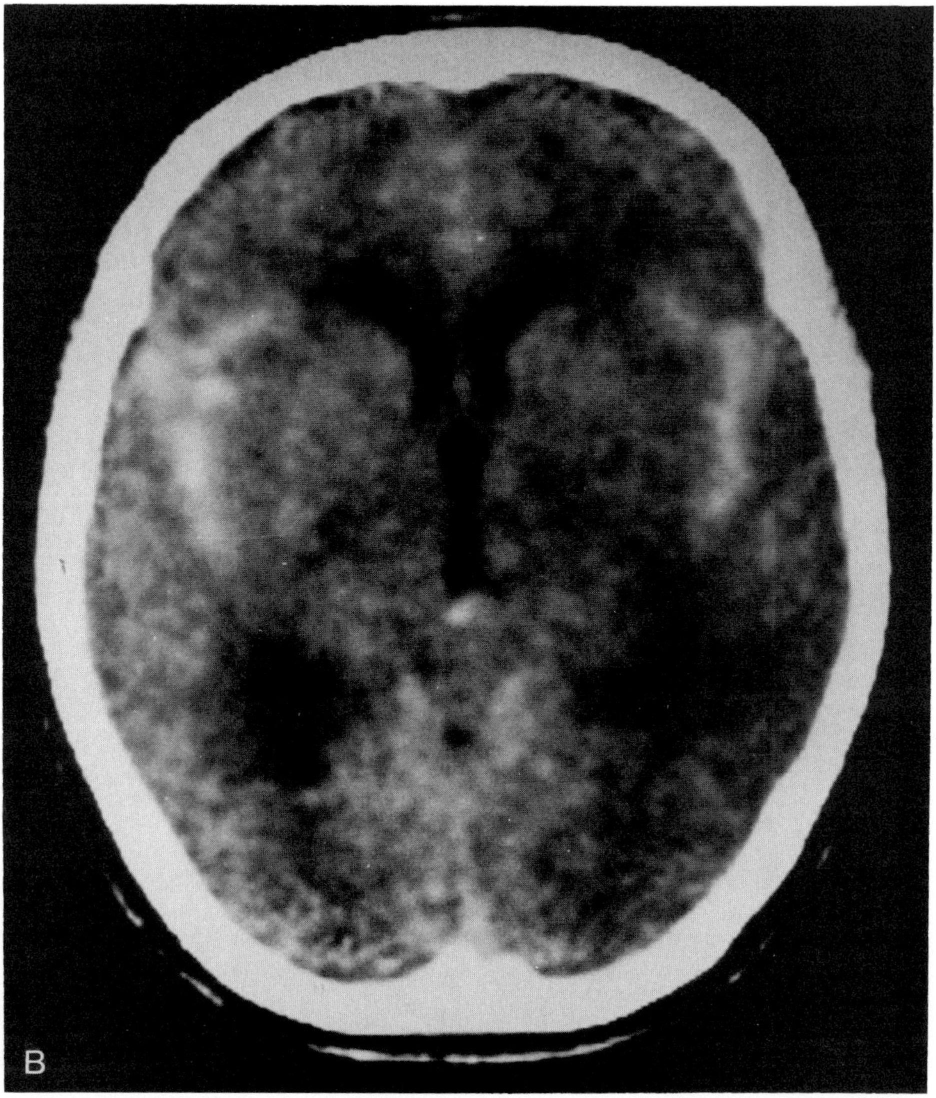

FIG. 2.1. (*B*)

According to the Cooperative Study in the United States from 1955 to 1966 (32), the rate of rebleeding is highest around 7 days after the onset of SAH. However, the so-called rebleeding in these statistics may partly include aggravation of the neurological status due to cerebral vasospasm.

According to Jane and others (25), for a patient with an anterior

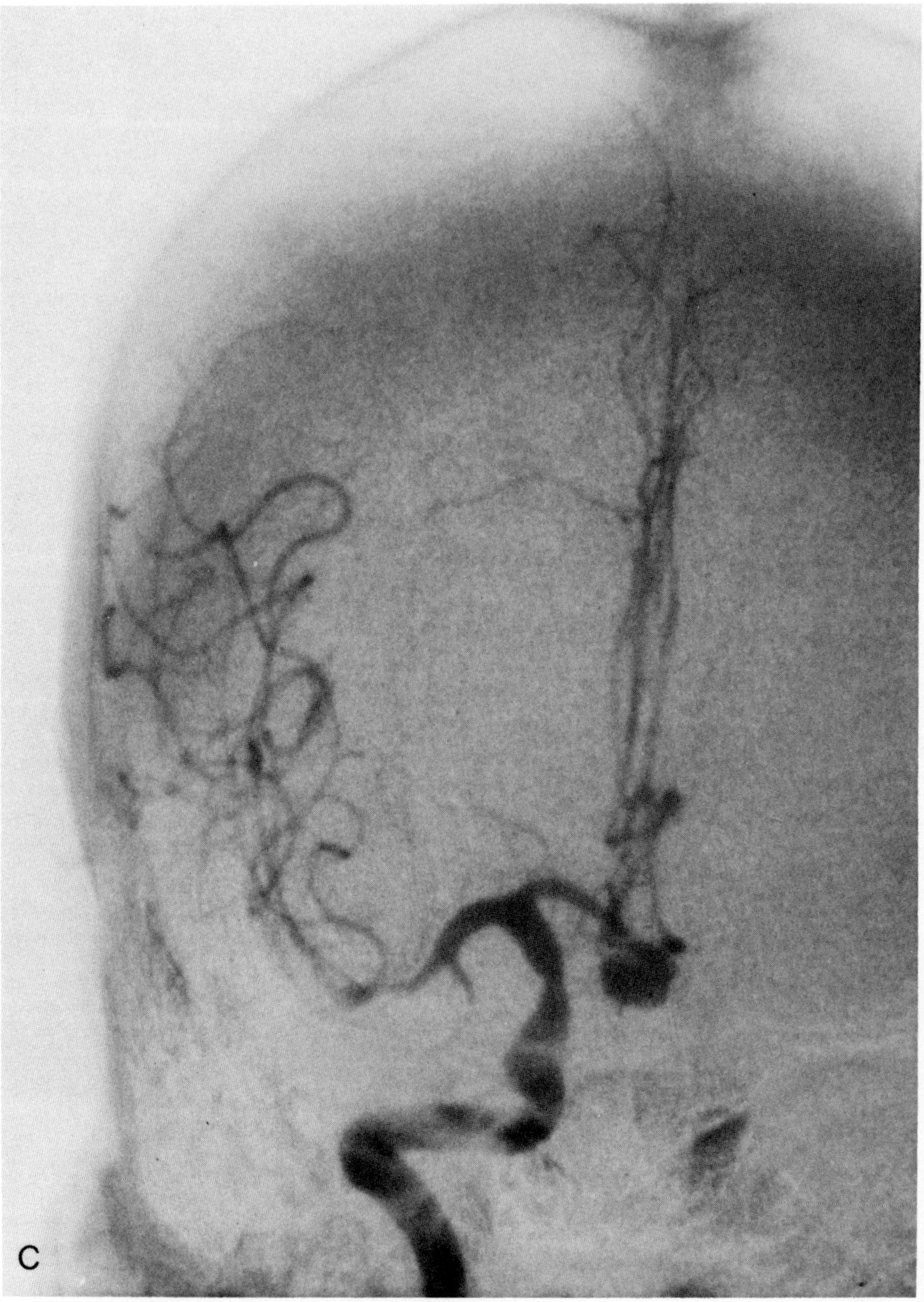

FIG. 2.1. (*C* and *D*) The same case. Angiograms on Day 4. An anterior communicating aneurysm and narrowing of the anterior and middle cerebral arteries on the right side are shown.

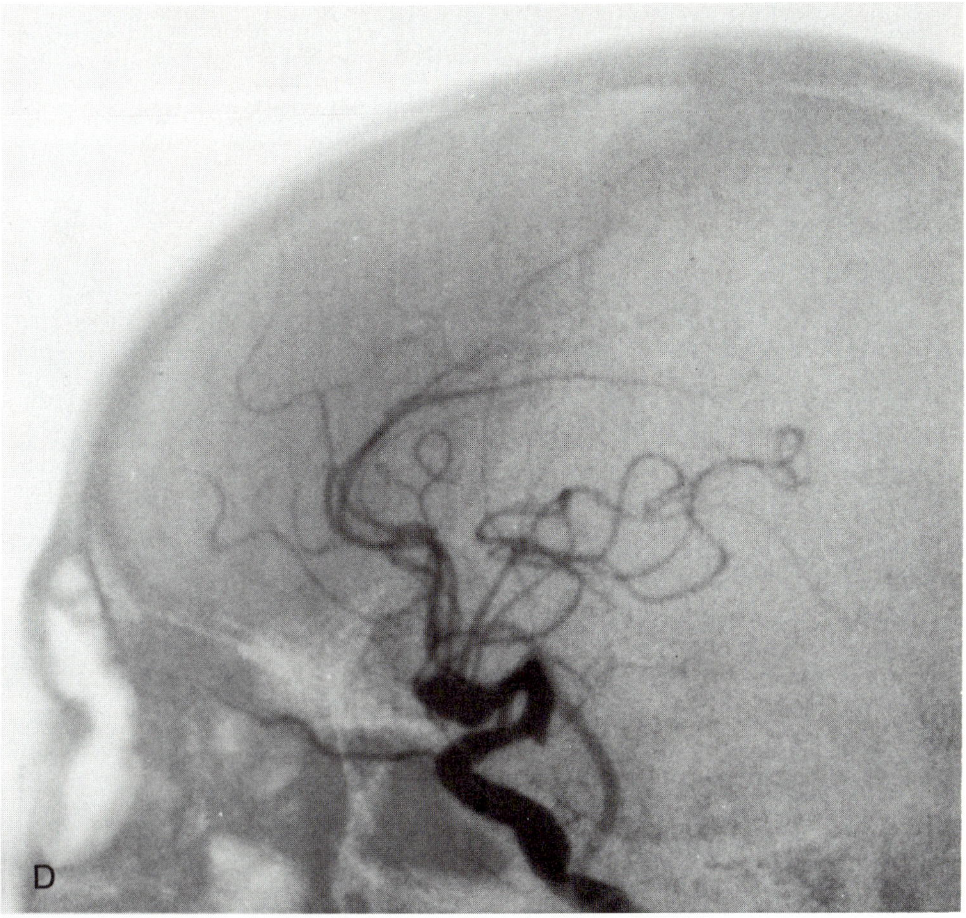

FIG. 2.1. (*D*)

communicating aneurysm or a posterior communicating aneurysm seen on the first day, namely, on the day of rupture, the chance he will rebleed within 6 months is about 50 to 60%. This rebleed rate rapidly diminishes, and on the 10th day the rate is approximately 35 to 50%. After 6 months this rate is about 3%/year; two-thirds of these late hemorrhages, however, result in mortality.

In the most recent Cooperative Study published in 1981 (2), rebleeding within 14 days after SAH occurred in 13% (33/249) of patients (9.6% occurred in good condition patients and 25% in poor condition patients), despite of high dose antifibrinolytic therapy.

Therefore, theoretically, surgery of ruptured aneurysms should be done as early as possible after SAH. This has rarely been practiced, however,

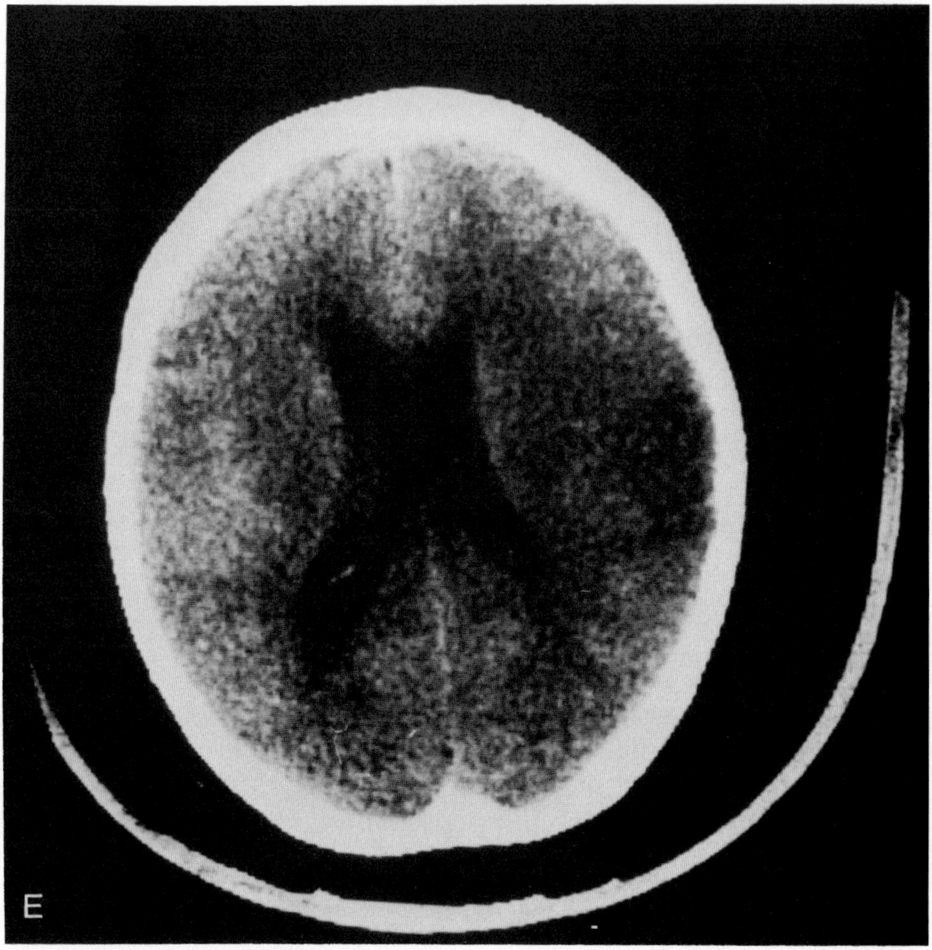

FIG. 2.1. (*E*) The same case. CT on Day 9. Semicomatose. Left hemiparesis developed. Low density in the right hemisphere. (*F*) The same case. CT on Day 10. Semicomatose. Left hemiplegia. Low density in the right hemisphere became more marked.

and has been in dispute in most neurosurgical centers around the world because of the reportedly poor results of surgery done in the early stage of SAH (11). Review of the author's series of microsurgery (Table 2.1) done on 730 consecutive cases of ruptured aneurysms of various locations experienced in the past 12 years (from December 1969 to December 1981) shows that the operative mortality of surgery done within the first week of SAH (249 cases) was 10.0%, whereas that of surgery done later than the first week (481 cases) was as low as 3.5%; the total operative mortality in 730 cases was 5.8%. Therefore, the operative mortality of surgery done

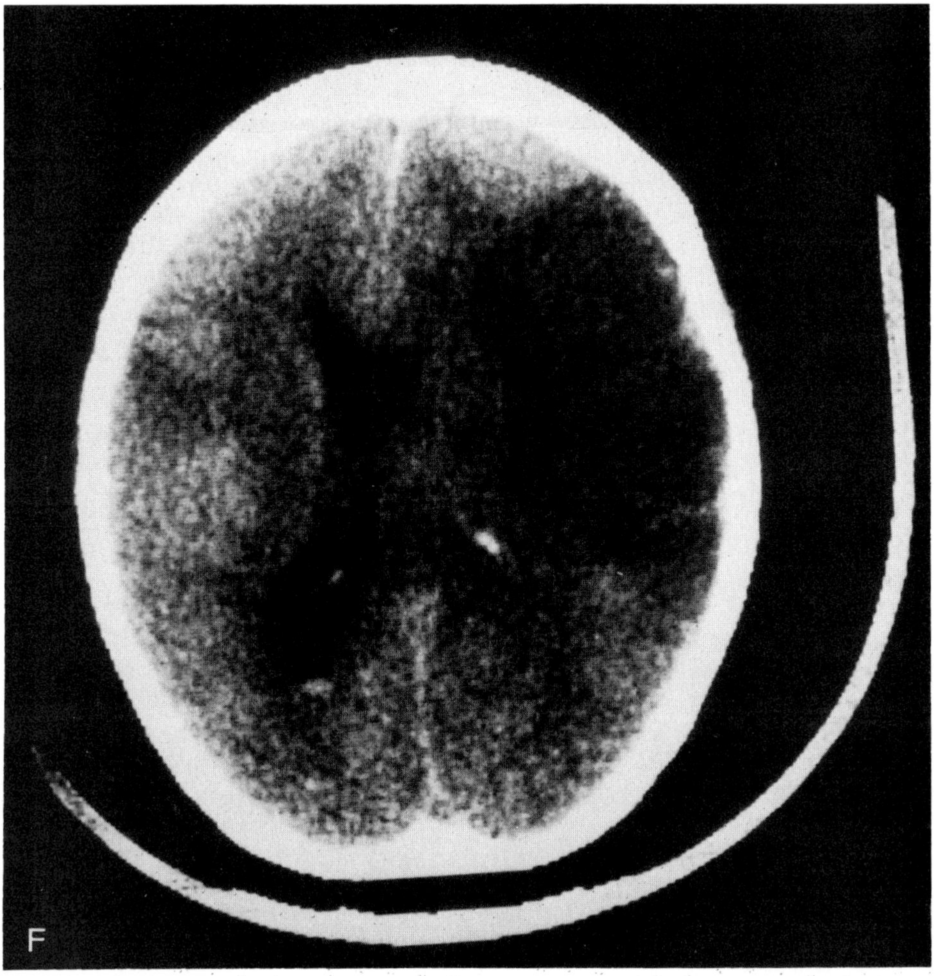

FIG. 2.1. (*F*)

within the first week was about 2.8 times as high as that of surgery done later than the first week. This was mainly due to two reasons: one was the general condition of a patient, which can be expressed as a grade (22), and the other was cerebral vasospasm which developed later after surgery.

GRADING OF RISK

Grading of risk or classification of patients according to their general condition was done by Botterell, Hunt, and others (7, 22, 31). Hunt has stressed the importance of the general condition of patients rather than the timing for surgery of aneurysms (23), and he established criteria for the grading of risk (22) which is now widely used.

Table 2.2 demonstrates the operative mortality and morbidity of the author's series classified according to the grading of Hunt (Grade Ia was included in Grade I). The lower the grade was, the lower was the operative mortality (*e.g.*, 1.4% in Grade I) and the better the follow-up results were (*e.g.*, 89.1% of Grade I patients were able to work). As a whole, 78.9% of the aneurysm cases that underwent surgery were well and working in the follow-up from 9 months to 12 years and 9 months, 8.9% were able to care for themselves (namely, the patient needs no help to wash, to eat, or to go to the toilet, but he is unable to work), and 6.4% were either bedridden or died of other diseases. Considering the mortality and morbidity together, the U-test revealed that Grade I and Grade II cases were not statistically different. Both Grades I and II cases had significantly better mortality and morbidity than Grade III ($p < 0.01$) which

TABLE 2.1

Timing of Microsurgery of Ruptured Aneurysms

Location of Aneurysms	Cases	Within 1 wk from the Last SAH	Later than the 1st wk	Operative Mortality
ICPcom[a]	159	44 (7)⁺	115 (3)⁺	10 = 6.3%
IC-bif	20	5 (3)	15 (1)	4 = 20.0%
Ant. chor.	34	12 (2)	22 (2)	4 = 11.8%
Acom	209	71 (6)	138 (6)	12 = 5.7%
A_1, A_2	39	14 (1)	25 (1)	2 = 5.1%
MC	133	60 (3)	73 (1)	4 = 3.0%
V-B	39	5 (1)	34 (2)	3 = 7.7%
Multiple	97	38 (2)	59 (1)	3 = 3.1%
Total	730	249 (25 = 10.0%)	481 (17 = 3.5%)	42 = 5.75%

ICPcom, internal carotid-posterior communicating (here including ophthalmic); IC-bif, internal carotid bifurcation; Ant. chor., anterior choroidal; Acom, anterior communicating, A_1,A_2, A_1 and A_2 portions of the anterior cerebral artery; MC, middle cerebral; V-B, vertebrobasilar; Multiple, multiple aneurysms; $( )^+$, operative death.

TABLE 2.2

Operative Mortality and Morbidity of Cases with Ruptured Aneurysms according to Grading

	Cases	Op. Mortality	Working	Caring for Self	BD[a]
Grade I	350	5 (1.4%)	312 (89.1%)	23 (6.6%)	10 (2.9%)
II	175	5 (2.9%)	156 (89.1%)	8 (4.6%)	6 (3.4%)
III	132	12 (9.1%)	85 (64.4%)	18 (13.6%)	17 (12.9%)
IV	63	13 (20.6%)	23 (36.5%)	16 (25.4%)	11 (17.5%)
V	10	7 (70.0%)	0	0	3 (30.0%)
Total	730	42 (5.75%)	576 (78.9%)	65 (8.9%)	47 (6.4%)

[a] BD, bedridden (33 cases) or died of other diseases after discharge (14 cases).

TABLE 2.3

Operative Mortality and Morbidity according to Grading

	Cases	Op. Mortality	Working	Caring for Self	BD[a]
Grade I[b]	423	6 (1.4%)	382 (90.3%)	25 (5.9%)	10 (2.4%)
II	175	5 (2.9%)	156 (89.1%)	8 (4.6%)	6 (3.4%)
III	132	12 (9.1%)	85 (64.4%)	18 (13.6%)	17 (12.9%)
IV	63	13 (20.6%)	23 (36.5%)	16 (25.4%)	11 (17.5%)
V	10	7 (70.0%)	0	0	3 (30.0%)
Total	803	43 (5.4%)	646 (80.4%)	67 (8.3%)	47 (5.9%)

[a] BD, bedridden (33 cases) or died of other diseases after discharge (14 cases).
[b] Grade I includes 73 cases of Grade 0.

was better than Grade IV ($p < 0.01$) which was, in turn, significantly better than Grade V ($p < 0.01$).

If Grade 0 cases were included in Grade I, as in Hunt's series (22), then the total number of aneurysm cases became 803, and the operative mortality was lowered to 5.4%, and the working rate in the follow-up increased to 80.4%, as shown in Table 2.3.

In the early stage of SAH, patients are usually of higher grades, which seems to explain the higher operative mortality in early surgery. Both the grade of patients and cerebral vasospasm are closely related to the amount of subarachnoid bleeding. In this sense, the mortality and the morbidity of SAH patients may be said to already be determined to a considerable degree at the time of bleeding. In early surgery of ruptured aneurysms, all these factors, especially the vasospasm which may later develop if subarachnoid blood is of a considerable quantity, regardless of surgical or conservative treatments, will influence the operative results—in addition to the surgeon's technique. In surgery of aneurysms in the later period, *e.g.*, more than 2 weeks after SAH, the surgeon's technique is almost the sole factor influencing the results.

TIMING OF SURGERY

The surgeon can prevent ruptured aneurysms from rebleeding by early surgery, but then he must encounter the problem of cerebral vasospasm which may develop later. Then, he must decide when to do surgery. In order to solve the problem of timing of surgery, the author's own series of 730 cases of ruptured aneurysms submitted to microsurgery was analyzed.

The first week after SAH was divided into two periods: from Day 0 (the day of aneurysmal rupture) to Day 2 (48 hours after SAH), and from Day 3 to Day 7. In the first week, of 249 cases that underwent microsurgery, Grade I cases were only 27 (10.8%), Grade II cases were 120 (48.2%), Grade III cases were 64 (25.7%), Grade IV cases were 30 (12.1%), and

Grade V cases were 8 (3.2%), *i.e.*, Grade III through V cases occupied 41.0% of the total. (Note: in previous communications (43, 44, 47, 48), the author counted the day of rupture as Day 1. Therefore, Day 2 in this article corresponds to Day 3 in these previous communications.)

The operative mortality in 153 cases that underwent surgery on Day 0 through Day 2 (that is, within 48 hours after SAH) and the mortality in 96 cases submitted to surgery on Day 3 through Day 7 were relatively high (9.8 and 10.4%, respectively) as compared to that in 96 cases submitted to surgery in the second week after SAH (4.2%) and that in 385 cases operated on later than the second week (3.4%), as seen in Table 2.4. If only Grade I to III cases were considered, however, the operative mortality in cases submitted to surgery on Days 0 through 2 was 4.8% (6/125) and that in cases submitted to surgery on Days 3 through 7 was 7.0% (6/86), as shown in the lowermost row of Table 2.4 although this difference was statistically not significant.

There was no statistically significant difference by χ^2 test in the operative mortality between Grade I and Grade II cases submitted to surgery in the first and second weeks. The same was true with both Grade I and Grade II cases for all timing of surgery. In Grade III cases, however, the operative mortality in surgery done on Days 3 through 7 (6/20, 30%) was relatively higher ($p < 0.1$) than that on Days 0 through 2 (4/44, 9.1%).

The operative mortality in cases submitted to surgery on Days 0 through 2 was not significantly different among Grade I, Grade II, and Grade III cases; it was, however, significantly ($p < 0.001$) different among Grade I, Grade II, and Grade IV cases. From these data, it may well be said, at least as far as the operative mortality is concerned, that Grade I and Grade II cases can be operated on at any time after SAH. Grade III cases may be submitted to surgery on Days 0 through 2 but not on Days 3 through 7. For Grade IV cases, surgery had better be postponed to a later time, awaiting improvement of general conditions.

For timing of surgery, age should also be considered. In Table 2.5, Grade I to IV cases (Grade V cases were excluded because, as is universally recognized, surgery is not indicated for Grade V cases) were divided into two groups, one below 60 years of age and one 60 years of age and older. There was a significant difference ($p < 0.005$) in the operative mortality between the group younger than 60 years old (3.2%) and the group 60 years and older (11.3%). In the first group, there was no significant difference by χ^2 test in the operative mortality at any timing of surgery. In the second group, however, the operative mortality in cases submitted to surgery on Days 0 through 2 (21.4%) was significantly higher than that in the second week ($p < 0.1$) or that later than the

TABLE 2.4

Microsurgery of Ruptured Aneurysms—Timing, Grade at Operation and Follow-up Results (730 cases)

	1st wk after SAH										2nd week after SAH					Later than 2nd wk				
	0 (SAH day) to 2nd day					3rd to 7th days														
Grade	Cases	Op.[a] Mt.	Working	Caring for Self	BD	Cases	Op. Mt.	Working	Caring for Self	BD	Cases	Op. Mt.	Working	Caring for Self	BD	Cases	Op. Mt.	Working	Caring for Self	BD
I	14	0	14	0	0	13	0	12	1	0	24	0	22	2	0	299	5	264	20	10
II	67	2	59	5	1	53	0	47	3	3	24	0	24	0	0	31	3	26	0	2
III	44	4	27	7	6	20	6	7	6	1	33	1	29	3	0	35	1	22	2	10
IV	23	7	7	5	4	7	1	3	3	0	14	2	9	1	2	19	3	4	7	5
V	5	2	0	0	3	3	3	0	0	0	1	1	0	0	0	1	1	0	0	0
Total	153	15	107	17	14	96	10	69	13	4	96	4	84	6	2	385	13	316	29	27
		9.8%	69.9%	11.1%	9.2%		10.4%	71.9%	13.5%	4.2%		4.2%	87.5%	6.3%	2.1%		3.4%	82.1%	7.5%	7.0%
N.B. Grades I to III cases	125	6	100	12	7	86	6	66	10	4	81	1	75	5	0	365	9	312	22	22
		4.8%	80.0%				7.0%	76.7%				1.2%	92.6%				2.5%	85.5%		

[a] Op. Mt., operative mortality; BD, bedridden (33 cases) or died of other diseases after discharge (14 cases).

TABLE 2.5

Grade I to IV Cases of Ruptured Aneurysms—Timing of Microsurgery and Results

Age	Timing of Operation	Cases	Op. Mortality	Working	Caring for self	BD[a]
↓	1st wk					
	0 (SAH) to 2nd day	106	4 (3.8%)	89 (84.0%)	9 (8.5%)	4 (3.8%)
	3rd to 4th days	72	5 (6.9%)	52 (72.2%)	11 (15.3%)	4 (5.6%)
	2nd wk after SAH	73	2 (2.7%)	66 (90.4%)	4 (5.5%)	1 (1.4%)
59 yrs	Later than 2nd wk	318	7 (2.2%)	267 (84.0%)	22 (6.9)	22 (6.9%)
	Subtotal	569	18 (3.2%)	474 (83.3%)	46 (8.1%)	31 (5.4%)
60 yrs	1st wk					
↓	0 (SAH) to 2nd day	42	9 (21.4%)	18 (42.9%)	8 (19.0%)	7 (16.7%)
	3rd to 7th days	21	2 (9.5%)	17 (81.0%)	2 (9.5%)	0
	2nd wk after SAH	22	1 (4.5%)	18 (81.8%)	2 (9.1%)	1 (4.5%)
	Later than 2nd wk	66	5 (7.6%)	49 (74.2%)	7 (10.6%)	5 (7.6%)
	Subtotal-	151	17 (11.3%)	102 (67.5%)	19 (12.6%)	13 (8.6%)
Grand Total		720	35 (4.9%)	576 (80.0%)	65 (9.0%)	44 (6.1%)

[a] BD, bedridden (32 cases) or died of other diseases after discharge (12 cases).

second week ($p < 0.05$), but not significantly higher than that on Days 3 through 7 (9.5%). This high mortality in early surgery in the higher age group was probably because these mortality cases belonged to the higher grades (among nine cases in the Day 0 through 2 subgroup, five belonged to Grade IV and two to Grade III, and both cases in the Day 3 to 7 subgroup belonged to Grade III). From these data, one may conclude that for cases 60 years of age or older, surgery may better be postponed to the second week or later.

To evaluate the mortality and morbidity together, the U-test may be suitable. According to this test, there was no difference in the mortality and morbidity between Grade I and Grade II cases, at any timing of surgery. The same was true for Grade IV and V cases. The results in Grade III cases, however, were different for different timing of surgery, *e.g.*, the results were better in cases submitted to surgery in the second week than in later timing ($p < 0.05$) or in the first week ($p < 0.01$) (this is in accordance with Pia (40)), and the results were better in cases submitted to surgery on Days 0 through 2 than on Days 3 through 7 ($p < 0.05$) (in accordance with Suzuki (55) and Hugenholtz and Elgie (20)). In the group younger than 60 years of age, cases that underwent surgery on Days 3 through 7 showed poorer results, as compared to cases operated on in all other periods of timing ($p < 0.05$) whereas, in the group 60 years or older, cases submitted to surgery on Days 0 through 2 showed poorer results than the others ($p < 0.01$).

These differences in the operative mortality and postoperative morbidity in the different grading, timing, and age groups were mostly due to the amount of subarachnoid bleeding and the consequential cerebral vasospasm. Probably, surgery on aneurysms and removal of subarachnoid clots within 48 hours after SAH (if at all possible) can decrease the amount of subarachnoid blood clots before their degradation occurs so as to decrease the extent of, or hopefully to prevent, development of the vasospasm. After Day 3, degradation of clots may have already occurred to produce vasoactive substances or to initiate free radical reactions, so that surgery can not prevent development of cerebral vasospasm. In the second week or later, if a case develops cerebral vasospasm, the grading becomes higher, and surgery may have to be postponed. Because of this inadvertent selection, the results of delayed surgery may seem to be better than those of early surgery. This observation is shared by other authors (20, 55, 56).

Pathogenesis of Cerebral Vasospasm and Its Treatment

Late or chronic cerebral vasospasm, or more exactly, the arterial spasm which appears in 40–50% of SAH (38), or in about 45% of the cases remaining through the second week of SAH of the author's series (43), exerts a crucial influence on the mortality and morbidity of the patients (38, 44, 47). Yet, its pathogenesis still remains unclear, although there have been many theories proposed about it.

It has several characteristics (38, 42, 44). (1) It usually appears after some time lag from the onset of subarachnoid hemorrhage (SAH). In the author's studies, it appeared first on Day 4 (the day of SAH being Day 0) and, on the average, on Day 7.6 ± 2.5 in the natural course. Even postoperative vasospasm appeared with nearly the same interval from the onset of SAH, namely, on the average, on Day 6.7 ± 1.6. (2) There is a close correlation between the development of vasospasm and subarachnoid clots, as pointed out by many investigators (15, 42, 49). One may say, "Without subarachnoid clots, no vasospasm" (Table 2.6). (3) In arteries of the other parts of the body which have bled, there is no sustained arterial contraction comparable to chronic cerebral vasospasm.

Any theory concerning the pathogenesis of the vasospasm should be able to explain these characteristics. The following theory, the author thinks, fulfills this requirement.

Free Radical Reactions and Lipid Peroxidation

All aerobic animals, including human beings, live using oxygen molecules as the main oxidant of energy substrate. They are provided with double or triple defense mechanisms against active oxygen species (hydrogen peroxide, H_2O_2; hydroxy radical, $\dot{O}H$; superoxide anion, $\dot{O}_2^-$; singlet oxygen, $^1O_2$) which are generated in the reduction process of the oxygen molecules and also have mechanisms to protect against the

TABLE 2.6

Subarachnoid Blood Clots on CT and Development of Vasospasm[a]

Preop. CT[b]		Postop. CT	Vasospasm (+)	Slight narrowing of artery	Vasospasm (−)
Blood clots (high density)	(+) 54	(+) 34	19	8	7
		(−) 20	1	2	17
	(−) 12	(−) 12	0	0	12

[a] In 66 cases submitted to surgery within 5 days after SAH.

[b] CT scans performed on Days 0 to 4 (*Preop. CT*) were divided into two groups: Group I with high density (blood clots) in the subarachnoid space (54 cases) and Group II without such high density (12 cases). In Group II, no high density and no cerebral vasospasm developed postoperatively. Among cases of Group I, 20 cases in which subarachnoid clots could be removed by surgery and postoperative CT showed no high density, only one case developed vasospasm, 2 cases showed a slight narrowing of arteries (less than 40% reduction of the caliber), and the other 17 cases developed no vasospasm. In the other 34 cases of Group I, subarachnoid clots could not be removed by surgery (high density remained on CT), and 19 of them developed vasospasm, 8 showed a slight narrowing of arteries, and only 7 had no vasospasm.

oxidation-peroxidation of body constituents by these active oxygen species. Existing animals are those which have thus survived the several million year process of evolution. These defense mechanisms, however, are very poor or almost undetectable in the cerebrospinal fluid (CSF) of the higher mammals, including man.

For instance, the glutathione peroxidase (GSHpx) level in the human serum is 0.126 ± 0.014 unit/ml, whereas that in the human CSF is 0.003 ± 0.001 unit/ml. Vitamin E is measured as 0.77 mg/dl in the human serum and is undetectable in the human CSF; catalase is 0.054 unit/min/ml in the human serum and undetectable in the CSF. These substances are known as potent free radical scavengers, or antioxidants, found in most tissues. One of the adverse phenomena caused by this lack of free radical scavengers in the CSF is, the author thinks, chronic or delayed cerebral vasospasm here discussed. Therefore, cerebral vasospasm can be regarded as a sort of deficiency disease—due to deficient defense mechanisms in the CSF.

When bleeding occurs in the subarachnoid space, hemolysis soon occurs, and oxyhemoglobin (oxyHb) is liberated. OxyHb itself has a prominent vasocontractile action (24, 39) which is not mediated by biogenic amines such as norepinephrine, serotonin, or histamine (61). Since, according to Tanishima, aspirin does not block contraction, the participation of prostaglandins seems unlikely (61). The contraction is almost completely blocked by nifedipine, indicating that oxyHb causes a real contraction of the vascular smooth muscle (63). As compared to oxyHb, methemoglobin (metHb) shows only a mild vasocontractile activity. Since oxyHb differs from metHb only by one electron, the particular molecular configuration of oxyHb as superoxo-heme ($Fe^{3+}O^{\cdot -}_2$) may be related to its potent vasocontractile activity.

Upon conversion of oxyhemoglobin to methemoglobin, superoxide anion is released (34) which, in turn, directly or indirectly as described below, through hydroxy radical, singlet oxygen, or alkoxy radical (28, 29, 33, 65), initiates free radical reactions such as peroxidation of polyunsaturated fatty acids (PUFAs) in the biomembrane (46). PUFAs are known to be most susceptible to free radical attacks (16) (Fig. 2.2). It is also known that some degradation products of hemoglobin such as hematin, iron ions, and methemoglobin possess a powerful catalytic action in the conversion of PUFAs to their peroxidized forms, hydro- and endoperoxides (64). Besides, leukocytes, which usually are found in and around subarachnoid clots, may also produce activated oxygen species such as superoxide. Therefore, it seems reasonable to assume that hemolysis triggers free radical reactions leading to lipid peroxidation.

As is well known, superoxide is converted by superoxide dismutase (SOD) to hydrogen peroxide in normal conditions. Hydrogen peroxide is

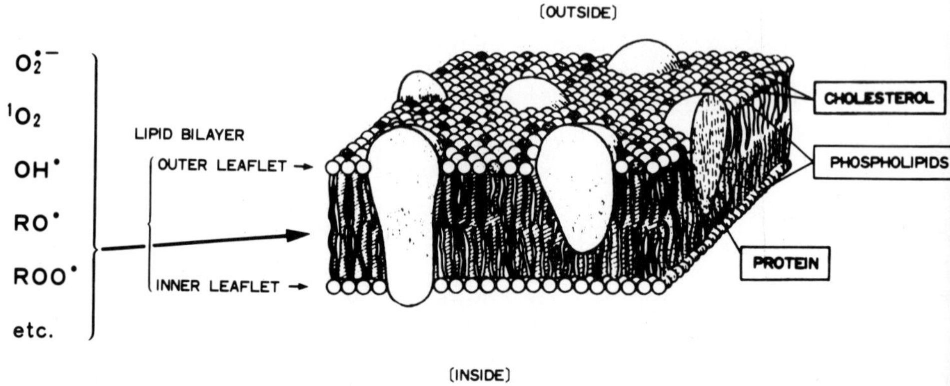

FIG. 2.2. Structure of the biomembrane and free radicals.

finally inactivated by catalase or glutathione peroxidase. If, however, these enzymatic activities are lowered or if iron (Fe^{2+}, Fe^{3+}) complexes are present, superoxide and hydrogen peroxide produce very active singlet oxygen and hydroxy radical by the so-called Haber-Weiss reaction (33). Superoxide may also react with PUFA hydroperoxides that are present as impurities in PUFAs to produce alkoxy radical (65). These active free radicals, such as hydroxy radical, singlet oxygen, and alkoxy radical, are known to react with PUFAs in the biomembrane and produce fatty acid free radicals (Fig. 2.3). These organic free radicals easily combine with oxygen to become lipid peroxide. This step of the reaction produces more free radicals which propagate new reactions. Thus, a chain reaction of lipid peroxidation is initiated (46).

Unlike other parts of the body, cerebrospinal fluid (CSF) is almost lacking in defense mechanisms (vitamin E, glutathione peroxidase, etc.) against free radicals. During SAH, these defense mechanisms are at first supplied by the extravasated blood itself but rapidly decrease and after 3 days become insufficient to prevent the free radical chain reactions from propagating (Figs. 2.4 and 2.5).

In the CSF of patients with SAH (32 in number), it was found that TBA (thiobarbituric acid)-reactive substances had increased, especially in cases which developed vasospasm (6, 46, 62). The presence of TBA-reactive substances (TRS) is regarded as representing the presence of lipid peroxides (67). The average TRS value of all the samples obtained from patients with SAH (N = 128) was 0.053 ± 0.003 nM/ml (mean ± SE), whereas in the control group (N = 10) it was 0.02 ± 0.003 nM/ml (6, 46, 62). The TRS value for patients with vasospasm was clearly higher than for those without vasospasm. When the TRS values for each group of patients were gathered every 3 days after onset of SAH, a statistically

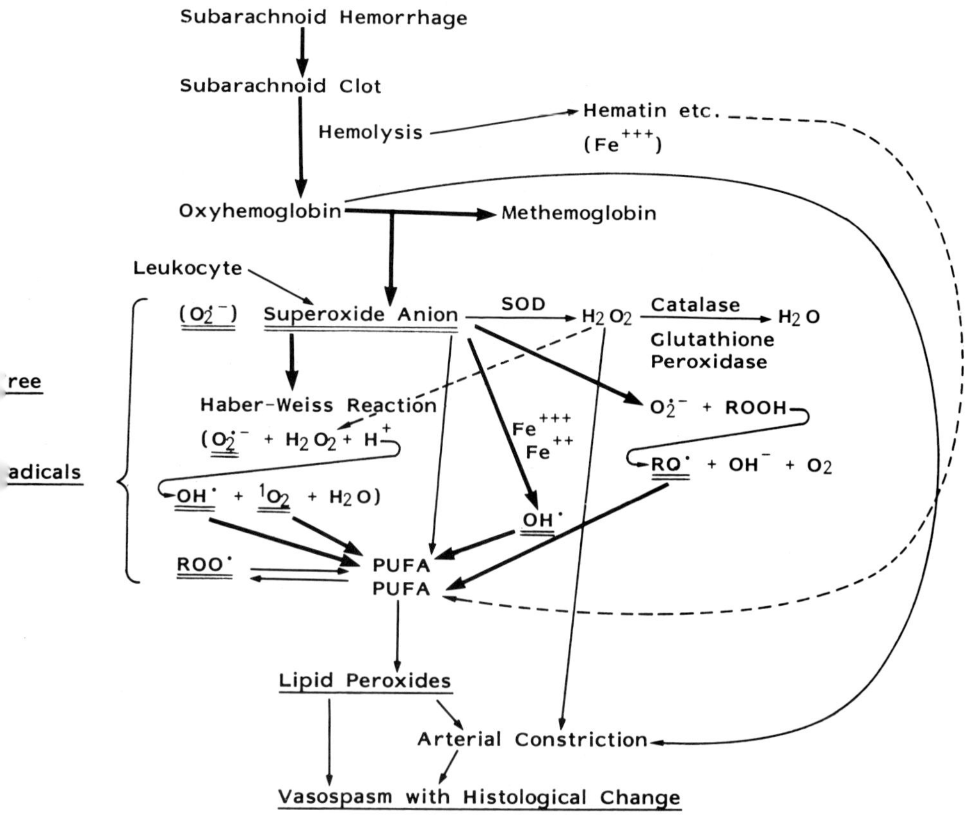

FIG. 2.3. Free radical reactions leading to lipid peroxidation in SAH.

significant difference was revealed on Days 7 to 9 ($p < 0.001$), as seen in Figure 2.6 (Note: the day of SAH is counted as Day 1 in this figure).

Gas-liquid chromatographic examination of the CSF fatty acid profile revealed that the ratio of PUFAs to the total lipid decreased just before the increase of TRS. A representative pattern is shown in Figure 2.7. The result suggests that the increase of TRS may be due to peroxidation of PUFAs of the biomembrane, such as arachidonate and linoleate.

The TRS value is, however, an indirect index of lipid peroxides. In order to directly prove lipid peroxidation in SAH, the CSF of a patient with SAH was periodically collected and fractionated using an octadecylsilyl silica column. The fraction eluted with 15% ethanol-water was analyzed by high-performance liquid chromatography (HPLC) detecting at 238 nm (conjugated diene). Several peaks were recognized in accordance with the occurrence of angiographic and symptomatic vasospasm.

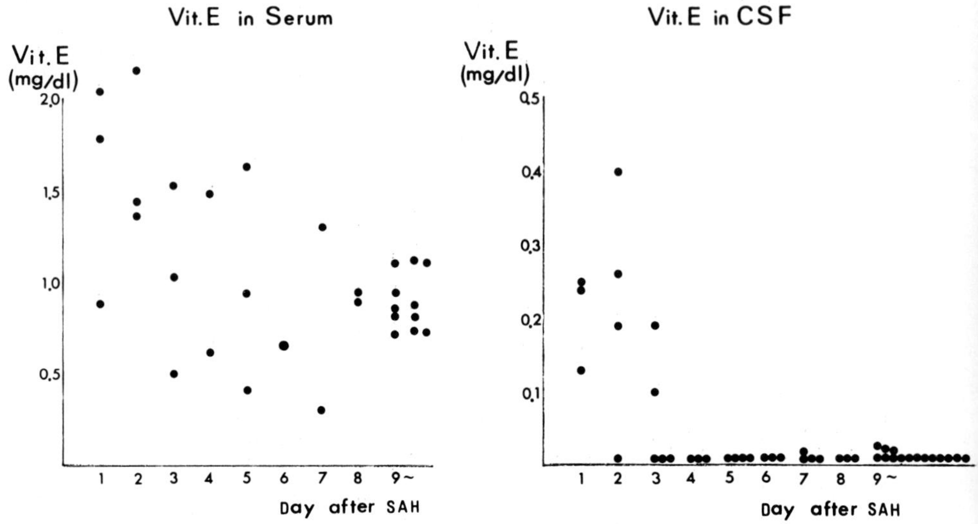

FIG. 2.4. Changes of vitamin E in serum and in CSF after SAH.

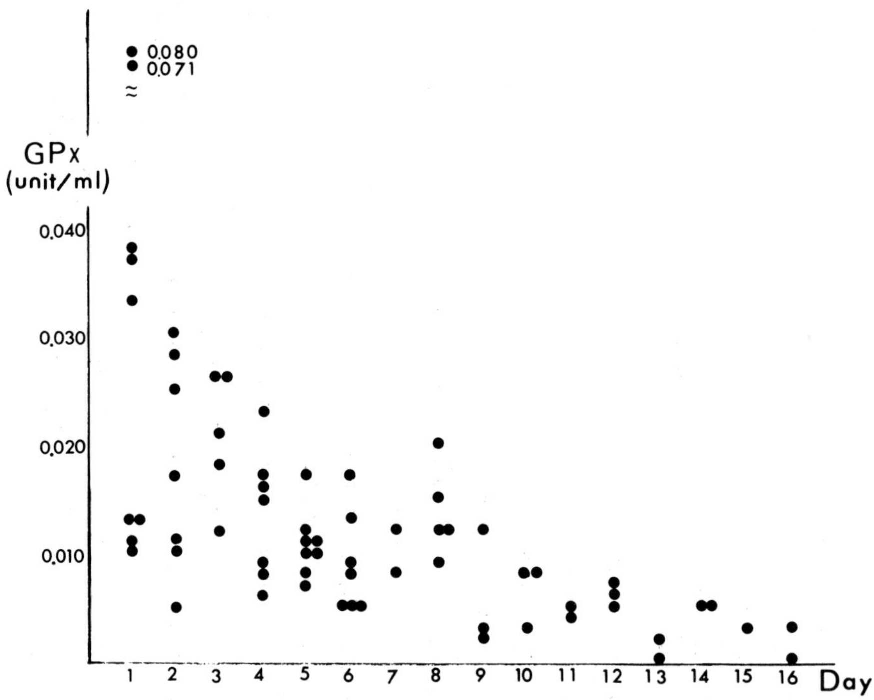

FIG. 2.5. Changes in glutathione peroxidase activity (GPx) in CSF after SAH.

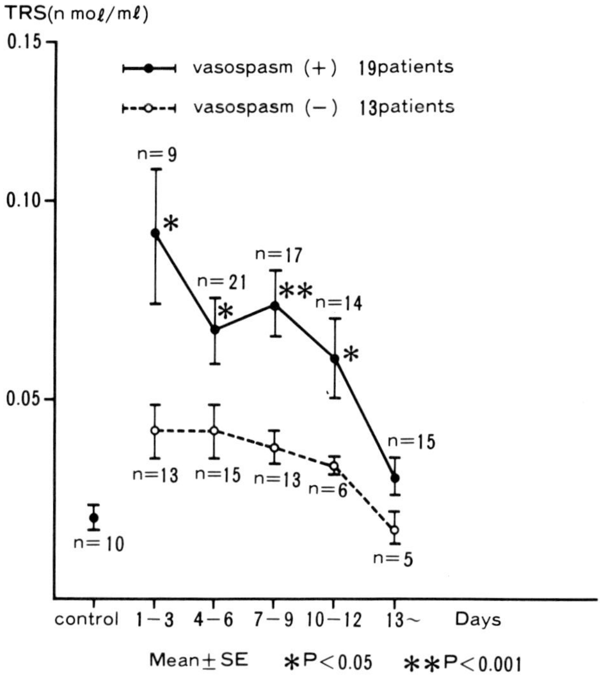

FIG. 2.6. Changes of TBA-reactive substances in CSF of patients with SAH. (Modified from K. Sano *et al.* (46).)

One of the peaks which appeared on Day 7 after SAH was identified as 5-hydroxyeicosatetraenoic acid (5-HETE) (see Fig. 2.12). with the aid of HPLC and gas chromatography-chemical ionization mass spectrometry (GC-MS) by the author's collaborators, Nakamura et al. (35, 50). No peak was observed, with HPLC corresponding to hydroxyeicosatetraenoic acids (HETEs) or hydroperoxy eicosatetraenoic acids (HPETEs) in the CSF obtained from normal controls (patients with cervical spondylosis).

In 10 patients with SAH, semiquantitative analysis of 5-HETE in the CSF was performed by measuring the peak identified as 5-HETE on HPLC (Fig. 2.8). A close correlation was observed between the occurrence of cerebral vasospasm and the appearance of 5-HETE in the CSF (in lumbar CSF obtained by lumbar puncture and cisternal CSF obtained by cisternal drainage, especially in the latter).

As is seen in Fig. 2.8, 5-HETE appeared in the CSF with some time lag after SAH. Identification of 5-HETE indicates formation of its precursor, 5-hydroperoxyeicosatetraenoic acid (5-HPETE), and proves the occurrence of lipid peroxidation in the CSF of SAH. This, however,

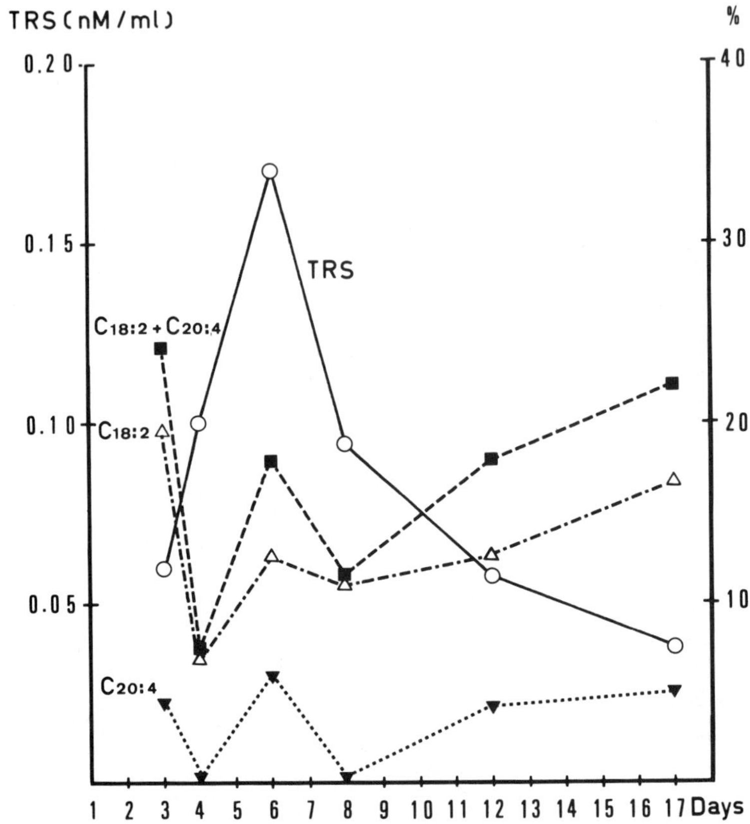

FIG. 2.7. A representative pattern of the fatty acid profile and TBA-reactive substances (TRS) in CSF after SAH. In this case, the high value of TRS was associated with development of vasospasm. Note the inverse relationship between the PUFAs and the TRS. The decrease of PUFAs preceded the increase of TRS. (Modified from K. Sano *et al.* (46).)

does not exclude the possibility of formation of H(P)ETEs other than 5-HETE or of prostaglandin endoperoxides and their derivatives since, in the above examination, analysis of these substances was not technically feasible. These facts, together with rapid decreases of GSHpx and vitamin E in the CSF of SAH patients, and a decrease of prostacyclin (PGI_2) in the artery (see below) may well explain the time lag in the appearance of cerebral vasospasm.

As reported elsewhere (6, 46, 61), the vasocontractile capacities of some of the possible constituents of free radical reactions initiated by clot lysis were evaluated using the basilar artery of dogs as described by Allen *et al.* (4). It was shown that oxyHb (10^{-4}M), hydrogen peroxide (10^{-4}M), linoleic acid hydroperoxide (10^{-4}M), and 15-hydroperoxyarachidonic acid (15-HPAA or 15-HPETE) (10^{-4}M) all possess significant vasocontractile

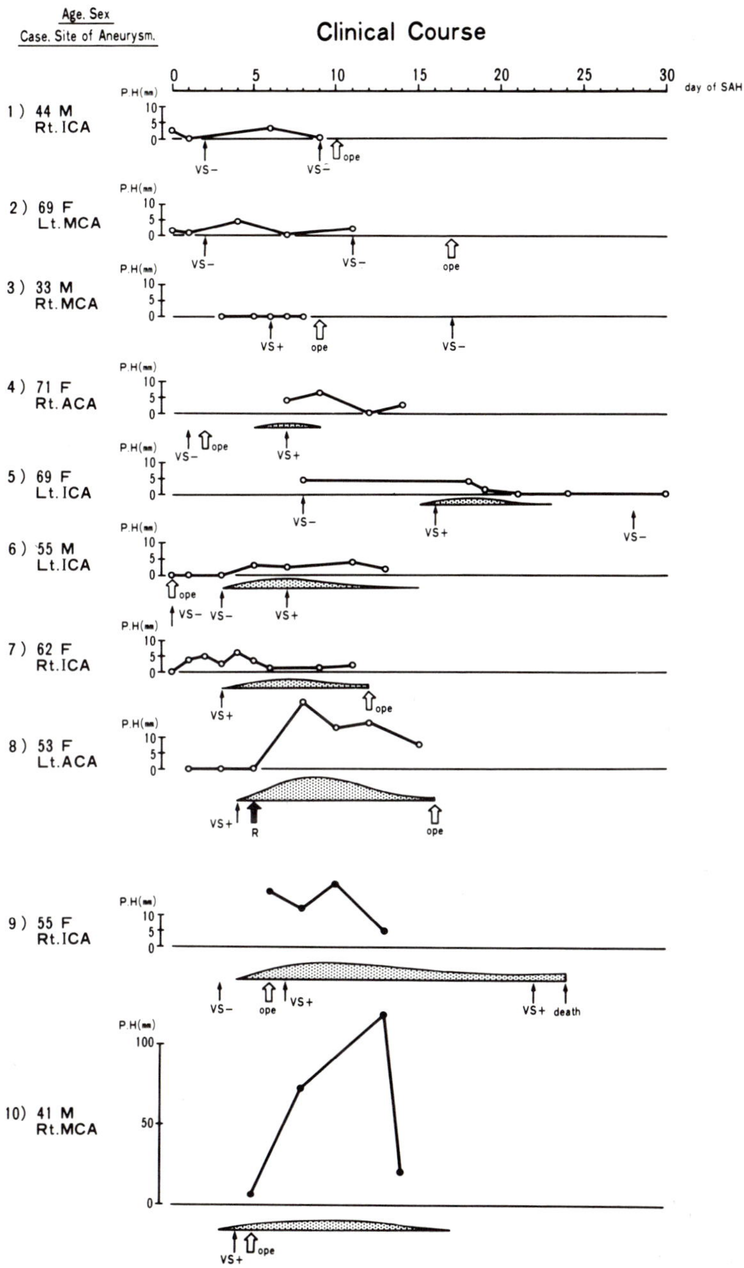

FIG. 2.8. Semiquantitative analysis of 5-HETE in CSF after SAH. CSF obtained by lumbar puncture (○). CSF obtained by cisternal drainage (●). Height of the peak identified as 5-HETE on high-performance liquid chromatography (*PH*). VS, vasospasms; R, rebleeding from aneurysms; *ope*, operation on aneurysm. *Dotted area* shows appearance of neurological deficits due to cerebral vasospasm.

capacity of varying potencies. Dose-response curves were obtained for all of them.

There must be, however, species differences in responsiveness of the artery to various vasocontractile substances. For instance, the human basilar and middle cerebral arteries do not respond to oxyHb (63). According to Kajikawa *et al.* (26), there is no definite correlation, in human cases, between the presence or absence of vasospasm and the amount of hemoglobin in the CSF. The presence of vasospasm does not have any apparent relation to the appearance of oxyHb in the CSF. Furthermore, the incidence of vasospasm is high when metHb is identified in the CSF. Therefore, it seems that the occurrence of vasospasm is more closely related to the amount of lipid peroxides than to the oxyHb itself in the CSF, at least in human SAH.

Morphological Changes of Cerebral Arteries with Spasm

Recently, Eldevik and others (13) expressed doubts about the existence of morphological changes in cerebral arteries with spasm, based on animal experiments and human autopsies. There have been, however, many reports on morphological (histological and ultrastructural) changes in those arteries fallen in vasospasm (3, 10, 14, 21, 59, 60), both in experimental and in clinical SAH.

Histological examinations by Hughes and Schianchi (21) of vasospastic large cerebral arteries in autopsy of human cases which died within 3 weeks after SAH revealed "a range of changes which were interpreted as necrosis of the smooth muscle" and the presence of plump cells, probably macrophages, in parts of the tunica media, and the swollen tunica intima, with the tunica elastica being corrugated and often disrupted. Arteries from autopsy of cases which died later than 3 weeks after SAH disclosed atrophy of the tunica media and a marked subendothelial thickening of the intima with an irregular and sometimes disrupted tunica elastica. The subendothelial thickening was especially stressed by Conway and McDonald (10), who examined autopsies of SAH patients.

The author has observed similar changes in cases who died of vasospasm following rupture of intracranial aneurysms, namely, subendothelial thickening (the endothelium must have also been damaged, but this was difficult to confirm because of a dropping out of the endothelium) and myonecrotic changes in parts of the media. In experimental models of vasospasm, the most striking changes seen by electron microscopy were also intimal or endothelial changes and some myonecrotic changes in the tunica media. As a matter of fact, the earliest morphological change in experimental SAH was the endothelial damage (granules and vesicles) which appeared one to several hours after injection of blood into the cistern (see below). Therefore, in the knowledge and experience of the author, the contention of Eldevik's group seems untenable.

Effects of Lipid Hydroperoxide on the Cerebral Artery

The question remains as to whether it is possible to produce chronic vasospasm and similar histological changes by a chemically known lipid peroxide.

Cisternal injection of 15-HPAA or 15-HPETE (0.2 and 2.0 mg dissolved in bovine serum albumin) caused a mild initial contraction of the basilar artery of the dog which lasted about 7 hours (46, 53). On Day 2, a stronger contraction recurred, persisting thereafter until sacrifice. An example is shown in Figure 2.9. Electronmicrography of those arterial samples revealed disappearance of myofibrils, pyknotic changes of nuclei, and the appearance of vacuoles as well as of electron-dense granules in scattered parts of the tunica media (Fig. 2.10) and, above all, a remarkable destruction of the endothelial cells (Fig. 2.11) with thickening of the subendothelial layer and corrugation of the elastic lamina (46, 53).

These histological changes, especially the endothelial damage, can be regarded as the toxic effects of lipid peroxides or free radical injury or free radical vasointoxication, because the endothelial changes appear before arterial constriction becomes manifest, and free oxygen radicals,

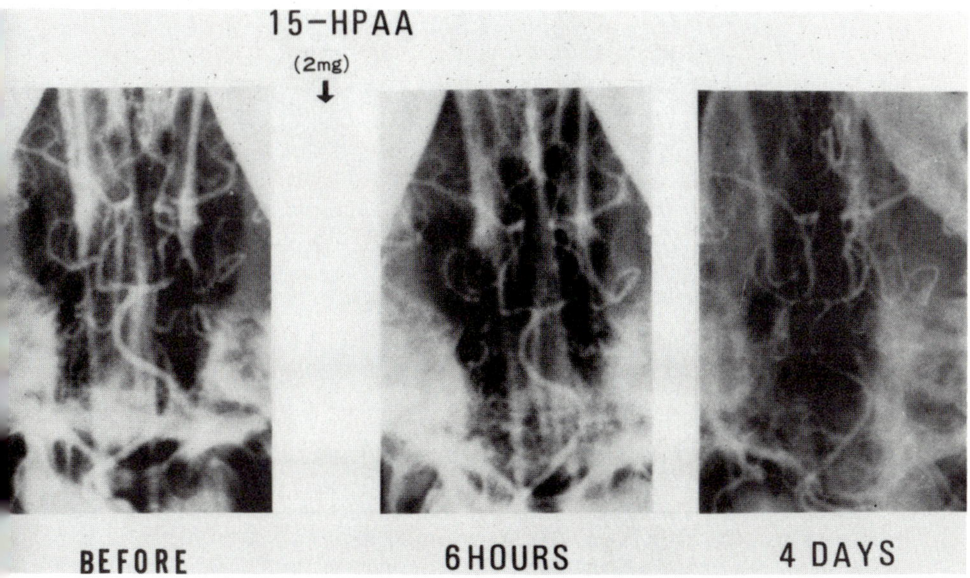

FIG. 2.9. Angiograms before (*left*) and after (*center* and *right*) intracisternal injection of 2 mg of 15-HPAA. (Modified from T. Sasaki *et al.* (53).)

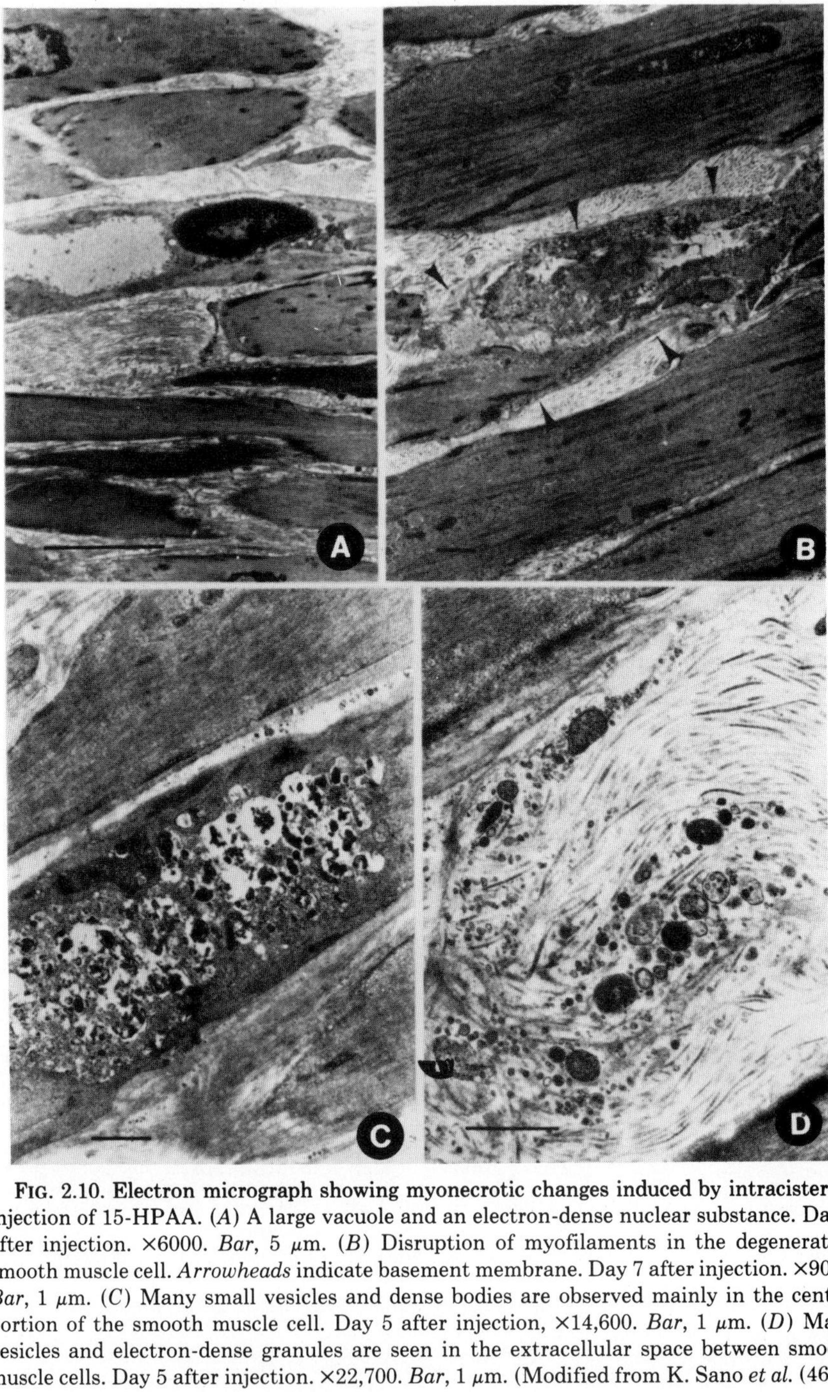

FIG. 2.10. Electron micrograph showing myonecrotic changes induced by intracisternal injection of 15-HPAA. (*A*) A large vacuole and an electron-dense nuclear substance. Day 4 after injection. ×6000. *Bar*, 5 μm. (*B*) Disruption of myofilaments in the degenerating smooth muscle cell. *Arrowheads* indicate basement membrane. Day 7 after injection. ×9000. *Bar*, 1 μm. (*C*) Many small vesicles and dense bodies are observed mainly in the central portion of the smooth muscle cell. Day 5 after injection, ×14,600. *Bar*, 1 μm. (*D*) Many vesicles and electron-dense granules are seen in the extracellular space between smooth muscle cells. Day 5 after injection. ×22,700. *Bar*, 1 μm. (Modified from K. Sano *et al.* (46).)

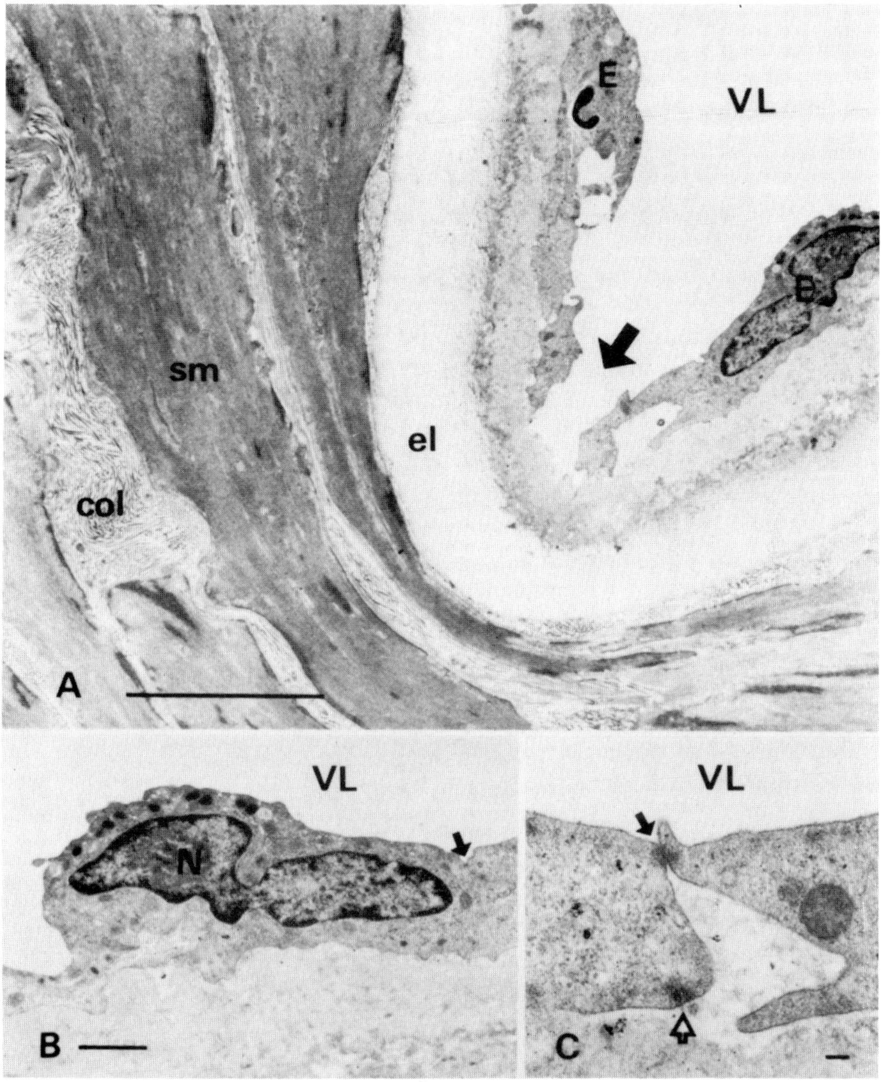

FIG. 2.11. Electron micrograph of the basilar artery from a dog sacrificed 10 hours after intracisternal injection 2 mg of 15-HPAA. (*A*) Degenerating endothelial cells (*E*) are completely separated from each other, resulting in denudation of the elastic lamina (*arrow*). Smooth muscle cells (*sm*) are markedly stretched. The internal elastic lamina (*el*) appears normal. Collagen figers (*col*). ×5700. *Bar* = 5 μm. (*B*) Degenerative changes of the endothelial cell are shown. Dense bodies and small vesicles in the cytoplasm are increased. *Arrow* indicates tight junctions, which seem to be nearly normal. Nucleus (*N*). ×9825. *Bar* = 1 μm. (*C*) Tight junctions connecting adjacent endothelial cells are observed only at the luminar side (*closed arrow*). Dense cytoplasmic meshwork of the tight junctions still remains at the abluminar side of the junctional zone of the separated endothelial cells (*open arrow*). ×3150. *Bar* = 0.1 μm. Vascular lumen (*VL*). (Modified from T. Sasaki *et al.* (53).)

especially hydroxy radicals, are known to cause endothelial lesions (28). According to Koide *et al.* (27), not only 15-HPAA but also 13-hydroperoxylinoleic acid, showed a potent vasocontractile capacity. The maximal artery response to each of these lipid hydroperoxides was almost 1.4 times stronger than that obtained with serotonin.

Prostacyclin (PGI_2) synthesis in the endothelium must be impaired by this endothelial damage. In addition, lipid hydroperoxides, *e.g.*, 15-HPAA (15-HPETE), are well known to inhibit synthesis of PGI_2 from endoperoxides (12). As stated earlier, peroxidation of PUFAs is increased in SAH. This means an increase in the endoperoxides and hydroperoxides of PUFAs. Endoperoxides become sources of prostaglandin synthesis and from these, vasoconstrictive thromboxane A_2 (TXA_2), $PGF_{2\alpha}$, D_2, E_2, etc. will be produced (Fig. 2.12). Hydroperoxides inhibit PGI_2 synthesis, resulting in decreases of PGI_2 in the vessel wall (Fig. 2.12). If there is endothelial damage, platelets in the blood stream come there to adhere and aggregate, producing TXA_2 and other vasoconstrictive substances.

Zervas and his collaborators showed that feline cerebral arteries, which are devoid of vasa vasorum, contained a rete vasorum in the adventitia that was permeable to large proteins and was in continuity with the subarachnoid space through stomata studding the adventitial surface. Horseradish peroxidase which was injected into the subarachnoid space could reach the media and the endothelial cells through the rete (68). Therefore, it is reasonable to assume that vasoactive substances in the subarachnoid space can easily penetrate the cerebral arteries. Then the cerebral artery will incur the effects of vasoconstrictive substances from the lumen side as well as from the side of the subarachnoid space.

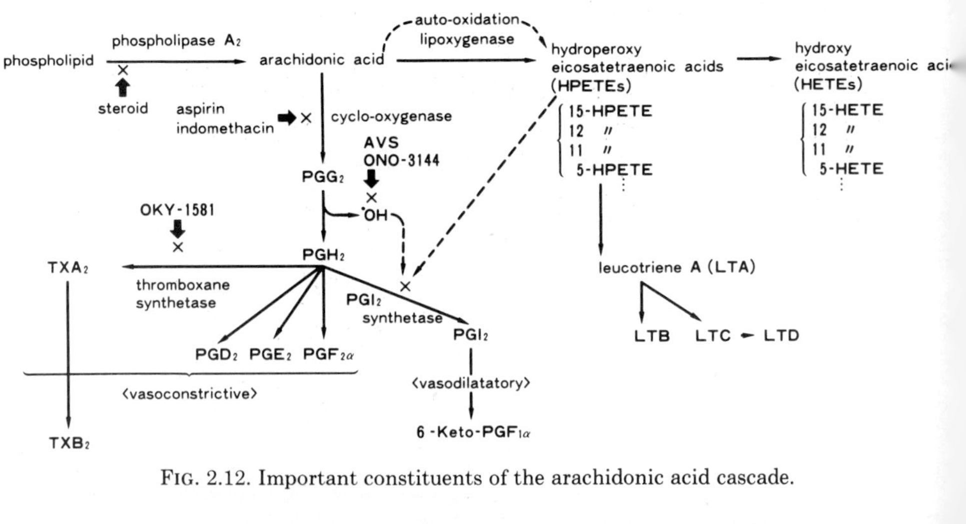

FIG. 2.12. Important constituents of the arachidonic acid cascade.

Furthermore, PGI_2, which inhibits these vasoconstrictive effects, is decreased in the arterial wall. It is no wonder that the artery becomes spastic.

Biosynthesis of PGI_2 in the Cerebral Artery and Its Change in SAH

Another question to be answered is whether prostacyclin (PGI_2) in the arterial wall decreases in cases of SAH.

However, first we must know whether PGI_2 is produced in the normal cerebral artery. Using canine basilar artery segments incubated with C-14 arachidonic acid, Sasaki and the author's group (45, 51) have observed by thin layer radiochromatography that the normal canine artery transformed the arachidonic acid mainly or solely to 6-keto $PGF_{1\alpha}$, the spontaneous metabolite of PGI_2 (51). ($PGF_{2\alpha}$ may be produced but in very small amounts.) This thin layer radiochromatographic pattern was essentially similar to that of the arteries of SAH dogs. Therefore, it can be concluded that in canine basilar arteries, there is only one product transformed from arachidonic acid and that this product is PGI_2.

Isovolemic injection of 6 to 7 ml of autologous blood into the canine great cistern caused vasospasm from Day 2 on (Fig. 2.14, *upper row*). The time course of PGI_2 synthetic activity following this experimental SAH is shown in Figure 2.13. (Note that in this figure, the day of subarachnoid blood injection was counted as Day 1, so that Days 3 and 8 in the figure correspond to Days 2 and 7 in the text, respectively.) The amounts of PGI_2 produced by incubation of each arterial specimen are shown with respect to the incubation time. The production rate of PGI_2 in the arterial segments obtained 2 hours after SAH was the same as that of the control. Seven hours after SAH, the initial rate of PGI_2 synthesis was slightly greater than that of the control, although not statistically significant. The arterial segments obtained on Days 2 and 7 revealed a pronounced and progressive diminution of PGI_2 synthesis (45, 51).

In this experiment, PGI_2 was assayed by its antiaggregatory activity on adenosine diphosphate (ADP)-induced platelet aggregation. That this activity was really that of PGI_2 was shown by its inactivation by acidification of the incubation medium, and also by the disappearance of activity when aspirin, a cyclooxygenase inhibitor, was added to the medium (51).

Prostaglandin synthesis in the artery may differ in animal species. A recent report by Abdel-Halim *et al.* (1) showed that PGI_2 is predominantly synthesized in the human cerebral artery. Thus, the human and the canine cerebral arteries are similar in prostaglandin synthesis. PGI_2 inhibits platelet adhesion and aggregation and also has remarkable

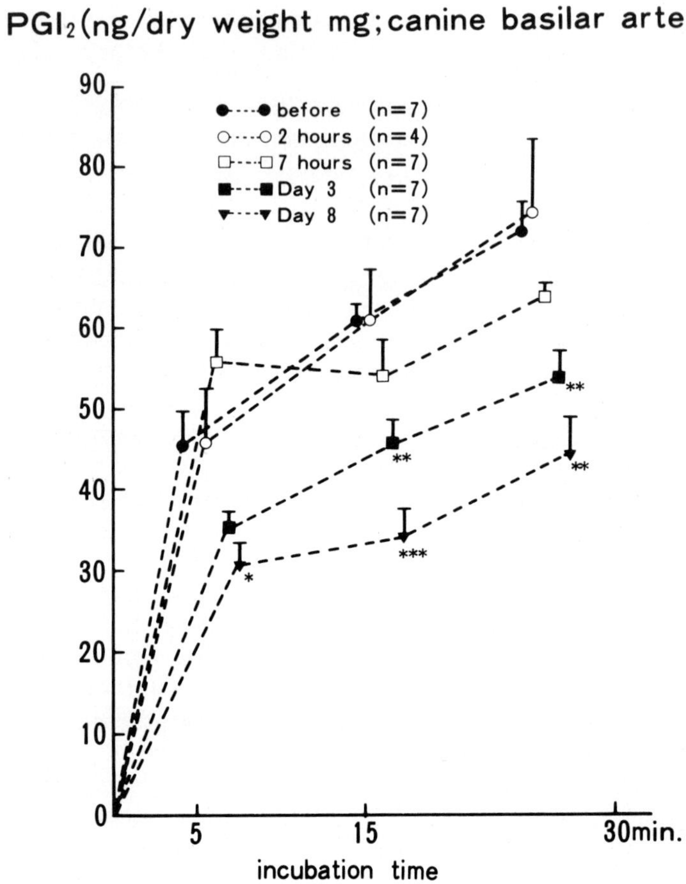

FIG. 2.13. The changes of PGI_2 biosynthetic activity of the canine basilar artery following subarachnoid blood injection. Arterial specimens were incubated in borate-buffered saline at 20°C. The amount of PGI_2 produced by the arterial specimen was bioassayed by measuring the inhibitory activity of the product on adenosine diphosphate (ADP)-induced platelet aggregation. Values are means ± SE of the means. The significant difference from control group by Student's *t*-test was $^*p < 0.05$; $^{**}p < 0.01$; $^{***}p < 0.001$. The arterial specimens obtained on Day 3 and Day 8 of subarachnoid blood injection showed remarkable diminution of PGI_2 synthesis. (Modified from T. Sasaki *et al.* (51).)

vasodilatatory action (8, 19). PGI_2 has been shown to be a potent inhibitor of the vasocontraction (8) induced by various substances, such as PGF_2, PGD_2, and PGE_2.

In the presence of endothelial damage, the artery, being devoid of or deficient in PGI_2 synthesis, would be exposed to the unopposed vasocontractile action of thromboxane A_2 (TXA_2) and of other vasocontractile substances released from the aggregated platelets. Assuming that the

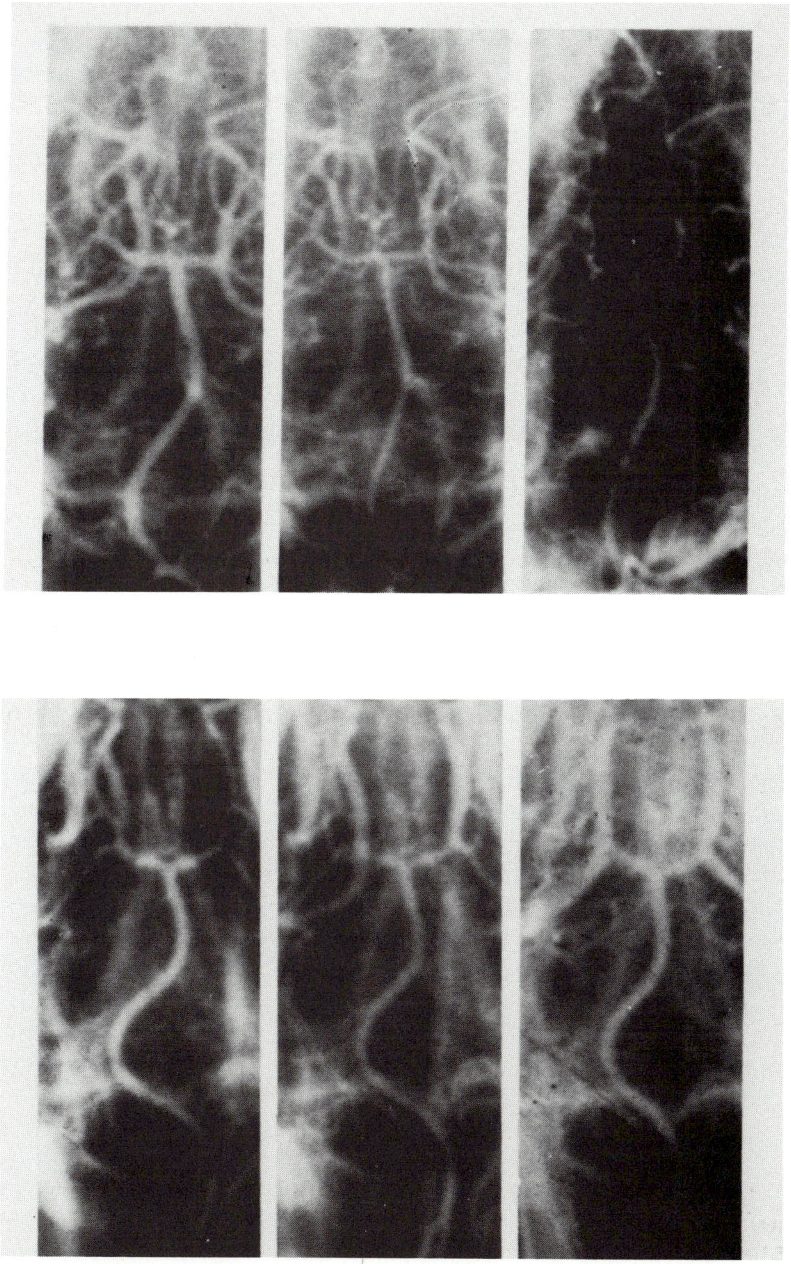

FIG. 2.14. Angiograms before (*left*), 15 minutes after (*center*), and 3 days after (*right*) cisternal blood injection. (*Upper*) Angiograms of a dog without treatment of OKY-1581, showing constriction of the basilar artery. (*Lower*) Angiograms of a dog treated with OKY-1581. Note absence of late spasm. (Modified from T. Sasaki *et al.* (52).)

dual control system of vessel tonus, as proposed by Gorman (19), is operative in cerebral vessels, the sustained elevation of TXA_2 in the face of decreased PGI_2 will inevitably result in a prolonged contraction of cerebral arteries.

Prevention of Experimental Vasospasm following SAH by Thromboxane Synthetase Inhibitor

The decreased synthesis of PGI_2 would shift the reciprocal relationship between TXA_2 and PGI_2 toward a disproportionate synthesis of TXA_2, which further leads to the release of ADP and serotonin from the platelets, to platelet aggregation, and finally to local vasoconstriction. Therefore, it may well be expected that correction of the imbalance between TXA_2 and PGI_2 would be useful in therapy for cerebral vasospasm. In order to clarify this, the following experiments were performed (52).

Sodium(E)-3-(4(-3-pyridylmethyl)phenyl)-2-methylacrylate (OKY-1581) was used as a thromboxane synthetase inhibitor. Dogs received intravenous injections of 160 mg of OKY-1581 dissolved in 2 ml of physiological saline immediately after isovolemic injection of autologous blood (7 ml) into the great cistern. Subsequently, the animals received continuous intravenous infusion of the drug at the rate of 400 mg to 4000 mg/50 ml/24 hours until sacrifice 4 days after induction of SAH. The control dogs received subarachnoid blood injection without treatment with OKY-1581.

In the control dogs, severe vasospasm lasted until sacrifice was produced, as seen in the upper row of Figure 2.14. The mean constriction levels of the basilar artery in relation to time after cisternal injection of blood in six dogs are shown in Figure 2.15 (*lowermost curve*). The diameter of the basilar artery in the angiogram before cisternal blood injection was taken as 100%. A biphasic constriction of the basilar artery was observed. The constriction up to 30 minutes after the induction of SAH was regarded as the early spasm and that after the second day as the late spasm. The mean constrictions for the early and late spasms were $35.9 \pm 3.1\%$ and $35.7 \pm 2.8\%$ (mean $\pm$ SE) of the arterial diameter (before cisternal blood injection), respectively.

The time courses of the basilar artery constriction in the dogs treated with OKY-1581 are shown in Figure 2.15 (the upper curve showing the time course of the 4000 mg/day group and the middle curve showing that of the 400 mg/day group). Although a mild early spasm was observed, the late spasm was almost completely abolished by the intravenous infusion of 4000 mg/day of OKY-1581. There was a statistically significant difference when the mean constriction levels for the early and late

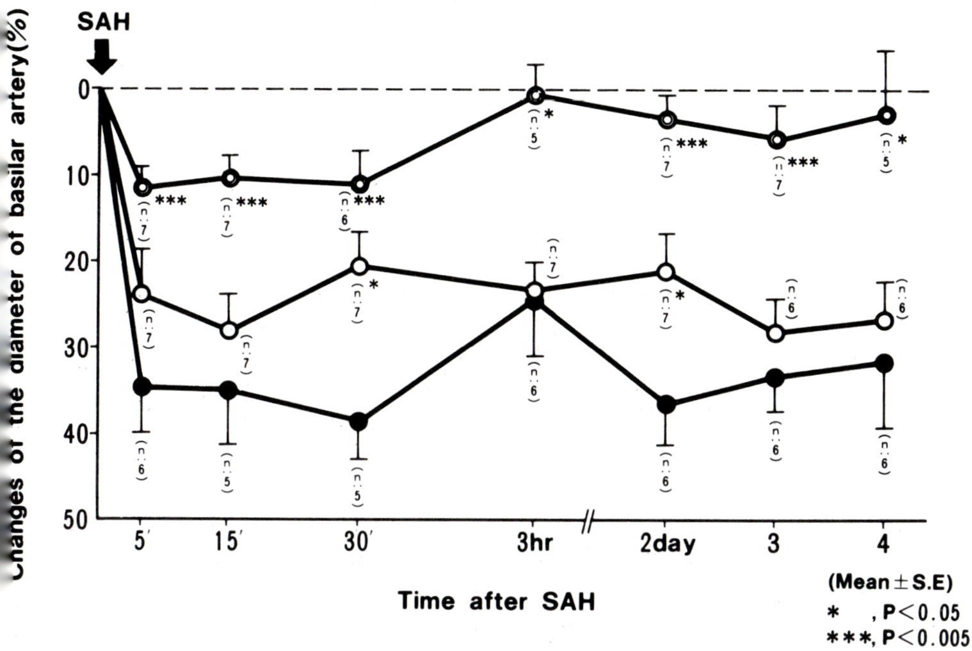

FIG. 2.15. Changes in diameter of the basilar artery after cisternal blood injection are plotted with respect to time. In the control group (●), biphasic constriction of the basilar artery is observed. In the dogs treated with 4000 mg/day of OKY-1581 (◎), no late spasm is present. The effect of the drug is not so marked in the dogs treated with 400 mg/day of the drug (○). Number of arteries tested (*n*). $*p < 0.05$; $***p < 0.005$. (Modified after T. Sasaki *et al.* (52).)

spasms were compared between the control and the OKY-1581 groups. As compared to the control, the early and late spasms in the 4000 mg/day group were, on the average, suppressed by 69.3 and 88.1%, respectively. Dose dependency of the effects of the drug was also noted, as shown in the upper and middle curves in Figure 2.15.

In the control dogs, degenerative changes in the endothelium were revealed by both transmission and scanning electron microscopical observations (52). There was an increase in the cytoplasmic density and the appearance of many small vesicles in the endothelium. In places, the endothelial cells were partially separated from each other, probably at the tight junctions. These changes indicate degeneration of the endothelium. These degenerative changes in the endothelium were observed sometimes as early as 1 hour after the blood injection and were invariably observed by the time of sacrifice on the fourth day. On the other hand, myonecrotic changes were limited to a small number of smooth muscle cells. These changes consisted of disruption of myofilaments, the appearance of many small vesicles and vacuoles in the smooth muscle cells, and pyknotic changes in the nuclei of the smooth muscle cells. Marked corrugation of the internal elastic lamina was invariably observed at the period of the late spasm.

In the dogs treated with 4000 mg/day of OKY-1581, degenerative changes of the endothelial cells and myonecrotic changes in the tunica media similar to those in the control were observed. However, corrugation of the internal elastic lamina was almost completely absent on the 4th day in 5 of 7 dogs, a finding compatible with the absence of late spasm in these dogs. The two remaining dogs showed mild corrugation of the internal elastic lamina on the 4th day (52).

As a possible explanation for these findings, the free radical hypothesis concerning the pathogenesis of vasospasm (46, 53) seems useful. As stated previously, free radical reactions associated with lysis of subarachnoid clots are involved in the genesis of vasospasm following SAH. Free radicals are known to damage the vascular endothelium (28). Assuming that the endothelial damage following SAH is caused by free radicals, it is expected that OKY-1581, which does not possess any radical scavenging action, would not inhibit the endothelial damage, regardless of its preventive action against vasoconstriction.

The results also indicate that a disproportionate synthesis of thromboxane A_2 plays an important role in the evolution of chronic cerebral vasospasm following SAH and that drugs such as OKY-1581 that selectively inhibit thromboxane synthetase might be useful in the prevention of vasospasm.

Vasoconstrictor Agents in the CSF of SAH Patients

It is well documented that CSF from patients with aneurysmal SAH may induce smooth muscle contraction (9). However, development of symptomatic vasospasm is not paralleled by an increase in vasoconstrictor activity in the CSF; such activity was shown to be highest in the early stage of SAH when vasospasm had not yet developed. This finding led Brandt *et al.* to hypothesize that cerebral vasospasm may be due to a disturbance of the protective mechanisms in the arterial wall maintaining normal vessel tone (PGI_2 or its metabolite), even in the presence of vasoconstrictor substances in the perivascular space (9). In their experiments using human cerebral artery strips, indomethacin, which inhibits cyclo-oxygenase and consequently inhibits PGI_2 synthesis (see Fig. 2.12), increased the CSF-induced contraction. On the other hand, PGI_2 and its metabolite, 6-keto-PGE_1 reversed the contractions induced by CSF, as well as by norepinephrine, serotonin, and $PGF_{2\alpha}$ (9). These findings are in accordance with the above-mentioned view of the author.

Sasaki tried to identify the vasoconstrictor agents in CSF from patients with SAH in his unpublished experiments. When the CSF of cases with or without vasospasm was applied to isolated canine basilar artery strips, the artery segments showed contraction. In order to identify the vasoconstrictor agents, experiments were done to reverse the CSF-induced contraction with specific pharmacological antagonists. The contraction was not reversed by methysergide (serotonin blocker), mepyramine (histamine blocker), phenoxybenzamine (blocker of alpha action of norepinephrine), proparanol (blocker of beta action of norepinephrine), or atropine (acetylcholine blocker). Therefore, serotonin, histamine, norepinephrine, and acetylcholine were eliminated as the prime vasoconstrictor agents in the CSF.

Since vasocontractile activity of lipid peroxides or prostaglandins has been said to be related to the disulfide form of the normal sulfhydryl structure of the biomembrane (5), Sasaki investigated action of two disulfide-reducing agents, dithiothreitol (DTT) and dithioerythritol (DTE). Both of these chemicals inhibited the CSF-induced contraction (Figs. 2.16 and 2.17). Furthermore, 1,2-*bis*(nicotinamido)-propane (AVS), which is a hydroxy radical scavenger and an inhibitor of contraction induced by lipid hydroperoxides, also showed an inhibitory effect on the CSF-induced contraction (Fig. 2.18).

These results speak for lipid peroxides or prostaglandins as the prime vasoconstrictor agents in the CSF of SAH patients. Contraction induced by potassium application was not inhibited by DTT or by DTE, both of which had inhibited the CSF-induced contraction. Therefore, potassium has little to do with the vasocontractile activity of CSF.

Summary of the Pathogenesis of Vasospasm

The pathogenesis of cerebral vasospasm in SAH may be summarized as follows. Free radical reactions, especially lipid peroxidation, are initiated by clot lysis because of insufficient defense mechanisms in the CSF against free radicals. These defense mechanisms are especially insufficient after Day 3. Each constituent of these free radical reactions (such as lipid hydroperoxides) has vasocontractile capacity. Furthermore, the endothelium and the media of the artery incur free radical injury (toxic effects of free radicals). Because of endothelial damage and inhibitory effects of the lipid hydroperoxides on PGI_2 synthesis, the arterial wall PGI_2 drops to a very low value. Vasoconstrictive substances act on the arterial wall not only from the side of the subarachnoid space, but also from the lumen side as well, because there is constant adhesion and aggregation of platelets to the damaged endothelium, and these platelets produce thromboxane A_2 and other vasoconstrictive substances which are unopposed by PGI_2.

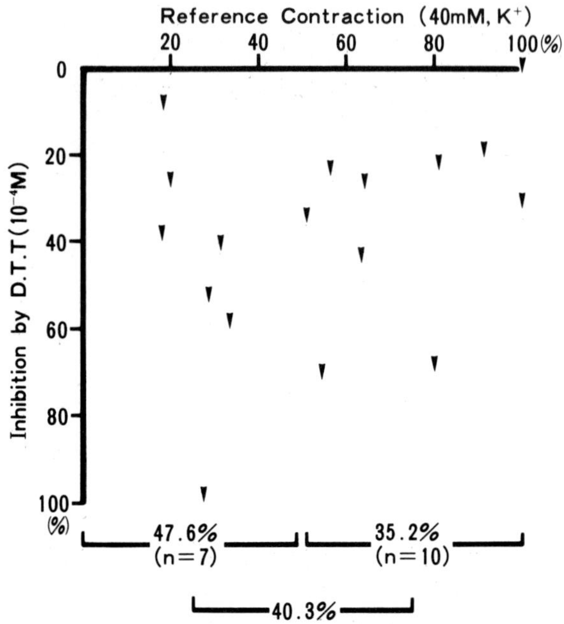

FIG. 2.16. Influence of DTT on CSF-induced contraction. Incubation (20 minutes) of canine basilar artery strips with DTT (10^{-4}M) suppressed the contraction induced by CSF (17 samples) obtained from 13 SAH patients, on the average, by 40.3%. The *ordinate* shows the inhibitory effect of DTT on CSF-induced contraction, and the *abscissa* the contractile capacity of each patient's CSF using the contraction induced by potassium (40 mM) as the reference (100%). Contraction by the CSF samples having a contractile capacity of more than 50% of the reference was suppressed by DTT by 35.2%, and that by CSF samples having contractile capacity of less than 50% was suppressed by 47.6%. (Courtesy of Drs. T. Sasaki and T. Asano.)

Thus, the artery falls into the state of chronic vasospasm with characteristic histological changes (Fig. 2.19). The pathogenesis of vasospasm, however, is not yet completely elucidated. Many things remain to be clarified. Probably, Winston Churchill's famous words which he delivered after the victory in Egypt in November 1942, may rightly be applied to the present status of studies on vasospasm: "This is not the end. It is not even the beginning of the end. But it is, perhaps, the end of the beginning."

Treatment of Cerebral Vasospasm

The cause of cerebral vasospasm is, in this way, multifactorial. Therefore, prevention or treatment of the vasospasm will be multifarious.

Various treatments are summarized in Tables 2.7 and 2.8. In Table 2.8, the therapies reviewed by Norwood *et al.* (36, 37) and Wilkins (66),

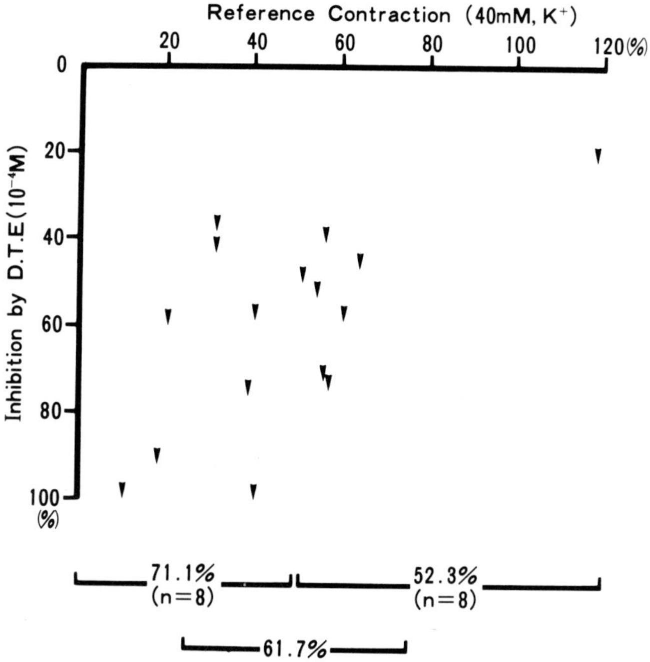

FIG. 2.17. Influence of DTE on CSF-induced contraction. Incubation (20 minutes) of canine basilar artery strips with DTE (10^{-4}M) suppressed the contraction induced by CSF (16 samples) obtained from 15 SAH patients, on the average, by 61.7%. The *ordinate* shows the inhibitory effect of DTE on CSF-induced contraction, and the abscissa the contractile capacity of each patient's CSF using the contraction induced by potassium (40 mM) as the reference (100%). Contraction by the CSF samples having contractile capacity of more than 50% of the reference was suppressed by DTE by 52.3%, and that by CSF samples having contractile capacity of less than 50% was suppressed by 71.1%. (Courtesy of Drs. T. Sasaki and T. Asano.)

perhaps a little bit too conventional, are listed from No. 8 to No. 12. The combination therapy of No. 13 was recently published by Levy *et al.* (30). Angiotensin-converting enzyme inhibition in No. 14 was also recently published by Gavras *et al.* (17). Topical application of lidocaine on the spastic artery proposed by Giannotta *et al.* (18) is different from the use of isoproterenol and lidocaine by Sundt *et al.* (54) and has been sometimes effective at operation also in the author's hands.

In Table 2.7, the therapies which seem promising or worthy of discussion are listed and are discussed briefly below.

1. Early surgery of aneurysms and removal of subarachnoid clots and setting cisternal drainage before free radical reactions advance are of primary concern (49). Removal of all clots is, on many occasions, very

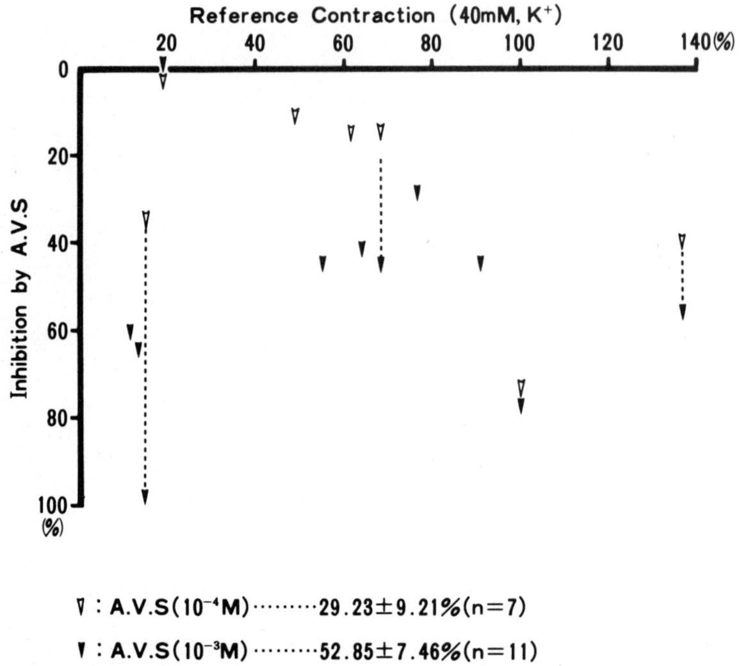

FIG. 2.18. Influence of 1,2-*bis*(nicotinamido)-propane (AVS) on CSF-induced contraction. Incubation (2 minutes) of canine basilar artery strips with 10^{-4}M or 10^{-3}M of AVS suppressed the contraction induced by CSF (18 samples) obtained from 11 SAH patients, on the average, by 29.23% and by 52.85%, respectively. Dose dependency of the effect was noticed in 3 CSF samples (increase of the inhibitory effect is shown by dotted lines according to increase in concentration of AVS). (Courtesy of Drs. T. Sasaki and T. Asano.)

difficult. This may be the reason why vasospasm may later develop even in cases undergoing early surgery (Table 2.6).

2. Hemodynamic improvement of cerebral circulation (by raising blood pressure, hypervolemia, etc.) is, of course, necessary after aneurysm clipping.

3. Protection of the brain against ischemia by barbiturates or Y-9179 (58) is important. Y-9179 (nizofenone), a cerebral protector and a free radical scavenger, had fewer side effects than barbiturates. A recent cooperative double-blind clinical trial showed that the group treated with this drug (administration of the drug was initiated before vasospasm developed and was continued for 5 days and, if vasospasm developed, was continued for an additional 5 days) was superior to the placebo group ($p < 0.05$) in the "disability status scale" 1 month after development of vasospasm, although development of vasospasm was not prevented by this drug.

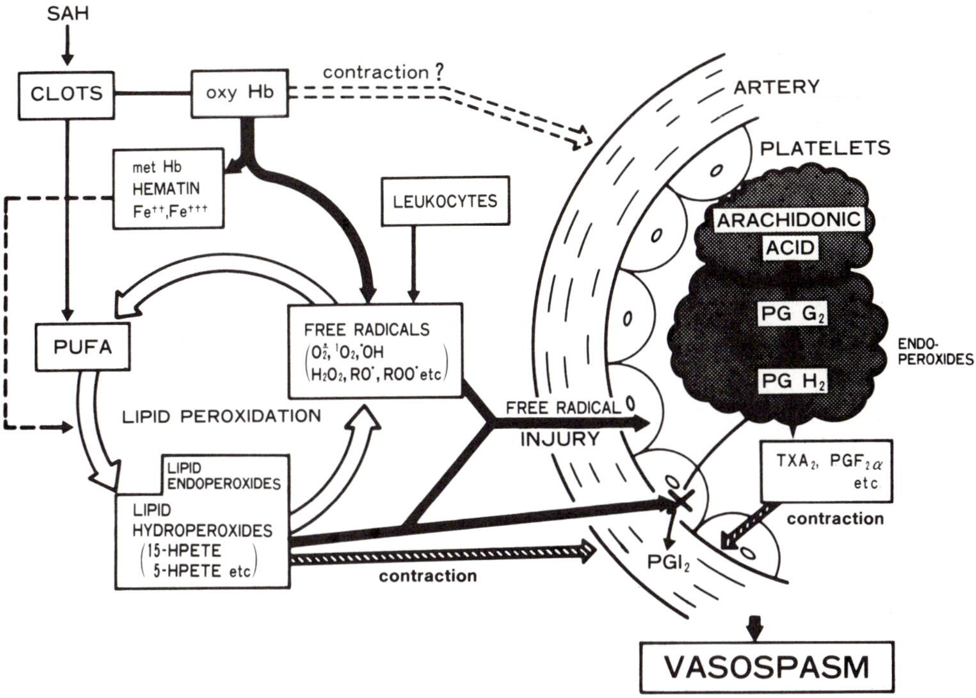

FIG. 2.19. A suggested mechanism for the pathogenesis of chronic cerebral vasospasm in SAH. (Modified from K. Sano *et al.* (46).)

4. Use of free radical scavengers such as vitamin E, barbiturates, Y-9179, AVS, ONO-3144 (a hydroxy radical scavenger), mannitol, etc. seems very important, especially in the early stage of SAH, from the viewpoint of the pathogenesis of vasospasm described above.

5. Suppression of platelet aggregation and pharmacological modification of prostaglandin synthesis are considered to be also important. Phosphodiesterase inhibitors which are thought to increase cyclic AMP are often used. Lipoxygenase inhibitors, if available, may be promising. Cyclooxygenase inhibitors and phospholipase A_2 inhibition, however, may aggravate vasospasm because these inhibit not only vasoconstrictive but also vasodilatatory prostaglandins (Fig. 2.12).

6. Inhibition of thromboxane A_2 synthesis, *e.g.*, by administration of OKY-1581 or ONO-3144 or, to a lesser extent, by trapidil (57) or Y-9179, should be very important. Use of prostacyclin or its analogues (8) may also be useful.

7. Calcium can be considered as the final common pathway for muscle contraction. Therefore, use of the so-called calcium antagonists may be of additional value in the treatment of vasospasm.

TABLE 2.7

Possible Modes of Therapy Against Vasospasm (1)

1. Removal of perivascular clot by early surgery and cisternal drainage of CSF
2. Hemodynamic improvement of impaired cerebral circulation
   - Elevation of systemic arterial pressure (dopamine, etc.)
   - Hypervolemia
   - Dextran, mannitol, etc.
3. Cerebral protection against ischemia by drugs
   - Barbiturates
   - Y-9179 (nizofenone)
4. Use of free radical scavengers
   - Vitamin E
   - Barbiturates
   - Y-9179 (nizofenone)
   - 1,2-*bis*(nicotinamido)-propane(AVS)
   - ONO-3144 (2-aminomethyl-4-tert-butyl-6-propionylphenol hydrochloride)
   - Mannitol, etc.
5. Suppression of platelet aggregation and pharmacological modification of prostaglandin synthesis
   - Phosphodiesterase inhibitors (papaverine, phthalazinol, etc. (9))
   - Cyclo-oxygenase inhibitors (indomethacin, aspirin, etc.)
   - Lipoxygenase inhibitors
   - Phospholipase A_2 suppression (steroids)
6. Inhibition of thromboxane-A_2 synthesis and/or stimulation of prostacyclin synthesis
   - OKY-1581 (sodium(E)-3-(4(-3-pyridylmethyl)phenyl)-2-methylacrylate)
   - ONO-3144 (2-aminomethyl-4-tert-butyl-6-propionylphenol hydrochloride)
   - Y-9179 (nizofenone)
   - Trapidil
   - Prostacyclin and its analogues
7. Calcium antagonists
   - Nimodipine
   - Nifedipine
   - Diltiazem
   - Cinnarizine
   - Verapamil
   - Perdipine

One of the main reasons why many neurosurgeons hesitate to perform early surgery (which is the best means to prevent rebleeding of aneurysms) is fear of postoperative vasospasm, which is actually only remotely related to surgery itself. Therefore, if some of these lines of investigation yield effective drugs for prevention or cure of chronic cerebral vasospasm in the near future, the treatment of ruptured intracranial aneurysms will be changed so that very early surgery to prevent rebleeding of aneurysms, combined with removal of as much subarachnoid clot as possible and fashioning of cisternal drainage, will be performed—accompanied by ample administration (systemic or topical) of such drugs. Then the results

TABLE 2.8

Possible Modes of Therapy Against Vasospasm (2)

8. Adenyl cyclase stimulation
    - $beta_2$-adrenergic drugs
        - isoproterenol ($beta_1$ + $beta_2$) (+lidocaine)
        - salbutamol (mainly, $beta_2$)
9. Phosphodiesterase inhibition
    - Papaverine, methylxanthines, ascorbic acid, aminophylline, diazoxide, chlorpromazine, reserpine, hydralazine
10. Combination of 8 and 9
    - salbutamol + aminophylline
11. Use of exogenous cyclic AMP or one of its congeners
    - dibutyryl cyclic AMP
12. Guanyl cyclase inhibition
    - phenoxybenzamine (blocking serotonin, alpha-adrenergic drugs, and cholinergic drugs)
    - phentolamine (alpha blocker)
    - methysergide, reserpine, kanamycin (serotonin blocker)
    - atropine (cholinergic blocker)
    - prostaglandin $F_{2\alpha}$ blocker (?)
    - sodium nitroprusside (alpha blocker) +
    - phenylephrine (alpha stimulator with little effect on the cerebral vessels)
13. Combination of 9 and 12
    - aminophylline + nitroprusside + dopamine
14. Angiotensin-converting enzyme inhibition
    - teprotide
15. Topical application of local anesthetics
    - lidocaine

of treatment of ruptured intracranial aneurysms will be greatly ameliorated.

PREOPERATIVE VASOSPASM AND TIMING OF SURGERY

There were 132 cases with preoperative vasospasm in the author's series (Table 2.9). In these cases, the vasospasm was always accompanied by the neurological signs and symptoms previously reported (44, 47), provided that a slight, reversible narrowing of the cerebral arteries was not counted as vasospasm. There was no case in which vasospasm was identified during the first 4 days after SAH (namely, before Day 4 after SAH). Two thirds of the cases first demonstrated symptoms of vasospasm between Days 5 and 8 (with the day of SAH counted as Day 0). The latest appearance of preoperative vasospasm was Day 15. The average interval between SAH and the onset of preoperative vasospasm was 7.6 ± 2.5 days. (This interval seems, as stated before, almost the same as that in the postoperative vasospasm, which was 6.7 ± 1.6 days.) That is, when the vasospasm occurred following SAH, the patient, after recover-

TABLE 2.9

Preoperative Vasospasm (132 cases)

Group	
1	Progressing vasospasm → Brain edema → Death 24 cases (9 AC aneurysms, 8 ICPC aneurysms, 3 basilar, 4 MC)
2	Rebleeding while waiting, mostly when vasospasm began to subside (7–17 days after the onset) 13 cases died 6 cases (2 A_2, 1 MC, 3 AC aneurysms) well and working after op.
3	Operation performed after vasospasm had subsided (duration of vasospasm, 8–24 days) Op. 3–8 wk after SAH 42 cases: working, 22 cases (52.4%); caring for self, 9 (21.4%); op. mortality, 4 (9.5%)
4	Operation performed while vasospasm was still present E, op. performed (3.1 ± 2.5) days after the onset of vasospasm 22 cases: working, 14 cases (63.6%); op. mortality, 2 (9.1%) L, op. performed (7.5 ± 2.5) days after the onset of vasospasm 25 cases: working, 18 cases (72.0%); op. mortality, 0

ing from the attack of SAH, began to show symptoms due to vasospasm around the end of the 1st week or the beginning of the 2nd week after SAH.

It is generally conceded that cases of ruptured aneurysms with vasospasm have a bad prognosis and are poor candidates for surgical treatment. For instance, 24 cases of Group 1 in Table 2.9 showed progressively deteriorating courses leading to death. In 19 cases of Group 2 in which rebleeding occurred while waiting, 13 cases died, and 6 cases that could fortunately undergo surgery were well and working. The rebleeding occurred, in most cases, when vasospasm began to subside. In 42 cases of Group 3 in which operation was performed after vasospasm subsided and rebleeding fortunately did not occur during the period, 22 cases (52.4%) were well and working, and 4 cases (9.5%) died. In 22 cases of Group 4E in which operation was performed relatively early (3.1 ± 2.5 days) after the onset of vasospasm, 14 cases (63.6%) were well and working, and 2 cases (9.1%) died. In these cases vasospasm was still present.

It is interesting to note that, in 25 cases of Group 4L in which operation was performed around 1 week (7.5 ± 2.5 days) after the onset of vasospasm, the results were good; 18 cases (72%) were well and working, and no case died. In these cases, vasospasm was still present but was beginning to subside.

Based on these data, the author has tried to operate on such cases that still demonstrated vasospasm when their disturbance of consciousness began to improve, usually more than 1 week after the onset of vasospasm, that is, when vasospasm began to subside. It was found that operative interventions did not aggravate the vasospasm that was already present and yet beginning to subside, although vasospasm may have migrated from the affected proximal portions of the arteries to more distal portions. In other words, vasospasm did not recur at the same portion of the cerebral arteries once it began to subside. This could be because the vascular components were disorganized following prolonged vasospasm (myonecrosis of the media of the arterial wall), and so were not able to produce contraction.

The author's policy of surgical treatment of cases with vasospasm is as follows. Operation on an aneurysm is indicated when disturbance of consciousness due to vasospasm begins to improve, even if the vasospasm is still noted in angiograms, or if vasospasm is of a quite local type (type 3 of the author's classification (44, 47)). Operation should be postponed when the extensive type of vasospasm is still in its initial stage. Therefore, the optimal time of direct operation on aneurysms with vasospasm will be the 2nd week after the onset of vasospasm (not the onset of SAH) if the patient's condition is improving. Rebleeding may occur when vasospasm is relieved. Therefore, the danger of rebleeding should always be taken into considereation if the operation has to be postponed beyond this optimal time.

PRINCIPLE OF SURGERY OF ANEURYSMS IN THE ACUTE STAGE OF SAH

The author's principle for the surgical treatment of ruptured aneurysms in the acute stage is now as follows.

1. During the first 3 days (48 hours) of SAH, namely, on Days 0 through 2, microsurgery of aneurysms with removal of subarachnoid blood clots is indicated for any case, except for Grade IV and V cases. Surgery should also probably be delayed in patients 60 years or older. Additional use of medicaments such as free radical scavengers is recommended.

2. After Day 3, surgery for cases in Grades III, IV, and V should be postponed until they show improvement of neurological conditions by various conservative treatments. Microsurgery is indicated for cases in Grades I and II.

3. Any case showing neurological deterioration (to higher grades) should be submitted to computerized tomography (CT) and angiographical examinations to detect vasospasm, which is the most probable cause of the deterioration. If vasospasm is present, surgery should be postponed until vasospasm begins to subside and disturbance of consciousness begins to improve, but not for too long, because rebleeding of aneurysms

may occur when vasospasm begins to subside. The optimal timing of surgery for cases with vasospasm may be the 2nd week after the onset of vasospasm.

In addition to this principle, the following should be added. If CT demonstrates an intracerebral hematoma caused by ruptured aneurysm, immediate surgery (clipping of the aneurysm and removal of the hematoma) is indicated for that case. In the author's series, 32 cases had intracerebral hematomata. Seven cases died before this definitive surgery was done. Twenty-five cases were submitted to surgery (aneurysmal neck clipping and removal of hematoma), of which 3 cases (12%) died, 12 cases (48%) were well and working, and 6 cases (24%) were caring for themselves, and 4 cases (16%) were bedridden. Therefore, surgery was able to achieve a useful social life for 48% of these cases.

In summary, among 798 consecutive cases of SAH admitted to the author's clinic in the past 12 years: 63 cases died before surgery; 5 cases were discharged without surgery (2 cases had spontaneous obliteration of aneurysms, and 3 cases did not want to have surgery); 730 cases were submitted to microsurgery, and the operative mortality was 5.8%. Total case mortality, *i.e.*, mortality of all admitted patients, was 13.2%. The working rate in the follow-up was 72.8%; that of the cases submitted to surgery was 78.9%. These results are better than other reports of delayed surgery (41) and will be ameliorated when the above-mentioned principle is more strictly observed.

ACKNOWLEDGMENTS

The author is most grateful for the assistance of Drs. Takao Asano, Tomio Sasaki, Takashi Watanabe, Chikayuki Ochiai, Kintomo Takakura (University of Tokyo), Akira Tamura, Takeo Tanishima (Teikyo University), Isamu Saito (Fuji Brain Institute Hospital), Takanori Fukushima (Mitsui Memorial Hospital), and many of his former assistants.

REFERENCES

1. Abdel-Halim, M. S., von Holst, H., Meyerson, B. *et al.* Prostaglandin profiles in tissue and blood vessels from human brain. J. Neurochem., *34:* 1331–1333, 1980.
2. Adams, H. R., Jr., Kassell, N. F., Torner, J. C., Nibbelink, D. W., and Sahs, A. L. Early management of aneurysmal subarachnoid hemorrhage. A report of the Cooperative Aneurysm Study. J. Neurosurg., *54:* 141–145, 1981.
3. Alksne, J. F., and Branson, P. J. Pathogenesis of cerebral vasospasm. Neurol. Res., *2:* 273–282, 1980.
4. Allen, G. S., Henderson, L. M., Chou, S. N., and French, L. A. Cerebral arterial spasm. Part 1. *In vitro* contractile activity of vasoactive agents on canine basilar and middle cerebral arteries. J. Neurosurg., *40:* 433–441, 1974.
5. Asano, M., and Hidaka, H. Contractile response of isolated rabbit aortic strips to unsaturated fatty acid peroxides. J. Pharmacol. Exp. Ther., *208:* 347–353, 1979.
6. Asano, T., Tanishima, T., Sasaki, T., and Sano, K. Possible participation of free radical reactions initiated by clot lysis in the pathogenesis of vasospasm after subarachnoid

hemorrhage. *In* Cerebral Arterial Spasm, edited by R. H. Wilkins, pp. 190–201. Baltimore and London, Williams & Wilkins, 1980.

7. Botterell, E. H., Lougheed, W. M., Scott, J. W., and Vandewater, S. L. Hypothermia and interruption of carotid or carotid and vertebral circulation, in the surgical treatment of intracranial aneurysms. J. Neurosurg., *13:* 1–42, 1956.
8. Boullin, D. J., Bunting, S., Blaso, W. P., Hunt, T. M., and Moncada, S. Responses of human and baboon arteries to prostaglandin endoperoxides and biologically generated and synthetic prostacyclin: Their relevance to cerebral arterial spasm in man. Br. J. Clin. Pharmacol., *7:* 139–147, 1979.
9. Brandt, L., Ljunggren, B., Andersson, K., Hindfelt, B., and Uski, T. Effects of indomethacin and prostacyclin on isolated human pial arteries contracted by CSF from patients with aneurysmal SAH. J. Neurosurg., *55:* 877–883, 1981.
10. Conway, L. W., and McDonald, L. W. Structural changes of the intradural arteries following subarachnoid hemorrhage. J. Neurosurg., *37:* 715–723, 1972.
11. Drake, C. G. Management of cerebral aneurysm. Stroke, *12:* 273–283, 1981.
12. Dusting, G. J., Moncada, S., and Vane, J. R. Prostacyclin (PGX) is the endogenous metabolite responsible for relaxation of coronary arteries induced by arachidonic acid. Prostaglandins, *13:* 3–15, 1977.
13. Eldevik, O. P., Kristiansen, K., and Torvik, A. Subarachnoid hemorrhage and cerebrovascular spasm. Morphological study of intracranial arteries based on animal experiments and human autopsies. J. Neurosurg., *55:* 869–876, 1981.
14. Fein, J. M., Flor, W. J., Cohan, S. L., and Parkhurst, J. Sequential changes of vascular ultrastructure in experimental cerebral vasospasm. Myonecrosis of subarachnoid arteries. J. Neurosurg., *41:* 49–58, 1974.
15. Fisher, C. M., Kistler, J. P., and Davis, J. M. Relation of cerebral vasospasm to subarachnoid hemorrhage visualized by computerized tomographic scanning. Neurosurgery, *6:* 1–9, 1980.
16. Flamm, E. S., Demopoulos, H. B., Seligman, M. L., Poser, R. G., and Ransohoff, J. Free radicals in cerebral ischemia. Stroke, *9:* 445–447, 1978.
17. Gavras, H., Andrews, P., and Papadakis, N. Reversal of experimental delayed cerebral vasospasm by angiotensin-converting enzyme inhibition. J. Neurosurg., *55:* 884–888, 1981.
18. Giannotta, S. L., Kindt, G. W., and Haar, F. L. Topical lidocaine in treatment of cerebral vasospasm. Surg. Neurol., *4:* 13–16, 1975.
19. Gorman, R. R. Prostaglandins, thromboxanes, and prostacyclin. Biochemistry and mode of action of hormones. Int. Rev. Biochem., *20:* 81–107, 1978.
20. Hugenholtz, H., and Elgie, R. G. Considerations in early surgery on good-risk patients with ruptured intracranial aneurysms. J. Neurosurg., *56:* 180–185, 1982.
21. Hughes, J. T., and Schianchi, P. M. Cerebral artery spasm. A histological study at necropsy of the blood vessels in cases of subarachnoid hemorrhage. J. Neurosurg., *48:* 515–525, 1978.
22. Hunt, W. E., and Kosnik, E. J. Timing and perioperative care in intracranial aneurysm surgery. Clin. Neurosurg., *21:* 79–89, 1974.
23. Hunt, W. E., and Miller, C. A. The results of early operation for aneurysm. Clin. Neurosurg., *24:* 208–215, 1977.
24. Ishii, S., Ito, M., Miyaoka, M., and Nonaka, T. The causative factors of vasospasm and its treatment. *In* Cerebral Arterial Spasm, edited by R. H. Wilkins, pp. 556–565. Baltimore and London, Williams & Wilkins, 1980.
25. Jane, J. A., Winn, H. R., and Richardson, A. E. The natural history of intracranial aneurysms: Rebleeding rates during the acute and long-term period and implication for surgical management. Clin. Neurosurg., *24:* 176–184, 1977.

26. Kajikawa, H., Ohta, T., Yoshikawa, Y., Funatsu, N., Yamamoto, M., and Someda, K. Cerebral vasospasm and hemoglobins: Clinical and experimental studies. Neurol. Med. Chir. (Tokyo), *19:* 61–71, 1979.
27. Koide, T., Noda, Y., Hata, S., Sugioka, K., Kobayashi, S., and Nakano, M. Contraction of the canine basilar artery following linoleic, arachidonic, 13-hydroperoxylinoleic, or 15-hydroperoxyarachidonic acid (41294). Proc. Soc. Exp. Biol. Med., *168:* 399–402, 1981.
28. Kontos, H. A., Wei, E. P., Povlishock, J. T., Dietrich, W. D., Magiera, C. J., and Ellis, E. F. Cerebral arteriolar damage by arachidonic acid and prostaglandin G_2. Science, *209:* 1242–1245, 1980.
29. Lai, C-S., Grover, T. A., and Piette, L. H. Hydroxyl radical production in a purified NADPH-cytochromec (p-450) reductase system. Arch. Biochem. Biophys., *193:* 373–378, 1979.
30. Levy, W. J., Bay, J. W., Sawhny, B., and Tank, T. Aminophylline plus nitroprusside and dopamine for treatment of cerebral vasospasm. J. Neurosurg., *56:* 646–649, 1982.
31. Lindsay, K. W., Teasdale, G., Knill-Jones, R. P., and Murray, L. Observer variability in grading patients with subarachnoid hemorrhage. J. Neurosurg., *56:* 628–633, 1982.
32. Locksley, H. B. Report on the cooperative study of intracranial aneurysms and subarachnoid hemorrhage. Section V, Part II. Natural history of subarachnoid hemorrhage, intracranial aneurysms and arteriovenous malformations based on 6368 cases in the cooperative study. J. Neurosurg., *25:* 321–368, 1966.
33. McCord, J. M., and Day, E. D., Jr. Superoxide-dependent production of hydroxyl radical catalyzed by iron-EDTA complex. FEBS Lett., *86:* 139–142, 1978.
34. Misra, H. P., and Fridovich, I. The generation of superoxide radical during the autoxidation of hemoglobin. J. Biol. Chem., *247:* 6960–6962, 1972.
35. Nakamura, T., Suzuki, N., Imabayashi, S., Ishikawa, Y., Sasaki, T., and Asano, T. Lipid Peroxides in the Cerebrospinal Fluid after Subarachnoid Hemorrhage. In *Oxygenases and Oxygen Metabolism,* edited by M. Nozaki *et al.*, pp 611–617. Academic Press, New York, 1982.
36. Norwood, C. W. A review of recent advances in vascular smooth muscle pharmacology. Surg. Neurol., *7:* 91–94, 1977.
37. Norwood, C. W., Poole, G. J., and Moody, D. Treatment of experimental delayed cerebral arterial spasm with a $beta_2$-adrenergic stimulator and a phosphodiesterase inhibitor. J. Neurosurg., *45:* 491–497, 1976.
38. Odom, G. L. Cerebral vasospasm. Clin. Neurosurg., *22:* 29–58, 1975.
39. Osaka, K. Prolonged vasospasm produced by the breakdown products of erythrocytes. J. Neurosurg., *47:* 403–411, 1977.
40. Pia, H. W. Grading of cerebral aneurysms and the timing of operation. Neurosurg. Rev., *4:* 143–150, 1981.
41. Post, K. D., Flamm, E. S., Goodgold, A., and Ransohoff, J. Ruptured intracranial aneurysms. Case morbidity and mortality. J. Neurosurg., *46:* 290–295, 1977.
42. Saito, I., and Sano, K. Vasospasm following rupture of cerebral aneurysms. Neurol. Med. Chir. (Tokyo), *19:* 103–107, 1979.
43. Saito, I., and Sano, K. Vasospasm after aneurysm rupture: Incidence, onset, and course. *In* Cerebral Arterial Spasm. edited by R. H. Wilkins, pp. 294–301. Williams & Wilkins, Baltimore and London, 1980.
44. Saito, I., Ueda, Y., and Sano, K. Significance of vasospasm in the treatment of ruptured intracranial aneurysms. J. Neurosurg., *47:* 412–429, 1977.
45. Sano, K. Cerebral vasospasm: The result of lipid peroxidation leading to inhibition of prostacyclin biosynthesis in the cerebral artery. Neurosurgeons (Tokyo), *1:* 105–111, 1981.

46. Sano, K., Asano, T., Tanishima, T., and Sasaki, T. Lipid peroxidation as a cause of cerebral vasospasm. Neurol. Res., *2:* 253–272, 1980.
47. Sano, K., and Saito, I. Timing and indication of surgery for ruptured intracranial aneurysms with regard to cerebral vasospasm. Acta Neurochir. *41:* 49–60, 1978.
48. Sano, K., and Saito, I. Timing of microsurgical treatment of ruptured intracranial aneurysms. *In* Cerebral Arterial Spasm, edited by R. H. Wilkins, pp. 447–454. Williams & Wilkins, Baltimore and London, 1980.
49. Sano, K., and Saito, I. Early operation and washout of blood clots for prevention of cerebral vasospasm. *In* Cerebral Arterial Spasm, edited by R. H. Wilkins, pp. 510–513, Williams & Wilkins, Baltimore and London, 1980.
50. Sasaki, T., Asano, T., Takakura, K., Sano, K., Nakamura, T., Suzuki, N., Imabayashi, S., and Ishikawa, Y. Cerebral vasospasm and lipid peroxidation.—Lipid peroxides in the cerebrospinal fluid after subarachnoid hemorrhage. Brain and Nerve (Tokyo), *34:* 1191–1196, 1982.
51. Sasaki, T., Murota, S., Wakai, S., Asano, T., and Sano, K. Evaluation of prostaglandin biosynthetic activity in canine basilar artery following subarachnoid injection of blood. J. Neurosurg., *55:* 771–778, 1981.
52. Sasaki, T., Wakai, S., Asano, T., Takakura, K., and Sano, K. Prevention of cerebral vasospasm after SAH with a thromboxane synthetase inhibitor, OKY-1581. J. Neurosurg., *57:* 74–82, 1982.
53. Sasaki, T., Wakai, S., Asano, T., Watanabe, T., Kirino, T., and Sano, K. The effect of a lipid hydroperoxide of archidonic acid on the canine basilar artery. An experimental study on cerebral vasospasm. J. Neurosurg., *54:* 357–365, 1981.
54. Sundt, T. M., Jr., Onofrio, B. M., and Merideth, J. Treatment of cerebral vasospasm from subarachnoid hemorrhage with isoproterenol and lidocaine hydrochloride. J. Neurosurg., *38:* 557–560, 1973.
55. Suzuki, J. Grading and timing of the operation on cerebral aneurysms. In: *Cerebral Aneurysms: Advances in Diagnosis and Therapy,* edited by H. W. Pia, C. Langmaid, and J. Zierski, pp. 201–208. Springer, Berlin, Heidelberg and New York, 1979.
56. Suzuki, J., Onuma, T., and Yoshimoto, T. Results of early operations on cerebral aneurysms. Surg. Neurol., *11:* 407–412, 1979.
57. Suzuki, S., Sobata, E., and Iwabuchi, T. Prevention of cerebral ischemic symptoms in cerebral vasospasm with trapidil, an antagonist and selective synthesis inhibitor of thromboxane A_2. Neurosurgery, *9:* 679–685, 1981.
58. Tamura, A., Asano, T., Sano, K., Tsumagari, T., and Nakajima, A. Protection from cerebral ischemia by a new imidazole derivative (Y-9179) and pentobarbital. A comparative study in chronic middle cerebral artery occlusion in cats. Stroke, *10:* 126–134, 1979.
59. Tanabe, Y., Sakata, K., Yamada, H., Ito, T., and Takada, M. Cerebral vasospasm and ultrastructural changes in cerebral arterial wall. An experimental study. J. Neurosurg., *49:* 229–238, 1978.
60. Tani, E., Yamagata, S., and Ito, Y. Intercellular granules and vesicles in prolonged cerebral vasospasm. J. Neurosurg., *48:* 179–189, 1978.
61. Tanishima, T. Cerebral vasospasm: Contractile activity of hemoglobin in isolated canine basilar arteries. J. Neurosurg., *53:* 787–793, 1980.
62. Tanishima, T., Asano, T., Sasaki, T., and Sano, K. Role of peroxidation in the genesis of cerebral arterial spasm. Acta Neurol. Scand. (Suppl.), *60:* 484–485, 1979.
63. Tanishima, T., Sano, K., and Fukushima, T. Studies on Contractile Activity of Human Cerebral Arteries. Presented at the 40th Annual Meeting of the Japan Neurosurgical Society, Kyoto, October 1981.
64. Tappel, A. L. The mechanism of the oxidation of unsaturated fatty acids catalyzed by

hematin compounds. Arch. Biochem. Biophys., *44:* 378–395, 1953.

65. Thomas, M. J., Mehl, K. S., and Pryor, W. A. The role of the superoxide anion in the xanthine oxidase-induced autoxidation of linoleic acid. Biochem. Biophys. Commun. *83:* 927–932, 1978.
66. Wilkins, R. H. Attempted prevention or treatment of intracranial arterial spasm: A survey. *In* Cerebral Arterial Spasm, edited by R. H. Wilkins, pp. 542–555. Williams & Wilkins, Baltimore and London, 1980.
67. Yagi, K. A simple fluorometric assay for lipoperoxide in blood plasma. Biochem. Med., *15:* 212–216, 1976.
68. Zervas, N. T., Liszcak, T. M., Mayberg, M. R., and Brack, P. M. Cerebrospinal fluid may nourish cerebral vessels through pathways in the adventitia that may be analogous to systemic vasa vasorum. J. Neurosurg., *56:* 475–481, 1982.

CHAPTER

3

Pineal Region Tumors: Problems in Pathology and Treatment

KEIJI SANO, M.D., D.M.Sc., F.A.C.S.(HON).

Like—but oh, how different! (Yes, it was the mountain Echo)
William Wordsworth (1770–1850)

Tumors in the pineal region occupy 4% of all intracranial primary neoplasms in Japan (583 of 14,672 cases) (9) (Table 3.1). This is definitely a higher incidence than in any other country (1, 45, 46). This high incidence is mostly comprised of the so-called germinoma or pinealoma of the two-cell pattern type (PTC), which forms 2.6% of all intracranial primary neoplasms according to the most recent statistics (9). In these same statistics, pineocytoma occurs at a rate of 0.2%, pineoblastoma at 0.1%, and teratoma, including malignant teratoma at 0.7%. In Cushing's series (10), pinealoma is found in 0.7% of the cases studied and in the Chinese statistics (8), it appears in 0.9%. Most of the European and American statistics show a lower incidence of this tumor than these figures (8).

Table 3.2 shows 125 cases of tumors in the pineal region (excluding falcotentorial meningiomas) experienced until 1981 in the author's clinic. All these tumors were histologically verified. In this table, "pinealoma and germinoma" include PTC and pineoblastoma (PB). The problem of nomenclature as to pinealoma or germinoma will be discussed later. In this text, PTC comprises pinealoma of Krabbe (25) or Horrax and Bailey (16, 17), and germinoma of Friedman (12) or Russell and Rubinstein (42–44); pineoblastoma corresponds to medulloblastoma of the pineal of Zülch (61). Mixed germ cell tumors in Table 3.2 were composed of various combinations of 2 or 3 of germinoma (seminoma), teratoma, teratocarcinoma, embryonal carcinoma, choriocarcinoma, and endodermal sinus tumor (see below). Eight cases of PTC in the previous communications of the author (45–47) were reclassified into this category after reexamination of their histologies.

TABLE 3.1

Incidence of Tumors in Pineal Region[a]

	Male	Female	Total
Pinealoma	192	22	214
Pineocytoma	7	2	9
Pineoblastoma	8	4	12
Teratoma	29	1	30
Malignant teratoma	15	1	16
Choriocarcinoma	4	0	4
Dermoid	3	0	3
Epidermoid	1	1	2
Gliomas	17	12	29
Others	226	38	264
Total (in parens)	(502)	(81)	(583)

[a] Data taken from 583 of 14,672 cases (4%) of brain tumors. Calculated from the data of Brain Tumor Registry in Japan (9).
[b] "Others" include meningioma (6 cases), unverified tumors, etc.

TABLE 3.2

Tumors in the Pineal Region—Histologically Verified (125 Cases)

	Age (below 20 yr old)	Age (20 yr old and older)
Pinealoma and Germinoma	44 < 41 M (39 PTC[a] + 1 PB); 3 F (3 PTC) (Including pineal + suprasellar 1)	21 < 19 M (16 PTC + 3 PB); 2 F (1 PTC + 1 PB)
Teratoma mature	15 (15 M)	1 (1 M)
Epidermoid	1 (1 M)	2 (2 F)
Teratocarcinoma	1 (1 M)	0
Mixed germ cell tumors	14 (14 M)	4 (4 M)
Unclassified germ cell tumor	2 (2 M)	0
Ependymona	3 (3 M)	5 (1 M + 4 F)
Other gliomas	4 (2 M + 2 F)	8 (6 M + 2 F)
Totals	84 (79 M + 5 F)	41 (31 M + 10 F)

[a] PTC, pinealoma of two-cell pattern type, often called germinoma; M, male; F, female; PB, pineoblastoma.

For PTC, regardless of its location, radiation therapy is regarded as the established standard therapeutic means. There have been many reports as to the effectiveness of radiotherapy and the follow-up results (4, 6, 21, 32, 49, 51, 56, 57). In most of these reports, however, histological verification of the tumor is almost lacking or insufficient. For example, in the most recent report of Ueki and Tanaka (54), of 88 cases of tumors in the pineal region (the report included, besides these 88 cases, 22 cases of "germinoma" of other locations), probably the largest series so far published, they analyzed the follow-up results of 61 cases of germinoma, among which only 20 cases were histologically verified and 41 cases were diagnosed as germinoma "only clinically by cerebrospinal fluid cytology, by computerized tomography (CT), or by recognition of prompt and distinct response to radiotherapy in ventriculography or CT." Therefore, the present series of the author may probably be the largest series of histologically verified tumors in this region.

Among 59 cases of PTC in the pineal region in Table 3.2, 32 cases were treated in the period from 1962 to 1981. In addition to these, 13 cases of PTC were found in the suprasellar region, and 9 cases were found in other locations during the same period. These were all treated by direct surgery (hence, histologically verified) and postoperativve irradiation. Cases treated by irradiation only (with or without shunt) were excluded. Here, direct surgery means total or partial removal of tumors.

In the following sections, PTC in the pineal region and PTC in the other regions (Table 3.3) will be compared as to their nature and the follow-up results of the treatment done in this period. All pineoblastoma cases (PB in Table 3.2) were treated before 1962, except one case which died before surgery and radiotherapy. Other so-called germ cell tumors will also be dicussed in relation to PTC. Symptomatology of pineal region tumors will be omitted because it is too well known. First, however, the author wants to discuss the old controversial problem as to the origin of PTC and its nomenclature and classification.

HISTOGENESIS OF THE SO-CALLED PINEALOMA OF THE TWO-CELL PATTERN TYPE (PTC)

PTC, as its name implies, is composed of two distinct cell types. Groups of large polygonal cells with frequently clear cytoplasms are

TABLE 3.3

Location, Sex, and Age of PTC (Pinealoma and Germinoma)—Histologically Verified (83 Cases)

	Age: under 20 yr old	Age: 20 yr old and older
Pineal region	42 (39 M, 3 F) (inc. pineal + suprasellar 1)	17 (16 M, 1 F)
Suprasellar region	10 (4 M, 6 F)	5 (4 M, 1 F)
Basal ganglia	3 (3 M)	1 (1 M)
Lateral ventricle	1 (1 M)	1 (1 M)
Cerebellopontine angle	0	1 (1 M)
Parietal	0	1 (1 F)
Frontal	0	1 (1 M)
Total	56 cases	27 cases

[a] M, male; F, female.

TABLE 3.4
Location, Sex, and Age of Pinealoma and Germinoma

		Pinealoma (24)	Seminoma (Germinoma) (24)
Location	Pineal region	19	9
	Suprasellar-hypothalamus	2	9
	Other locations	3	6
Sex	Male	20	21
	Female	4	3
Age	Under 20 yr	17	16
	20 Yr and over	7	8

separated by fibrous strands with perivascular lymphocytic infiltration, displaying a "mosaic pattern." Because of its morphologic similarity to seminoma or dysgerminoma, the terms germinoma (Friedman (12) and later Russell and Rubinstein (42–44)) and atypical teratoma (Russell and Rubinstein (44)) have now received wide acceptance.

In principle, the term pinealoma should be restricted to the tumors that arise from the parenchyma cells of the pineal gland. However, various different conceptions of the term used by different authors created chaos. Once PTC is excluded from the category of pineal gland tumors, a true neoplasm of the pineal gland becomes a curiosity.

For reevaluation of the histogenesis of PTC (tumors with mosaic pattern), 48 surgical specimens, a number sufficient for the present study, were selected and carefully reviewed by both light and electron microscopic examinations.

Of the total 48 cases of PTC, 28 cases were located in the pineal body, 11 were in the suprasellar-hypothalamic area, and the remaining 9 were in other sites (Table 3.4). They consisted of 41 males and 7 females, indicating marked preponderance of males over females. Thirty-three patients were younger than 20 years old and 15 patients were 20 years old and older.

The pineal organ of lower vertebrates functions as a photoreceptor that transduces an exteroceptive input (light) into neural signals. In birds, the pineal is not a true photoreceptor, but as a response to light, it changes the rate of synthesis of hormonal products like melatonin (photoendocrine transducer). In mammals the pineal gland is an *endocrine organ* with some of the properties of a "neuroendocrine transducer"; one of its major functions is to convert an input of neural signals to a hormonal output, *i.e.*, melatonin and other methoxyindoles and probably polypeptides (7).

In the normal pineal gland, lobules consisting of pineal parenchyma cells are incompletely separated by irregular trabeculae and fibrous septa carrying blood vessels along with them (24). Like all other endocrine organs, the pineal gland has a very rich capillary blood supply (sinusoids). The parenchyma cells closely attach to the sinusoidal sheaths. The intimate proximity of the cells to the sinusoids is regarded as one of the common features of endocrine glands. Thus, it might be expected that true tumors originating from the pineal parenchyma cells would show a close relationship between the tumor cells and the sinusoids as the tumor stroma. That the cell clusters of the pineal parenchyma are not enclosed with connective tissues and that the capillaries are often found in the midst of the cell clusters without accompanying connective tissues was already noticed by Knud Krabbe in his classic thesis (24). In one of Hortega's silver impregnation specimens (19), one can see the pineal parenchyma cells attaching to a capillary with their processes and end bulbs.

The seminiferous tubules constitute the exocrine portion of the testes. There is no direct interrelationship between the tubules and blood vessels from the tunica vasculosa testis (3). Typical microscopic pictures of seminoma reveal regular fibrous supporting stromata containing capillaries and lymphocytes which divide the tumor into lobules. There is no evidence of tumor cells attaching to the capillaries (33, 48).

Based on this new criterion that in a true tumor of the pineal origin, tumor cells should be, as in any endocrine neoplasms, in close proximity to the capillaries (sinusoids) without intervening mesenchymal tissues, histological reevaluation of 48 specimens was performed. Figure 3.1 shows an example of a tumor considered to be the true pineal origin. The characteristics mentioned above can easily be noticed. Besides this fundamental finding, the pattern of lymphocytic infiltration is different between tumors of pineal origin and seminoma. In the former, lymphocytes are mainly seen along the margins of tumor nests or clusters with occasional sparse scattering in tumor cell clusters. In the latter, lymphocytes are seen mainly in fibrous septa with occasional granulomatous reaction, something never noticed in the tumor of pineal origin. In addition, tumor cells in seminoma are somewhat larger than those of pineal origin tumor.

According to the criterion, PTC can be divided into two groups: one corresponds to the true tumor of pineal origin, which may be called *pinealoma*, and the other to the above described seminoma which, according to Friedman (12), may be called *germinoma*.

Figure 3.2 is a typical example of germinoma. Figure 3.3 demonstrates schematically this germinoma and the above-described pinealoma.

In some parts of pinealoma, transition from the main component of

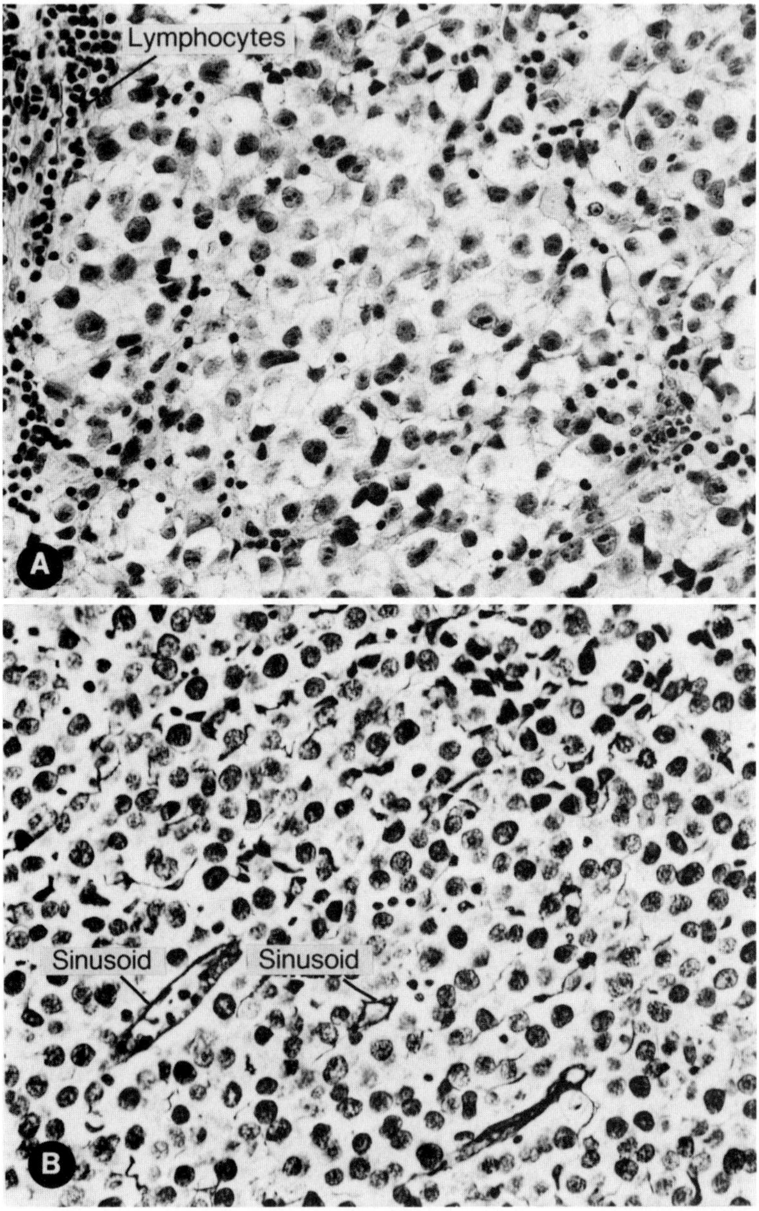

FIG. 3.1. Pinealoma of pineal origin. (*A*) Fairly uniform clear cells are closely packed together. Distinct supporting stromata are not noticed in the medullary tumor nest, which shows a pavement arrangement. In the tumor cell cluster, a few fine blood channels are seen. Lymphocytes mainly aggregate along the margin of the tumor cell cluster. H & E, ×532. (*B*) Silver reticulin impregnation outlines the sinusoidal sheaths. The tumor cells are in close proximity to the sinusoids.

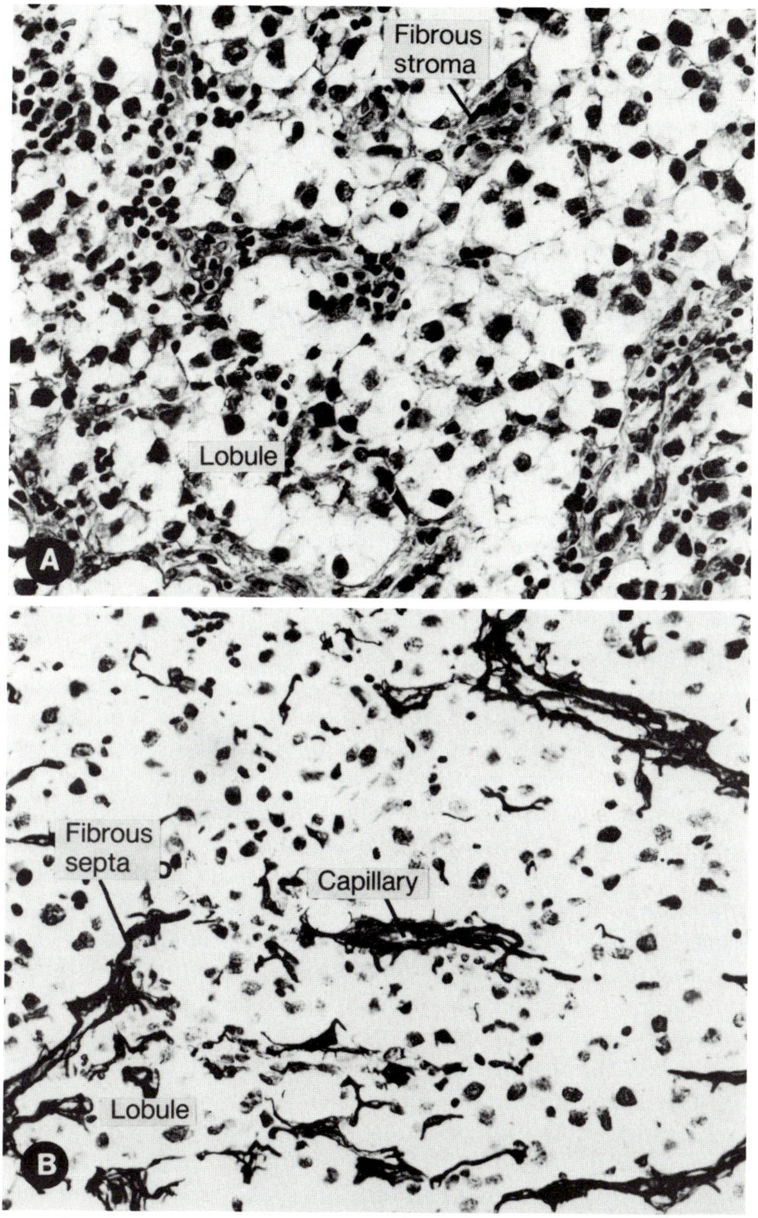

FIG. 3.2. Germinoma (seminoma). (*A*) The fibrocollagenous stromata divide the tumor into lobules, although incompletely. Perivascular lymphocytic infiltration is noticed in the fibrous septa. H & E, ×532. (*B*) Silver reticulin impregnation exhibits sparse fine fibers within the tumor cell cluster. Note that there is no direct relationship between the tumor cells and the blood vessels.

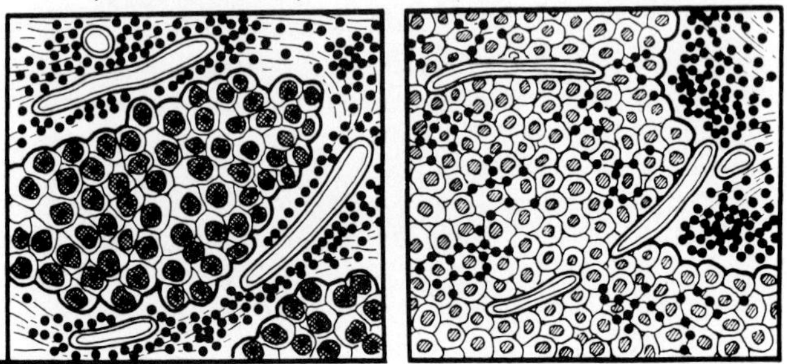

	Seminoma (Germinoma)	Pinealoma
Tumor architecture	Lobular pattern	Medullary growth
Tumor stroma	Fibrous septa	Sinusoid (Capillary)
Lymphocytic infiltration	intra-septal	mainly marginal tumor nests

FIG. 3.3. Differences between pinealoma and germinoma (seminoma).

large ovoid cell with a central vesiculated nucleus to rather smaller cells with an eccentric dark staining nucleus and eosinophilic cytoplasm is frequently observed, as shown in Figure 3.4.

The cytologic features of these smaller cells are just compatible with those of pineocytoma postulated by Russell and Rubinstein (15, 42, 44). Therefore, the available evidence strongly favors Russell's pineocytoma to be regarded as a mature type of pinealoma here described.

Ultrastructural observations of this pinealoma (30, 31) also support the concept of its endocrine properties. The cytoplasmic process of the tumor cell extends into the perivascular interstices, and the tumor cell remains closely adjacent to the fenestrated pores of the endothelium. The tumor cell extensively has smooth-surfaced endoplasmic reticula in the tubular and vesicular forms of cisternae, which may represent their secretive phase. Also, microtubules, as one of the characteristics of pineal cells, are noticed in the cytoplasm of the tumor cell (Fig. 3.5).

According to the recent study of Yamamoto (58), in 4 cases of pinealoma in the pineal region, cellular melatonin was measured using a spotting irradiated helium neon laser beam (633 nm). The diameter of the beam was 10^{-3} cm and its power (output) was either 1, 7, or 25 mWatts. All cases examined showed fluorescence in the range of 633 + (40 ± 25) nm, which corresponds to melatonin. Astrocytoma cells and fibroblast cells did not show such fluorescence.

According to the formulated criterion, 24 of the 48 cases could be attributed to the category of pinealoma (Table 3.4). In these 24 cases

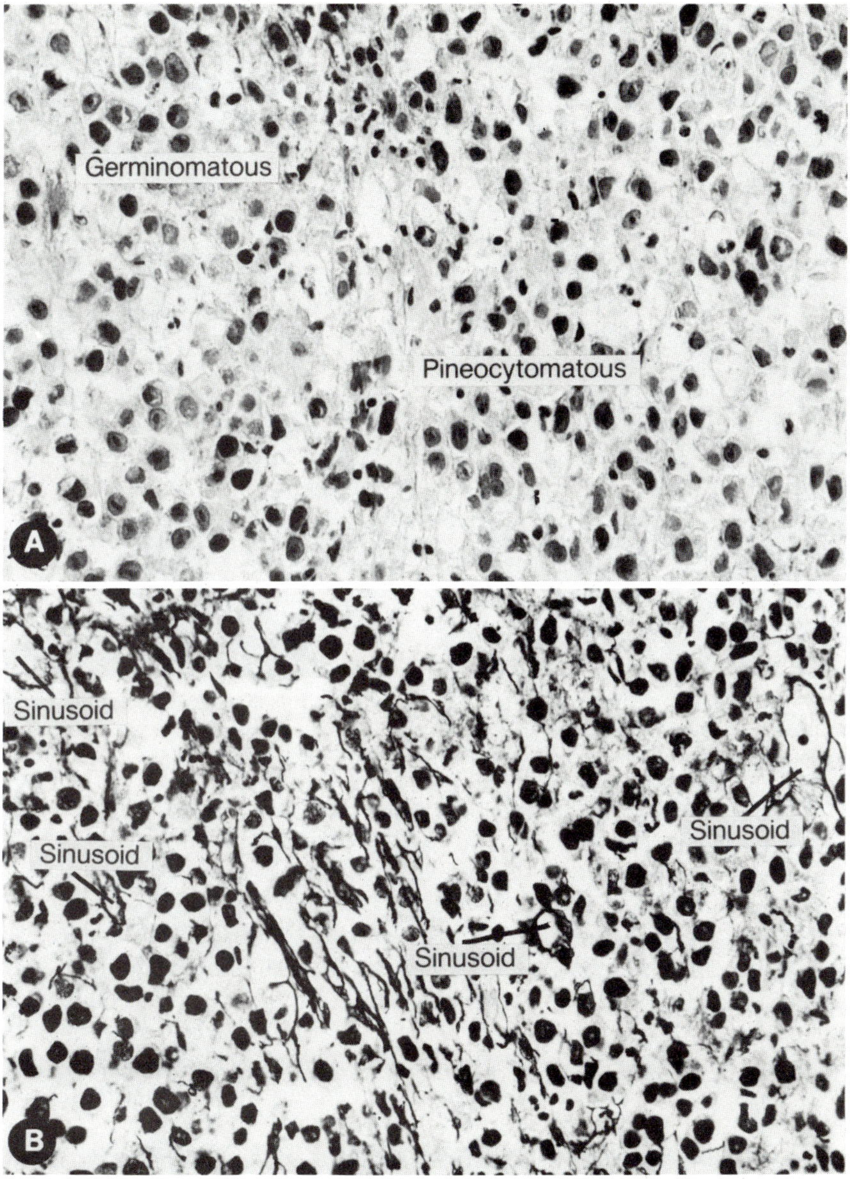

FIG. 3.4. Pinealoma. Transition from a large cell to a smaller cell of pineocytoma. (*A*) The photograph shows transition from germinomatous pinealoma (*upper left*) to pineocytomatous elements (*lower right*). The latter area is composed of carrot-shaped cells with darkly stained spheroid nuclei, which eccentrically locate in the pale eosinophilic cytoplasms. H & E, ×532. (*B*) With a silver impregnation the sinusoids are well discernible in both areas, suggesting that pineocytomatous differentiation is retained in pinealoma.

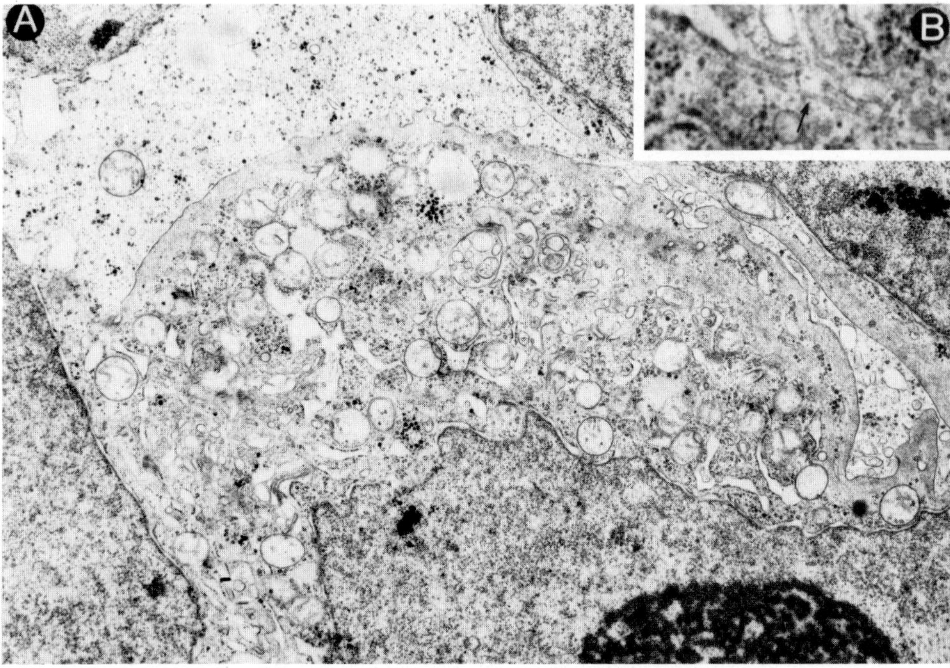

FIG. 3.5. Electron micrograph of a pinealoma. (*A*) The tumor cell extensively has smooth surfaced endoplasmic reticula in the tubular and vesicular forms of cisternae. ×27,000. (*B*) Microtubules (*arrow*) are seen in the cytoplasm of the tumor cell. ×45,000.

with pineloma, 19 were found in the pineal region, 2 in the suprasellar-hypothalamic area, and 3 in other sites. The sites of the other 24 cases with germinoma included the pineal region in 9 cases, the suprasellar-hypothalamic area in 9, and the other sites in 6. Of tumors involving the pineal region, pinealoma accounted for two-thirds of the 28 cases (19 cases); in contrast, 80% of suprasellar-hypothalamic neoplasms were germinoma (Table 3.4). In both pinealoma and germinoma, males were predominant (83–88%). However, 2 pinealoma cases in the suprasellar region and 3 of 9 germinoma cases in the suprasellar region were females. Therefore, in pinealoma and germinoma in the suprasellar region, the male predominance was not marked.

The results found in earlier ultrastructural studies (53) supporting the close resemblances between pineal tumors with mosaic pattern and testicular seminomas may be because those specimens had been mostly obtained from suprasellar-hypothalamic tumors.

Riverson and Zülch (40) maintained that germinoma and pineal parenchymatous tumors can be differentiated by de Girolami stain and PAS stain. This, however, was not confirmed by the author's hands.

Problems of Nomenclature

The term "pinealoma" was introduced by Krabbe in 1923 (25) in a very casual way as "an adenoma, or more exactly, 'pinealoma'" and was adopted by Horrax and Bailey (16, 17) and has since been generally used. It is held to signify a tumor of the pineal parenchyma cells. The tumor is composed essentially of masses of large spherical epithelial cells separated by a reticular connective tissue containing lymphoid cells. Because of these two types of cells, the tumor is often called the two-cell-pattern type pinealoma. Both Bailey (2, 16, 17) and Zülch (61) regarded these epithelial cells as originating from the parenchyma cells of the pineal body. However, the resemblance among this tumor, seminoma of the testis, and dysgerminoma of the ovary has often been pointed out and was emphasized by Friedman (12), who proposed the term "germinoma" for this type of pineal tumor. Russell and Rubinstein (42–44) were of the same opinion and called this tumor "atypical teratoma" or "germinoma."

There are, less frequently, tumors composed of a homogeneous mass of smaller epithelial cells without lymphoid cells. Horrax and Bailey (2, 16, 17) called this tumor "pinealoma of spongioblastic type" or 'pineoblastoma." Russell and Rubinstein (44) regarded this type of tumor as the true pinealoma of pineal parenchyma origin and divided it into "pineocytoma" and malignant "pineoblastoma" (44). Zülch named these two "isomorphic pinealoma" and "medulloblastoma of the pineal," respectively, and called the two-cell-pattern type tumor "anisomorphic pinealoma" (61). These nomenclatures are tabulated in Table 3.5.

Cushing (10) caused another confusion by stating that "from a surgical standpoint it seems better therefore to let the term 'pinealoma' for the time being represent an anatomical place-name rather than to have it connote any particular type of tumour." Pinealoma, however, should be applied to the specific type of tumor of pineal parenchyma origin with the mosaic pattern above mentioned, and germinoma should be applied to seminoma.

TABLE 3.5
Nomenclature of PTC and Teratoid Tumors

Bailey	Zülch	Russell (and Rubinstein)	
Teratoma and Teratoid	Teratoma and teratoid	(Typical) teratoma and teratoid	
Pinealoma (25)	Anisomorphic pinealoma	Atypical Teratoma (*Germinoma* (12))	
Spongioblastic type of pinealoma or pineoblastoma	{ Isomorphic pinealoma	Pineocytoma	} Pinealomas
	Medulloblastoma of the pineal	Pineoblastoma	

AGE DISTRIBUTION OF CASES WITH PINEALOMA AND GERMINOMA

Figures 3.6 and 3.7 show age distribution of pinealoma and germinoma. The age of predilection of patients with pinealoma involving the pineal region ranged from 12 to 20 years, with the average age 16.4 ± 4.8. Suprasellar-hypothalamic germinomas mostly appeared between the ages of 8 and 12, with the mean age 10.4 ± 2.5—a little bit younger than the age of patients with pinealoma. However, germinomas of the pineal region did not show such a predilection for younger ages. The average age of pineoblastoma cases was 13.8 ± 10.9 (15), *i.e.*, younger than that of pinealoma cases. According to Herrick and Rubinstein (15), the average age of pineocytoma cases was 42.6 ± 20.6. As for age, therefore, pinealoma is found in patients between those with immature pineoblastoma and those with mature pineocytoma. Neoplasms of endocrine organs usually appear after endocrine functions develop to some extent, so the average age of 16 years for pinealoma seems compatible with this. As for the sex distribution, pinealoma, pineoblastoma, and probably pineocytoma, as well as germinoma, showed a male predominance (Tables 3.2–3.4).

INTRACRANIAL GERM CELL TUMORS

Table 3.6 shows cases of the so-called intracranial germ cell tumors experienced in the author's clinic. All these tumors were located in the

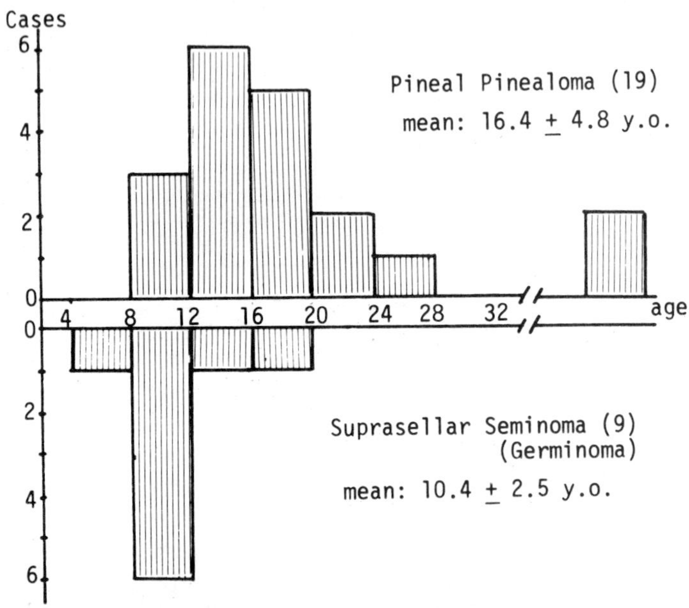

FIG. 3.6. Age distribution of pineal pinealoma and suprasellar germinoma. Two pinealoma cases on the extreme right were males, 34 and 43 years old.

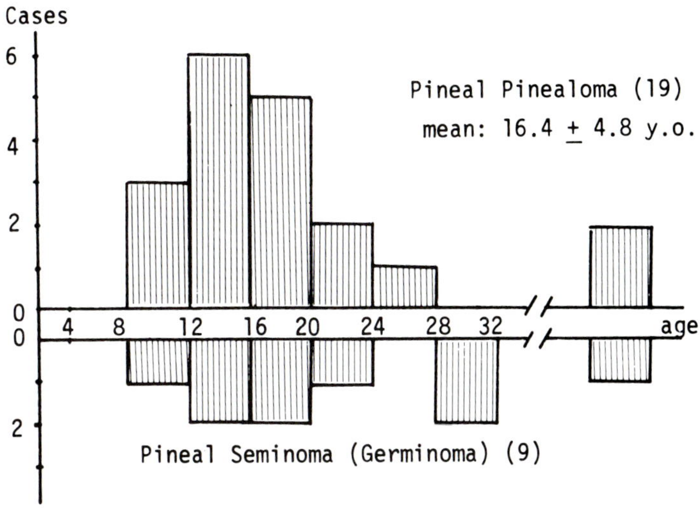

FIG. 3.7. Age distribution of pineal pinealoma and pineal germinoma. One germinoma case on the extreme right was a 34-year-old male.

TABLE 3.6
Intracranial Germ Cell Tumors

	No. of Cases	Under 20 yr old		20 yr and older	
		M	F	M	F
Teratoma	16	15	0	1	0
Teratocarcinoma	2	2	0	0	0
Germinoma (seminoma)	24	13	3	8	0
Endodermal sinus tumor	0	0	0	0	0
Embryonal carcinoma	1	1	0	0	0
Choriocarcinoma	1	1	0	0	0
Unclassified	2	2	0	0	0
Mixed germ cell tumors	25	18	3	4	0
Total	71	52	6	13	0

area of the third ventricle, including the pineal and suprasellar regions. Germinoma is included in this list; pinealoma, however, is excluded. All mature teratoma cases (16 cases), one of 2 teratocarcinoma cases, 18 of 25 mixed germ cell tumor cases, and 2 cases of unclassified germ cell tumor were located in the pineal region (see Table 3.2). Table 3.7 shows histological components of the mixed germ cell tumors above described. As seen in Table 3.7, two or three components can be noted.

Among 71 cases of germ cell tumors, 58 (81.6%) were under 20 years of age, and 13 (18.4%) were 20 years or older. There were 65 (91.5%) males and only 6 (8.5%) females (Table 3.6). This age and sex distribution of intracranial germ cell tumors is essentially similar to that of germ cell tumors of other organs.

TABLE 3.7

Histological Components of Mixed Germ Cell Tumors (25 Cases)

Tumor Type	No. of Cases
Germinoma (seminoma) + teratoma[a]	6
Germinoma + teratoma + embryonal carcinoma	1
Germinoma + teratoma + choriocarcinoma	1
Germinoma + endodermal sinus tumor	3
Germinoma + choriocarcinoma	1
Germimoma + ?	2
Endodermal sinus tumor + teratoma	5
Choriocarcinoma + teratocarcinoma	2
Choriocarcinoma + ?	2
Embryonal carcinoma + teratoma	2

[a] Including 1 case of teratocarcinoma.

Surgical Approaches and Techniques for Pineal Region Tumors

There have been several approaches proposed and tried for pineal region tumors (39, 59): I—the parietal transcallosal approch of Dandy (11), Kunicki (27), Suzuki and Iwabuchi (52), and others; II—the occipital or parietooccipital transtentorial approach: Brunner (5), Pratt and Brooks (37), Heppner (14), Poppen and Marino (36), Kempe (23), Glasauer (13), Jamieson (20), Lazar and Clark (29), Sano and Matsutani (47), Lapras (28), and others. III—the infratentorial supracerebellar approach: Horsley (18), Rorschach (41), Krause (26, 34), Zapletal (60), Stein (50), Pendl (35), Sano (47), and others; IV—the posterior transventricular approach: van Wagenen (55). V—the frontal or anterior transcallosal approach.

As previously reported (45–47), the author has been performing direct surgery on teratoid tumors and on pinealoma or germinoma in the pineal region. In case of pinealoma or germinoma, postoperative irradiation always followed.

For the occipital transtentorial approach to a pineal tumor, the author prefers the incision (usually on the nondominant side) illustrated in Figure 3.8. The midline portion of the incision can be elongated to the suboccipital region if it is necessary to open the posterior fossa.

Craniotomy is close to the superior sagittal sinus and the transverse sinus. The patient is either in the prone position or the lounging position, as seen in Figure 3.8. The occipital lobe is punctured through the dura, and a silicone rubber tube is inserted into the posterior portion of the lateral ventricle and secured to the dura. The tube drains the cerebrospinal fluid during the operation and makes lateral retraction of the occipital lobe easier. The tentorium is split close to the sinus rectus, and the superior surface of the cerebellum is exposed. The operating microscope

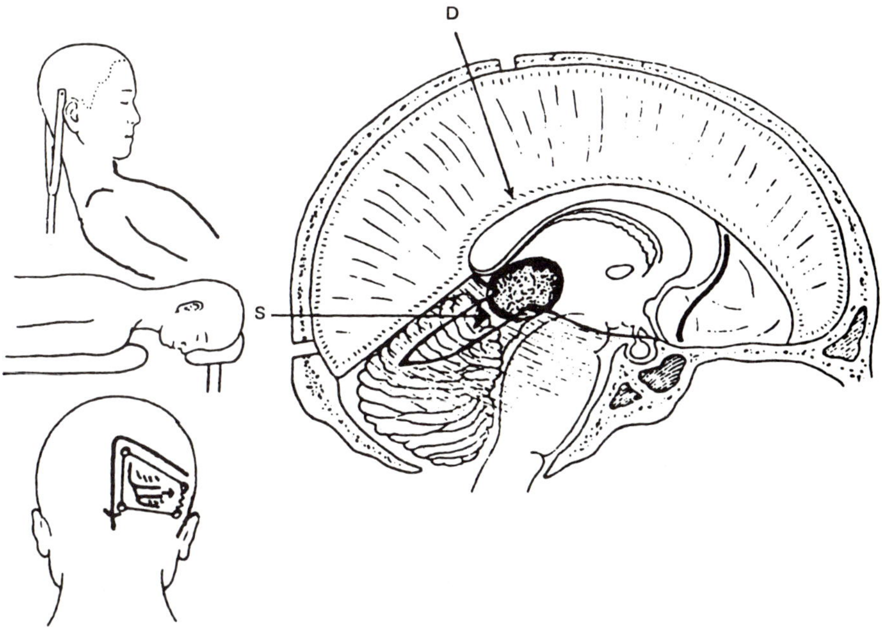

FIG. 3.8. Occipital transtentorial approach.

is used from this stage. A pineal tumor is often visible rostral to the vermis, underneath the vein of Galen (Fig. 3.9). If the tumor is located further rostrally, the splenium of the corpus callosum is split by suction to expose the tela chorioidea of the third ventricle. If the tumor is large, it is often already breaking through the tela chorioidea; if not, the tela is incised in the midline or is close to the nondominant occipital lobe after cauterization with a bipolar coagulator.

Therefore, this approach enables the operator to use the low (parieto) occipital (as proposed by Poppen and Marino (36) and others) approach and, if necessary, the high parietooccipital (as proposed by Dandy (11) and others) approach as well.

If the tumor is a pinealoma or a germinoma (a germinoma is usually a little bit tougher), the tumor is removed piecemeal (Fig. 3.10). If the tumor is a teratoma, removal en bloc will often be feasible. After removal of the tumor, the other end of the silicone rubber tube (which has been inserted into the lateral ventricle) is brought into the lateral cistern or the pontine cistern in order to secure the cerebrospinal fluid pathway. This is done because the rostral portion of the aqueduct is often compressed by the tumor, and even after removal of the tumor the effect of the compression may remain for a certain period.

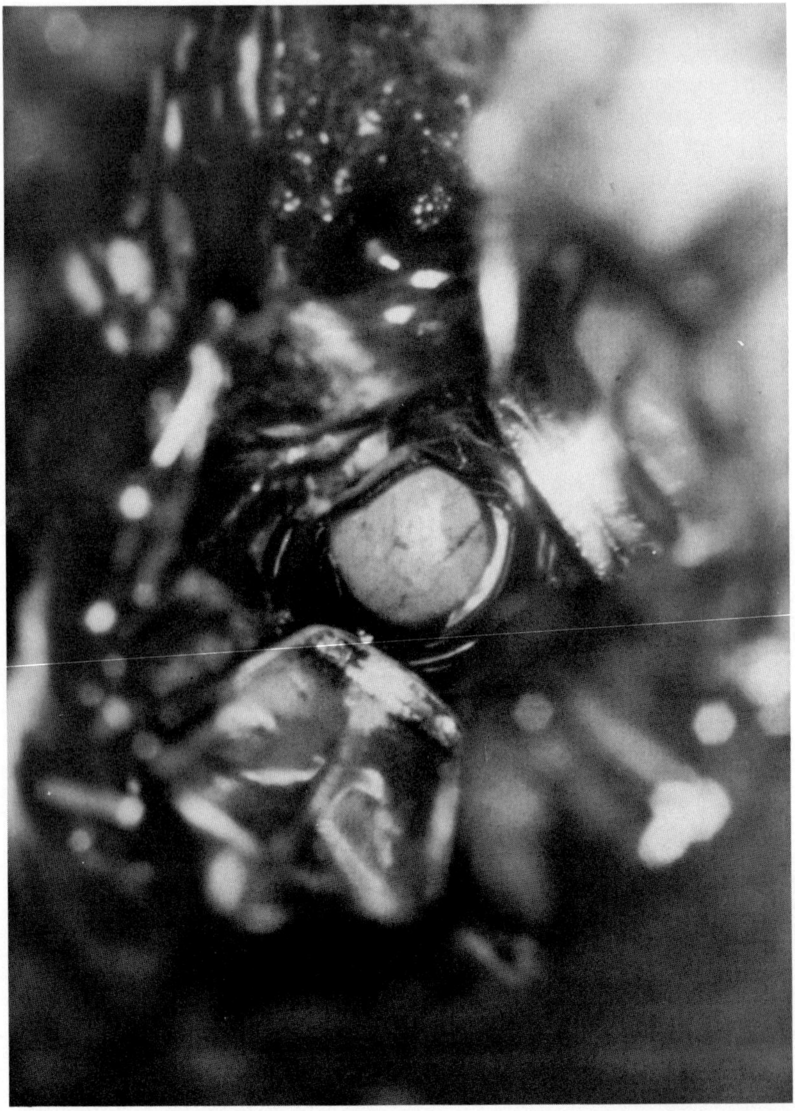

FIG. 3.9. A 19-year-old female. Occipital transtentorial approach. A tumor is seen rostral to the vermis, underneath the vein of Galen.

The infratentorial supracerebellar approach, as tried by Krause (26, 34) and revived by Zapletal (60) and Stein (50) through a midline suboccipital incision, is utilized when the pineal tumor is not too large. The superior surface of the cerebellum is pressed down after electrocauterizing and severing the bridging veins between the cerebellum and the

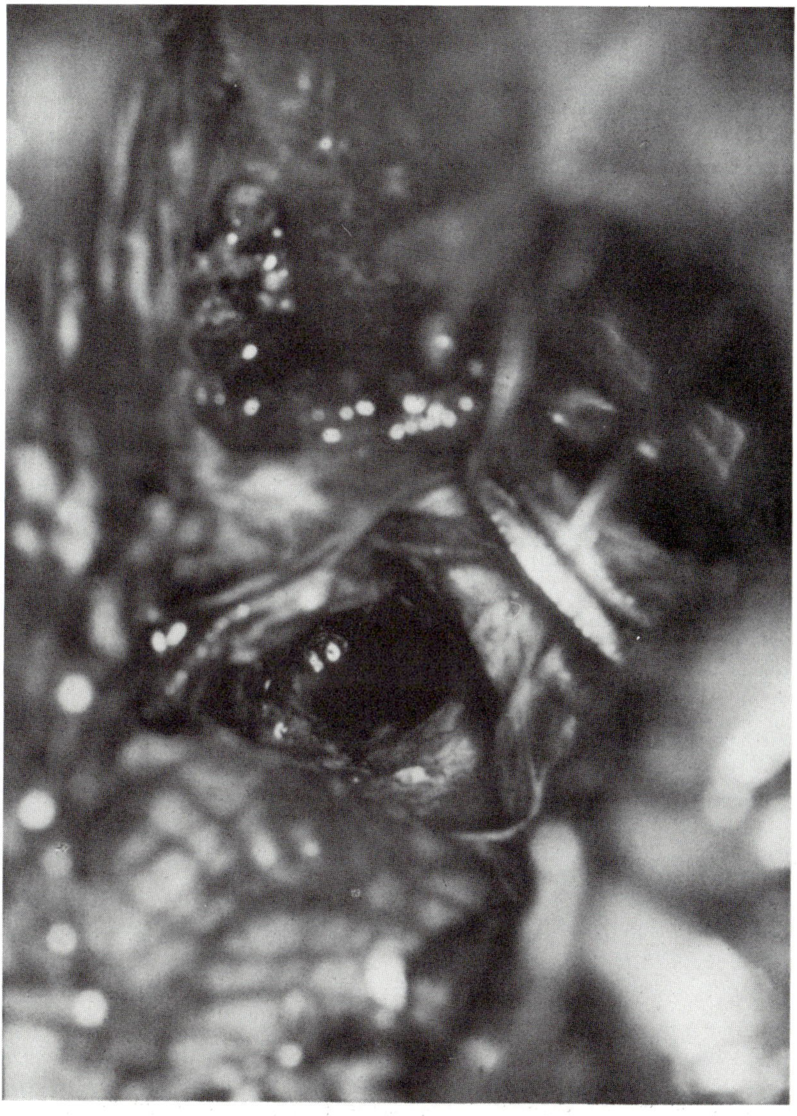

FIG. 3.10. The tumor is removed *in toto*. Histology: pinealoma.

tentorium (Fig. 3.11). The tumor can be seen beneath the vein of Galen and between the basal veins of Rosenthal. The precentral cerebellar vein and the superior vermian vein are identified and severed. The tumor is usually removed piecemeal. Figure 3.12 shows computed tomography (CT) of a 7-year-old boy with a rather small tumor in the pineal region which was removed by this approach. Figure 3.13 is a postoperative CT

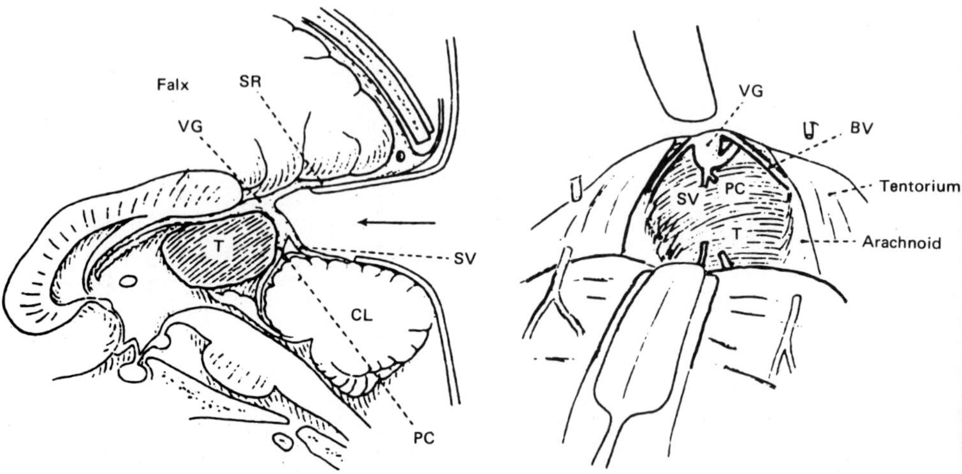

FIG. 3.11. Infratentorial supracerebellar approach. *SR*, sinus rectus; *VG*, vein of Galen; *T*, tumor; *SV*, superior vermian vein; *BV*, basal veins; *PC*, precentral cerebellar vein; *CL*, cerebellum.

scan (1 week after the operation). The tumor is totally removed. This tumor turned out to be a teratocarcinoma. The patient is well and going to school a little more than 2 years postoperatively.

The author has experienced no operative mortality either by the occipital or by the infratentorial approach. Steroid is administered before, during, and after the operation.

Postoperative irradiation for pinealoma or germinoma was done with Co-60 or LINAC, with the total dose 5000–6000 rad (the daily dose, 100–200 rad). The field of irradiation was 6 × 6 cm to 8 × 8 cm, centering either on the pineal region or on the suprasellar region. In recent cases, whole brain irradiation and spinal cord irradiation were added, but even in these cases the total dose did not exceed 5000–6000 rad.

In 1980, the author experienced 2 cases (boys 4 and 7 years old, respectively) of huge malignant pineal teratoma with an endodermal sinus tumor element which showed increased serum alpha-fetoprotein. The author thought that these were both too large to attack either by the occipital transtentorial approach or by the infratentorial supracerebellar approach. He decided to remove the tumors en bloc by a frontal transcallosal approach. Frontal craniotomy was fashioned, as shown in Figure 3.14*A* and *B*. The corpus callosum was longitudinally split, about 4 cm in length, at its junction with the nondominant cingulate gyrus. The tumor was easily identified and gently detached from the surrounding tissues under the microscope, and then was removed en bloc (Figs.

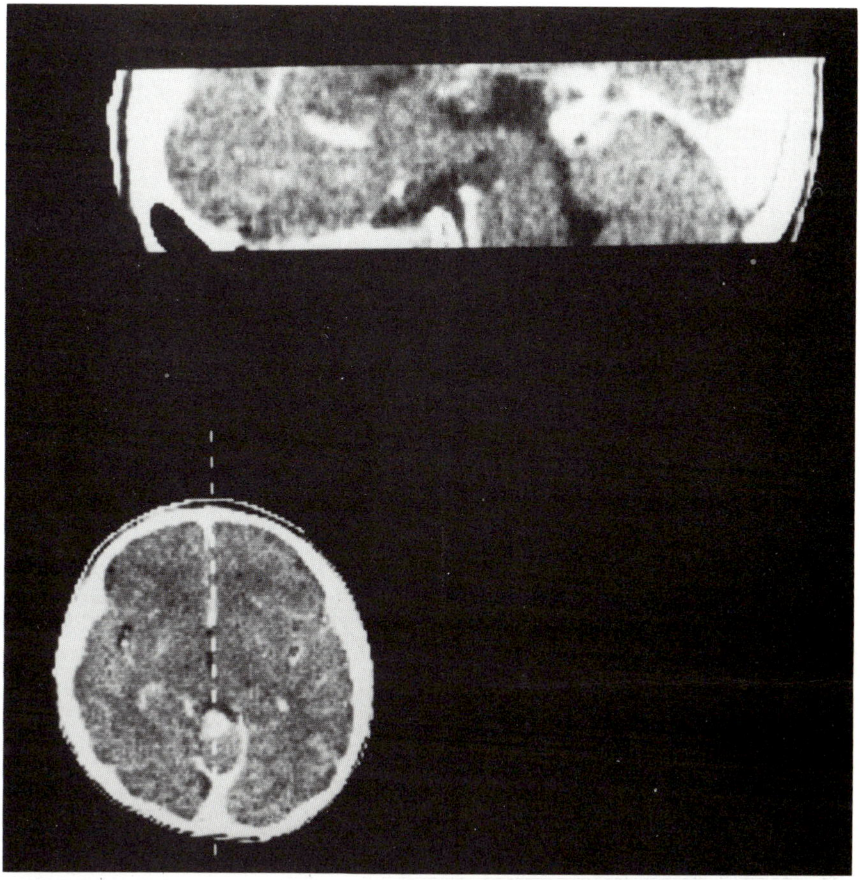

FIG. 3.12. A 7-year-old boy with a rather small teratocarcinoma in the pineal region.

3.15–3.17). The tumors were 4.5 cm and 5 cm in diameter. After the operation, a marked decrease of alpha-fetoprotein was noted. The postoperative course was uneventful, and the patients returned to school. The 4-year-old boy is still healthy 2 years postoperatively. The 7-year-old boy, however, later developed metastases diffusely in the body and died 1½ years later.

Among various approaches to the pineal region, the author prefers the occipital transtentorial approach or the infratentorial supracerebellar approach if the tumor is located posterior to the adhesio interthalamica. If the tumor is too large and reaches anterior to the adhesio interthalamica, the transcallosal, especially the frontal transcallosal, approach may be recommended.

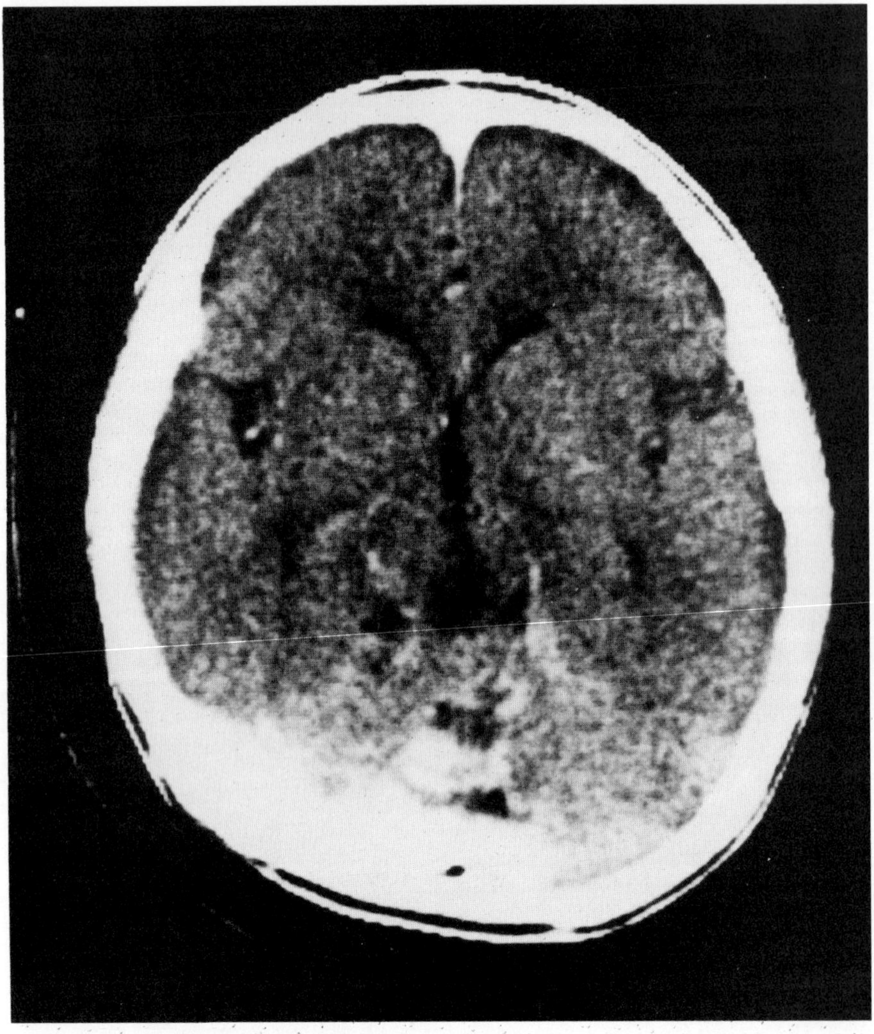

FIG. 3.13. Postoperative CT (1 week after the operation). No tumor can be noticed. A small amount of blood clot is seen on the cerebellum.

Follow-up Results

The survival rates (calculated by the Kaplan-Meyer method (22)) of pinealoma and germinoma cases treated by direct surgery and postoperative irradiation are tabulated in Table 3.8. This table includes not only 32 cases of tumor involving the pineal region but also 13 cases of tumor in the suprasellar region and 9 cases of tumor in other locations.

There was no operative mortality. The 1-year survival rate (1 YSR),

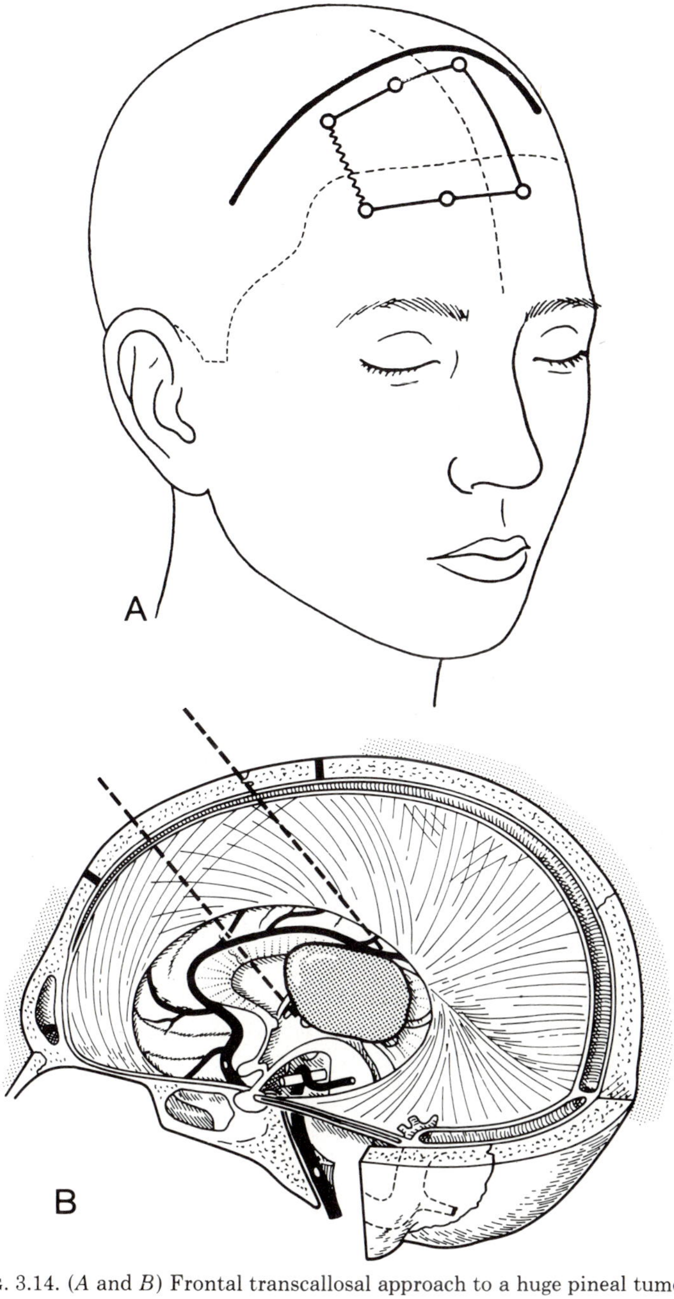

FIG. 3.14. (*A* and *B*) Frontal transcallosal approach to a huge pineal tumor.

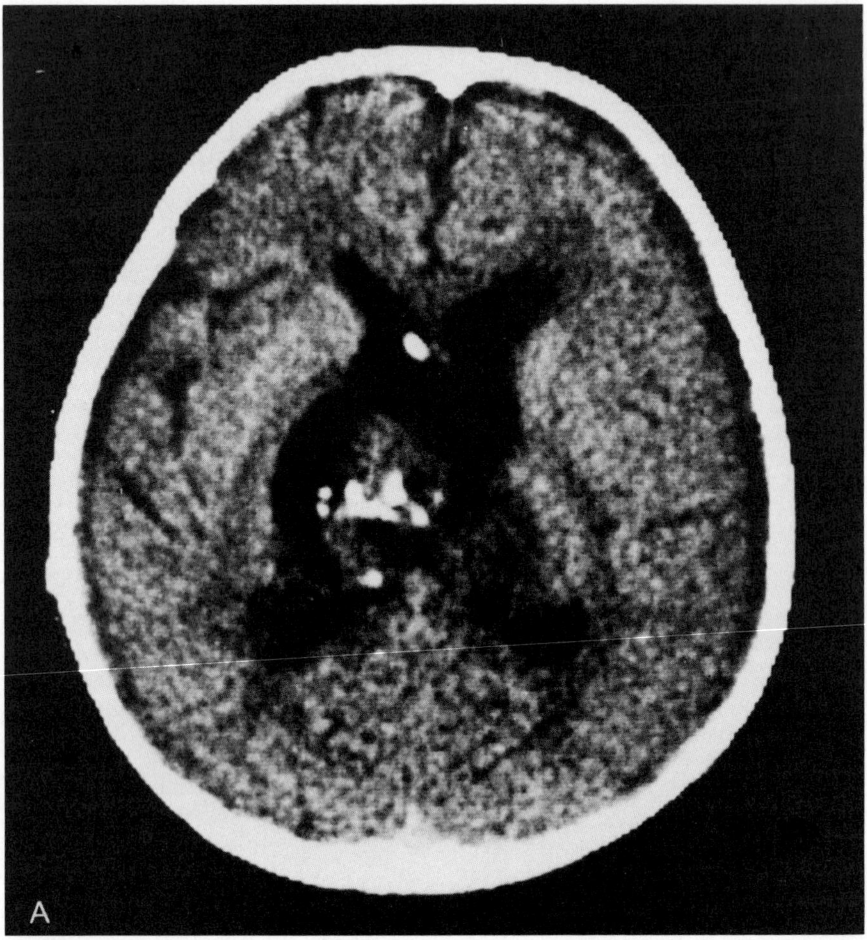

FIG. 3.15. (*A*) A 4-year-old boy. Plain CT.

the 3-year survival rate (3 YSR), the 5-year survival rate (5 YSR), and the 10-year survival rate (10 YSR) were 98.1%, 83.8%, 83.8%, and 78.9%, respectively. Cases under 20 years of age showed better results than those 20 years old or older, with the 10 YSR at 82.7% in the former and 72.4% in the latter group. Suprasellar pinealoma (or germinoma) cases showed better results than pineal pinealoma (or germinoma) cases, with the 10 YSR 100% in the former and 74.9% in the latter. In pineal pinealoma (or germinoma), cases younger than 20 years old showed better results than cases 20 years old or older, with the 10 YSR at 78.3% in the former and 71.4% in the latter.

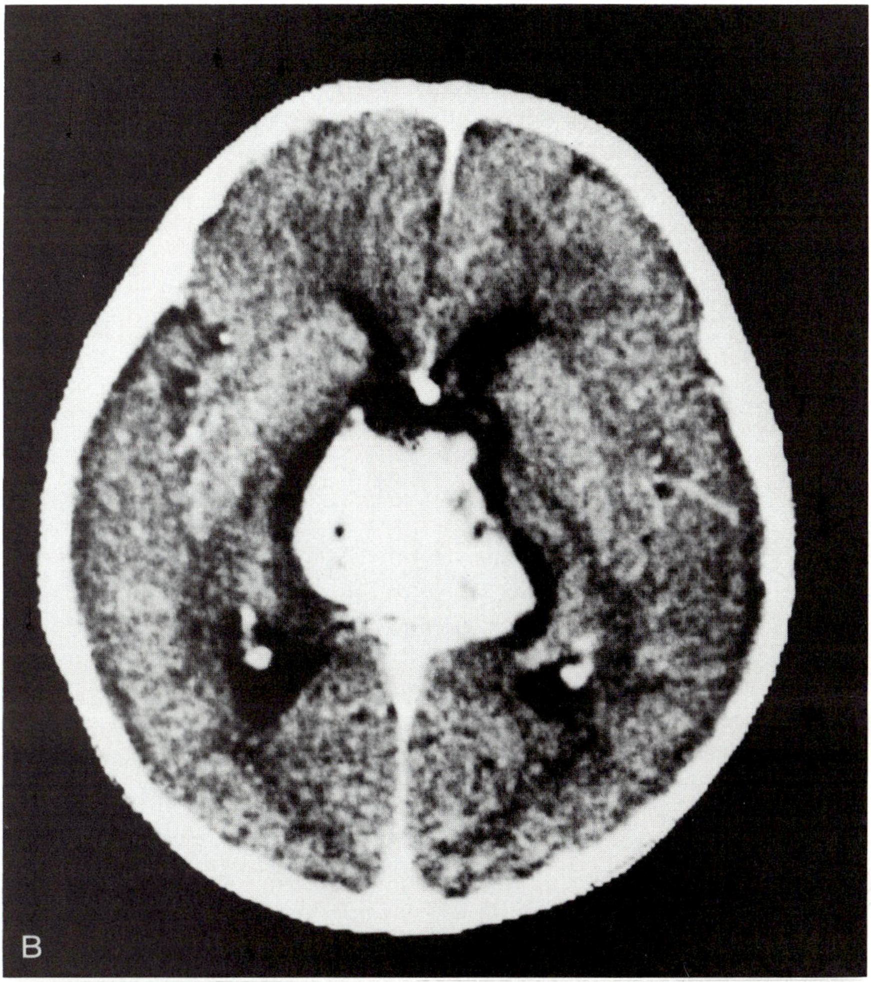

FIG. 3.15. (*B*) The same case. Contrast enhancement. A huge tumor in the pineal region occupying the third ventricle.

When survival rates of cases with germinoma and pinealoma were separately compared, germinoma cases showed slightly better results than pinealoma cases (Fig. 3.18 and *lowermost values* of Table 3.8), namely, 10-year survival rates were 85.6% in the former and 66.9% in the latter (4 cases of pinealoma and 2 cases of germinoma could not be followed up.). These results may reflect the fact that germinoma was mostly found in the suprasellar region and pinealoma mostly in the pineal region.

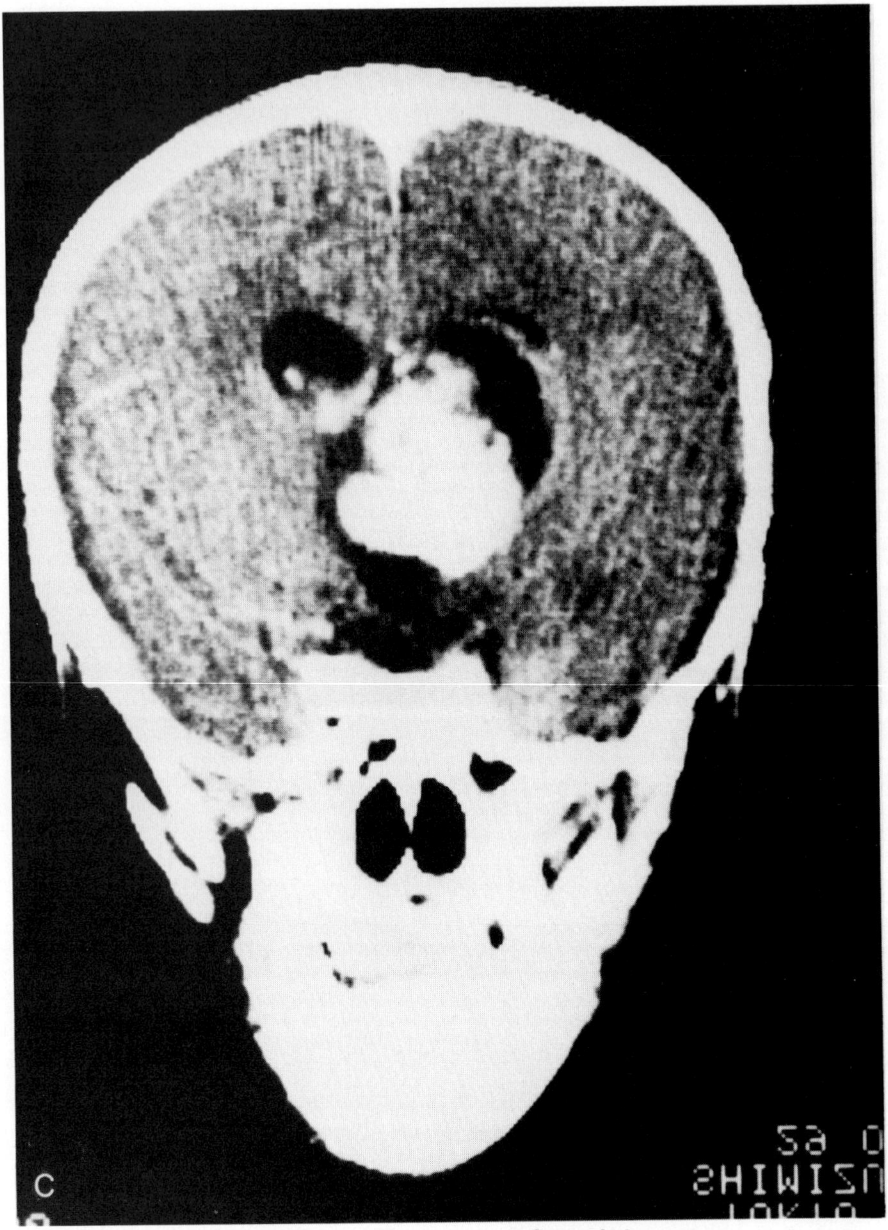

FIG. 3.15. (*C*) The same case. Coronal view.

Among these 54 cases of pinealoma and germinoma, 42 cases are alive at present, and 12 cases are dead. Of those 42 cases, 36 of them could be followed up to ascertain their present functional status. The results are listed in Table 3.9. Of those 36 cases, 80.7% were well and working or

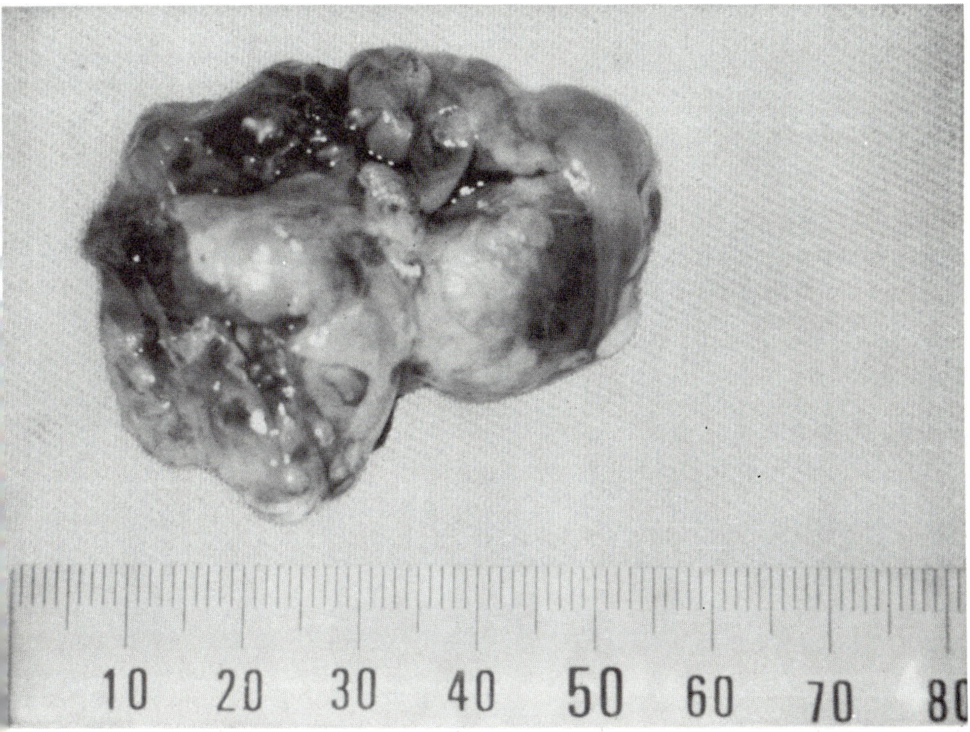

FIG. 3.16. The same case. The tumor is removed *in toto*. A teratoma with an endodermal sinus tumor element.

going to school, and 8.3% were not working but were able to care for themselves without help. Some (2.7%) were bedridden. Of the suprasellar germinoma cases, 25% were well but were unable to work because of visual disturbance. This visual disturbance seems closely related to the preoperative status of visual acuity.

If a patient with suprasellar germinoma had visual acuity of 0.2 or less, the patient never regained his useful vision. If he had visual acuity of 0.4 or more, he regained his useful vision (*e.g.*, to 0.8–1.0). The borderline of the preoperative visual acuity was 0.3, namely, the patient with this vision either regained or lost his useful vision after the treatment. (Note: 1.0 correspond to 20/20 and 0.1 to 20/200.)

The causes of death in the above-mentioned 12 cases are shown in Table 3.10. It should be noted that 2 cases, namely, 3.7% of 54 cases, died of dissemination metastases in the cerebrospinal fluid space and 1 case, namely, 1.9%, died of recurrence of the neoplasm.

These results are better than the results of radiotherapy without direct surgery. Patients harboring mixed germ cell tumors are usually of poor prognosis, even if their tumors are totally removed and followed by

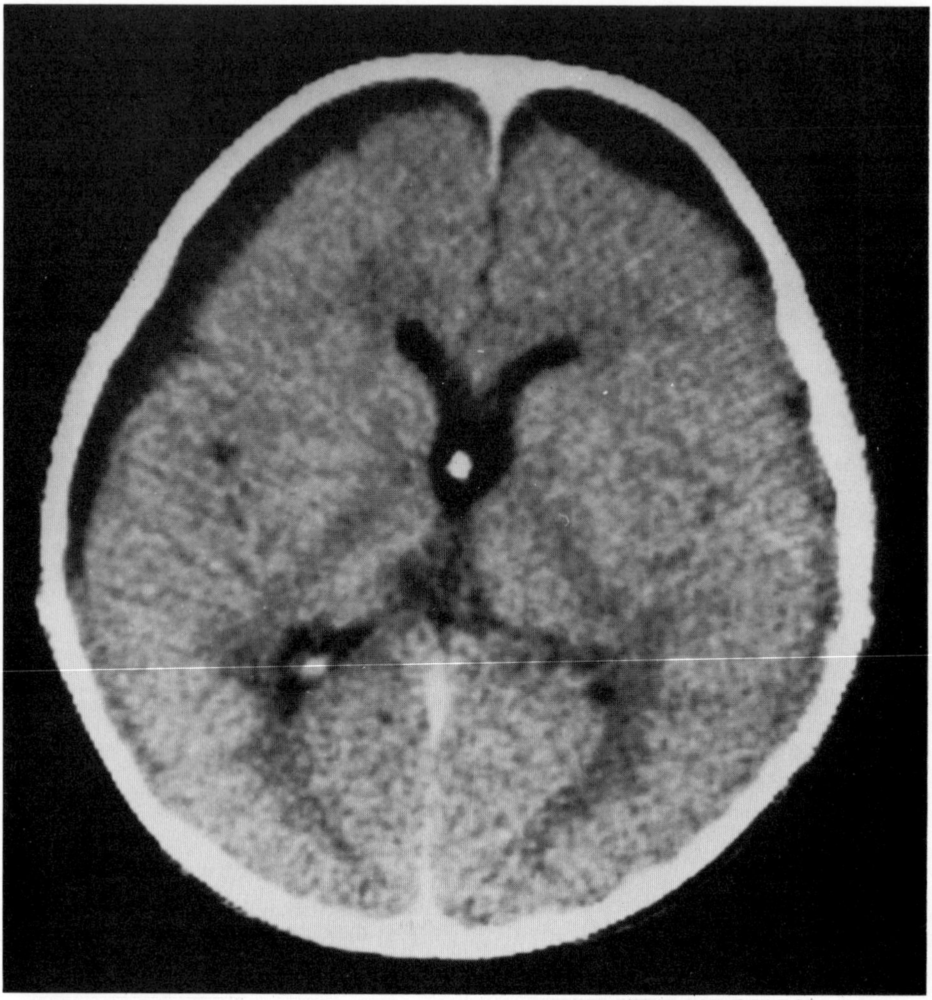

FIG. 3.17. The same case. Ten weeks after the operation. No tumor is seen, even with contrast enhancement.

radiotherapy. Cases of mature teratoma, on the contrary, showed good outcome in the follow-up. Table 3.11 shows survival rates of cases with tumors other than pinealoma and germinoma.

Radiotherapy or Surgery

Both pinealoma and germinoma are radiosensitive. Therefore, radiation alone or radiation plus ventriculoperitoneal shunting are prevailing as the established treatment. The greatest criticism against direct surgery

TABLE 3.8

Survival Rates of Cases with Pinealoma and Germinoma Treated by Direct Surgery and Postoperative Irradiation

Total No. of Cases: 54		1-yr (98.1%)	3-yr (83.8%)	5-yr (83.8%)	10-yr (78.9%)
Location					
Pineal	32	96.9[a]	83.3[a]	79.6[a]	74.9[a]
Suprasellar	13	100	100	100	100
Other	9	100	57.1	57.1	
Age					
All Locations ≥ 20 yr old	19	94.7	78.0	72.4	72.4
All Locations < 20 yr old	35	100	87.1	87.1	82.7
Pineal ≥ 20 yr old	14	92.9	78.6	71.4	71.4
Pineal < 20 yr old	18	100	87.1	87.1	78.3
Suprasellar ≥ 20 yr old	1	100	100	100	
Suprasellar <20 yr old	12	100	100	100	100
Histologically verified cases					
Pinealoma	20	100	76.5	76.5	66.9
Germinoma	22	95.5	85.6	85.6	85.6

[a] Values are expressed as percentages.

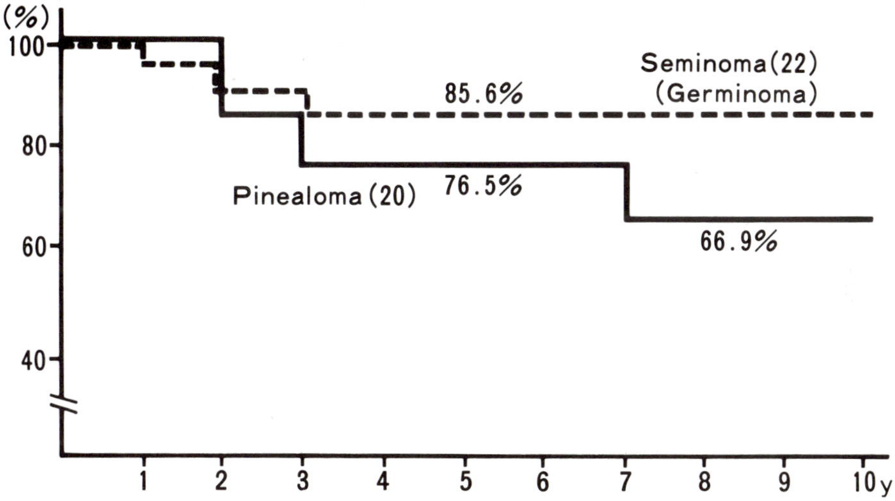

FIG. 3.18. Survival rates of germinoma cases and pinealoma cases treated by direct surgery and postoperative irradiation.

is the anticipated significant operative mortality and the increased probability of dissemination metastases in the cerebrospinal fluid space.

However, there was no operative mortality in the author's series. He believes meticulous surgical maneuvers, especially microsurgical ones, do not carry a significant operative risk. He also believes that reduction of

TABLE 3.9

Functional Status of Patients with PTC (Pinealoma and Germinoma) Treated by Direct Surgery and Postoperative Radiotherapy

	Total: 42	Pineal: 23	Suprasellar: 13	Other regions: 6
Unable to follow-up	6	3	1	2
Able to work or go to school	29/36 (80.7%)	16/20 (80%)	9/12 (75%)	4/4 (100%)
Well, but unable to work because of visual disturbance	3/36 (8.3%)	0	3/12 (25%)	0
Able to care for self	3/36 (8.3%)	3/20 (15%)	0	0
Bedridden	1/36 (2.7%)	1/20 (5%)	0	0

TABLE 3.10

Causes of Death in 12 Cases of PTC (Pinealoma and Germinoma)

Location	Recurrence	CSF Dissemination	Hormonal Insufficiency	Other Disease	Unknown
Pineal (9)	1	1	1	1	5
Suprasellar (0)	0	0	0	0	0
Other sites (3)	0	1	0	1	1
Total	1	2	1	2	6

TABLE 3.11

Follow-up Results of Tumors Other than PTC (Pinealoma and Germinoma)

	Cases	1-yr Survival (%)	3-Yr Survival (%)	5-Yr Survival (%)	10-Yr Survival (%)
Teratoma (mature)	16	93.7	87.1	78.3	78.3
Germ cell tumors other than mature teratoma and germinoma	29	55.2	39.2	33.6	
Epidermoid in the pineal region	2	100.0	100.0	100.0	100.0
Ependymoma in the pineal region	8	63.0	50.0	0	0

the bulk of a neoplasm by direct surgery, even if that neoplasm is radiosensitive, is important for the effectivenss of radiotherapy.

This may be clearly demonstrated if one compares the results of treatments of pineal pinealoma-germinoma with those of suprasellar pinealoma-germinoma, wherein reduction of the bulk of the tumor is easier and more extensive. The 10 YSR of suprasellar pinealoma-germinoma cases was 100%, whereas that of pineal pinealoma-germinoma cases was 74.9% in the author's series.

In the literature, the incidence of dissemination metastases of PTC in the cerebrospinal fluid space ranged from 8% to 20% (47); in the author's series it was 3.7%. Therefore, one cannot say that direct surgery of the tumor will increase the probability of dissemination metastases.

In Japan, the general trend now is first to irradiate the tumor with 2000 rad. If the tumor disappears on the CT scan, radiation therapy is continued; if not, direct surgery is performed, because in that case the tumor is most probably a neoplasm other than pinealoma or germinoma.

However, when a pinealoma or a germinoma is of considerable size, it may recur even if the tumor disappears on the CT scan after radiotherapy. Therefore, the author recommends direct surgery and postoperative radiotherapy for pinealoma-germinoma cases (except for cases with small or multiple tumors).

WHY IS PINEALOMA OR GERMINOMA RADIOSENSITIVE?

In autopsies of pinealoma-germinoma cases treated by irradiation, one will often find the tumor has completely disappeared. This is in contrast with the coagulation necrosis (ischemic necrosis) one usually finds in gliomas treated by irradiation. One cannot, however, come to the conclusion that pinealoma is not of glial origin.

In radiotherapy of cancer of the other parts of the body, neutrophils appear around the 4th day in the necrotic area of the tumor and, furthermore, macrophages and histiocytes join in scavenging of the necrotic area, thus forming granulation in about 4 weeks. In radiotherapy of gliomas, however, such mesenchymal and reticuloendothelial reactions are scarce because of the anatomical specificities of the central nervous system, the radiation-induced necrotic area will remain to be found at autopsy and, furthermore, tumor cells surrounding the necrotic area will become of decreased radiosensitivity because of poor blood supply and lack of oxygen.

In pinealoma or germinoma, on the contrary, mesenchymal and reticuloendothelial reactions, which are represented by lymphocytes or small lymphoid cells, are active and so scavenge radiation-induced necrotic epithelial cells. This phenomenon may partly explain the radiosensitivity of the tumor, and also may explain why the tumor tissue completely disappears after effective radiotherapy.

Both pinealoma and germinoma are small, as compared to gliomas of the cerebrum or the cerebellum. Therefore, from the dose relationship between one neoplastic cell and photons of radiation energy, it is no wonder that the tumor is radiosensitive, especially when as soon as the neoplastic cells die, they are rapidly scavenged.

PRINCIPLES OF TREATMENT OF PINEALOMA AND GERM CELL TUMORS

If a patient is suspected of having pinealoma or any of the germ cell tumors, it is recommended to examine the so-called tumor markers, especially alpha-fetoprotein (AFP) and human chorionic gonadotrophins (HCG) (38). If AFP and HCG are negative, the tumor may be a pinealoma, germinoma, embryonal carcinoma, teratocarcinoma, or mature teratoma. If 2000 rad of local radiation effectively abolishes the tumor on CT, it may be a pinealoma or a germinoma, and radiotherapy should be continued. However, if the size of the tumor is more than 2 cm or, sometimes, more than 1.5 cm in diameter, direct surgery and removal of the tumor, followed by radiation (for pinealoma and germinoma, usually local radiation will be sufficient), should be recommended. Mature teratoma can be cured only by removal of the tumor, and its prognosis is good. Embryonal carcinoma and teratocarcinoma show usually poor prognosis, even after surgical removal and postoperative radiotherapy of the whole neuraxis. Recently, chemotherapeutic agents, such as actinomycin D and *cis*-platinum, have been reported to be worthy of use.

If HCG is positive, the tumor must be choriocarcinoma or a mixed germ cell tumor with choriocarcinomatous elements. If AFP is positive, the tumor must be endodermal sinus tumor or a mixed germ cell tumor with endodermal sinus elements. In both cases, prognosis is rather poor even after surgical removal of the tumor and postoperative radiotherapy of the whole neuraxis. The above-mentioned chemotherapeutic agents are also recommended to be worth while administering.

These principles are schematically illustrated in Figure 3.19.

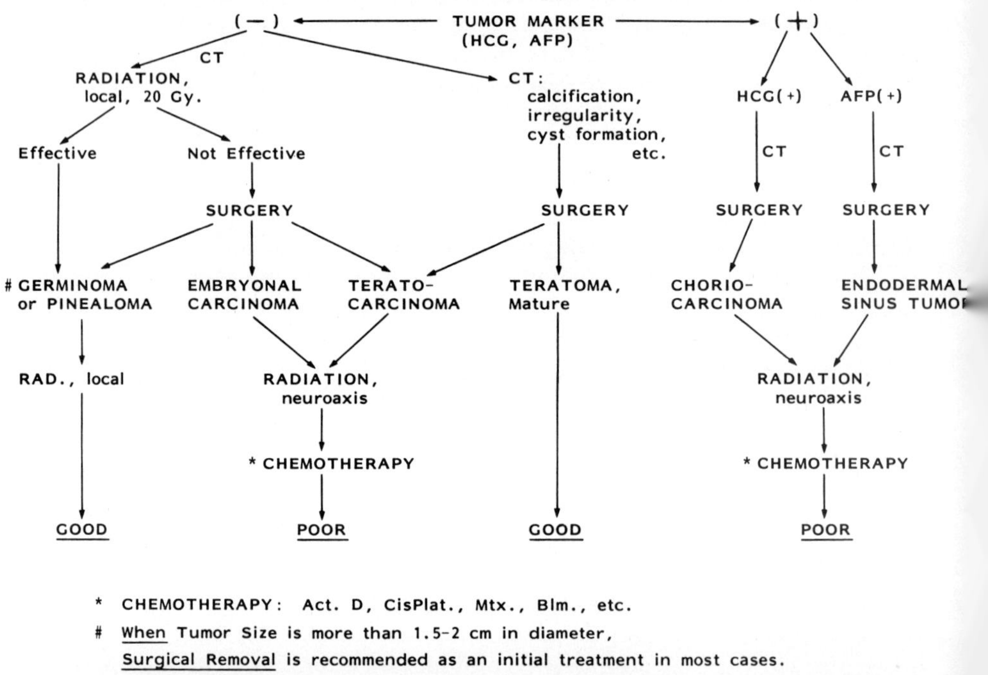

FIG. 3.19. Principles of treatments of germ cell tumors and pinealoma. *Act.D*, actinomycin D; *Cis Plat.*, cis-platinum; *Mtx*, methotrexate; *Blm*, bleomycin.

CONCLUSION

There are various kinds of tumors in the pineal region, even without considering falcotentorial meningiomas. Among them, the so-called two-cell pattern tumor is most frequent. This tumor can be divided, in the author's opinion, into the tumor of pineal parenchyma origin (pinealoma) and the tumor of germ cell origin (germinoma or seminoma). This tumor and germ cell tumors are also found in other areas of the brain; most frequently, however, they are found in the area of the third ventricle. Pinealoma and germ cell tumors are grossly divided into two groups by the tumor markers AFP and HCG. However, exact diagnosis can be made only by surgery and histological examination of the surgical specimens.

As for treatment, mature teratoma should be surgically removed because it is not radiosensitive. Pinealoma and germinoma are radiosensitive; if they are of a considerable size, however, surgical removal and postoperative radiotherapy should be recommended (for these tumors, local radiation may be sufficient in usual cases, since dissemination metastases are not frequent). Embryonal carcinoma, teratocarcinoma, endodermal sinus tumor, or their combinations (mixed germ cell tumors) should be submitted to surgery and postoperative radiation (whole neuraxis) combined with chemotherapy. Except for pinealoma, germinoma, and mature teratoma, which show a good prognosis, other tumors show a rather poor prognosis.

ACKNOWLEDGMENTS

The author is most grateful for the assistance and guidance of Dr. Masao Matsutani (University of Tokyo) and Prof. Terukazu Seto (Teikyo University).

REFERENCES

1. Araki, C., and Matsumoto, S. Statistical re-evaluation of pinealoma and related tumors in Japan. J. Neurosurg., *30:* 146–149, 1969.
2. Bailey, P. *Intracranial Tumors.* Charles C Thomas, Springfield, Ill., 1948.
3. Bloom, W., and Fawcett, D. W. *A Textbook of Histology*, Ed. 10, pp. 805–851. W. B. Saunders, Philadelphia, London, and Toronto, 1975.
4. Bradfield, J. S., and Perez, C. A. Pineal tumors and ectopic pinealomas. Analysis of treatment and failures. Radiology, *103:* 399–406, 1972.
5. Brunner, C. Cited by Rorschach, H., in this chapter.
6. Camins, M. B., and Schlesinger, E. B. Treatment of tumours of the posterior part of the third ventricle and the pineal region: A long-term follow-up. Acta Neurochir., *40:* 131–143, 1978.
7. Cardinali, D. P. Melatonin. A mammalian pineal hormone. Endocrine Rev., *2:* 327–346, 1981.
8. Cheng, M-K. Brain tumors in the People's Republic of China: A statistical review. Neurosurgery, *10:* 16–21, 1982.
9. Committee of Brain Tumor Registry in Japan. Brain Tumor Registry in Japan, Vol. 4, 1982.
10. Cushing, H. *Intracranial Tumors: Note Upon a Series of 2000 Verified Cases with*

Surgical Mortality Pertaining Thereto, pp. 62–65. Charles C Thomas, Springfield, Ill., 1932.

11. Dandy, W. An operation for the removal of pineal tumors. Surg. Gynecol. Obstet., *33:* 113–119, 1921.
12. Friedman, N. B. Germinoma of the pineal. Its identity with germinoma ("seminoma") of the testis. Cancer Res., *7:* 363–368, 1947.
13. Glasauer, F. E. An operative approach to pineal tumors. Acta Neurochir., *22:* 177–180, 1970.
14. Heppner, F. Zur Operationstechnik bei Pinealomen. Zentralblatt. Neurochir., *19:* 219–224, 1959.
15. Herrick, M. K., and Rubinstein, L. J. The cytological differentiating potential of pineal parenchymal neoplasms (true pinealomas): Clinicopathological study of 28 tumours. Brain, *102:* 289–320, 1979.
16. Horrax, G., and Bailey, P. Tumors of the pineal body. Arch. Neurol. Psychiatry, *13:* 423–270, 1925.
17. Horrax, G., and Bailey, P. Pineal pathology. Further studies. Arch. Neurol. Psychiatry, *19:* 394–414, 1928.
18. Horsley, V. Discussion. Proc. R. Soc. Med., *3:* (PT2) 77, 1910.
19. Hortega, Del Rio P. Cited by Horrax and Bailey (16) in this chapter.
20. Jamieson, K. G. Excision of pineal tumors. J. Neurosurg., *35:* 550–553, 1971.
21. Jenkin, R. D. T., Simpson, W. J. K., and Keen, C. W. Pineal and suprasellar germinomas. Results of radiation treatment. J. Neurosurg., *48:* 99–107, 1978.
22. Kaplan, E. L., and Meier, P. Non-parametric estimation for incomplete observations. J. Am. Stat. Assoc., *53:* 457–481, 1958.
23. Kempe, L. G. *Operative Neurosurgery.* Vol. 1. Springer-Verlag, New York, 1968.
24. Krabbe, K. H. Histologische und embryologische Untersuchungen über die Zirbeldrüse des Menschen. Anat. Hefte, *54:* 187–319, 1916.
25. Krabbe, K. H. The pineal gland, especially in relation to the problem of its supposed significance in sexual development. Endocrinology, *7:* 379–414, 1923.
26. Krause, F. Operative Freilegung der Vierhügel Nebst Beobachtungen über Hirndruck und Dekompression. Zentralbl. Chir., *53:* 2812–2819, 1926.
27. Kunicki, A. Operative experience in 8 cases of pineal tumor. J. Neurosurg., *17:* 815–823, 1960.
28. Lapras, C. Experience with the direct surgical approach in 52 tumors of the pineal region. In: *Multidisciplinary Aspects of Brain Tumor Therapy*, edited by P. Paoletti, M. D. Walker, G. Butti, and R. Knerich, pp. 173–176. Elsevier/North Holland Biomedical Press, Amsterdam/New York/Oxford, 1979.
29. Lazar, M. L., and Clark, K. Direct surgical management of masses in the region of the vein of Galen. Surg. Neurol., *2:* 17–21, 1974.
30. Matsutani, M. Ultrastructural study of pinealoma in view of its histogenesis. Brain Nerve (Tokyo), *28:* 41–56, 1976 (in Japanese).
31. Matsutani, M., Sano, K., Seto, T., and Takakura, K. A new proposal regarding histogenesis of intracranial germinoma. Ninth International Congress of Neuropathology, Sept. 5–10, Vienna, Austria, 1982.
32. Mincer, F., Meltzer, J., and Botstein, C. Pinealoma. Cancer, *37:* 2713–2718, 1976.
33. Mostofi, F. K., and Price, E. B. Jr. Tumors of The Male Genital System. In: *Atlas of Tumor Pathology*, Ser. 2, Fasc. 8, pp. 7–84, 21–39. AFIP, Washington, D.C., 1973.
34. Oppenheim, H., and Krause, F. Operative Erfolge bei Geschwülsten der Sehhügel- und Vierhügelgegend. Berl. Klin. Wochenschr. *50:* 2316–2322, 1913.
35. Pendl, G. Infratentorial approach to mesencephalic tumors. In: *Clinical Microneurosurgery*, edited by W. T. Koos and F. W. Böck, pp. 143–150. Georg Thieme, Stuttgart, 1976.

36. Poppen, J. L., and Marino, R. Jr. Pinealomas and tumors of the posterior portion of the third ventricle. J. Neurosurg., *28:* 357–364, 1968.
37. Pratt, O. W., and Brooks, E. F. Successful excision of a tumour of the pineal gland. Can. Med. Assoc. J., *39:* 240–243, 1938.
38. Raimondi, A. J., and Tomita, T. Pineal tumors in childhood. Epidemiology, pathophysiology, and surgical approaches. Child's Brain, *9:* 239–266, 1982.
39. Rhoton, A. L. Jr., Yamamoto, I., and Peace, D. A. Microsurgery of the third ventricle. Part 2. Operative approaches. Neurosurgery, *8:* 357–373, 11981.
40. Riverson, E. A., and Zülch, K. J. Pineal parenchymal tumours and germinomas (the problem of the so-called pinealomas). Neurosurg. Rev., *1:* 3–11, 1979.
41. Rorschach, H. Zur Pathologie der Tumoren der Zirbeldrüse. Beitr. Klin. Chir., *83:* 451, 1913.
42. Rubinstein, L. J. Tumors of the central nervous system. In: *Atlas of Tumor Pathology*, Ser. 2, Fasc. 6, pp. 269–284. AFIP, Washington, D.C., 1972.
43. Russell, D. S. The pinealoma: Its relationships to teratoma. J. Pathol. Bacteriol., *56:* 145–150, 1944.
44. Russell, D. S., and Rubinstein, L. J. *Pathology of Tumours of the Nervous System*, Ed. 4. Arnold, London, 1977.
45. Sano, K. Pinealoma in children. Child's Brain, *2:* 67–72, 1976.
46. Sano, K. Diagnosis and treatment of tumours in the pineal region. Acta Neurochir., *34:* 153–157, 1976.
47. Sano, K., and Matsutani, M. Pinealoma (germinoma) treated by direct surgery and postoperative irradiation. A long-term follow-up. Child's Brain, *8:* 81–97, 1981.
48. Scully, R. E. Tumors of the ovary and maldeveloped gonads. In: *Atlas of Tumor Pathology*, Ser. 2, Fasc. 16, pp. 226–299. AFIP, Washington, D.C., 1978.
49. Smith, N. J., El-Mahdi, A. M., and Constable, W. C. Results of irradiation of tumors in the region of the pineal body. Acta Radiol. Ther. Phys. Biol. *15:* 17–22, 1976.
50. Stein, B. M. The infratentorial supracerebellar approach to pineal lesions. J. Neurosurg., *35:* 197–202, 1971.
51. Sung, D., II, Harisiadis, L., and Chang, C. H. Midline pineal tumors and suprasellar germinomas: Highly curable by irradiation. Radiology, *128:* 745–751, 1978.
52. Suzuki, J., and Iwabuchi, T. Surgical removal of pineal tumors (pinealomas and teratomas): experience in a series of 19 cases. J. Neurosurg., *23:* 565–571, 1965.
53. Tabuchi, K., Yamada, O., and Nishimoto, A. The ultrastructure of pinealomas. Acta Neuropathol. (Berl.), *24:* 117–127, 1973.
54. Ueki, K., and Tanaka, R. Treatments and prognosis of pineal tumors—Experience of 110 cases. Neurol. Med. Chir. (Tokyo),. *20:* 1–26, 1980.
55. van Wagenen, W. P. A surgical approach for the removal of certain pineal tumors. Report of a case. Surg. Gynecol. Obstet., *53:* 216–220, 1931.
56. Wara., W. M., Fellows, C. F., Sheline, G. E., Wilson, C. B., and Townsend, J. J. Radiation therapy for pineal tumors and suprasellar germinomas. Radiology, *124:* 221–223, 1977.
57. Wara, W. M., Jenkin, R. D. T., Evans, A., Ertel, I., Hittle, R., Ortega, J., Wilson, C. B., and Hammond, D. Tumors of the pineal and suprasellar region: Children's Cancer Study Group Treatment Results 1960–1975. Cancer, *43:* 698–701, 1979.
58. Yamamoto, H., Personal communication, 1982.
59. Yamamoto, I., Rhoton, A. L. Jr., and Peace, D. A. Microsurgery of the third ventricle. Part 1. Microsurgical anatomy. Neurosurgery, *8:* 334–356, 1981.
60. Zapletal, B. Ein neuer operativer Zugang zum Gebiet der Incisura Tentorii. Zentralbl. Neurochir., *16:* 64–69, 1956.
61. Zülch, K. J. *Brain Tumors: Their Biology and Pathology.* Springer, New York, 1957.

CHAPTER

4

Integrative Treatment of Gliomas

KEIJO SANO, M.D., D.M.Sc., F.A.C.S.(HON.)

Selbst der Arzt muß produktiv sein, wenn er wahrhaft heilen will; ist er es nicht, so wird ihm nur hin und wieder wie durch Zufall etwas gelingen, im ganzen aber wird er nur Pfuscherei machen—Even the doctor must be productive if he really wants to cure. If not, though he may succeed by chance, in general, he will only bungle things.

Gespräche mit Goethe in den letzten Jahren seines Lebens.
J. P. Eckermann
March 11, 1828

Percival Bailey wrote in 1948 in his classic monograph (5) that "There is only one rational treatment of intracranial neoplasm and this is to remove it by operation as soon as the diagnosis can be established. Alas, it is easier said than done! Although easier now than half a century ago, there are many intracranial tumors which it is still impossible to remove . . . ." Most gliomas, namely, neuroectodermal tumors of the brain parenchyma, belong in this category.

Thus, we have to resort to means other than surgery, at least as an adjunct to surgery, such as radiotherapy, chemotherapy, or immunotherapy. Radiotherapy is effective for some kinds of glioma, such as medulloblastoma. It is difficult, however, to cure patients with glioma by radiotherapy alone. The same is true for chemotherapy or immunotherapy. All these modalities of therapy should be *integrated* for the sole purpose of curing patients.

Glioma occupies 34.7% of 14,672 cases of primary intracranial neoplasms in Japan (7)—the percentage is a little bit lower than those of American and European statistics, which are a little more than 40%. As seen in Figure 4.1, more than one-half of gliomas (5091 cases) are pathologically malignant.

CELL KINETICS OF GLIOMAS AND ITS CLINICAL IMPLICATION

Before discussing the integrative treatment of gliomas, it may be better to recapitulate the cell kinetics of gliomas. Every neoplasm (including glioma) has a proliferating pool and a nonproliferating pool (Fig. 4.2). In the former, tumor cells are proliferating, that is, dividing with a certain cell cycle time ($M + G_1 + S + G_2$ phases). In the latter, tumor cells are

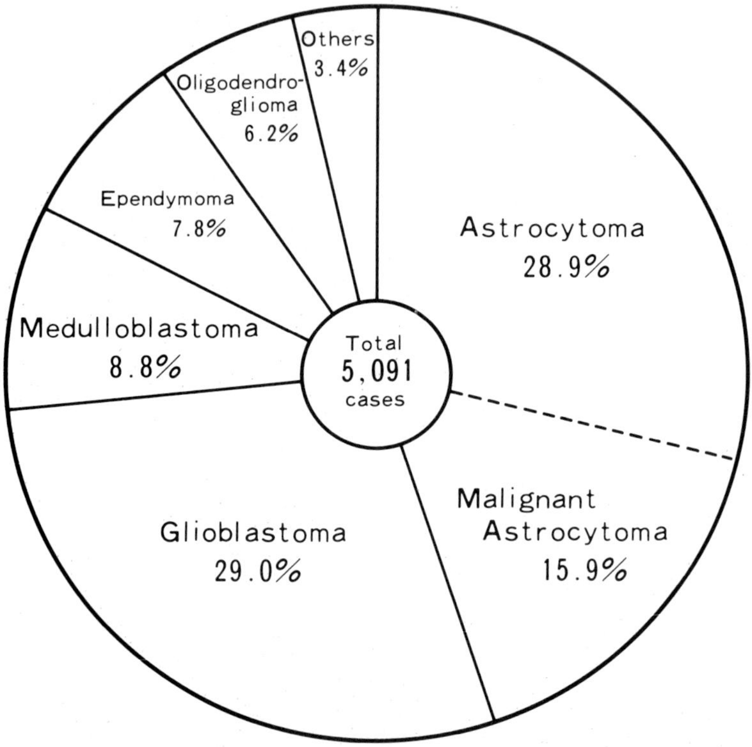

FIG. 4.1. Incidence of gliomas by histological type (total: 5091 cases) in Japan. (Reproduced with permission from the Brain Tumor Registry in Japan (7).)

temporarily resting (G_0 cells). The ratio of proliferating pool cells to the total tumor cell population is called the growth fraction. Cell loss is also an important feature of tumor tissue. The rate of cell loss represented as a fraction of the rate at which cells are added to the total tumor cell population by mitosis is called the cell loss factor.

According to Hoshino and his collaborators (15, 18), in glioblastoma, the cell cycle time is approximately 57.3 ± 6.1 hours, or 2–3 days, the S phase is 7–10 hours, and the growth fraction in a viable part (excluding the nonviable part) of the tumor is about 0.3–0.4 (30–40%), and the cell loss factor is about 80–85 percent. In astrocytoma, the S phase is the same (7–10 hours); however, the cell cycle time is probably longer than that in glioblastoma, and the growth fraction is markedly low.

In malignant gliomas, especially glioblastoma, G_0 cells in the nonproliferating pool rapidly move into the proliferating pool to repopulate the tumor when the tumor tissue is partly removed or destroyed. On the other hand, in benign gliomas, movement of G_0 cells into the very small nonproliferating pool is insignificant. This means that if surgical removal or radiotherapy or their combination effectively reduce the number of both proliferating and nonproliferating pool cells in benign gliomas, a patient's survival time can be increased significantly, whereas this is not the case with malignant gliomas because of the rapid transition of G_0 cells into proliferating cells.

In 7 cases of malignant gliomas which were macroscopically totally removed in the author's clinic and recurred, Matsutani and Hoshino (25) calculated the cell cycle time from the following equation. In these cases, the cell loss factor may be regarded as 0 because the recurrent tumors could freely expand in ample space without compression.

$$N_o(1 + GF)^{t/T} = N_t$$

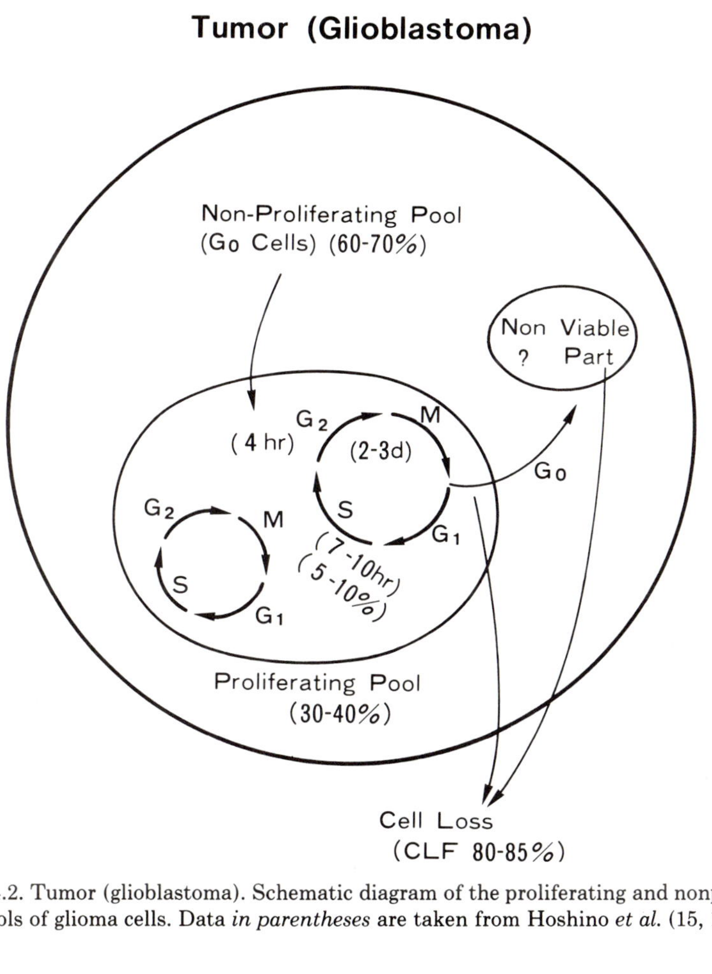

FIG. 4.2. Tumor (glioblastoma). Schematic diagram of the proliferating and nonproliferating pools of glioma cells. Data *in parentheses* are taken from Hoshino *et al.* (15, 18).

Here N_o is the number of tumor cells which were the source of recurrence. GF is the growth fraction, T is the cell cycle time, and N_t is the number of tumor cells t days after removal (calculated as 1 gm = 1 cm^3 = 10^9 cells). If one assumes N_o is 10^8 (equivalent to a tumor residue of 0.1 gm or 0.1 cm^3) and the growth fraction is 0.3, 3 of 4 glioblastoma or malignant astrocytoma cases treated by surgery (without radiation or chemotherapy) showed cell cycle times of 2–3 days. This is in accordance with the values obtained by Hoshino *et al.* (15, 18).

Schiffer *et al.* estimated the growth fraction in murine tumors by the primer-available DNA-dependent polymerase activity (PDP), based on the fact that the ratio of PDP-positive cells could be regarded as representing the growth fraction (32). According to Schiffer (31), the PDP index and consequently the growth fraction in a case of glioblastoma was 0.308, and the calculated cell cycle time was 43.9 hours, while in a case of medulloblastoma, the former was 0.347 and the latter was 57.9 hours—similar to the values obtained by Hoshino.

Figure 4.3 shows the theoretical proliferation curves of glioma cells and the effects of therapeutic interventions. Presumably, when the size of a tumor reaches 10 gm (*i.e.*, the number of tumor cells is ca 10^{10}),

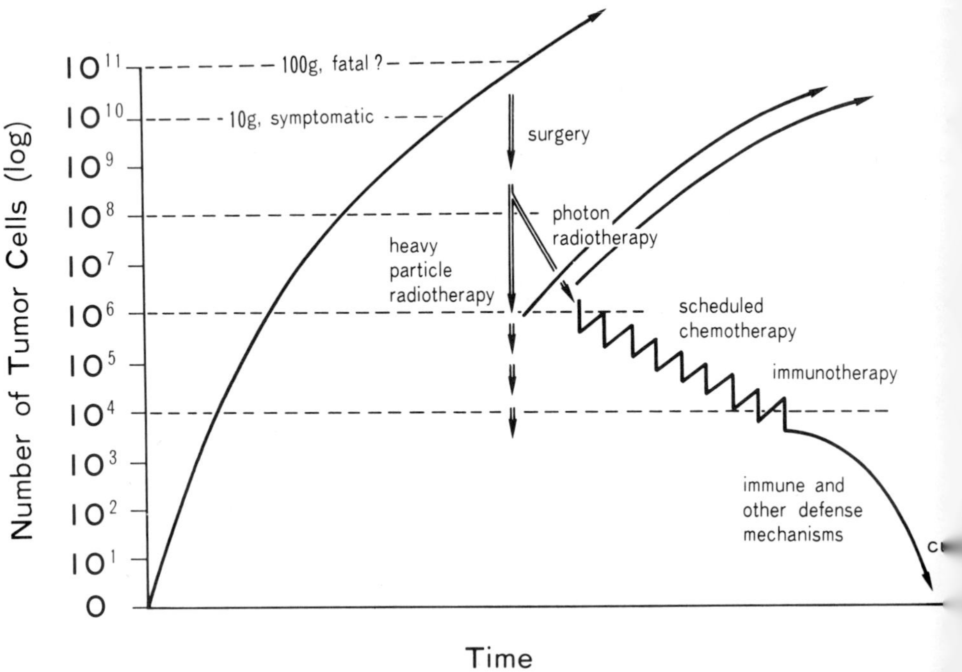

FIG. 4.3. Tumor growth and therapeutic interventions. *Ordinate*, number of tumor cells (log); *Abscissa*, time. See the text.

some symptoms may appear. If the tumor is assumed to be spherical in shape, this means that the tumor diameter on CT (computed tomography) is approximately 2.72 cm. If the tumor size reaches 100 gm (*i.e.*, the number of tumor cells is ca 10^{11}, or the tumor diameter on CT is ca 5.85 cm), the patient's life may be in danger. Treatments are usually started between these two stages of tumor growth. If it is located in the brain stem, however, even a 1 gm tumor (with the number of tumor cells at 10^{9}) may well be symptomatic or fatal.

Even if 99% of the tumor cells are removed by surgery, there still remain a little more than 10^{8} tumor cells. If subsequent radiotherapy kills 99% of the remaining tumor cells (2 log kill), there still may be a little more than 10^{6} tumor cells which can become the source of recurrence. To cure the patient, probably, the remaining tumor cells should be less than 10^{4} or less than 10^{3}. To achieve this last 2 or 3 log kill in a stepwise fashion is the task of the scheduled chemotherapy, immunotherapy, or other adjuvant therapies. Once this task is achieved, the remaining small number of cells will hopefully be managed by the immune and other defense mechanisms of the body.

In most cases of glioma, especially glioblastoma, surgery alone can achieve only 0.5 log kill (50% of tumor cells are removed) or 1 log kill (90% of tumor cells are removed). If we assume that the cell cycle time is 3 days, that the growth fraction is 0.3, and that there is no spontaneous cell loss in that tumor, the time necessary for the tumor to regain its original size will be 8 days in cases with 0.5 log kill and 27 days in cases with 1 log kill. If we can fortunately kill 99% of the tumor cells (2 log kill) by surgery and postoperative radiation, that time will be 53 days. If we very fortunately destroy 99.9% of tumor cells (3 log kill) by a combination of surgery and radiation therapy, then the time for the tumor to regain its original size will be 78 days. This means that even if we can reduce the number of glioma cells to 1/100 to 1/1000, the tumor will regain its original size in 8–11 weeks. Therefore, the second adjuvant treatment should be administered repeatedly within an interval less than this period or, if there is spontaneous cell loss, at least equal to this period.

Another difficulty we must encounter in malignant gliomas is the heterogeneity of ploidy and the heterogeneity of ploidy in different populations within different areas of the same tumor. This can be revealed by flow cytometry (FCM), which is a technique that measures the quantity of DNA contained in individual nuclei and records a frequency distribution of the DNA content per nucleus in the sampled cell population. In Figure 4.4, the first peak represents the diploid chromosomal complement (2C) of nondividing (G_0) and postmitotic (G_1) cells. The DNA content increases during the DNA synthetic phase (S) to

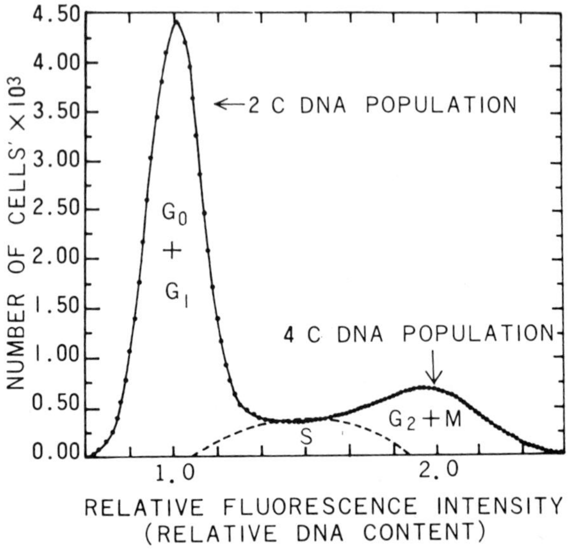

FIG. 4.4. A diagrammatic flow cytometry profile of brain tumor cells. The relative fluorescence intensity values of 1.0 and 2.0 correspond to the nuclei with a 2C and 4C DNA content, respectively. G_0, nondividing cells; G_1, postmitotic cells; G_2, premitotic cells; *M*, mitotic cells; *S*, DNA synthesizing cells.

double that amount (4C, tetraploid), as seen in premitotic (G_2) and mitotic (M) cells represented by the second peak. Cells that register either between these two peaks or partially overlap with these peaks are considered to be cells in the process of DNA synthesis (S phase). According to Hoshino *et al.* (16), profiles of DNA distribution in histologically benign tumors, such as low-grade astrocytomas, revealed a large diploid population (2C) of G_0–G_1 cells, with very few cells in DNA synthesis, as well as a small population of G_2 (-M) phase cells that contained a 4C DNA complement. There was little variability within one tumor. In contrast, in malignant gliomas including glioblastoma, there was a substantial population of cells in DNA synthesis, and a highly variable distribution of nuclear DNA complement, consisting not only of diploid, or aneuploid, but also of triploid, tetraploid and, possibly, octaploid populations. In addition, there was a large variability in FCM profiles between different regions of the same tumor. In such tumors consisting of heterogeneous cell populations, each cell type may show varied responses to various chemotherapeutic agents. Therefore, a combination of several drugs may be necessary as the use of multiple antibiotics to treat mixed bacterial infections (16).

THE THERAPEUTIC PRINCIPLE OF GLIOMAS

In Table 4.1, the therapeutic principles of neoplasms of the central nervous system (CNS) in general are described. These also hold for gliomas. If, by some means, *a peaceful coexistence with neoplasms* is brought to fruition, that is, if tumor cells do not proliferate any more, do not divide, and do not metastasize, then the only procedure needed is to relieve intracranial or intraspinal pressure, and the patient may lead a normal or nearly normal life until he dies of natural causes. This peaceful coexistence, however, has not been actualized yet.

Then, *extermination of neoplasms* should be performed to cure patients of them. This includes three stages or steps. The *first step* is to induce the state of remission. As many of the tumor cells as possible should be removed by surgery, radiotherapy (either conventional or special), or chemotherapy, or by a combination of all these. If the reduction of tumor cells is 100%, *e.g.*, by total surgical removal without neurological deficits, there is a complete remission or a complete cure. The *second step* is to maintain the state of remission. This may be achieved by potentiation of the immune and other defense mechanisms of the body and by scheduled chemotherapy. The latter consists of administration of chemotherapeutic agents within various scheduled intervals. For instance, if 2 log kill of tumor cells is achieved by surgery and radiotherapy and the time for the tumor to regain the original size is calculated from its cell kinetics to be 8 weeks, administration of single or, more often, multiple chemotherapeutic agents with a potency of 1 log kill every 7 weeks will

TABLE 4.1

Therapeutic Principles (CNS Neoplasms)

I. Extermination of Neoplasms
   1. Remission induction
      Surgical removal (partial, extensive, total)
      Radiation therapy
         Conventional
         Special: BAR therapy
            Cellular synchronization-radiation therapy
            Boron-neutron capture therapy, etc.
      Chemotherapy
   2. Remission maintenance
      Scheduled chemotherapy
      Potentiation of immune and defense mechanisms:
         BCG, Krestin. picibanil, levamisole, etc.
         Interferon
   3. Eradication of neoplastic cells
      Immune and defense mechanisms

II. Peaceful Coexistence with Neoplasms?

gradually decrease the number of tumor cells until finally they reach less than 10^4 or 10^3, as illustrated in Figure 4.3. During the procedure, the immune and defense mechanisms should be potentiated. The *third step* is the eradication of tumor cells by the potentiated immune-defense mechanisms of the body.

In the following, the author will discuss each of these three steps.

Remission Induction

The most effective means to reduce the number of tumor cells is, of course, surgical removal. In most glioma cases, total surgical removal is only rarely feasible, with the exception of benign cerebellar astrocytoma or benign gliomas located in the frontal or temporal tips. Conventional photon radiation is usually not so effective for gliomas, except for medulloblastoma. There is a need for special kinds of radiotherapy other than conventional irradiation to treat gliomas, especially malignant gliomas.

BAR THERAPY OR BUdR-RADIATION THERAPY

In order to improve the results of radiotherapy, several attempts have been made to enhance the radiosensitivity of tumors. According to Bagshaw (4), these are classified into four categories, namely, sensitization, augmentation, potentiation, and additivities.

The author's group has been interested in one of the agents belonging to the category of sensitization: namely, one of the synthesized thymidine analogues, 5-bromo-2′-deoxyuridine, commonly called broxuridine or BUdR (Fig. 4.5). According to the basic studies of many authors, BUdR is incorporated into the DNA of dividing cells in place of thymidine and is capable of increasing radiosensitivity of the cells by a factor of 2 to 3 (8, 9).

The difference between thymidine and BUdR is the difference between a methyl radical and bromine in the 5th position on the pyrimidine ring. The Van der Waals radius of the methyl radical is 2.0 Å, and that of the bromine is 1.95 Å. This difference is so slight that the cells may not recognize it and so incorporate BUdR as if it were thymidine. Perhaps because the Van der Waals radius of iodine is 2.15 Å and that of chlorine is 1.80 Å, incorporation of BUdR into DNA is better than that of IUdR or CUdR. 5-fluoro-2′-deoxyuridine, namely, FUdR, is not incorporated into DNA but into RNA. This may be because the Van der Waals radius of fluorine is 1.35 Å and that of the hydrogen on the 5th position of uridine is 1.2 Å.

Another characteristic of BUdR is its systemic fate. As reported by Kriss and others (20), more than 90% of BUdR is degraded by the liver within 1 hour after intravenous administration.

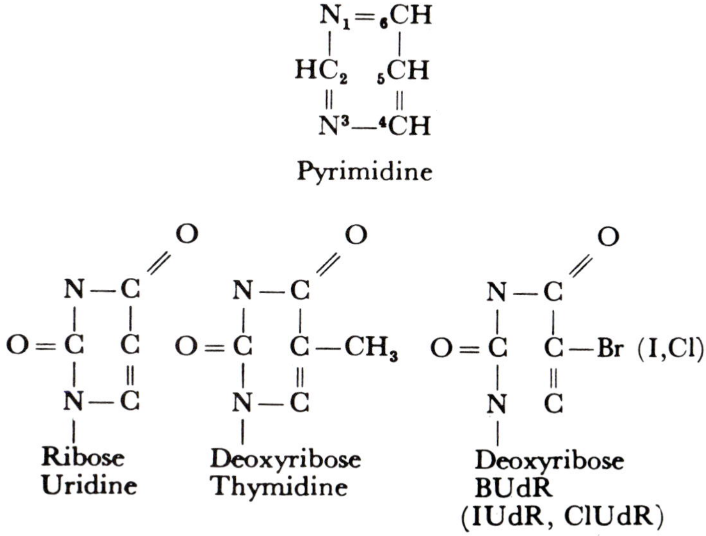

FIG. 4.5. Pyrimidine, uridine, thymidine, and BUdR.

This BUdR seems especially promising as an adjuvant to radiotherapy of brain tumors for the following reasons: (a) most brain tumors are solitary and rarely metastasize; (b) since the surrounding normal nerve cells have no mitotic activity, they would not incorporate BUdR into their DNA; (c) the normal brain tissue is usally protected from administered chemicals by the blood-brain barrier whereas at least the majority of the tumor cells are exposed to them because of breakdown of the barrier; (d) BUdR is incorporated into neoplastic vessels which are richly formed in malignant tumors. Intraarterial or intrathecal infusion may be recommended to obtain a high amount of BUdR in the tumor tissue and to avoid too rapid degradation of BUdR by the liver. This rapid degradation is advantageous, however, in that the side effects of BUdR are thus minimized when it reaches the general circulation.

The author's group found that a very small amount of antimetabolite such as methotrexate, 5-FU, or FUdR, increased the uptake of BUdR into the cell nuclei *in vitro* (17, 28, 29). This can be explained in the following way. Presumably, not all tumor cells take up BUdR during mitosis because they can synthesize the thymidine necessary for duplicating their DNA. However, if this biosynthetic mechanism is inhibited by a small amount of an antimetabolite, the dividing tumor cells will be forced to incorporate exogenous thymidine, in this instance the analogue BUdR, in order to duplicate their DNA.

From 1965 to 1977, the author's group used the following regimen to treat patients with brain tumors. BUdR (600–1000 mg/day) was administered together with a small amount of antimetabolite (for example, 0.5–3 mg/day of methotrexate or 1–5 mg/day of 5-FU) by means of continuous intraarterial infusion. When intrathecal infusion was done, the dosage was about ⅕ to ⅒ of this regimen. Radiation therapy was started 7–14 days after commencement of the infusion and was repeated every day. The daily dose of irradiation was about 150–200 rads, for a total tumor dose of 4500–6000 rads. For brevity, the author called this "BAR therapy," taking the B of BUdR, the A of antimetabolite, and the R of radiation (27, 28).

Usually, BUdR was infused for a period of 4–7 weeks. The total amount of BUdR administered to each patient averaged 25,000 mg, with the maximum 45,000 mg (with intraarterial infusion). Radioactivation analysis proved in one case of glioblastoma who received intraarterial infusion of BUdR for 5 weeks (38,500 mg of BUdR) that the bromine content of the tumor tissue was at least 4 to 6 times as high as that of the surrounding brain or the bone marrow.

Until February 1977, the author's group performed this BAR therapy in 184 cases. The pathological classification is shown in Table 4.2. The observed survival rates (3) of glioma cases as of 1977 are shown in Figure 4.6. The 1-year survival rate, the 2-year-survival rate, the 3-year-survival rate, the 5-year-survival rate, and the 8-year-survival rate of cases with moderately malignant gliomas were high, 94.7%, 82.2%, 64.0%, 48.0%, and 40.5%, respectively. The survival rates of cases with highly malignant gliomas were 62.1%, 35.6%, 20.8%, 14.9%, and 14.9%, respectively.

TABLE 4.2

Malignant Brain Tumors Treated by BAR Therapy (February 1977)

Tumor	No. of Cases
Highly malignant gliomas	77
Glioblastoma multiforme	53
Malignant oligodendroglioma	10
Malignant ependymoma	6
Medulloblastoma	7
Pineoblastoma	1
Moderately malignant gliomas	58
Astrocytoma	35
Oligodendroglioma	10
Ependymoma	5
Pinealoma	8
Unverified gliomas (brainstem, thalamus)	14
Sarcomas	10
Metastatic tumors	16
Others	9
Total	184

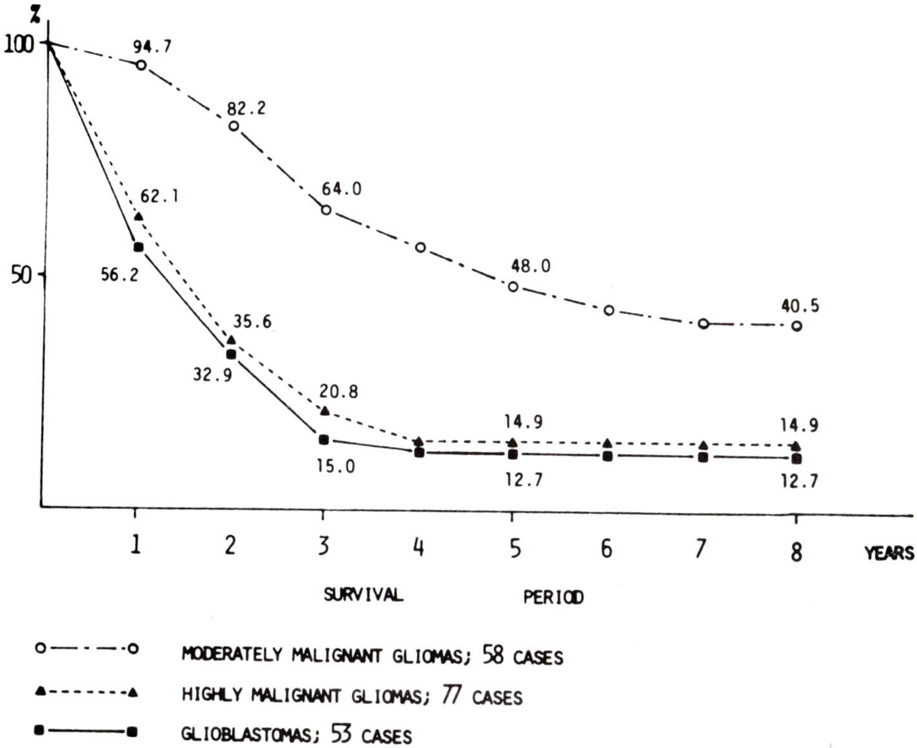

FIG. 4.6. Survival rates of gliomas treated by BAR therapy. (Reproduced with permission from K. Sano (27).)

Among malignant gliomas, glioblastoma cases showed slightly lower values than these rates, namely, 56.2% (1-year survival), 32.9% (2-year), 15.0% (3-year), 12.7% (5-year), and 12.7% (8-year), respectively. These survival rates were significantly better than those of other reports (6, 19), even though these results were obtained before adopting the scheduled chemotherapy accompanied by immunopotentiating agent administration.

BAR therapy was not only effective for prolongation of survival time, but also because many of the treated cases could lead a useful life; for example, even among the cases of highly malignant gliomas, the quality of survival was excellent (complete recovery to social life) in 14.3% and good (incomplete recovery to social life) in 26%, so that about 40% of the cases could lead a useful life.

Intraarterial infusion of BUdR, however, caused occlusion of the carotid in 20 cases, although many of them were asymptomatic. Partly because of this and partly because of the intricacy of intraarterial or intrathecal infusion techniques, the author's group discontinued the BAR therapy in 1977. Recently, however, the author's group revived the therapy in a different form. BUdR (1000 mg/m^2) was intravenously injected during the night and conventional fractionated irradiation was done the following morning. This injection was continued for about 20 days, and the total radiation doses were from 4000 to 7000 rads. Figure 4.7 is a contrast-enhanced CT (computed tomograph) of a 32-year-old

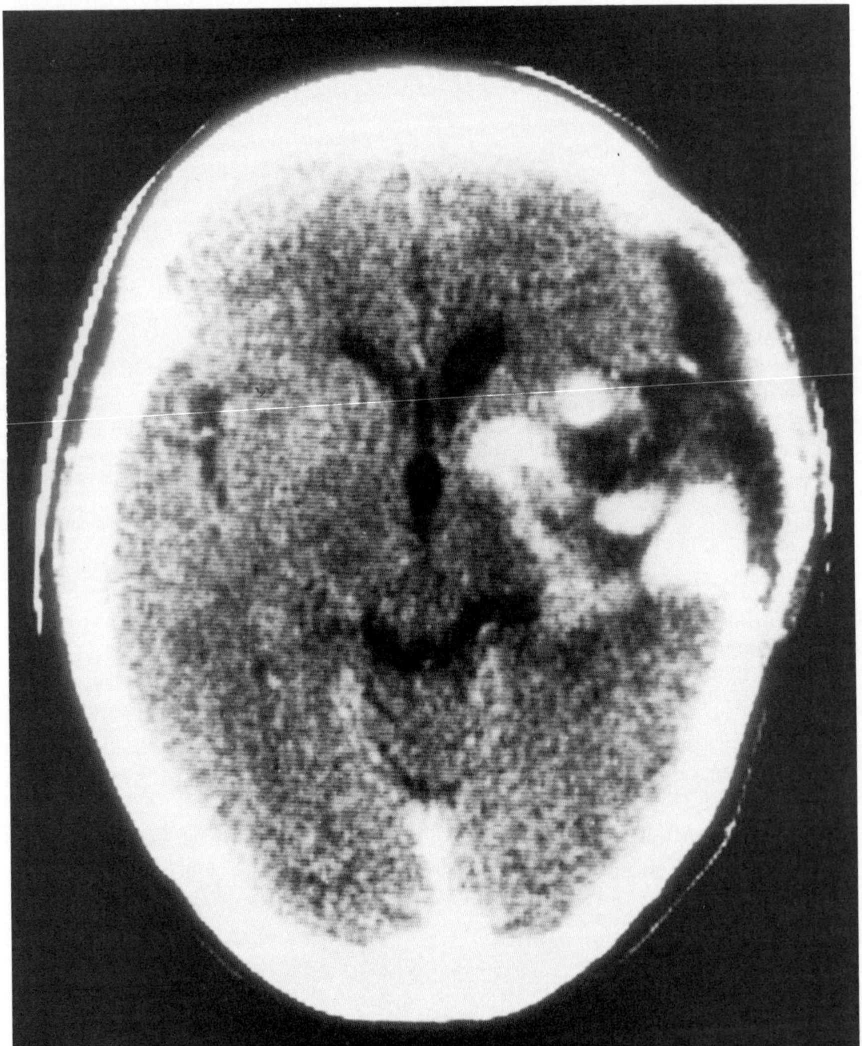

FIG. 4.7. A 32-year-old woman with a glioblastoma in the right hemisphere. Postoperative CT scan.

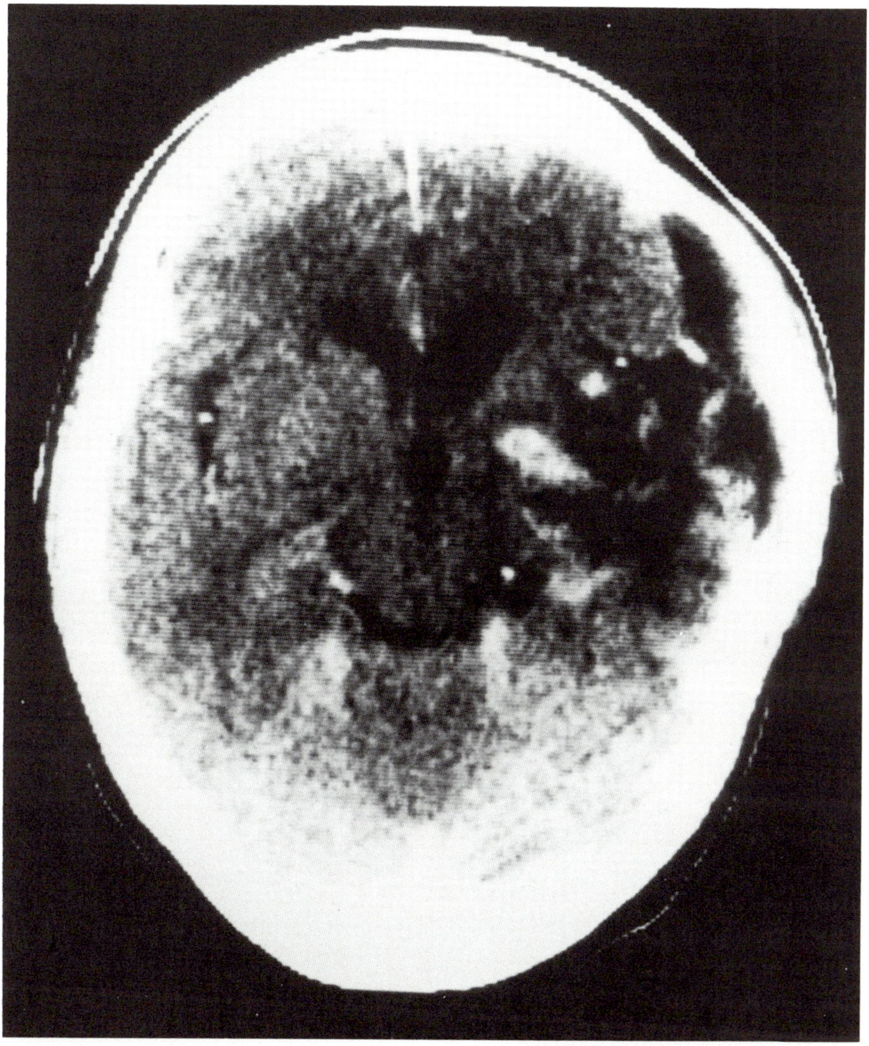

FIG. 4.8. The same case, 3 weeks later. In the middle of the radiotherapy course (2600 rad).

woman with a glioblastoma in the right hemisphere, 2 weeks after the operation. Figure 4.8 is the CT 3 weeks later (2600 rads), and the tumor can be still noticed. Figure 4.9 is the CT 2 months after the second CT; by this time, 26,000 mg of BUdR had been injected, and 5000 rads of conventional radiation and 2000 rads of local radiation had been administered. As seen in Figure 4.9, the tumor completely disappeared, and the condition of the patient was markedly ameliorated. This intravenous

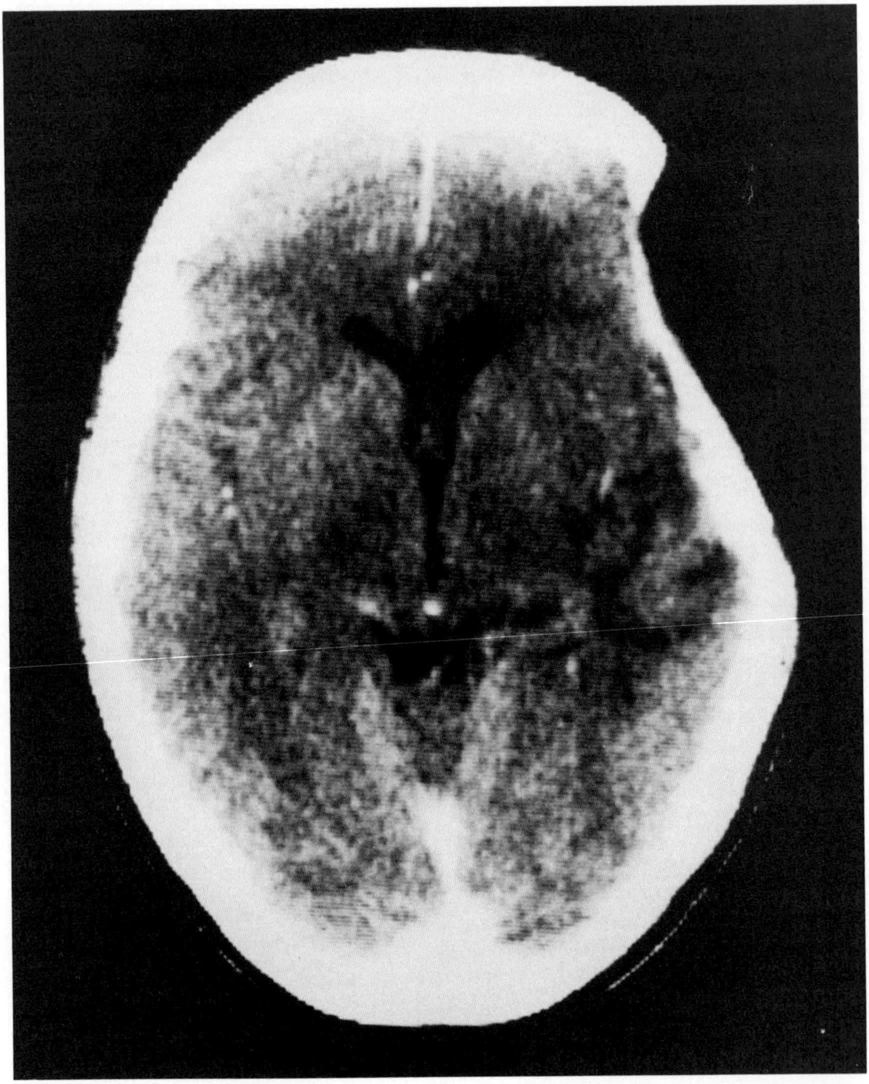

FIG. 4.9. The same case 2 months after the CT scan of Figure 4.8. The total amount of BUdR injected intravenously was 26,600 mg (radiation, 7000 rad). The tumor has disappeared on CT scan.

injection (ordinary drip infusion) of a larger amount of BUdR combined with radiation seems promising because of few side effects and the simplicity of the procedure. Unlike the previous BAR therapy, antimetabolite is not infused so that the side effects are practically negligible. In this sense, BUdR radiosensitization is better than misonidazole (33).

CELLULAR SYNCHRONIZATION-RADIATION THERAPY

It has been noted that the radiosensitivity of tumor cells is dependent on the cell cycle phases, of which the G_2–M phases are the most sensitive (35, 36, 40). However, 60–70% of the tumor cells are in the G_0 phase, and as this is a dormant nonproliferating cell population, it is not sensitive to radiation. Among dividing cells, the cell populations of the G_2 and M phases are less than 10% and as the cell populations in the G_2 and M phases are approximately only 3–4% of *all* tumor cells, simple radiation is considered quite inefficient. Therefore, if one could synchronize tumor cell division and increase the fraction of cells in the G_2 and M phases, the effects of radiotherapy would be greatly enhanced. Shitara *et al.* (34) verified such a synchronizing effect of colcemid (desacetylmethyl colchicine) on cultured glioma cells of the rat C6-cell line. They and Yamamoto *et al.* (43) further advanced the study and found similar synchronizing effects of vincristine (a metaphase stopper), ACNU (1-(4-amino-2-methylpyrimidin-5-yl)methyl-3-(2-chlorethyl)-3-nitrosourea hydrochloride), and VM26 (epipodophyllotoxin) on cultured cells (27, 43). The analysis of cell cycle phase is easily and rapidly obtained with the aid of flow cytometry.

Figure 4.10 is such an example. Figure 4.10*A* is a histogram of cultured C6 rat glioma. The abscissa is the relative fluorescent intensity of ethidium bromide stain proportional to the nuclear DNA content, and the ordinate shows the cell number per channel. As stated before, the first large peak represents cells of the G_0–G_1 phase with 2C DNA content, and the second small peak shows cells of the G_2—M phase with 4C DNA content. The cells of the S phase lie between these two peaks. The ratio of cells in each cell cycle phase to total cells can be calculated. The

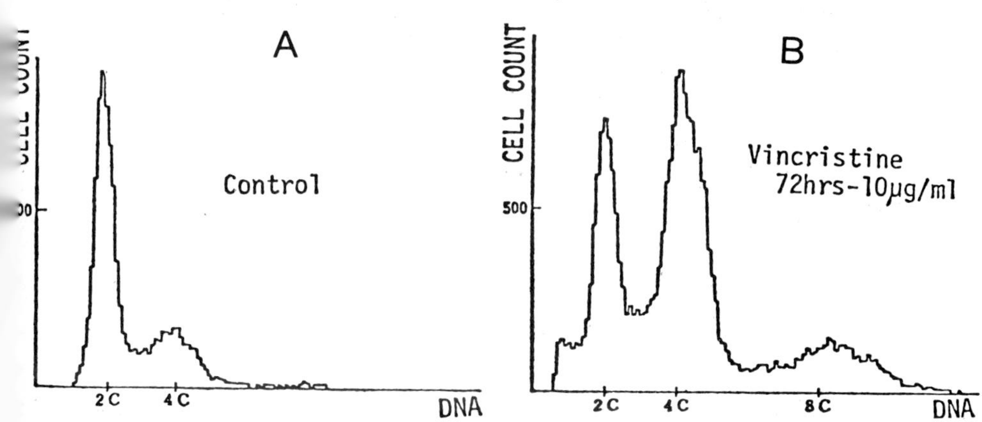

FIG. 4.10. FCM analysis of the effects of vincristine on C6 glioma cells. (*A*) Before adding vincristine (10 μg/ml) to the culture medium. (*B*) 72 Hours after adding vincristine.

fraction of $G_0 + G_1$ cells is 74%, that of S cells is 17%, and that of G_2–M phase cells is 9%. Figure 4.10*B* is a histogram of the cell populations 72 hours after adding vincristine (10 μg/ml) to the culture medium. Seventy-two hours after adding vincristine, G_0 cells (G_1 cells already divided) are 26%, S phase cells are 26.4% and G_2–M phase cells are 47.6%—a remarkable increase.

In Table 4.3, the synchronizing effects of several chemotherapeutic agents on cultured C6 glioma cells are listed. VM26 (24 hours after addition to the culture medium), vincristine (72 hours), and ACNU (72 hours) seemed suitable for the purpose of synchronization.

For clinical application of this cellular synchronization, the following regimen has been used. Vincristine (0.025 mg/kg body weight) or VM26 (1 mg/kg body weight) was given intravenously on Days 1, 2, and 3 of the treatment, and ACNU (1 mg/kg body weight) was given intravenously on Days 2 and 3, as illustrated in Figure 4.11. Radiation started on the same day that therapy began. On days 4 and 5, the radiation dosage was increased to 300 rads (3 Gy) per day and was then reduced to a daily dose of 150 rads for two or three weeks. In the 3rd or 4th weeks, the same course of chemotherapy was repeated. After 2 or 3 weeks rest, a similar boost course was repeated. The total dose of radiation was about 5000 to 6000 rads.

Leukocyte and thrombocyte counts and liver function were examined every week, and if severe side effects of chemotherapy were noticed, the second or third course of chemotherapy was skipped, or the dosage of

TABLE 4.3

Effect of Chemotherapeutic Agents on Cell Cycle Distribution of C_6 Glioma Cells Treated In Vitro[a]

	Concentration (μg/ml)	Time (hr)	Ratio of Cells in G_2 and M Phases
Control			9.0
Vincristine	10	24	19.9
		72	47.6
VM26	1	24	71.1
		72	43.4
BCNU	10	24	38.6
		72	Cell death
ACNU	10	24	30.1
		72	47.2
5-FU	10	24	17.5
		72	25.9
Bleomycin	10	24	26.7
		72	33.0

[a] Accumulation of cells in G_2 and M phases are demonstrated.

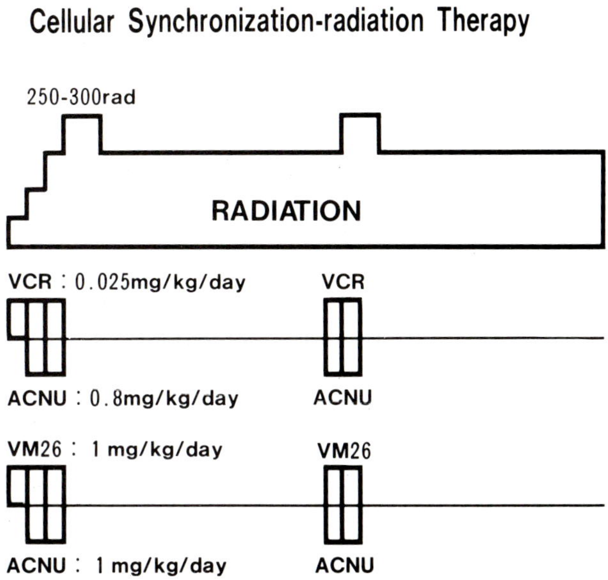

FIG. 4.11. Cellular synchronization-radiation therapy with vincristine and ACNU or VM26 and ACNU.

drugs was reduced. Supratentorial glioblastoma (56 cases) were treated with vincristine plus ACNU and 35 cases with VM26 plus ACNU.

Responses to the therapy were evaluated by measuring tumor size on CT (contrast-enhanced) scans with a planimeter before the therapy and one month after completion of the therapy. According to the criteria advocated by the Ministry of Health and Welfare, the responses were classified as follows: complete response (CR)—no visible tumor, with disappearance of secondary changes due to tumor (the state should last more than 4 weeks); partial response (PR)—more than 50% reduction of tumor area on CT (or more than 65% reduction of tumor volume) without aggravation of secondary changes due to tumor (the state should last more than 4 weeks); stable (ST)—less than 50% reduction of tumor area on CT (or less than 65% reduction of tumor volume) or less than 25% increase in tumor area (less than 35% increase in tumor volume) without aggravation of secondary changes due to tumor (the state should last more than 4 weeks); and progression (PG)—more than 25% increase in tumor area (or more than 35% increase in tumor volume) with aggravation of secondary changes due to tumor or appearance of new neoplasmic changes.

If CR and PR are defined as "effective," the therapy with vincristine plus ACNU was effective in 34% of the cases, with ST of 52% and PG of 14%. The therapy with VM26 plus ACNU was effective in 49%, with ST of 45% and PG of 6%.

Figure 4.12 shows survival rates of glioma cases treated by this therapy followed by the scheduled chemotherapy (see below), as compared with those treated by BAR therapy or by the simple irradiation with or without chemotherapy. Survival rates of those patients treated with vincristine plus ACNU at 12 and 24 months were 64 and 42%, respectively. The survival rates of patients who were treated with VM26 plus ACNU were 67 and 44%, respectively. Forty-three percent of patients who were treated by simple radiation with or without chemotherapy survived at 12 months, and 23% had survived at 24 months (42). The difference between survival rates at 12 and 24 months of patients who were treated by cellular synchronization-radiation therapy and those treated by simple radiation was significant ($p < 0.02$ and $p < 0.01$, respectively).

Eighty percent of patients treated by this therapy with either vincristine plus ACNU or VM26 plus ACNU complained of nausea. All patients who received vincristine and ACNU experienced constipation. Thirty-three percent of the patients who received vincristine and ACNU and 20% of the patients who received VM26 and ACNU experienced delayed myelosuppression in the form of leukopenia (leukocyte count nadir < 3000/cmm), thrombocytopenia (platelet count nadir < 100,000/cmm), or both, between the 3rd and the 5th weeks after the drug administration.

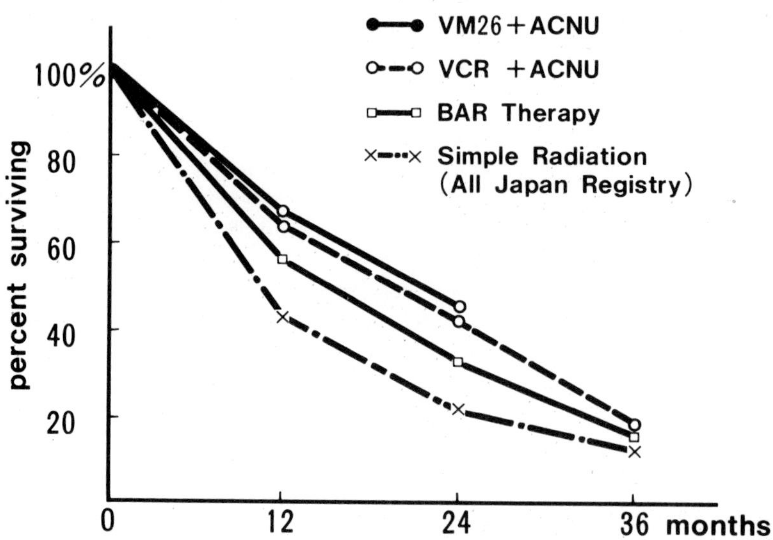

FIG. 4.12. Survival rates of glioblastoma treated by cellular synchronization-radiation (VM26 + ACNU, or vincristine + ACNU) followed by scheduled chemotherapy, as compared with those by BAR therapy or simple radiation.

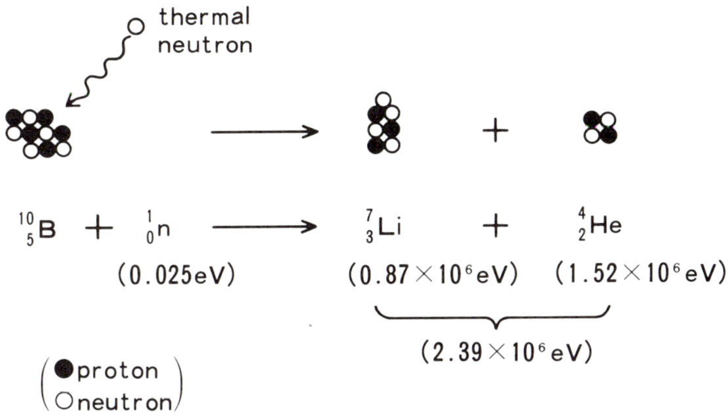

FIG. 4.13. Principle of boron-neutron capture therapy.

BORON-NEUTRON CAPTURE THERAPY

Boron-neutron capture therapy is based on the three major facts: (a) a nonradioactive isotope of boron (boron-10) reacts with a slow or thermal neutron that has a low energy of 0.025 electron V and produces lithium and a nucleus of helium, an α-particle. A huge energy of about 2.4 mega electron V, almost 100,000,000 times more than the original energy of the neutron, is produced, and most of the energy is consumed by the α-radiation (Fig. 4.13). (b) In treating a brain tumor, the normal brain is not seriously affected by the slow neutron because the normal constituent elements of the tissue, H, N, Cl, O, C, etc., barely react with the neutrons owing to the extremely small "cross-section" (barn) of these nuclides. (c) An α-particle does not have a range of more than 10 μm in tissue. This means that if Boron-10 compounds are selectively located in the tumor tissue, the normal brain tissue will not be affected by α-radiation.

Brain tumors are suited to this boron-neutron capture therapy, because most of the normal brain tissue does not take up boron owing to the so-called blood-brain barrier, as contrasted to the brain tumor.

These qualities of boron-neutron capture therapy constitute a selective heavy particle radiation of brain tumors that preserves normal brain tissues.

We owe much of the development of this treatment to Dr. William H. Sweet (37). The author sent his pupil, Hiroshi Hatanaka, to Dr. Sweet to learn this therapy. When he returned to Japan, Dr. Hatanaka started this therapy in the author's clinic in 1968.

The revised technique of boron-neutron capture therapy of Hatanaka and the author's group (12–14, 26) is based on the following four major changes: (a) A direct intraarterial infusion into the carotid or vertebral artery to obtain a higher concentration of boron in the tumor. (b) a new compound, $Na_2{}^{10}B_{12}H_{11}$ SH (sodium mercaptoundecahydrododecaborate), which gives a high and long-lasting boron concentration in the tumor. The brain only takes up less than 1/10 or 1/20 of the amount of the compound taken up by the tumor, namely, this new compound gives a large tumor-brain ratio. The boron compound stays in tumor tissue long enough to wait for the boron clearance from the blood. The tumor-blood ratio, at the time of neutron radiation, will be larger than 1 (usually 1–4), as compared to that of 0.3–0.4 of classical compounds like paracarboxyphenylboronic acid. (c) Administration of large doses of adrenocorticosteroid is important to prevent radiation damage to the normal cerebral blood vessels. (d) Rather modest doses of neutron have been used to avoid brain damage which might be caused by more than 2000 rads of single dose radiation. By the new method, the normal brain receives much less radiation (usually no more than 1400 rads at the surface), and the cerebral vascular walls receive extremely smaller radiation doses than in the classical therapy of about 20 years ago. This vascular wall dose is usually less than 2000 rads, even at the surface of the brain (Table 4.4).

Neutron-induced α-autoradiography by Amano and Sweet (2) demonstrated that α-particles produced by the neutron capture reaction made innumerable holes and indentations on the surface of a cellulose nitrate film which were made visible by an etching process with NaOH. Where there was more boron-10, there was a proportionately higher density of α-tracks. Tumors of experimental animals as well as patients showed much higher concentrations of boron-10 than in the normal brain tissue (Fig. 4.14). Under the microscope, these α-tracks were grouped in the tumor tissue, whereas in the normal brain tissue as well as on the capillary walls there were very few α-tracks. Using the same technique, Abe (1) found that boron-10 accumulated in transplanted brain tumors as well as in those induced by ethylnitrosourea in SD rats.

One or two weeks after a craniotomy for tumor excision or biopsy, the patient underwent an intraarterial infusion of isotonic boron-10 solution in the evening before the scheduled neutron irradiation and then was

TABLE 4.4

Schematic Dose Schedule—Revised Boron-Neutron Capture Therapy[a]

nvt[b]	Revised (8–10 × 10^{12})	Classical (18 × 10^{12})
Tumor	3800 rad (2100)	6600 rad (3400)
Brain	1200 rad (900)	2600 rad (1400)
Vessel lumen	2000 rad (1200)	15,500 rad (7800)

[a] Numbers in parentheses represent doses at 1.8 cm below the surface.
[b] Neutron fluence (neutron flux × time).

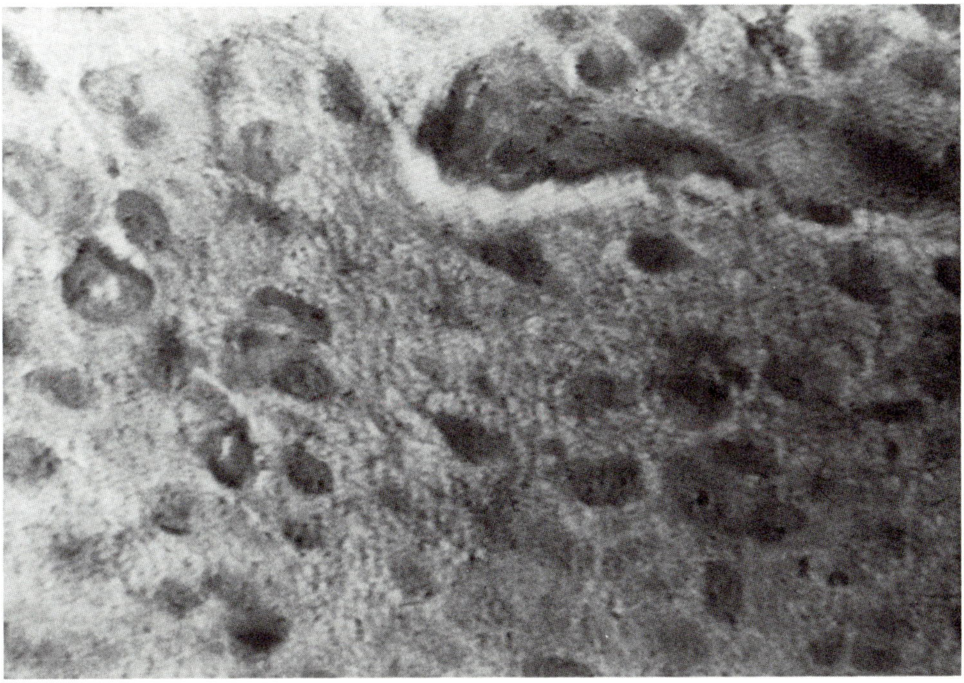

FIG. 4.14. Neutron-induced α-autoradiography. A 52-year-old woman with glioblastoma. α-Tracks (holes) can be seen in tumor tissue. (Courtesy of Dr. K. Amano).

ambulated to the nuclear reactor where the scalp was reopened to appose that part of the brain which harbored the tumor to the thermal neutron collimator. Reflection of the scalp was necessary to prevent a boron-10 neutron-capture reaction in the skin that contained a fairly large amount of boron-10. The scalp was shielded against the neutron beam to avoid skin necrosis, while the brain matter was exposed. After the neutron irradiation, if the neutron fluence delivered to the tumor bed was satisfactorily large, the tumor underwent a gradual degeneration, depending on the amount of neutron capture reaction which was in direct proportion to neutron flux and the boron-10 concentration. If everything went well, a patient could go home within 3 weeks after the first surgical intervention. The infused boron-10 dose was 30–50 mg [^{10}B]/kg of body weight. The boron-10 concentration attained in the tumor at the time of neutron irradiation was 13–60 μg/gm of tumor, while its concentration in the normal brain matter was not measurable.

The neutron flux from Musashi Institute of Technology reactor at its medical port is 1.5×10^9 n/cm^2/sec. The actual flux can vary, depending on the shape of the craniotomy, the shape of the patient's head, and the depth of the tumor bed. The neutron flux delivered to the tumor bed can be improved, despite the rapid attenuation of the thermal neutron, through the use of certain surgical techniques, such as wider exposure of the skull or a larger craniotomy, and with multidirectional irradiation.

Length of survival (counting from the date of the first surgery) and quality of survival (as measured by the performance status scale after Karnofsky) are listed in Table 4.5. The mean length of survival after boron-neutron capture therapy (BNCT) for Grades III to IV glioma patients was 657 (plus) days as of August 1982 and was superior to the conventional photon treatment result of 388 days. Those patients treated by BNCT only after the failure of previous treatments with photon lived 531 days. It should be noted that when BNCT was conducted by the same surgeon who had performed the initial surgical operation, the result was even better, and the mean survival has exceeded 934 days, or 31.1 months. The reasons for better results are: (a) precise topography of tumor; (b) appropriately wide skin flap and craniotomy which warrant large depth dose of neutron flux; (c) good prevention of tumor dissemination; (d) satisfactory recovery of blood circulation which guarantees a good repair of the blood-brain barrier mechanism in the normal brain matter and a satisfactory transport of boron-10 to the tumor. The longest surviving patient is in full working condition, even after 10 years, and is now at the age of 60. The speech disturbance and the right-sided motor weakness which had been noted before BNCT are not recognized.

Similar results were noted with Grade II glioma patients. However, owing to the more benign nature of the tumor, the difference between the BNCT and photon groups was less than in the case of Grades III to IV tumors.

Brain stem tumors (pons-medulla) are clinically more malignant because of the more lethal site of these tumors. Because of the deep location of this tumor and the poor penetration of the thermal neutron, the depth dose of neutron was insufficient to expect a therapeutic effect. However, only in one patient, who was the youngest case in all the BNCT series and, so, had a small head (3 years old), could one expect a rather sufficient depth dose. Despite recurrence after photon radiation, she tolerated the BNCT and survived 5 years without any sign of recurrence.

Twelve patients were autopised after their death. The data will be reported by Hatanaka and are summarized as follows: (a) The causes of death indicate that all patients died from causes irrelevant to neutron capture treatment itself. (b) No brain damage attributable to neutron capture treatment was proved at autopsy, except when the brain had been repeatedly operated on due to recurrence or had been repeatedly radiated. A patient treated with 3 courses of BNCT still did not prove any damage in brain areas that had not been surgically intervened upon;

TABLE 4.5

Mean Survival of Glioma Patients and the Type of Initial Radiotherapy

Tumor / Initial Radiation	Neutron Capture (Nuclear Reactor)	Photon (Cobalt 60/Accelerator) + Chemo-Immuno	Photon (Cobalt 60/Accelerator) + Neutron Capture
Supratentorial Glioma, grades III–IV (68 cases)	>21.9 ± 7.1 mos; Karnofsky 73% (18 cases) >31.1 ± 11.1 mos (10 cases operated on by the same surgeon) 10.4 ± 2.4 mos (8 cases operated on by different surgeons)	12.9 ± 1.6 mos; Karnofsky 56% (41 cases)	17.7 ± 4.1 mos (9 cases)
Supratentorial Glioma, grade II (30 cases)	>46.6 ± 1.4 mos; Karnofsky 92% (5 cases)	>41.2 ± 10.5 mos; Karnofsky 67% (25 cases)	
Pons medulla astrocytoma, Grades II–III/or unverified (21 cases)	8.7 ± 1.5 mos; Karnofsky 45% (4 cases)	8.2 ± 2.2 mos; Karnofsky 39% (16 cases)	60.4 mos; Karnofsky 80% (1 case)

(c) Most of the adequately radiated area of the brain at autopsy did not contain any viable tumor cells. Here "adequately radiated" means that RBE doses of 2000 to 12,000 had been delivered to the tumor cells (cf RBE of 3.7 by Michael Davis). No tumor was confirmed in 3 patients at autopsy. At least 4 of 8 others proved a local cure, excluding 2 cases whose adequately radiated areas were considered premature for evaluation.

One of the problems of BNCT yet to be solved is that thermal neutron attenuates promptly in the brain tissue, with a half-value layer of 1.8 cm. If one can use epithermal neutrons with slightly higher energy that are thermalized after traveling some distance to the brain tissue, tumor cells in the depths of the brain can be destroyed. When a nuclear reactor with facilities for both thermal and epithermal neutrons is available, the scope of treating malignant brain tumors will be enormously expanded.

CHEMOTHERAPY

For remission induction, chemotherapy is not as effective as surgery and/or radiotherapy. Even intraarterial infusion of chemotherapeutic agents, such as BCNU, has rarely achieved the same results as the above-mentioned remission-inducing treatments (11) have at present.

Remission Maintenance

All the initiating treatments described lack the finishing touch unless followed by procedures to maintain the state of remission. Except for total surgical removal, all other initial therapeutic modalities are usually unable to eradicate all neoplastic cells. Therefore, maintenance therapies to keep the induced state of remission or to gradually decrease the number of tumor cells must follow.

For this purpose, at present, the scheduled chemotherapy which decreases the number of tumor cells in a stepwise fashion, and the use of immunopotentiators or interferon, may well be useful.

SCHEDULED CHEMOTHERAPY

There are many chemotherapeutic agents currently available (Table 4.6). None are very effective and free of side effects. Selection of drugs and the design of drug schedules should be based on tumor cell kinetics and the pharmacokinetics of the drugs.

In general, in tumor tissue, one capillary can nourish tumor cells within the distance of 70–150 μm, and tumor cells which proliferate outside of this limit will die because of malnutrition or hypoxia (39). Therefore, in tumor tissue without necrotic area, the distance between two capillaries is thought to be 100–300 μm. An effective cytocidal drug should reach the necessary farthest point from a capillary, and its transportation from

TABLE 4.6
Chemotherapeutic Agents

	Molecular Weight	CCNS[a] or CCS	BBB[a]
1. Alkylating agents			
Cyclophosphamide	279	CCNS	−
Endoxan (Ex)			
Nitrosoureas			
BCNU	214	CCNS	+
CCNU	234	CCNS	+
Methyl-CCNU	248	CCNS	+
Me-CCNU			
PCNU	263	CCNS	+
ACNU	309	CCNS	+
Procarbazine[b] (PCZ)	258	CCNS	+
Imidazol carboxymide[b]			
DTIC, DIC	182	CCNS	+
BIC	279	CCNS	+
Dianhydrogalactitol[b] (DAG)	146	CCNS?	+
2. Antimetabolites			
Methotrexate (MTX)	454	CCS	−
5-Fluorouracil (5-FU)	130	CCS	−
Futraful (FT-207)	200	CCS	+
Cytarabin (Ara-C)	243	CCS	−
3. Antibiotics			
Mitomycin C (MMC)	334	CCNS	−
Bleomycin (BLM)	1550	CCS	−
Daunomycin (DM)	564	CCNS	−
Adriamycin (ADM)	580	CCNS	−
Mithramycin	1084	CCNS	−
4. Plant alkaloids			
Vincristine (VCR)	923	CCS	+
VM-26 (PTG)	657	CCS	+
5. Miscellaneous agents			
Hydroxyurea	76	CCS	+

[a] BBB, blood-brain barrier; +, cross BBB; −, do not cross BBB; CCNS, cell cycle-nonspecific; CCS, cell cycle-specific.
[b] Probable alkylating agent.

the capillary should not be too slow, because the drug may be degraded on its way to the distant target cells. Also, if the affinity of the drug to tumor cells is too large, the drug may be incorporated into the cells nearest to the capillary only and may not travel the distance. All of these factors should be taken into consideration.

Tumor cells infiltrating the normal brain tissue where the blood-brain barrier is still preserved will often be the source of recurrence. Therefore, drugs that readily cross the blood-brain barrier are preferable to drugs which do not cross the blood-brain barrier or do so poorly (21). Hydrophilic drugs, such as methotrexate, 5-FU, procarbazine (PCB), and DAG, have difficulty crossing the blood-brain barrier unless their molecular weight is less than 180 (10). Therefore, most of the above-mentioned drugs do not cross the blood-brain barrier, except for PCB and DAG. In addition, the capillary permeability of these drugs, even if they can cross the blood-brain barrier, is slow, on the order of 1×10^{-5} cm/sec. Consequently, the concentration of hydrophilic drugs in the tumor tissue nearest to the capillaries is high, but that in distant tumor tissue or in the normal brain adjacent to tumor is very low (22).

Lipophilic drugs, such as nitrosoureas, namely, BCNU, CCNU, Me-CCNU (methyl-CCNU), ACNU (also partly hydrophilic), PCNU (also partly hydrophilic), etc., on the other hand, can easily cross the blood-brain barrier, even those of large molecular weight (around 450) (41). The capillary permeability of these drugs is about 1×10^{-4} cm/sec, which is 10 times as rapid as that of hydrophilic drugs (21). These lipophilic drugs are known to distribute evenly in tumor tissue as well as in normal brain tissue (22). The distribution and the diffusion distance of these drugs are influenced by local cerebral blood flow and by the "1-octanol/water partition coefficient" (log P) of the drugs (23). Levin and Kabra (23) found in intracerebral inoculated rat sarcoma 9L that the longest life span was obtained by administration of PCNU, with log P of 0.37. They believed that the optimal log P was this value, and the closer to this value log P of a drug was, the more effective was that drug. Log P of BCNU was 1.53; that of CCNU, 2.83; that of Me-CCNU, 3.30; and that of ACNU was 0.9. In this sense, ACNU which has less toxicity than PCNU, may be worthwhile to use.

These nitrosoureas incur degradation in the body and produce diazonium ions which last only several seconds. Alkylation of tumor DNA is due to the diazonium ions. Therefore, it is desirable that degradation of a drug does not occur until it reaches tumor cells. In this sense, the use of phenobarbital as an anticonvulsant drug in brain tumor patients should be avoided because it is known that phenobarbital enhances degradation of nitrosoureas (24).

As mentioned previously, no malignant glioma is truly homogeneous or truly monoclonal. Even if a tumor were monoclonal at the beginning of therapy, after a small number of drug treatments, the tumor will develop drug resistance, probably by selection or by mutation. Therefore, the combined use of three or four or more drugs is recommended.

Chemotherapeutic agents can also be divided into: (a) the cell cycle-specific or phase-specific drugs which affect only tumor cells in the proliferating pool; and (b) the cell cycle nonspecific drugs which affect cells both in the proliferating and in the nonproliferating pools. To the first group belong antimetabolites such as 6-MP, 5-FU, methotrexate, and vinca alkaloids. The second group comprises alkylating agents and the so-called DNA-binders, namely, adriamycin, daunomycin, bleomycin, etc. (Table 4.6).

Gliomas have small growth fractions (less than 0.3). Therefore the first group is not suitable for their chemotherapy. When drugs of this group are used, they should be administered in combination with drugs of the second group. In the last 5 years or so, the author's group has been using a combination of vincristine, Me-CCNU (or ACNU), and procarbazine with various immunopotentiators every 8 weeks for maintenance chemotherapy of malignant gliomas, as illustrated in Table 4.7. However, the results have been not so satisfactory. The search for new, more effective drugs or their combinations is badly needed.

IMMUNOPOTENTIATORS

Since it is suspected that the cellular immunocompetence of malignant brain tumor patients is deteriorated, certain immunopotentiators should normalize the immunocompetence, suppress the tumor, and contribute to the prolongation of life-span of the patients (38).

Peripheral lymphocyte counts of malignant glioma patients were decreased. The lymphocyte count of benign brain tumor patients showed no significant difference, as compared to that of control healthy adults, however. PPD skin reaction was negative in most cases of malignant brain tumor patients. Seventy-one percent of malignant glioma patients, in contrast to only 33% of benign brain tumor patients, showed a negative reaction.

The lymphocyte counts decreased with progression of the tumor, and they reached their lowest level with anergic PPD skin reaction in the terminal stage. On the contrary, the lymphocyte count was constant or increased with regression of the tumor. The positive PPD skin reaction roughly indicates remission of the tumor.

Serum complement CH 50 level indicates humoral immunity. The range of CH 50 in healthy adults was between 30 and 45 units with positive PPD skin reaction. It increased gradually with progression of

TABLE 4.7

Scheduled Chemotherapy

Day 1:	Vincristine (0.02 mg/kg, iv)
	Me-CCNU (100 mg/m^2, po or ACNU (100 mg/m^2, iv)
Days 2 to 15:	Procarbazine (60 mg/m^2/day, po)
Day 8:	Vincristine (0.02 mg/kg, iv)
Days 1 to 15:	Prednisolone (20 mg/day, po)

This regimen was repeated every 8 wk (with immunopotentiators: BCG (100 mg/wk, po) or Krestin (3.0 gm/day, po) or Picibanil (2–5 KE[a], im)

[a] Biological unit.

the tumor. In cases of malignant glioma patients, it increased to more than the normal range in the advanced stages, and the PPD skin reaction became negative. There was correlation between the immunoparameters of complement and PPD skin reaction, and the clinical grading of glioma patients (Fig. 4.15). With progression of the clinical grading, increased CH 50 level with anergic delayed hypersensitivity skin reaction was demonstrated.

The above results suggest that the general immunocompetence of malignant brain tumor patients is deteriorated and that the repair of the function might introduce a favourable effect on brain tumor therapy. Use of immunopotentiators such as BCG, levamisole, Krestin, and Picibanil should be recommended as adjuncts to the scheduled chemotherapy.

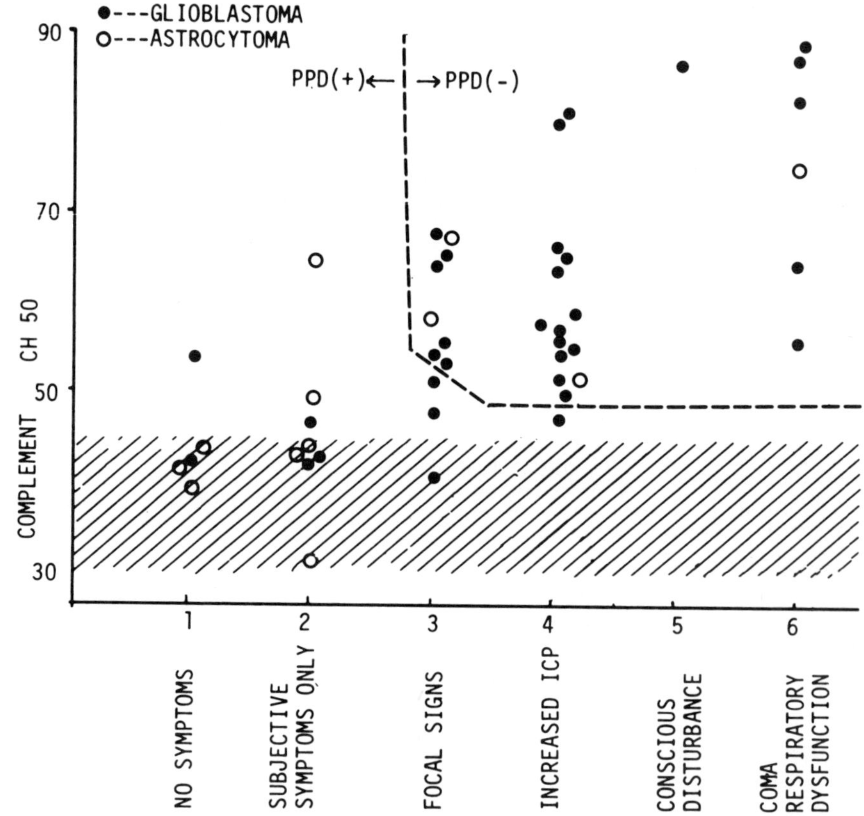

FIG. 4.15. Immunocompetence and clinical grading. (Reproduced with permission from K. Takakura and K. Sano (38).)

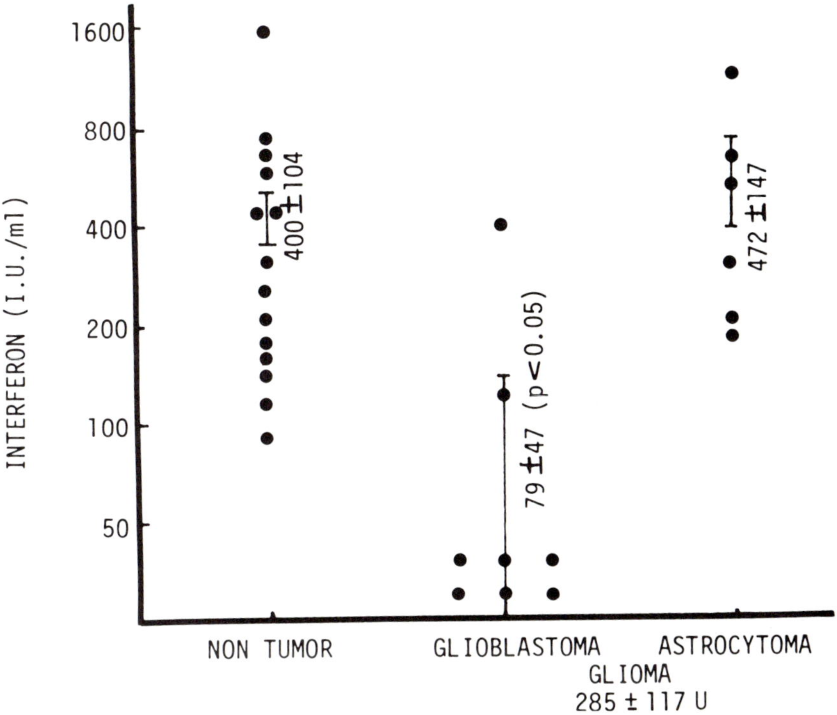

FIG. 4.16. Interferon-producing activity of lymphocyte in glioma patients. (Reproduced with permission from K. Takakura and K. Sano (38).)

INTERFERON

The interferon-inducing activity of lymphocytes under the stimulation of polyriboinosinic acid-polyribocytidylic acid (Poly I/C) *in vitro* was studied in 14 healthy control adults (8 glioblastoma and 6 astrocytoma patients). Interferon activity was 400 ± 104 IU/ml in the control group, and 285 ± 117 IU/ml in the glioma group. It was 79 ± 47 IU/ml in glioblastoma and 472 ± 147 IU/ml in astrocytoma patients. It is noted that the lymphocytes of benign glioma patients continued to produce interferon. Alternatively, the lymphocytes of glioblastoma patients lost most of this capability (Fig. 4.16) (30, 38).

Therefore, administration of Poly I/C or of interferon itself is recommended. In a recent cooperative study (unpublished) of effectiveness of human fibroblast interferon (HuIFN-β), it was demonstrated that about 22% of cases with gliomas (glioblastoma and malignant astrocytoma, 42; medulloblastoma, 7; other gliomas, 5) showed "complete response" or "partial response" (as for the criteria, see above).

Eradication of Neoplastic Cells

If we can maintain the state of remission for a long time, it may be possible to eradicate all neoplastic cells by potentiating the immune and other defense mechanisms of the body during the period. Researches along this line are still in their dawn, but can be expected to be fruitful. The author thinks that *integration* of all of the therapeutic means listed in Table 4.1 is necessary to cure ill-fated patients with malignant gliomas. As mentioned before, there must also be efforts to find a way of *peaceful coexistence with neoplasms.*

To achieve all these, doctors must be *productive* or creative, as old Goethe remarked to Eckermann 1½ centuries ago.

ACKNOWLEDGMENTS

The author is most grateful for the assistance of Drs. Kintomo Takakura, Nobuyuki Shitara, Hiroaki Yamamoto, Yoshihiko Tsujita, Masao Matsutani (University of Tokyo), Hiroshi Hatanaka, Kazuyoshi Amano (Teikyo University), Tako Hoshino (University of California), and many of his former assistants.

REFERENCES

1. Abe, M. ^{10}B compound distribution in rat tissue of transplanted and ethylnitrosourea-induced brain tumors. Fukuoka Acta Medica (Fukuoka), *73:* 250–271, 1982 (in Japanese).
2. Amano, K., and Sweet, W. H. Alpha-autoradiography of ^{10}B compound distribution in tissue by use of superimposition technique. Nippon Acta Radiol. (Tokyo), *33:* 267–272, 1973.
3. Axtell, L. M. Computing survival rates for chronic disease patients. A simple procedure. J.A.M.A., *186:* 1125–1128, 1963.
4. Bagshaw, M. A. Approaches for combined radiation and chemotherapy. Laval Méd., *34:* 124–133, 1963.
5. Bailey, P. *Intracranial Tumors*, Charles C Thomas, Springfield, Ill., 1948.
6. Bouchard, J. Radiation therapy in the management of primary brain tumors. Ann. N. Y. Acad. Sci., *159:* 563–570, 1969.
7. Committee of Brain Tumor Registry. Brain Tumor Registry in Japan, Vol. 4, 1982.
8. Djordjevic, B., and Szybalski, W. Genetics of human cell lines. III. Incorporation of 5-bromo- and 5-iododeoxyuridine into the deoxyribonucleic acid of human cells and its effects on radiation sensitivity. J. Exp. Med., *112:* 509–513, 1960.
9. Erikson, R. L., and Szybalski, W. Molecular radiobiology of human cell lines. V. Comparative radiosensitizing properties of 5-halodeoxycytidines and 5-halodeoxyuridines. Radiat. Res., *20:* 252–262, 1963.
10. Fenstermacher, J. D., and Johnson, J. A. Filtration and reflection coefficients of the rabbit blood-brain barrier. J. Physiol. (Lond.), *211:* 341–346, 1966.
11. Greenberg, H. S., Ensminger, W. D., Seeger, J. F., Kindt, G. W., Chandler, W. F., Doan, K., and Dakhil, S. R. Intra-arterial BCNU chemotherapy for the treatment of malignant gliomas of the central nervous system: A preliminary report. Cancer Treat. Rep. *65:* 803–810, 1981.
12. Hatanaka, H., Amano, K., Kamano, S., Tovaryš, F., Machiyama, N., Matsui, T., Fankhauser, H., Hanamura, T., Nukada, T., Kurihara, T., Ito, N., and Sano, K. Boron-neutron capture therapy *vs.* photon beam for malignant brain tumors—12

years' experience. In: *Modern Neurosurgery I*, edited by M. Brock, pp. 122–136. Springer, Berlin/Heidelberg, 1982.

13. Hatanaka, H., and Sano, K. A revised boron-neutron capture therapy for malignant brain tumors. In: *Present Limits of Neurosurgery*, edited by I. Fusek and Z. Kunc, pp. 83–85, Avicenum, Prague, 1972.
14. Hatanaka, H., and Sano, K. A revised boron-neutron capture therapy for malignant brain tumors. Z. Neurol., *204:* 309–332, 1973.
15. Hoshino, T., Barker, M., Wilson, C. B., Boldrey, E. B., and Fewer, D. Cell kinetics of human gliomas. J. Neurosurg., *37:* 15–26, 1972.
16. Hoshino, T., Nomura, K., Wilson, C. B., Knebel, K. D., and Gray, J. W. The distribution of nuclear DNA from human brain-tumor cells. Flow cytometric studies. J. Neurosurg., *49:* 13–21, 1978.
17. Hoshino, T., and Sano, K. Radiosensitization of malignant brain tumours with bromouridine (thymidine analogue). Acta Radiol., *8:* 15–26, 1969.
18. Hoshino, T., Wilson, C. B., Rosenblum, M. L., and Barker, M. Chemotherapeutic implications of growth fraction and cell cycle time in glioblastomas. J. Neurosurg., *43:* 127–135, 1975.
19. Jelsma, R., and Bucy, P. C. The treatment of glioblastoma multiforme of the brain. J. Neurosurg., *27:* 388–400, 1967.
20. Kriss, J. P., Maruyama, Y., Tung, L. A., Bond, S. B., and Révésez, L. The fate of 5-bromodeoxyuridine, 5-bromodeoxycytidine and 5-iododeoxycytidine in man. Cancer Res., *23:* 260–268, 1963.
21. Levin, V. A. Current trends in brain tumor therapy. In: *Multidisciplinary Aspects of Brain Tumor Therapy*, edited by P. Paoletti, M. D. Walker, G. Butti, and R. Knerich, pp. 165–172. Elsevier/North-Holland Biomedical Press, Amsterdam/New York/Oxford, 1979.
22. Levin, V. A., Freeman-Dove, M., and Landahl, H. D. Permeability characteristics of brain adjacent to tumors in rats. Arch. Neurol., *32:* 785–791, 1975.
23. Levin, V. A., and Kabra, P. Effectiveness of the nitrosoureas as a function of their lipid solubility in the chemotherapy of experimental rat brain tumors. Cancer Chemother. Rep., *58:* 787–792, 1974.
24. Levin, V. A., Stearns, J., Byrd, A., Finn, A., and Weinkam, R. J. The effect of phenobarbital pretreatment on the antitumor activity of 1,3-bis(2-chloroethyl)-1-nitrosourea (BCNU), 1-(2-chloroethyl)-3-cyclohexyl-1-nitrosourea (CCNU), and 1-(2-chloroethyl)-3-(2,6-dioxo-3-piperidyl)-1-nitrosourea (PCNU), and on the plasma pharmacokinetics and biotransformation of BCNU. J. Pharmacol. Exp. Ther., *208:* 1–6, 1979.
25. Matsutani, M., and Hoshino, T. Analysis of tumor growth in recurrent malignant gliomas. Brain Nerve, *27:* 277–281, 1975 (in Japanese).
26. Sano, K. Chemo-Radiotherapie der malignen Hirngeschwülste. Therapiewoche, 23, 50: 4939–4946, 1973.
27. Sano, K. Chemo-radiotherapy of malignant brain tumors. *In: Neurological* Surgery. Proceedings of the Sixth International Congress of Neurological Surgery, S Paulo, 1977, edited by R. Carrea and D. Le Vay, pp. 79–87, Excerpta Medica, Amsterdam, 1978.
28. Sano, K., Hoshino, T., and Nagai, M. Radiosensitization of brain tumor cells with a thymidine analogue (bromouridine). J. Neurosurg., *28:* 530–538, 1968.
29. Sano, K., Sato, F., Hoshino, T., and Nagai, M. Experimental and clinical studies of radiosensitizers in brain tumors, with special reference to BUdR-antimetabolite continuous regional infusion-radiation therapy (BAR therapy). Neurol. Med-Chir. (Tokyo), *7:* 51–72, 1965.

30. Sano, K., Shitara, N., and Takakura, K. Interferon productivity of human lymphocytes with the induction of Poly I:C in cases of malignant glioma. Adv. Neurol., *7:* 376–380, 1979.
31. Shiffer, L. M. Personal communication to Hoshino.
32. Schiffer, L. M., Markoe, A. M., and Nelson, J. S. R. Estimation of tumor growth fraction in murine tumors by the primer available DNA dependent DNA polymerase assay. Cancer Res., *36:* 2415–2418, 1976.
33. Sheline, G., Wasserman, T., Wara, W., and Phillips, T. The role of radiosensitizers in therapy of malignant brain tumors. In: *Multidisciplinary Aspects of Brain Tumor Therapy*, edited by P. Paoletti, M. D. Walker, G. Butti, and R. Knerich, pp. 197–208. Elsevier/North Holland Biomedical Press, 1979.
34. Shitara, N., Kohno, T., and Takakura, K. New approach to brain tumour chemoradiotherapy with cellular synchronization by colcemid. Acta Neurochir., *35:* 123–133, 1976.
35. Sinclair, W. Cell cycle dependence of the lethal radiation response in mammalian cells. Current topics. Radiat. Res., *7:* 264, 1972.
36. Sinclair, W. K., and Morton, R. A. Variations in X-ray response during the division cycle of partially synchronized Chinese hamster cells in culture. Nature (Lond.), *199:* 1158, 1963.
37. Sweet, W. H., Soloway, A. H., and Brownell, G. L. Boron-slow neutron capture therapy of gliomas. Acta Radiol., *1:* 114–127, 1963.
38. Takakura, K., and Sano, K. Role of immunopotentiators on brain tumor therapy. In: *Multidisciplinary Aspects of Brain Tumor Therapy*, edited by P. Paoletti, M. D. Walker, G. Butti, and R. Knerich, pp. 223–234, Elsevier/North Holland Biomedical Press, Amsterdam, 1979.
39. Tannock, I. F. The relation between cell proliferation and the vascular system in a transplanted mouse mammary tumor. Br. J. Cancer, *22:* 258–273, 1968.
40. Terashima, T., and Tomach, L. J. Variation in several responses of HeLa cells to X-irradiation during the division cycle. Biophys. J., *3:* 11, 1963.
41. Wright, E. M., and Diamond, J. M. Pattern of nonelectrolyte permeability. Proc. R. Soc. Biol. (Lond.), *172:* 227–271, 1969.
42. Yamamoto, H. Calculated from data of Brain Tumor Registry in Japan, 1981.
43. Yamamoto, H., Shitara, N., Takakura, K., and Sano, K. Recruitment-chemoradiotherapy with VM-26 (Epipodophyllotoxin) of malignant brain tumors. Acta Neurochir. (Suppl.), *28:* 616–618, 1979.

CHAPTER

5

Observations in the Study of T-Lymphocyte Subsets by Monoclonal Antibodies and Flow Cytometric Analysis in Intracranial Neoplastic Disorders

MERVIN P. KRIL, M.D., and MICHAEL L. J. APUZZO, M.D.

INTRODUCTION

The precise mechanism by which the immune response is rendered inadequate in its efforts to halt neoplastic transformation or progression in the host remains enigmatic. Recently, considerable interest has focused on antigen-antibody complexes and their role in the eliciting of T lymphocyte and macrophage subsets which effect immune suppressor mechanisms (1, 12, 23, 24). Over the past two decades a considerable body of data has emerged which indicates that intrinsic tumors of the central nervous system are moderately antigenic and that patients bearing such tumors demonstrate altered cellular competence as well as evidence of humoral responses to their neoplasms (1, 4, 19, 20, 27). Suppressor T cell subsets have been suggested as being one mechanism of immunosuppression in neoplasms of organ systems other than the central nervous system (5, 8), and recent studies have indicated that depressed levels of mitogenic responses are associated with significantly increased levels of suppressor cell activity in malignant glioma patients (3). It is therefore reasonable to postulate that this cellular group might play a role in the emergence of the compromised host status that has been apparent in studies related to immunocompetence in malignant central nervous system tumors. In addition, it is considered that another T cell subset, the helper inducer group, is critical for the emergence of T cells, B cells, and macrophages; regulation of this group is considered to be influenced by the suppressor T subset.

Comprehension of these and other issues concerning the complex interrelationships of immune responses and central nervous system neoplasms indicate that efforts to define T lymphocyte subsets in patients bearing central nervous system neoplasms would be a logical step in elucidation of basic mechanisms of host-tumor interrelationships.

We have employed two recent technological developments in the assessment of T lymphocyte subsets in patients with various types of intracranial neoplasms. The first, monoclonal antibody technique (6, 19), has enjoyed wide use as a means of marking various cellular components in particular and for our purpose phenotype components of T cell subsets; the second, flow cytometric cellular analysis (13), has combined laser technology with computer science to yield an instrument capable of rapidly counting and/or sorting various cell types in a mixed population. The accuracy, reliability, and reproducibility of data using these techniques have made them an ideal methodology to define, phenotypically, T cell subsets (12).

MATERIALS

Fifty-six patients providing material for these studies were recruited from a series of patients with various intracranial tumors treated at the University of Southern California Medical Center (Table 5.1). Preoperative blood samples were obtained following initial computerized tomographic disclosure of a probable neoplastic process and prior to initiation of any pharmacological agent with potential immune impact. Histological confirmation was ultimately obtained in all cases and reviewed by the Director of the Cajal Neuropathology Laboratory.

There were 22 patients with malignant primary intrinsic tumors which were histologically consistent with a diagnosis of malignant astrocytoma or glioblastoma multiforme. Of the 20 patients with primary extrinsic tumors, 10 were diagnosed as meningioma, 6 as pituitary adenoma, and 4 as acoustic neuroma. Seven patients had solitary metastatic cerebral lesions. A final group of 7 patients harbored nonneoplastic central nervous system lesions, including (totals in parentheses): brain abscess (3), intracerebral hemorrhage (2), subacute sclerosing panencephalitis (1), and cysticercosis (1).

TABLE 5.1

Individuals Serving as Sources of Case Material: Peripheral Blood Samples

1. Normal	25
2. Malignant primary intrinsic tumor	22
3. Benign primary extrinsic tumor	20
Meningioma (10)[a]	
Pituitary adenoma (6)	
Acoustic neuroma (4)	
4. Metastatic tumor	7
5. Nonneoplastic CNS	7
Brain abscess (3)	
ICH[b] (2)	
SSPE (1)	
Cysticercosis (1)	

[a] Numbers in parentheses represent number of cases of particular tumor in question.

[b] SSPE, subacute sclerosing panencephalitis; ICH, intracerebral hemorrhage.

Twenty five aged-matched individuals without evidence of either local or systemic disorders served as control donors.

METHODS

Peripheral blood (15 ml) was collected by direct venipuncture into heparinized tubes. This was transferred at room temperature and gently mixed with phosphate-buffered saline (PBS). Ficoll-Paque media (10 ml; Pharmacia Fine Chemicals, Piscataway, N.J.) were layered under the resultant suspension, and then the mixture was centrifuged at 1500 rpm for 25 minutes. The supernatant was discarded, and the buffy coat layer was carefully pipetted into a separate test tube. To this, 15 ml of PBS were added and gently mixed. The suspension was spun at 1800 rpm for 10 minutes. The supernatant was discarded, and the pellet was resuspended in 15 ml of PBS and again washed 2 times with PBS. The final pellet was resuspended in 1 ml of PBS and again washed 2 times with PBS. The final pellet was resuspended in 1 ml of PBS, and a total lymphocyte count was obtained with a hemocytometer. Lymphocyte suspensions were then made up to a final density concentration of 5×10^6 cells/ml.

Lymphocyte cell suspension (200 ml) was placed into each of 3 test tubes, to which 5 microliters of specific reconstituted murine monoclonal antibody (OKT3-total T; OKT4-helper-inducer T; OKT8-suppressor-cytotoxic T; Ortho Pharmaceuticals, Raritan, N.J.) were added to two of them; the third served as a control. These suspensions were mixed well and then incubated in an ice water bath for 30 minutes with gentle agitation applied every 10 minutes. PBS (10 ml) were added to each tube, which was then spun at 40°C at 1500 rpm for 10 minutes. The media was withdrawn and discarded, and the cell pellet was broken by gentle shaking. The wash process was repeated twice. To the resultant cell pellet, 100 microliters of fluorescein-labeled goat anti-mouse serum (Litton Bionetics, Kensington, Md.) was added in a dilution of 1:10 PBS to one tube and 1:20 PBS to the other two tubes. The suspension was reincubated and treated as the lymphocyte monoclonal antibody mixture had been. The resultant cell pellet (consisting of T lymphocyte monoclonal antibody and fluorescein-labeled goat anti-mouse serum) was resuspended in 1 ml of PBS, and the various lymphocyte subsets were determined by flow cytometric analysis using a fluorescein-activated cell sorter (Becton-Dickinson, Sunnyvale, Calif.).

RESULTS

The results are summarized in Table 5.2.

In consideration of the total lymphocyte population, *mean normal values* for total T (74% ± 9), helper-inducer T (47% ± 8), and suppressor-cytotoxic T (21% ± 11) were consistent with established norms in other

TABLE 5.2

T-Cell Population and Subsets as Defined by Monoclonal Antibody[a]

Group	Total T (OKT 3)	T Helper-Inducer (OKT 4)	T Suppressor-Cytotoxic (OKT 8)
Normal	74 ± 9	47 ± 8	21 ± 11
Malignant primary intrinsic tumor	56 ± 21	37 ± 17	21 ± 9
Benign primary extrinsic tumor	58 ± 19	43 ± 14	16 ± 7
Metastatic tumor	58 ± 23	51 ± 8	19 ± 5
Nonneoplastic CNS	55 ± 18	42 ± 17	21 ± 11

[a] Numbers represent percentage of total lymphocyte populations.

TABLE 5.3

Statistical Analysis of T-Cell and Subset Data[a]

Group Compared to Normals	T Total (OKT 3)	T Helper-Inducer (OKT 4)	T Suppressor-Cytotoxic (OKT 8)
Malignant primary intrinsic tumor	↓ ($p < 0.01$)	↓ ($p < 0.05$)	NS
Benign primary extrinsic tumor	↓ ($p < 0.01$)	NS	↓ ($p < 0.01$)
Metastatic tumor	↓ ($p < 0.01$)	NS	NS
Nonneoplastic CNS	↓ ($p < 0.01$)	NS	NS
Malignant *vs.* benign	NS	NS	NS

[a] By use of Student *t*-test.

laboratories (12, 17). Mean total T in intrinsic malignant (56% ± 21), extrinsic benign (58% ± 19), metastatic (58% ± 23), and nonneoplastic (55% ± 18) groups were significantly ($p < 0.01$) depressed when compared to normals (student *t*-test; Table 5.3).

In the *malignant* group, mean helper-inducer T values (37% ± 17) were significantly decreased ($p < 0.05$) while suppressor-cytotoxic T values (21% ± 9) showed no alteration from control values.

In the *benign* extrinsic group, suppressor-inducer T values (16% ± 7) were significantly ($p < 0.05$) depressed while helper-inducer T values were unchanged.

No significant alterations in either helper or suppressor populations were observed in either the *metastatic* or *nonneoplastic* groupings.

Control tubes consistently demonstrated values of less than 2% and data obtained by employing two different solutions of goat anti-mouse serum agreed within 5%, thereby providing evidence of adequate biological control in the design of the experiment.

DISCUSSION

In the past, antibodies have proven to be a useful tool in various fields of biology and medicine. However, by the very nature of their preparation, they demonstrated certain limitations in application to various research and clinical problems. These limitations were largely a reflection of lack of "purity" and specificity for "target" antigens. Thus an antibody, as previously prepared, would often cross react with "nontarget" antigens so that bioassays were inconclusive and inconsistent.

One of the first sources of "purified" antibody was that obtained from patients with multiple myeloma. Such sera often demonstrated "monoclonal" peaks containing an antigen-specific antibody. Unfortunately, the antigen, against which the antibody was directed, was more often than not of little primary interest. Thus, immunology awaited the arrival of a means to produce an antibody directed specifically against a "target" antigen.

Such a breakthrough soon occurred consequent to research in the field of genetics. In 1975, Kohler and Milstein (16) developed a culture medium which enhanced the rate of fusing two somatic cells to produce and recover a hybrid. The implications of this to immunologists were readily appreciated. By applying this method to B lymphocytes, it could be possible to produce a lineage of antibody-forming cells, so called "clones," which produced one and only one antibody specific for one antigen. Then by recloning this hybrid, a large quantity of purified antibody would be readily available, the so-called monoclonal antibody, since it was derived from one clone.

The basic technique of preparation is as follows. A mouse is immunized with the desired antigen, given a booster dose, and subsequently splenectomized. Spleen cells thus obtained from the immunized mouse are placed in suspension, then added to mouse myeloma cells which have already been grown in culture. To this resultant mixture, polyethylene glycol is added since it will increase the fusion of cell membranes. This mixture (of "immunized" spleen cells and myeloma cells) is then cultured in HAT medium. HAT, a selective growth media of *H*ypoxanthine, *A*minopterine and *T*hymidine, was developed by Kohler and Milstein and proved to be the major technological breakthrough necessary for mass production of hybridoma clones. Myeloma cells used for the formation of hybridomas are preselected so as to lack the enzyme hypoxanthine phosphoribyl transferase, and hence such "naked" myeloma cells cannot survive in HAT media. Although spleen cells are viable, they fail to grow, so that within 24–48 hours the media consists mainly of actively growing hybridoma cells (16).

Various screening methods are then available to determine which of the hybridomas is producing the desired antibody. Once selectively isolated, the desirable clonal line can be reinjected into a mouse whose ascitic fluid will then contain high levels of monoclonal antibody.

Although an exciting development, clonal production of monospecific antibody is not without its limitations. If the antigen is only weakly immunogenic, fewer clones are produced. As well, the use of human (instead of mouse) cells to produce clones is still relatively new, albeit promising. Hybrids, once formed, may not all be stable in their ability to express antibody, or they may do so only in small amounts. Unfortunately, the very specificity of the monoclonal antibody may limit its use because of an inability to form crystal lattices (necessary for precipitation and agglutination reactions) or an inability to bind complement (which may represent a crucial method of tumorolysis). Notwithstanding the aforementioned limitations of this method, the future of monoclonal antibody production is an exciting one. As a mnemonistic aid, Mitchell has categorized potential uses for monoclonal antibodies as 5 Ds: diagnosis, detection, delivery, destruction, and dissection (22).

By utilizing a panel of monoclonal antibodies it will likely be possible to classify tumors, incontrovertibly, with respect to their histology. Similarly, such a panel might be utilized as a screening method to detect tumor antigen in a patient's serum.

Tumor detection *in vivo* may be enhanced with monoclonal antibodies. Unlike radionuclide markers which localize to areas of inflammation, monoclonal antibodies localize to tumor cells themselves and thus may detect small amounts which would otherwise go unnoticed.

Because of such localization to tumor cells, monoclonal antibodies may serve as a transport vehicle to deliver various tumoricidal agents to precise areas of tumor involvement. Also, use of monoclonal antibodies to effect actual tumor destruction by themselves is currently being studied. In this respect, many problems must be overcome, but the potential for immunomanipulation is exciting. Such manipulation also raises the question, at least theoretically, as to whether the use of monoclonal antibodies for treatment might actually result in immunoenhancement and might thereby increase neoplastic growth.

Dissection of the various cellular elements involved in the immune response may soon be close at hand, since there are already available a wide range of monoclonal antibodies directed against these cells (such as T and B lymphocytes, macrophages, and NK cells).

Thus, by utilizing biotechniques developed in the field of genetics, immunologists now have the means to produce large amounts of monospecific antibody from hybrid cloning. Although not without limitations, this technique proves to have powerful and far-reaching applications both in immunology itself and tumor immunology in particular.

FACS, an eponym for fluorescent-activated cell sorter, represents a remarkable breakthrough in bioengineering and provides researchers with a new and powerful tool which gives rapid, accurate, and reproducible results (13). Derived from the same basic principals as a Coulter counter, it adds further refinements drawn from both laser and computer technology. As a first approximation to its understanding and appreciation, FACS may be thought of as an instrument capable of subserving simultaneous analysis and sorting of viable cellular subpopulations in a given specimen. These functions are achieved by utilizing principles of laser optics as well as computer programming to preselect, count, and sort cells of interest based upon their varied physiochemical parameters (such as size and granularity), as well as degree of fluorescence.

The basic elements of design fundamental to its understanding are: cell transport media, ultrasonic transducer, laser source, detectors, deflecting plates, and the concept of gating.

Cell transport is effected by laminar sheath flow technique which confines cells to the center of the flow of a liquid stream and thereby reduces clogging due to clumps. The diameter of the sheath can be regulated, as well as the flow rate, so that only 1 cell at a time is counted or measured.

The ultrasonic transducer is used for sorting. Basically, it subjects the cell stream to low intensity vertical vibration of 40,000 cps, thereby fragmenting the stream into droplets (40,000/sec) at a short but accurately predetermined distance.

A laser is used as a light source because of its high intensity and monochromatic properties. The beam excites fluorescence from cells (previously labeled with fluorochromes) as they traverse the beam.

Detectors consist of dichroic mirrors and filters which are used to select bands of fluorescence for measurement, as well as photomultiplier tubes which can convert impulses into electronic signals. Detection is usually of two types: (a) Low angle light scatter (0–14°) which is primarily a function of cell size and (b) large angle scatter (90°) or degree of fluorescence. Thus, it is possible to detect, count, and sort cells on the basis of their size and degree of fluorescence.

Deflection plates are electrically charged and can be used to sort cells into various collection containers. Basically, once the cell stream is fragmented by the ultrasonic transducer and the cells have been counted, it is possible, electronically, to set up a "sort signal" which produces an electrical pulse to charge the stream and then deflect the "desirable" cells into appropriate containers.

From studies on controls or known specimens, it is possible to sort cells which meet preselected criteria and therefore fall into a certain region (called a "window") of a particular feature distribution. Therefore, only those cells which meet these criteria (or can pass "through the window") are counted and sorted. Gated analysis combines measurement of light scatter and fluorescence to form a useful "window") of a particular feature distribution. Therefore, only those cells which meet these criteria (or can pass "through the window") are counted and sorted. Gated analysis combines measurement of light scatter and fluorescence to form a useful "window" in two dimensions. For example, it is possible to count cells of a certain size displaying a certain degree of fluorescence.

In practical application of these principles (called pulse processing), it is possible to count total lymphocytes as well as those which fluoresce. By using fluorochromes specific for a particular lymphocyte subset, it is easy to express cellular subpopulations as a ratio or percentage of the total number. Since gating represents a means of combining two parameters it is also possible to obtain frequency distributions of cells with different sizes residing within a population.

The human immune system consists of discrete subsets of T cells that are critical for immune homeostasis. It is the balance between effector and regulator subsets that governs the outcome of antigen triggering (7, 18, 24, 26).

The helper-inducer subset is central for the activation of other T cells, B cells, and macrophages. This inductive influence is regulated by the presence of suppressor T cells that function to activate the inducer subset or, alternatively, the effector population itself. Loss or activation of these subsets leads to a variety of immunologic disorders characterized by autoimmunity or immunodepression. Immunodeficiency may result from either a loss of helper-inducer T cell subsets or a relative activation of the suppressor cell population.

Employing cell surface antigen-specific monoclonal antibody and a fluorescent-activated cell sorter we have observed phenotypic compartments of T lymphocyte lineage in patients with various histological types of central nervous system neoplasia. This combined technique has not been applied to such patients in the past. Normal control values conformed to previously expected norms (12, 19), thus establishing credibility of the technique in our hands. In addition, the observation of general depression of total T cell numbers has been noted by a number of other investigators using alternative techniques (1). The overall interpretation of these data beyond these disclosures is problematical and must be approached with caution.

In the primary malignant group the helper-inducer population was significantly decreased, while the suppressor-cytotoxic subset was unchanged when compared to norms. Although no functional assays were obtained, these data suggest a relative suppressor influence in what has come to be recognized as a potentially critical immunoregulatory balance between helper-inducer and suppressor subsets (12, 24, 25). The helper-inducer subset, considered critical in the emergency of functional components of the effector arm of the immune response, was reduced in percentage related to the total lymphocyte pool.

Gerosa *et al.* (9) have recently observed significantly increased Tg or suppressor cells in the peripheral blood of patients with malignant intracranial gliomas using a Fc-IgG binding technique. However, in this study, Tm or helper cell numbers were approximately those observed in normal controls.

In the extrinsic benign group with the observation of depression of the mean suppressor-cytotoxic values and relative helper-inducer predominance, the data would be consistent with the concept of positive immune influence toward modulation of tumor burden. It is plausible then to entertain the idea of an extratumoral action modulating neoplastic progression along with an intrinsic biological preponderance of retarded cellular activity in benign neoplasms. However, it must be stressed that functional assays are required before such conclusions can be firmly considered.

No apparent alteration in percentages or ratios was observed in the solitary metastatic group. Other considerations may be pertinent to mechanisms of alterations in suppressor activity. Directed against tumor-associated antigen, these suppressor cells may form only a small subgroup of the total suppressor cell population. Thus, despite the lack of gross changes which we observed, a specific group of suppressor cells may prove to be most critical in regulating the response to the tumor itself.

Many models have been suggested which present potential causative initiators of immunosuppression. These include "blocking" antibody antigen complexes, substances, or hormones elaborated by tumor, and suppressor T-cells and macrophages (1). Absolute definition of each of these potential suppressor initiators is essential prior to rational embarcation toward therapeutic endeavors. Regarding suppressor cellular subsets, studies should monitor not only numbers but also functions of various cellular elements involved in the immune response and assays of serum antigen-antibody complexes. Further elucidation of the dynamics of the immune response would be well served by serial studies of various cellular and noncellular parameters involved in host response to tumor antigen. The importance of the dynamic nature of the immune response in relation to alterations in tumor burden and other variables has been stressed in the past (20) and remains a pertinent consideration in our comprehension of host-neoplasm interrelations. Braun *et al.* (3) and Gerosa *et al.* (9) have provided important but limited insight to such processes in a small number of glioma-bearing cases. The development of rapid and easily reproducible techniques which could comfortably be employed in serial fashion to assess the status of the immune system would be of great benefit to the clinician. Such techniques utilizing T-cells are being investigated with neoplastic and other nonneoplastic disorders such as multiple sclerosis, subacute sclerosing panencephalitis, and inflammatory bowel disorders (11, 14, 15, 25). The combination of monoclonal antibody application with flow cytometric analysis allows data retrival within 2 hours after blood samples are obtained, a significant improvement in the time of assay and a reduction in the overall complexity of the technique as compared to other methods. Further refinements of this method would allow a means of monitoring patient response to therapy as well as possibly serving a role in marking tumor recurrence. However, this work must be considered preliminary, with further functional definition required, before strict interpretation of data can be revealed.

SUMMARY

The combination of monoclonal antibody specific for lymphocyte cell surface determinants indicative of T cell subsets and flow cytometric analysis offers a rapid and reliable method for assessment of T cell populations in various states of health and disease. Applications of this technique to patients with various histological types of intracranial neoplasia has indicated:

1. A significant depression of the total T cell population
2. A relative suppressor-cytotoxic predominance in malignant intrinsic neoplasms
3. A relative helper/inducer predominance in benign extrinsic neoplasms.

Application of this rapid assay may offer a practical mode of serial assessment of immune responsivity in intracranial neoplastic processes. Further study with assays of immune complexes and suppressor functions are indicated to define the significance of these observations and to provide a more detailed data base for interpretation of results.

ACKNOWLEDGMENTS

The authors wish to thank John M. Weiner, Dr.P.W., for his statistical analysis of the data and Malcolm S. Mitchell, M.D., for his review of the manuscript.

REFERENCES

1. Apuzzo, M. L. J., Mitchell, M. S. Immunological aspects of intrinsic glial tumors. J. Neurosurg., *55:* 1–18, 1981.
2. Bradstock, K. F., Janossy, G., Pizzolo, G., *et al.* Subpopulations of normal and leukemic human thymocytes: An analysis with the use of monoclonal antibodies. J. Natl. Cancer Inst., *65* (1): 33–42, 1980.

3. Braun, D. P., Penn, R. D., Flannery, A. M. *et al.* Immunoregulatory cell function in peripheral blood leukocytes of patients with intracranial gliomas. Neurosurgery, *10:* 203–208, 1982.
4. Brooks, W. H., Roszman, T. L., Mahaley, M. S., *et al.* Immunobilogy of primary intracranial tumours. II Analysis of lymphocyte subpopulations in patients with primary brain tumours. Clin. Exp. Immunol. *29:* 61–66, 1977.
5. Cobleigh, M. A., Braun, D. P., and Harris, J. E. Quantitation of lymphocytes and T cell subsets in patients with disseminated cancer. J. Natl. Cancer Inst., *64:* 1041–1045, 1980.
6. Diamond, B. A., Yelton, B. A., and Scharff, M. D. Monoclonal antibodies. A new technology for producing serologic reagents. N. Engl. J. Med. *22:* 1344–1349, 1981.
7. Eardley, D. D., Hugenberger, J., McVay-Boudreau, L., *et al.* Immunoregulatory circuits among T-cell sets. I. T-helper cells induce other T-cell sets to exert feedback inhibition. J. Exp. Med., *401:* 1106–1115, 1978.
8. Engleman, E. G., Benike, C., Hoppe, R. T., *et al.* Suppressor cells of the mixed lymphocyte reaction in patients with Hodgkin's disease. Transplantation Proc. *11* (4): 1827–1829, 1979.
9. Gerosa, M. A., Olivi, A., Rosenblum, M. L., *et al.* Impaired immunocompetence in patients with malignant gliomas: The possible role of Tg-lymphocyte subpopulations. Neurosurgery, *10* (5): 571–573, 1982.
10. Gershon, R. K., Mokyr, M. B., and Mitchell, M. S. Activation of suppressor T cells by tumour cells and specific antibody. Nature, *250:* 594–596, 1974.
11. Gupta, S., Malaviya, A. N., Rajogopalan, P., *et al.* Subpopulations of human T lymphocytes. IX. Imbalance of T cell subpopulations in patients with progressive systemic sclerosis. Clin. Exp. Immunol. *38:* 342–347, 1979.
12. Hoffman, R. A., Kung, P. C., Hansen, W. P., *et al.* Simple and rapid measurement of human T lymphocytes and their subclasses in peripheral blood. Proc. Natl. Acad. Sci. USA *77:* 4914–4917, 1980.
13. Horan, P. K., Wheeless, Jr., L. L. Quantitative single cell analysis and sorting. Science, *198:* 149–157, 1977.
14. Huddlestone, J. R., Oldstone, M. B. A. T suppressor (T_g) lymphocytes fluctuate in parallel with changes in the clinical course of patients with multiple sclerosis. J. Immunol., *123:* 1615–1618, 1979.
15. Kay, N. E. Abnormal T-cell subpopulation function in CLL: Excessive suppressor (T_S) and deficient helper (T_H) activity with respect to B-cell proliferation. Blood, *57:* 418–420, 1981.
16. Kohler, G., and Milstein, C. Continuous cultures of fused cells secreting antibody of predefined specificity. Nature, *256:* 495–497, 1975.
17. Kung, P. C., and Goldstein, G. Functional and developmental compartments of human T lymphocytes. Vox Sang, *39:* 121–127, 1980.
18. Kung, P. C., Goldstein, G., Reinherz, E. L., *et al.* Monoclonal antibodies defining distinctive human T cell surface antigens. Science, *206:* 347–349, 1979.
19. LeBien, T. W., and Kersey, J. H. A monoclonal antibody (TA-1) reactive with human T lymphocytes and monocytes. J. Immunol., *125:* 2208–2213, 1980.
20. Mahaley, Jr., M. S., Brooks, W. H., Roszman, T. L., *et al.* Immunobiology of primary intracranial tumors. Part 1. Studies of the cellular and humoral general immune competence of brain-tumor patients. J. Neurosurg., *46:* 467–476, 1977.
21. Menzies, C. B., Gunar, M., Thomas, D. G. T., *et al.* Impaired thymus-derived lymphocyte function in patients with malignant brain tumour. Clin. Neurol. Neurosurg., *82* and *83:* 157–168, 1980.

22. Mitchell, M. S. *Hybridomas in Cancer Diagnosis and Treatment.* Raven Press, New York, 1982.
23. Rao, V. S., Bennett, J. A., Grodzicki, R. L., *et al.* Suppressor T cells induced by soluble immune complexes can adoptively transfer inhibition of cytophilic antibody receptors on macrophages. *Cell. Immunol. 46:* 227–238, 1979.
24. Reinherz, E. L., Schlossman, S. F. Current concepts in immunology. N. Engl. J. Med., *303:* 370–373, 1980.
25. Reinherz, E. L., Weiner, H. L., Hauser, S. L., *et al.* Loss of suppressor T cells in active multiple sclerosis. N. Engl. J. Med., *303:* 125–129, 1980.
26. Rice, L., Laughter, A. H., Twomey, J. J. Three suppressor systems in human blood that modulate lymphoproliferation. J. Immunol., *122:* 991–996, 1979.
27. Roszman, T. I., Brooks, W. H. Immunobiology of primary intracranial tumours. III. Demonstration of a qualitative lymphocyte abnormality in patients with primary brain tumours. Clin. Exp. Immunol., *39:* 395–402, 1980.

II

Congenital Malformations

CHAPTER

6

The Genetics of Congenital Malformations

ALASDAIR G. W. HUNTER, M.Sc., M.D. C.M., F.R.C.P.(C)

Malformations result from intrinsic derangement in embryologic pathways and may occur singly or multiply through a variety of underlying mechanisms that have their origins in genetic and environmental disturbances, acting alone or in concert. Embryologically, multiple malformations may arise in parallel, or as a series of interconnected events, and may present a recognizable pattern or syndrome. The physician has the responsibility to manage patients with malformations to allow for as normal a life as possible, which should include providing the patient or family with sufficient information to make a considered decision regarding future reproduction. A general knowledge of genetics and the information that applies to a particular condition is a prerequisite for the accomplishment of this aim.

In the 1970s we witnessed an explosion of understanding in human and medical genetics, both at the visible chromosomal level, with the advent of refined banding techniques, and at the molecular or gene level, through the application of bacterial endonucleases, DNA probes, and DNA sequencing techniques. While the revolution continues into the 1980s, a 1978 survey found that 50% of physicians who had been in practice for less than 6 years had not had any course in genetics, and 28% of medical schools still had no formal training in genetics (7). Furthermore, whereas certain subspecialties, such as pediatrics, medicine, and neurology, have had a natural affinity with genetics, this has not generally been so for neurosurgery. In McKusick's 1978 edition of *Mendelian Inheritance in Man*, neurology, neuroopthalmology, and mental retardation journals were the three most quoted sources and, whereas 2 neurological journals were among the top 20 most often quoted, there were no neurosurgical journals among the top 31 (22).

In this paper, I plan to review the standard mechanisms involved in the genetic causation and familial transmission of congenital malformations. As human development proceeds there is a continuous process of cell multiplication with the potential for error or change in the genetic material at any stage of cell division, be it DNA replication, meiosis, or mitosis. However, only when the germ cells are involved does the error carry the potential for transmission to the next generation. Genetic abnormalities may result from changes that are visible at the level of the chromosome and thus may involve large groups of contiguous genes, or they may result from changes at the invisible molecular level with one or a few genes involved.

CHROMOSOME ABNORMALITIES

Gametogenesis involves the specialized process of cell division called meiosis by which the chromosome number is halved. The normal complement of 46 chromosomes is comprised of 23 pairs, with one member derived from each parent, which are randomly separated in the first stage of meiosis, giving rise to gametes which have a haploid set of 23 chromosomes. Also, there is exchange of genetic material between the pairs of the same (homologous) chromosomes which align gene for gene during the process. The result is an important reassortment of genetic material from one generation to the next, thereby maintaining the variability of the species. This process of bringing 46 chromosomes together as 23 pairs and then separating the pairs equally into 2 cells which themselves subsequently divide to form 4 cells, each with half the number of chromosomes, is a very imperfect process, and errors occur frequently. The clinically most significant error is the failure of a homologous pair of chromosomes to separate (nondysjunction), thus producing gametes with a deficit or excess of a chromosome. The disordered development that results from this imbalance in genetic material will usually result in miscarriage but can result in the birth of a child with multiple malformations. Chromosomes 21, 18, and 13 are most notable in this regard. As well as these numerical abnormalities, there is also a diverse spectrum of rearrangements that may alter the structure of the chromosomes. If a break occurs in a chromosome, it can rejoin again normally, but it is also possible for a part to be lost altogether or for the "raw" ends to rejoin abnormally, either within itself or with another chromosome which has undergone breakage. In the latter case, material will be exchanged between nonhomologous chromosomes which do not normally pair or exchange material. The requirement of chromosome pairs to be aligned gene for gene during meiosis means that these chromosome exchanges (translocations), and certain other structural rearrangements, will bring nonhomologous chromosomes together at meiosis and thereby may disrupt the balanced separation of chromosomal material into daughter gametes. The result may be deficiency and/or duplication of significant and visible amounts of genetic material and consequent malformation of the embryo (Fig. 6.1*A*). Such structural changes originate as isolated *de novo* events but thereafter may become familial. If chromosome changes arise during early cleavage divisions of the zygote, the result may be

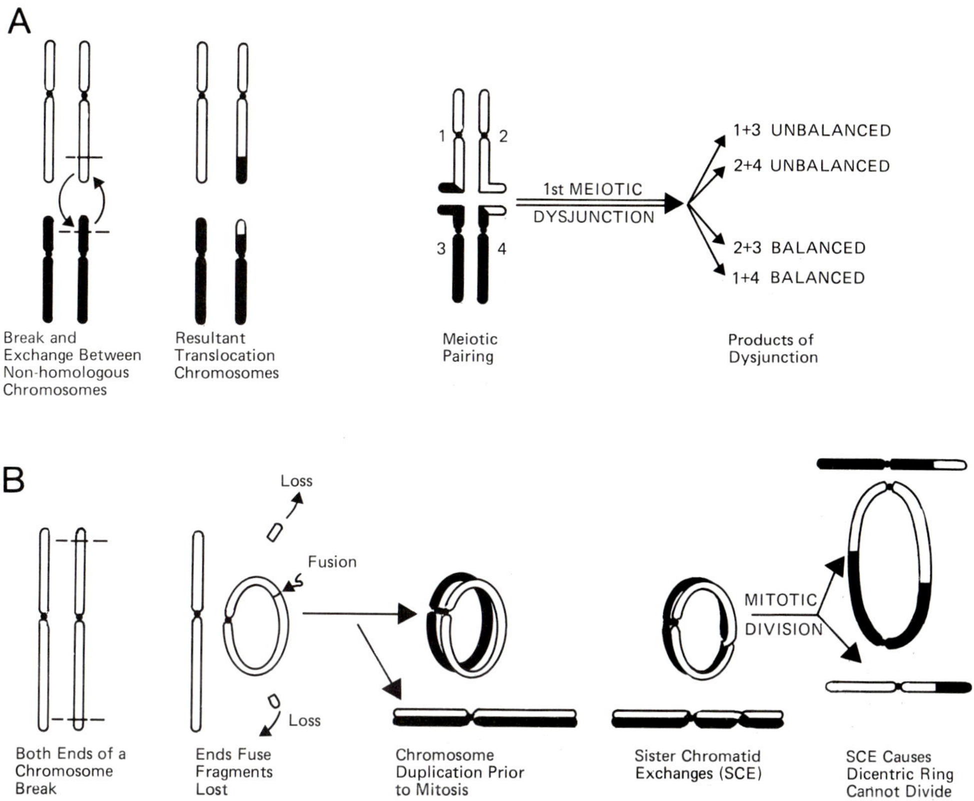

FIG. 6.1. (*A*) Reciprocal translocation. Diagrammatic representation of how the reciprocal exchange of material between a pair of nonhomologous chromosomes requires four chromosomes to align at meiosis and how the process of dysjunction may result in balanced or unbalanced gametes. (*B*) Ring chromosome. Diagrammatic representation of ring chromosome formation illustrating loss of chromosome material and how normal sister chromatid exchange leads to a dicentric ring with consequent abnormalities of dysjunction.

mosaicism, a mixture of cell lines with different chromosome complements derived from the same zygote. Advancing cytogenetic technology has enabled detection of even smaller abnormalities of chromosome position and content (Fig. 6.2), and progress may ultimately be limited only by the resolution of the light microscope.

The underlying mechanism whereby chromosome abnormalities cause congenital malformations is poorly understood. There is now a wide range of recognized patterns of malformations due to deletions or additions of specific chromosome segments (4, 9). However, it is clear that two individuals with the same chromosome abnormality may have a different constellation of malformations. Whatever the pathway involved

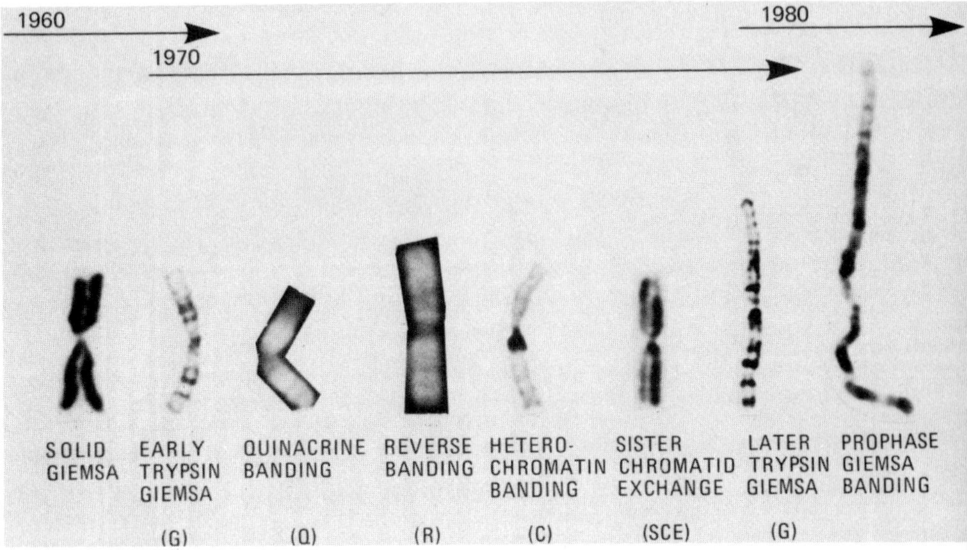

FIG. 6.2. Examples of chromosome no. 1, stained by a number of techniques, illustrating the evolution of cytogenetic technology over the past 2 decades.

in the chromosomal causation of congenital malformations, it is likely that there is interaction with the background susceptibility of the patient to each malformation and with the environment of the individual pregnancy. Conversely, it is clear that a number of different teratogens, be they drugs, chromosome anomalies, or single gene defects, may result in the same abnormality. For example, a variety of different chromosome abnormalities may cause craniosynostosis or holoprosencephaly (Table 6.1). This may result through interference with the same metabolic pathway or through action on different pathways that impinge upon the same embryologic field.

Deletion or duplication of chromosome material might result in the deficiency or excess of one or more enzymes, embryonic inducing substances, or structural proteins. In fact, in a number of instances of chromosome abnormality, the level of activity of an enzyme has been shown to be commensurate with the number of gene copies present (27). This gene-dosage relationship has been used to "map" a number of enzymes to particular chromosome sites (16). Congenital malformations might result from absence of a critical protein at a specific stage of development, or from disturbances in the critical coordination required between embryological events that is disrupted by abnormal levels of enzymes or inducing factors.

By definition, a balanced reciprocal translocation involves the exchange of chromosome material between nonhomologous chromosomes without visible loss of chromosome material; yet, there is evidence of an increased incidence of congenital malformations and retardation in some patients (12). Such developmental abnormalities might occur because of the loss of a technically undetectable chromosome segment, or because the chromosome break occurs through a gene which is rendered nonfunctional, or because the function of a gene is altered by its new location.

An unusual structural abnormality is formation of a ring chromosome. This involves breakage toward each end of a chromosome with loss of the chromosome segment from both of the ends, which then fuse to form a ring (Fig. 6.1*B*). In addition to causing malformations by deletion as described above, it allows for a possible additional interesting mechanism for producing congenital malformations. During somatic cell division (mitosis), sister chromatids, the duplicated chromosome arms that are destined to separate sending half to each daughter cell, may exchange material. This is normally of no consequence. However, in the case of a ring chromosome this type of exchange produces an interlocking of the chromatids so that both end up in one cell or, alternatively, the ring fails to migrate and is excluded from both daughter cells. If the chromosome involved is lethal when trisomic or monosomic, the result is cell death. Thus in an individual whose cells carry a large ring chromosome, cell death might become a significant factor in development. Meiosis can also be disturbed by the presence of a ring chromosome. This may account for some individuals who are small because of reduced cell number and who may be infertile (24, 28).

TABLE 6.1

Different Chromosome Abnormalities that May Result in Craniosynostosis or Holoprosencephaly[a]

Craniosynostosis (8)		Holoprosencephaly (15)	
1q−	Loss of part of long arm	Trisomy 13	Extra No. 13
3q+	Trisomy of part of long arm	Trisomy 18	Extra No. 18
5p−	Loss of part of short arm	Trisomy 21	Extra No. 21
6q+	Trisomy of part of long arm	13q−	Loss of part of long arm
7p−	Loss of part of short arm	18p−	Loss of part of short arm
7p+	Trisomy of part of short arm	r18	Loss from both ends—fuse to ring
9p−	Loss of part of short arm	Triploidy	Extra haploid set
11q−	Loss of part of long arm		
12p−	Loss of part of short arm		
13q−	Loss of part of long arm		
Triploidy total		69 chromosomes (extra haploid set)	

[a] Data in this table emphasize that genes from widely separated chromosomes sites may affect the same developmental pathway.

SINGLE GENE DEFECTS

As we look to the level of the gene, the defect in genetic material is no longer visible, and in most cases its presence must be implied from the characteristic Mendelian patterns of inheritance shown by single gene defects. More recently, it has become increasingly possible to document the presence of an abnormal gene through measurement of its protein gene product or its effect upon the action of bacterial endonucleases (6). An autosomal recessive gene requires that both copies of the gene be abnormal in order for the condition to occur, whereas an autosomal dominant gene requires that only a single abnormal copy be present. In many cases the explanation for this difference may be that autosomal recessive conditions involve enzymatic pathways with a high level of built in redundancy, whereas dominant genes involve structural proteins which have little tolerance for abnormalities of quantity or quality. As of 1978, 30% of 521 definitely established autosomal recessive conditions had an identifiable enzymatic defect (22). However, with few exceptions these established enzyme defects have caused disturbances in specific biochemical pathways and have thus provided ample postnatal clues to direct research. Progress has been slower with autosomal dominant conditions, partly because of the greater difficulty involved in the isolation and assay of structural proteins, and it has been relatively slight with respect to malformations where the gene defect possibly has a transitory expression in the first trimester and where the trail to the abnormal protein is cold by the time of birth. However, exciting progress both in embryology, combining the study of teratogens and mutant genes with the techniques of cell transplantation and scanning electromicroscopy, and in genetics, using a variety of new molecular methods, promises dramatic advances in understanding the pathophysiology of congenital malformations. Important among these has been the ability to use bacterial endonucleases to fractionate DNA at precise sites (25), to then isolate fragments with specific DNA probes (23), and finally to proceed to sequence the DNA base pairs with a facility that was unimagined a decade ago (11). Gradually, a map of these fragments is being constructed; it will be compared with the growing map of known single gene conditions and should eventually allow study of patients and families with specific malformation syndromes. In the interim our knowledge of the functioning and structure of the gene has increased rapidly (Fig. 6.3) and has provided great insight into a number of areas such as the disorders of globin chain synthesis (2). However, rather than attempt to review this rapidly changing area I should like to review some relevant questions that arise in the management of individuals and their families when affected by single gene-mediated congenital malformations.

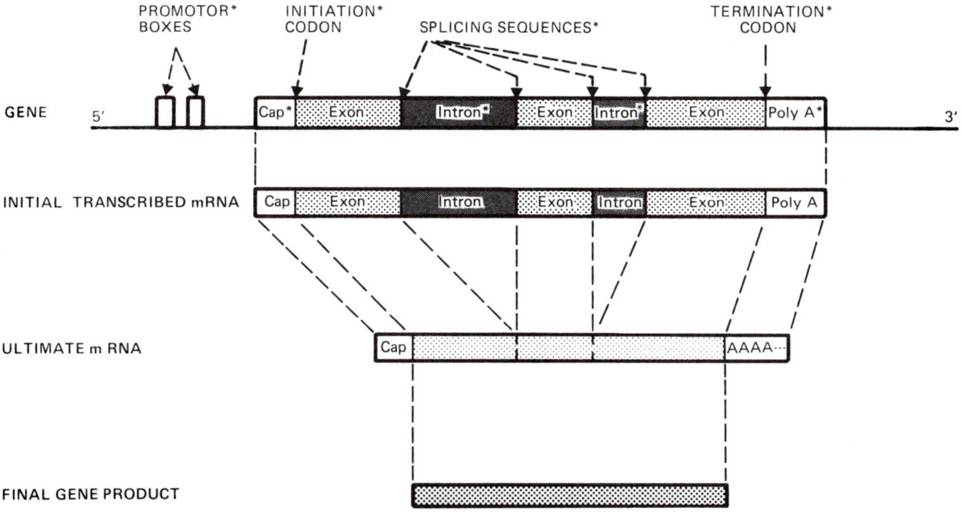

FIG. 6.3. Diagrammatic representation of the current concept of gene structure, emphasizing the several functional components that are not ultimately represented in the protein end product. The *asterisk* indicate the sites, of mutations in codons that would not be represented in the final gene product.

MUTATION AND SELECTION

Just as chromosome nondysjunction was evidence of the inefficiency of cell division, mutation is an ongoing reflection of errors in the copying of the DNA or genome that results in changes in the DNA coding sequence and thus may affect the quality or quantity of the protein gene product. A normal gene of several hundred DNA base pairs in length has many potential sites at which mutation to an abnormal state could occur, whereas to restore normal activity to the abnormal gene there would have to be a precise change at the specific site of the original mutation. Thus we should expect an ever increasing load of abnormal genes in the population. However, the rate of mutation at any one gene is low, and the preponderance of normally functioning genes in the population is maintained by the relatively powerful force of selection. The situation can be envisioned as a "seesaw," and in a stable population a balance is struck between the two opposing forces (Fig. 6.4). As deleterious genes arrive in the population through mutation, they are removed by selection when it acts to prevent the individual from reproducing and therefore contributing his or her genes to the next generation. Thus, a balance is reached wherein the rate at which abnormal genes are lost by selection equals the rate at which they are produced through mutation.

The impact of mutation is particularly visible when a child, with

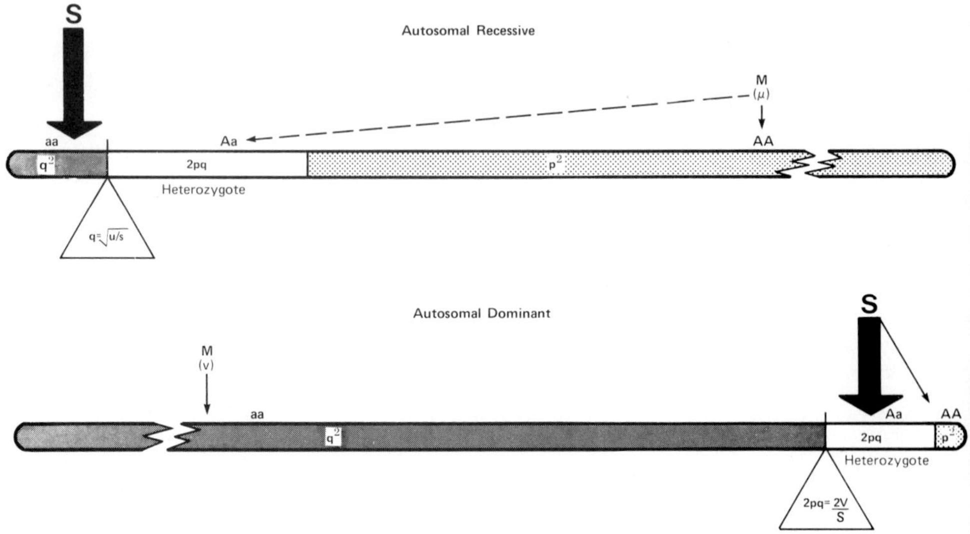

FIG. 6.4. A schematic "see-saw" representation of how the balance between the rate of mutation and force of selection determines gene frequency under conditions of autosomal recessive and autosomal dominant inheritance. The fulcra contain the mathematical expressions of the relationships (see text).

established paternity, is born with an autosomal dominant condition into a family with normal parents. The possibility that a mutation will occur is present with each cell division, and therefore, with increasing paternal age there is a cumulative risk of a germ cell mutation. This is in contrast to the aging ovum, which does not undergo repetitive divisions from puberty but rather remains suspended in first meiotic division and shows an increased risk of nondysjunction with age. A paternal age effect has been established for new mutations in a number of well-known autosomal dominant conditions, including Crouzon craniofacial dysostosis and Apert acrocephalosyndactyly (20).

The majority of abnormal genes are present in the individual together with a normal gene. By common definition such heterozygotes who carry an abnormal dominant gene demonstrate visible phenotypic expression of that gene which is thus exposed to the forces of selection, and sporadic cases can be attributed to a new mutation. This is not so for the sporadic occurrence of an autosomal recessive gene that requires the affected individual to have two defective copies of the gene in question. The likelihood that this homozygosity will arise from the chance mating of two normal but heterozygous ("carrier") parents is far greater than that of either one or both genes arising from a new mutation. For example, the frequency of heterozygotes in the population carrying a single copy of the gene for autosomal recessive Hurler mucopolysaccaridosis is perhaps 1 in 100; thus, 2 heterozygotes would mate by chance with a frequency of 1 in 10,000. This can be compared with the 1 in 10,000,000 chances of a heterozygote parent (1 in 100) mating with a spouse in which one new mutation occurs (1 in 100,000). This distinction between the likelihood of new mutation, with a low recurrence risk, in a sporadic dominant disease *vs.* a heterzygous mating, with a 25% recurrence risk, in a sporadic autosomal recessive case can pose difficult counseling problems where both autosomal recessive and dominant genes cause clinically indistinguishable conditions. X-linked genes may further complicate the picture.

At present we are unable to reduce the frequency of spontaneous mutation, although there is concern that the rate may increase due to greater exposure to irradiation and chemical mutagens from the environment. However, medical intervention can affect the force of selection by enhancing the potential for reproduction in the individual affected with a genetic disease. Thus, a proportion of abnormal genes that would normally be removed from the gene pool would be passed to the next generation, and it is pertinent to ask whether this could have any negative effects. Consider Apert acrocephalosyndactyly where, prior to the advent of modern corrective craniofacial surgery, less than 5% of patients were likely to have reproduced. The improved appearance resulting from surgery may substantially increase the potential for reproduction. Thus, there would be a significant reduction in the impact of selection, thereby increasing the frequency of this abnormal gene in the population and resulting in an increase in the incidence of the syndrome. For demonstration purposes let us assume that 50% of patients with Apert acrocephalosyndactyly now reproduce. For an autosomal dominant condition the balance between mutation and selection is represented by the expression "$H = 2v/s$," where "H" is the heterozygote frequency (disease frequency), "v" is the rate of mutation to the disease, and "s" is the coefficient of selection (10). Assuming a 1 in 100,000 mutation rate for Apert syndrome, the disease frequency would change in the next generation from 1 in 47,500 to 1 in 25,000. I have perhaps exaggerated the impact of treatment for purposes of illustration. It is possible that many patients with treated Apert syndrome, when informed of the 50 percent risk to their children would opt not to reproduce. However, as physicians, we should be aware that as we commit our resources to the treatment and reduction of selection against autosomal dominant diseases, we are committing an even greater proportion of our childrens' resources. For the present, the number of genetic syndromes that can be successfully treated is so small that the true impact on the incidence of malformations and genetic disease can be expected to be negligible for some time yet.

In a dominant disease, selection acts on the heterozygote which essentially represents the disease frequency, and so a change in selection is reflected in an immediate change to the new disease frequency in the next generation. In an autosomal recessive condition, the effect of a similar change in selection coefficient produces a much slower change in the population frequency of the gene because selection only acts on the relatively rare homozygous affected individual and not on the heterozygote carriers who are the major reservoir of the gene (Fig. 6.4). The expression representing the equilibrium among gene frequency (q), mutation rate (u), and selection (s) in this case is $q = \sqrt{u/s}$. The gene frequency (q) has a direct relationship to the frequency of an autosomal recessive disease which is represented by q^2. In this case with the same mutation rate and change in selection as in the Apert example, the disease frequency would go from 1 in 95,000 to 1 in 50,000, but the change would require about 85 generations (10). It is generally considered that changes in gene frequency of this order of magnitude and the relatively small number of abnormal genes involved are of minor importance when compared to the benefits of medical intervention for the affected individual.

Genetic Heterogeneity

Genetic heterogeneity describes a situation wherein what is initially considered to be a single genetic disease or syndrome is found, either on closer clinical scrutiny, pedigree analysis, or biochemical and/or cell studies to result from more than one abnormal gene. At the clinical level, and in the absence of pedigree or biochemical data to support genetic heterogeneity, there is a certain amount of subjectivity in deciding to what degree a condition is heterogeneous, which has led to Dr. McKusick's well known "Lumpers and Splitters" cartoon (21). An awareness that a syndrome may show heterogeneity is of paramount importance when counseling a family if the subtypes or variants of that syndrome have either a different prognosis or a different pattern of inheritance. It is also important to be aware when one is attempting to establish the biochemical basis for a condition, that there may be heterogeneity and that all the cases being studied may therefore not have precisely the same biochemical abnormality.

There are a variety of explanations for genetic heterogeneity. A number of embryological disturbances may converge upon the same malformation. For example, holoprosencephaly might arise from separate gene mutations affecting cell division, adhesion, migration, induction, and survival, whereas the end result of the different mutations would be clinically indistinguishable. Similarly, there could be a number of different genes involved in an embryonic pathway, and while a mutation of any one of them could result in the same syndrome, mutation of different genes would allow for variation in severity or different modes of genetic transmission. For instance one of the genes might be on the X chromosome and therefore might show an X-linked pattern of inheritance. At the molecular level, heterogeneity may arise from different mutations that involve the same gene. A mutation that changes the amino acid sequence of a protein may affect any amino acid. The codon at the site of the same amino acid may undergo different mutations and thus may result in different amino acid substitutions, as in the case at position 6 of the β-globin chain resulting in Hb-S (sickle cell disease) or Hb-C (hemoglobin C disease). Alternatively, different sites (codons) in the gene may be affected, causing amino acid substitution at different positions on the protein. Thus, an enzyme might be affected by mutations that affect either its tertiary structure, active site, cofactor binding site, protein binding site, or degradation rate. For example, Hurler and Scheie syndromes are both mucopolysaccharidoses that involve mutation of the gene for α-iduronidase, but they have quite different clinical features. In fact, as knowledge of gene structure at the DNA level has grown, it has become clear that there are a variety of potential types of mutations that involve codons that are not destined to be represented in the protein gene product but rather affect its transcription, or the translation or processing of the messenger RNA (Fig. 6.3) (2).

On the other hand, spurious heterogeneity may occur because of failure to appreciate the full spectrum and range of variability that a particular condition may show. This is especially true if only a few cases and/or small families are available for study. For example, study of only the right hand side of the pedigree in Figure 6.5 might lead to the diagnosis of familial renal carcinoma; the entire pedigree must be examined in order to establish the diagnosis of Von Hippel-Lindau disease.

Pleiotropy

The variability mentioned in Von Hippel-Lindau disease introduces the phenomenon of pleiotropy, which means that multiple phenotypic or clinical end effects may be the result of only a single gene mutation. This is central to the concept of single gene syndromes wherein multiple malformations, sometimes at distant body locations, occur together. There are a number of explanations for pleiotropy. For instance, as in classic phenylketonuria, a single enzyme defect may result in a cascade of biochemical defects. A deficiency of phenylalanine hydroxylase blocks formation of tyrosine, leading to hypopigmentation; failure to metabolize phenylalanine leads to increased use of other metabolic pathways with the resultant mousey odor due to phenylacetic acid, positive ferric chloride test due to phenylpyruvic acid, and mental retardation through an

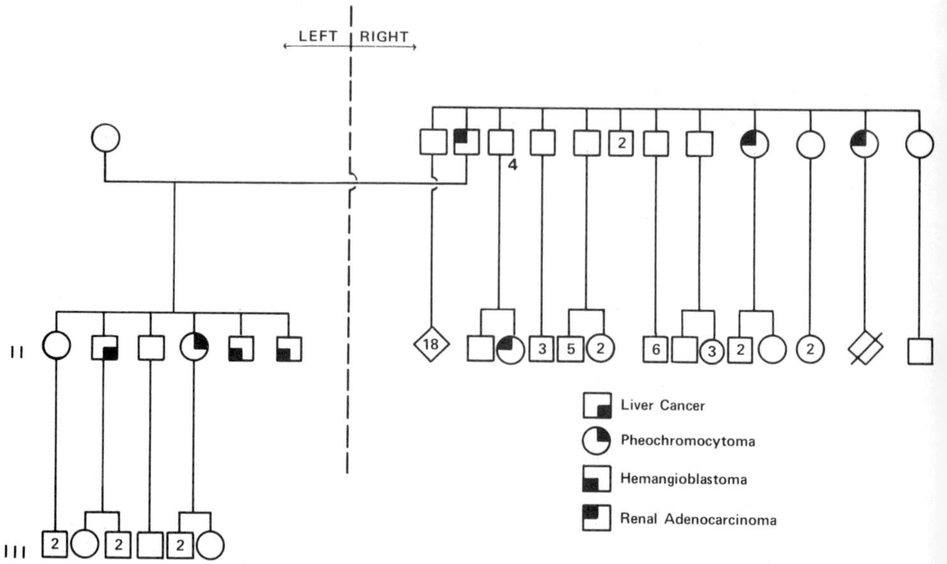

FIG. 6.5. A pedigree of Von Hippel-Lindau disease which illustrates variable expression, lack of penetrance, and pleiotropy, as well as the importance of studying large complete families in order to fully realize the range of variability a condition may show.

as yet poorly understood mechanism. Pleiotropy may also be understood in terms of a structural protein common to more than one tissue or organ. For example, the deficit of Type III collagen in Type IV Ehlers-Danlos syndrome leads to involvement of gut, blood vessels, and skin because that is the normal distribution of Type III collagen (5). These mechanisms may also be operative in the causation of malformation syndromes. Further understanding of the expression of malformations is also coming from advances in embryology and teratology. Thus, we can begin to investigate for a possible common origin of abnormal cells that ultimately arrive at diverse sites in the embryo producing apparently widespread foci of malformations. For example, Waardenburg syndrome includes patchy hypopigmentation of the hair, skin, and iris, deafness, dystopia canthorum, and an increased frequency of cleft lip. Cells derived from the neural crest form a common origin of the pigment cells, the melanosomes of the inner ear, which are involved in the regulation of endolymph, and the frontonasal mesenchyme, which has been shown in an analogous mutation in the mouse (Dancer mutant) to have a decreased level of cellular proliferation (19). Pleiotropy may also arise because different organs develop in closely contiguous areas in the embryo that fall under a common influence. The term developmental field has been applied to this concept, and an example would include the forelimb and kidney, which are both malformed in a number of acrorenal syndromes (29). Although far apart in the newborn, these organs are contiguous in the embryo and thus may be subject to the same disturbance in the embryonic area. Furthermore, their development may be interrelated, as in the production of an inducing substance, so that a mutation affecting one organ might secondarily affect the other.

VARIABLE EXPRESSIVITY

A characteristic of pleiotropic genes, especially those involved in malformation syndromes, is that the actual phenotypic (clinical) expression varies from patient to patient. Rarely, if ever, is a specific malformation pathognomonic of, or necessary for, the diagnosis of a particular syndrome. Not all patients with craniosynostosis and syndactyly have Apert syndrome; not all patients with tuberous sclerosis have intracranial calcification. Causes of variable expression may include environmental influences that vary from gestation to gestation and a differing genetic background that alters an individuals suceptibility to a mutant gene. Interfamily differences may also occur because of true heterogeneity at the level of the gene. For example, those families in which the manifestations of neurofibromatosis are limited to café au lait spots and acoustic neuromas probably have a different gene mutation than those families with the typical more generalized form of the disease (26).

One extreme of variable expression of a gene is no expression at all (nonpenetrance). Thus in Figure 6.5 there is apparent nonpenetrance of the gene for Von Hippel-Lindau disease in the individual (I-4) whose daughter has inherited the gene which is expressed as renal carcinoma. This lack of penetrance presumably shares causes in common with variable expression. However, an assumption of lack of penetrance must not be substituted for an adequate history and evaluation. Furthermore, a failure to appreciate the full spectrum of expressivity of a condition, including its age of onset, or minor expressions of the malformation, could lead to misinterpretation of a pedigree.

Pleiotropy, variable expression, and nonpenetrance are characteristic of the genes responsible for a number of conditions with which neurosurgeons are intimately involved, such as neurofibromatosis (26), tuberous sclerosis (3), Von Hippel-Lindau disease (14), craniosynostosis (8), and seizure disorders (1). Craniosynostosis and seizure disorders are already known to be heterogeneous, that is, they may be caused by a number of different gene mutations, and it is likely that, based on current clinical knowledge and our general experience from the discipline of biochemical genetics, that the others will also be found to be heterogeneous. The importance of knowing the range of variability of a syndrome cannot be overstated when one attempts to provide an accurate prognosis for the individual and family, both in the clinical and genetic sense. One must be aware of the questions to ask, investigations to suggest, and clinical signs to seek. As an example we have found it useful to look for minor dysmorphic features of the hands in an effort to distinguish patients at high risk for genetic transmission of craniosynostosis (17). Unfortunately, in many areas our knowledge is inadequate. For example, does a child with an astrocytoma and 2 café au lait spots and whose mother has 3 café au lait spots have neurofibromatosis? What is the risk that one of the clinically and radiologically normal parents of a child with tuberous sclerosis is a nonmanifestsing carrier of the gene. Fortunately, a number of investigators continue their efforts to resolve these questions (3, 26).

Multifactorial Inheritance

Passing reference was made to the influence of the environment and the individual's background genetic susceptibility as an explanation for the variable expression of a single gene. The concept of multifactorial inheritance, often with a superimposed "developmental time scale" threshold, has been proferred as an explanation for this background liability and for the embryopathology of certain congenital malformations. The most quoted example is that of cleft palate, but the theory can be developed for craniosynostosis. In the general population there is variation in the time of closure of the sagittal suture, but unless the suture closes or shows relatively poor growth well before brain growth has ceased, and thus leads to distortion of skull shape, it can be considered normal variation. Clearly, there are numerous influences, under both genetic and environmental control, that may effect the precise rate of suture growth and time of closure. Thus we can surmise that several genes have an impact upon skull shape and rate of skull growth. The result of the interaction of the various genes will be a distribution curve for the time of suture closure in the general population. The final shape of that curve will also reflect environmental influence (Fig. 6.6). Genes from relatively few different loci are required in order to visualize how a multiplicity of genes, each with a minor effect on the characteristic in question, can produce a range of normal response. For two alternative forms (alleles) of a single gene, "A" and "a," three possible gene combinations (genotypes) will result in the general population, viz., "AA," "Aa," and "aa". Two genes, each with 2 alleles, will give 5, and 3 genes, each with 2 alleles, will give 7 genotype combinations. For purposes of illustration let us assume that all alleles have a population frequency of 0.5. The different genotypes would then have the frequency distributions

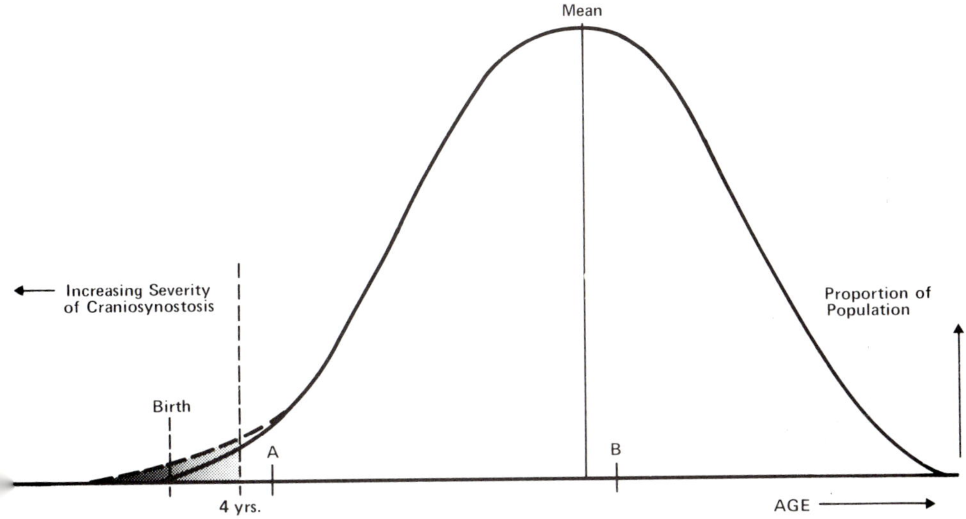

FIG. 6.6. A hypothetical distribution of age at closure of a cranial suture resulting from the interaction of the alleles of a number of genes affecting suture growth with relevant environmental effects. Only those whose suture growth is abnormally slow before brain growth is complete would have an abnormal skull shape. Individual A has a greater susceptibility than individual B to a secondary cause of craniosynostosis. *Dotted area* represents skew due to single major genes such as Apert syndrome.

shown in Figure 6.7. In the same sense that alleles of the gene at the ABO blood locus are responsible for different blood types which, although different and reflecting gene mutation, are not abnormal in the sense of causing a disease, then the different genes affecting suture closure will interact to produce the variation seen in Figure 6.6 without any one gene necessarily having a major enough effect so as to be called an abnormal gene. However, even in the absence of a single gene with a major impact on the time of suture closure, certain individuals may experience such a combination of genetic and environmental factors at the extreme of normal variation that the suture closes early enough to distort skull shape. In the case of sagittal synostosis, such individuals might be expected to come from families with a tendency to relatively reduced growth at this suture, and they might be identifiable by having relatively dolicocephalic parents. Indeed, we have found some support for this possibility through comparing the anteroposterior and lateral skull measurements of parents of children with sagittal synostosis to those of normal controls (18).

A proportion of patients suffering from a wide range of different conditions such as mucopolysaccharidosis, hypophosphatasia, and thal-

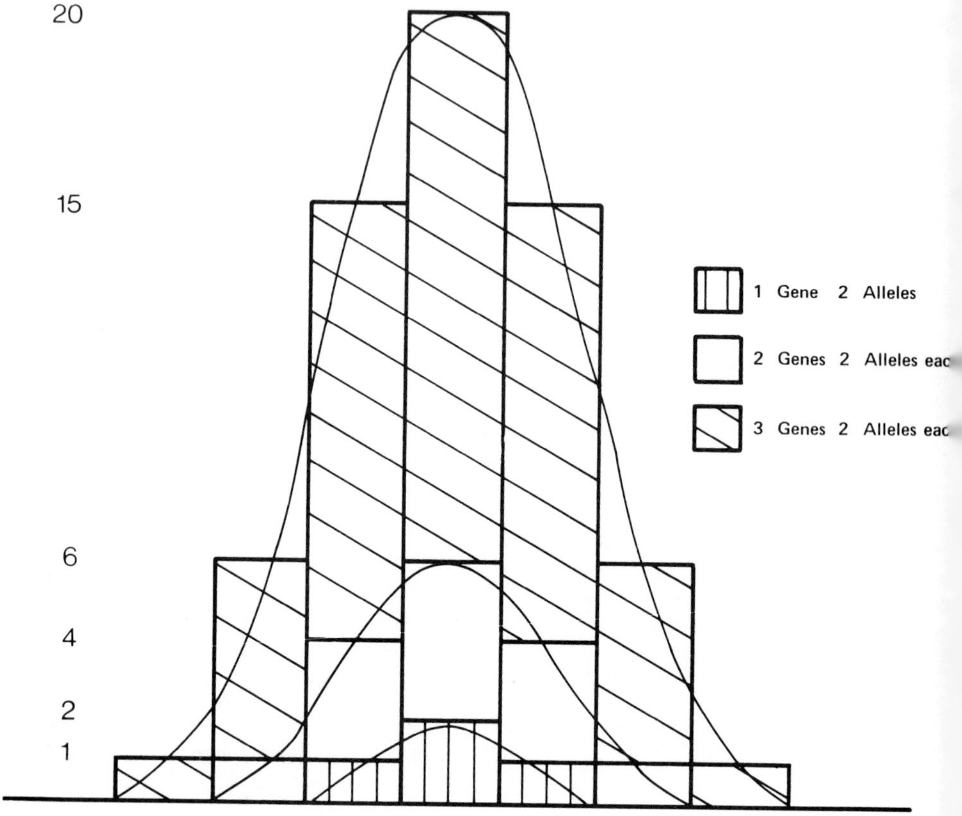

FIG. 6.7. Histogram of genotype frequencies resulting from differing numbers of genes, each of which have two alleles with frequencies of 0.5 in the population. The superimposed curves would result if the gene effects were additive, and the different alleles at each site had similar effects.

assemia may suffer craniostenosis. Consider patients "A" and "B" in Figure 6.6. If hypophosphatasia were to result in a 1-year advance in suture closure, then patient "A" would suffer premature synostosis and "B" would not. Thus the position of the individual on the liability curve, as determined by his or her genetic endowment, modified by the environment, will influence the response to secondary conditions including single major genes that may act on suture closure. Environmental causes, such as *in utero* constraint (13) or dietary rickets, would also act against this overall suceptibility. A further example of the environment interacting against the genetic background is seen in epilepsy, wherein patients who have seizures following trauma or tumor have a higher incidence of relatives with seizures than do controls, and patients who do not have seizures following insults sufficient to produce seizures have relatives with a lower incidence of seizures than in the general population (1).

SUMMARY

In this paper I have attempted to review briefly both how and why visible chromosome and invisible gene abnormalities may cause congenital malformations and syndromes. The causes may represent nonspecific disturbances in the timing of embryologic events or specific effects on a particular tissue, organ, or cell type. Several different biochemical pathways or structural proteins may impinge upon a single or several embryological events; several genes may be involved in a single pathway, and different changes may affect a single gene. The end result of many of these different processes may well be a similar morphological manifestation. An appreciation and understanding of the potential diversity of genetic causes for a malformation, and the wide variation in the phenotypic expression of malformations or syndromes that is typically seen, is essential if one is to provide adequate medical management to patients and their families.

The rapid advances being seen today in the fields of genetics and embryology hold great potential for a true understanding of the developmental biology of, and the ultimate prevention of, congenital malformations.

ACKNOWLEDGMENTS

Thanks to Dr. David Cox for his constructive suggestions and review of the manuscript; to CHEO Media Services for work on the figures; to Linda Pitcher for typing the paper in all its' revisions.

REFERENCES

1. Anderman, E. Multifactorial inheritance of generalized and focal epilepsy. In *Genetic Basis of the Epilepsies*, edited by E. Anderson, W. A. Hauser, J. K. Penry, and C. F. Sing, pp. 355–374, Raven Press, New York, 1982.
2. Benz, E. J., and Forget, B. G. The thalassemia syndromes: Models for the molecular analysis of human disease. Annu. Rev. Med. *33:* 363–373, 1982.
3. Berberich, M. S., and Hall, B. D. Penetrance and variability in tuberous sclerosis. Birth Defects, *15*(5B): 297–304, 1979.
4. Borgaonkar, D. S. *Chromosome Variation in Man. A Catalog of Chromosomal Variants and Anomalies*, Ed. 3. Alan R. Liss, New York, 1980.
5. Byers, P. H., Holbrook, K. A. McGillvray, B., MacLeod, P. M., and Lowry, R. B. Clinical and ultrastructural heterogeneity of type IV Ehlers-Danols syndrome. Hum. Genet., *47:* 141–150, 1979.
6. Chang J. C., and Kan, T. W. A sensitive new prenatal test for sickle cell anemia. N. Engl. J. Med., *307:* 30–31, 1982.
7. Childs, B., Huether, C. A., and Murphy, E. A. Human genetics teaching in U.S. medical schools. Am. J. Hum. Genet., *33:* 11–24, 1981.
8. Cohen, M. M. Craniostenosis and syndromes with craniostenosis: Incidence, genetics,

penetrance, variability, and new syndrome updating. Birth Defects *15*(5B): 13–63, 1979.

9. de Grouchy, J., and Turleau, C. *Clinical Atlas of Human Chromosomes.* John Wiley & Sons, New York, 1977.
10. Falconer, D. S. *Introduction to Quantitative Genetics*, pp. 23–46. The Ronald Press, New York, 1964.
11. Friedman, T. Rapid nucleotide sequencing of DNA. Am. J. Hum. Genet. *31:* 19–28, 1979.
12. Funderburk, S. J., Spence, M. A., and Sparkes, R. S. Mental retardation associated with "balanced" chromosome rearrangements. Am. J. Hum. Genet. *29:* 136–141, 1977.
13. Graham, J. M., de Saxe, M., and Smith, D. W. Sagittal synostosis: Fetal head constraint as one possible cause. J. Pediatr. *95:* 747–750, 1979.
14. Grossman, M., and Melmon K. L. Von Hippel-Lindau disease. In: *The Phakomatoses*, edited by P. J. Vinken and G. W. Bruyn, Chap. 8. American Elsevier, New York, 1972.
15. Gullotta, F., Rehder, H., and Gropp, A. Descriptive neuropathology of chromosome disorders in man. Hum. Genet., *57:* 337–344, 1981.
16. Human Gene Mapping 5. Edinburgh Conference: 5th International Workshop on Human Gene Mapping. Birth Defects, *11*(11): 1979.
17. Hunter, A. G. W., and Rudd, N. L. Craniosynostosis. II. Coronal synostosis: Its familial characteristics and associated clinical findings in 109 patients lacking bilateral polysyndactyly or syndactyly. Teratology, *15:* 301–310, 1977.
18. Hunter, A. G. W., and Rudd, N. L. Craniosynostosis. I. Sagittal synostosis: Its genetics and associated clinical findings in 214 patients who lacked involvement of the coronal suture(s). Teratology *14:* 185–194, 1976.
19. Johnson, M. C. The neural crest in abnormalities of the face and brain. Birth Defects, *11*(7): 1–18, 1975.
20. Jones, K. L., Smith, D. W. Harvey, M. A. S., Hall, B. D., and Quan, L. Older paternal age and fresh gene mutation: Data on additional disorders. J. Pediatr. *86:* 84–88, 1975.
21. McKusick, V. A. On lumpers and splitters, or the nosology of genetic disease. Birth Defects, *5*(1): 23–32, 1969.
22. McKusick, V. A. *Mendelian Inheritance in Man*, ed. 5. The Johns Hopkins University Press, Baltimore, 1978.
23. Miller, W. L. Recombinant DNA and the pediatrician. J. Pediatr., *99:* 1–15, 1981.
24. Moreau, N., and Teyssier, M. Ring chromosome 15: Report of a case in an infertile man. Clin. Genet., *21:* 272–279, 1982.
25. Nathans, D., and Smith, D. H. Restriction endonucleases in the analysis and restructuring of DNA molecules. Annu. Rev. Biochem. *44:* 273–293, 1975.
26. Riccardi, V. M. Neurofibromatosis: Clinical Heterogeneity. Curr. Prob. Cancer, 1982.
27. Rivera, H., Turleau, C., de Grouchy, J., Junien, C., Despoisse, S., and Lucker, J. M. Retinoblastoma—del (13q14): Report of two patients, one with a trisomic sib due to maternal insertion. Gene dosage effect for esterase D. Hum. Genet. *59:* 211–214, 1981.
28. Surama, R. B., Bailey, J. D., and Cohen P. E. A ring chromosome in a patient with normal intelligence and short stature. J. Med. Genet., *8:* 517–521, 1971.
29. Temtamy, S., and McKusick, V. A. *The Genetics of Hand Malformations*, pp. 157–169, 171–172. Alan R. Liss, New York, 1978.

CHAPTER

7

The Embryology and Neuropathology of Congenital Malformations

UROS ROESSMANN, M.D.

There are several crucial steps during development of the central nervous system which are directly related to the most important of the congenital malformations.

Neural induction takes place shortly after gastrulation. The cells that are destined to form neuroepithelium respond to a stimulus from the prospective chordomesoderm, the *inducer*, and begin to form the neural plate. In so doing, this tissue assumes a *potency*, the capability of developing into the highly specialized organ and, at the same time, *determination*, the restriction of the cells' ability to develop into any other tissue. Interference with induction results in a malformed organ, while loss or disruption of any part of the tissue with prospective potency and determination results in loss of the corresponding part of the organ.

Formation of the neural plate is followed within a few days by folding of the plate and then closing of the folds into the neural tube. This fusion begins around the 20th day and is accompanied with the beginning of the segmentation process. Failure of closure, or schisis, results in a large group of clinically important malformations, not only because of their incidence but also because some are amenable to surgical correction. These malformations have excited much interest and study; yet, they remain controversial. The very first question to be answered is whether they are caused by failure of closure of the neural tube or whether the neural tube has closed and later reopened through some factor such as hydrodynamic imbalance within the central nervous system.

The classic example of schisis malformation is myelomeningocele. As the layers of the malformation are examined from the spinal cord, corresponding in form to the neural groove, followed by the open neural arch and covered with highly deficient dermis with the flattened epidermal layer, it is feasible to propose that this condition is primary failure of the neural tube which, in turn, induces failure of the skeletal segments and the mesenchyme surrounding it. Since closure of the caudal neuropore is usually the last event in formation of the neural tube, it is likewise feasible that this should be the event that leads to the malformation.

Embryological studies, however, have shown that the lumbar and sacral segments of the spinal cord are formed from additional growth of the so-called end bud, which continues to grow after the caudal neuropore has closed (5). It is these segments, which arise from the end bud, that are most commonly involved in myelomeningoceles. Thus, primary failure of closure is not the best explanation for the malformation.

Failure of closure of the anterior neuropore should lead to deficient formation of the intracranial portion of the central nervous system. Clinically, this lesion is known as anencephaly. The eyes of all anencephalics are well formed, and the optic nerve can be found up to the point of entry into what should be the cranial cavity. In all anencephalics all of the cranial nerves are formed, although the efferent fibers are missing. Thus, the optic cups must have been formed and the neural crest derivatives must have proliferated uninhibitedly, while the remainder of the neural tube derivatives was destroyed. The anencephalic skull is not only deficient in the membranous portion covering the vault, but also the bones of the base are grossly deficient (6). Also, the amount of brain tissue corresponds directly to the amount of bony development (Fig. 7.1).

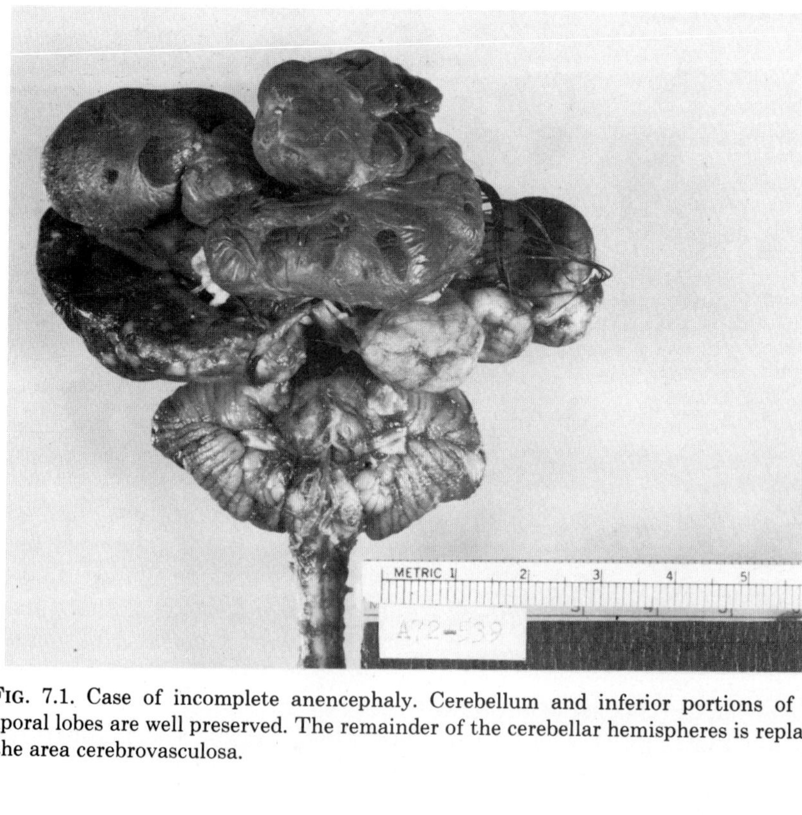

FIG. 7.1. Case of incomplete anencephaly. Cerebellum and inferior portions of the temporal lobes are well preserved. The remainder of the cerebellar hemispheres is replaced by the area cerebrovasculosa.

It is likely that the primary defect in anencephaly is one of skeletal development which, in turn, exposes the central nervous tissue. The lesion is an example of secondary destruction of the prospectively potent tissue through outside forces.

Bifid spinal cords and spines occur in cases in whom the outer coverings are intact. Such lesions are most commonly found in the cervical and thoracic regions and probably represent the purest forms of myeloschisis. The spinal cord shows good organization, with all the neuronal elements and fiber tracts preserved, except the dorsal arches are split and the dorsal columns are positioned laterally. Absence of neural arches usually relates perfectly to the extent of the cord lesion. Such malformations represent a true primary failure of neural tube closure, which induces the skeletal malformation. The malformation does not lead to destruction of tissue, and the organ may function normally despite its altered form; some individuals with such a lesion may grow and develop normally.

The Chiari complex is of greatest clinical interest, and many of its aspects are still puzzling. The changes are of two kinds: (a) myelomeningocele at the caudal end of the neuraxis; (b) the major malformation of the posterior fossa-foramen magnum region. This lesion cannot be fitted into the schisis scheme. Rather than failure of closure of the neural tube, there is a massive shift in the craniocaudal direction of the elements of the brain stem, cerebellum, and spinal cord (Fig. 7.2). Shift is complex and cannot be explained by simple mechanistic theories involving either push from above or pull from below. A recently proposed theory based on embryological observations offers a logical explanation (4). The authors identify the problem as arising during development of the brain cord transition zone, the area of junction between the tissues determined to form rhombencephalon and those that will form the upper segmental structured portion of the spinal cord. A downward shift of the induction for the rhombencephalic portion of the system relative to the mesodermal structures would lead to formation of the brain stem in the spinal canal, rather than being displaced at a later time. Such downward displacement of the transition zone would also lead to a proportionate shift in the neural tube closure, with the resulting defect at the caudal end leading to schisis. This theory is a logical explanation of the entire complex of the malformations, and it is founded on embryological observations.

The second problem with the Chiari malformation is its nomenclature. The lesion complex discussed above is usually called Chiari II (or Arnold-Chiari malformation, although Professor Arnold's contribution was virtually nonexistent). Many cases of less severity are observed clinically and pathologically and are classified as Chiari I. Chiari's original description included a mixed population, and our survey of the literature and of our material led us to propose a new classification (3). The population

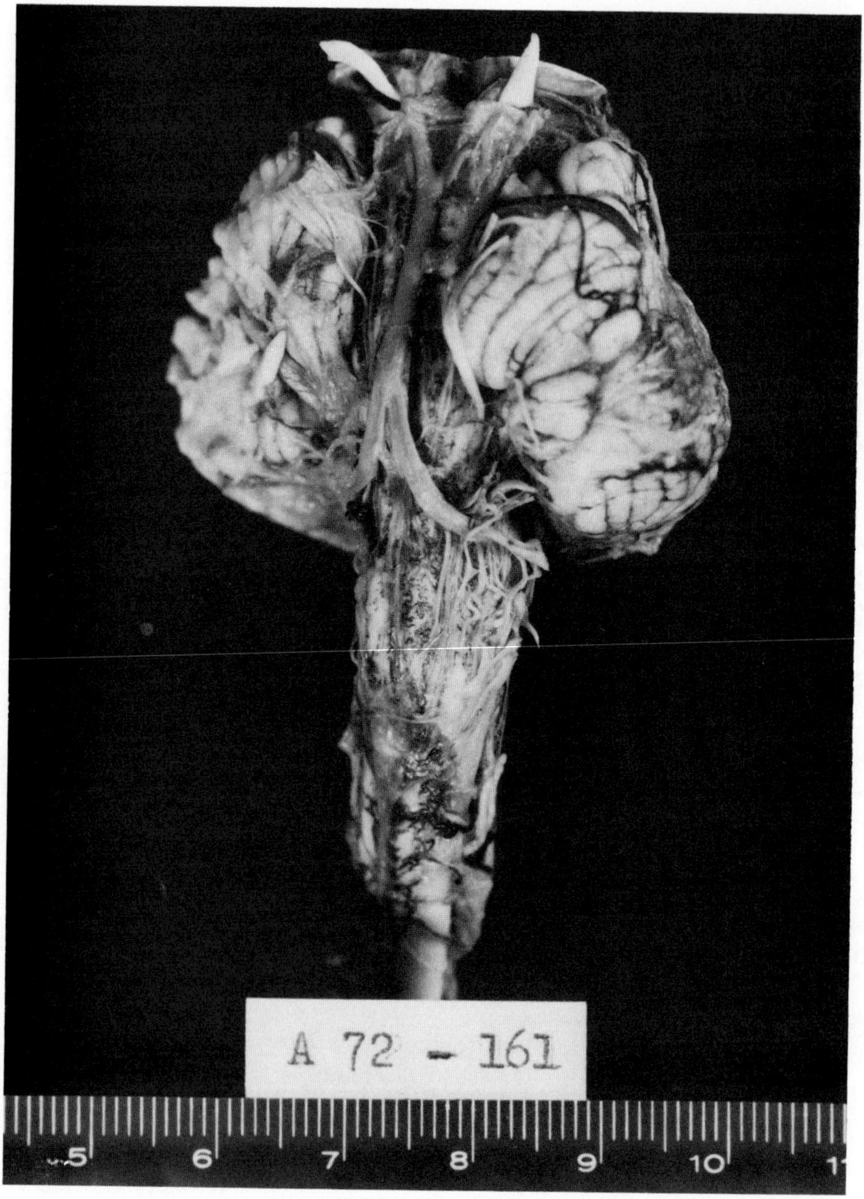

FIG. 7.2. Chiari II malformation. Of note is the elongation of the brain stem. Pons extends to the level of foramen magnum, and the entire medulla oblongata is displaced downward. The upward course of the cranial nerve roots indicates displacement of the stem with regard to the skeletal structures.

falls into two distinct groups, clinically and pathologically. The first is called Adult Chiari Malformation. It is characterized by normal survival of individuals into adult life before the symptoms manifest; anatomic examination discloses downward herniation of the cerebellar tonsils, medulla oblongata, and fourth ventricle (Fig. 7.3). The second group is called Chronic Tonsillar Herniation and shows only cerebellar tonsillar herniation. Neither group shows spinal dysraphism; both are frequently associated with syringomyelia and skeletal malformations such as abnormalities of segmentation and cervicooccipital misalignment (Fig. 7.4). Hydrocephalus is less frequent. Recognition of these two malformations is important, as they respond to simple posterior fossa decompression.

In addition to the dysraphic lesions discussed above, the spinal cord may show two other forms of longitudinal splitting. Diastematomyelia and diplomyelia tend to be confused, and the terms are used in the literature as synonyms. Diastematomyelia refers to splitting of the spinal cord into two distinct halves by an intervening mesodermal band which may occasionally contain bony spicules. It is often one component of the

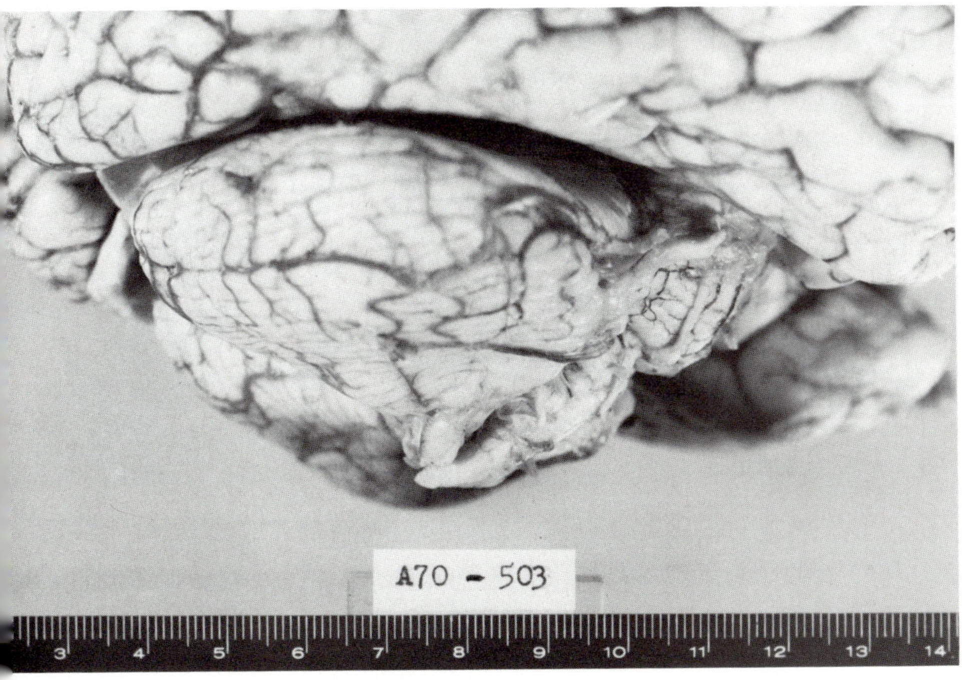

FIG. 7.3. Adult Chiari malformation. The cerebellum is flattened, the tonsils are herniated, and the medulla oblongata is elongated.

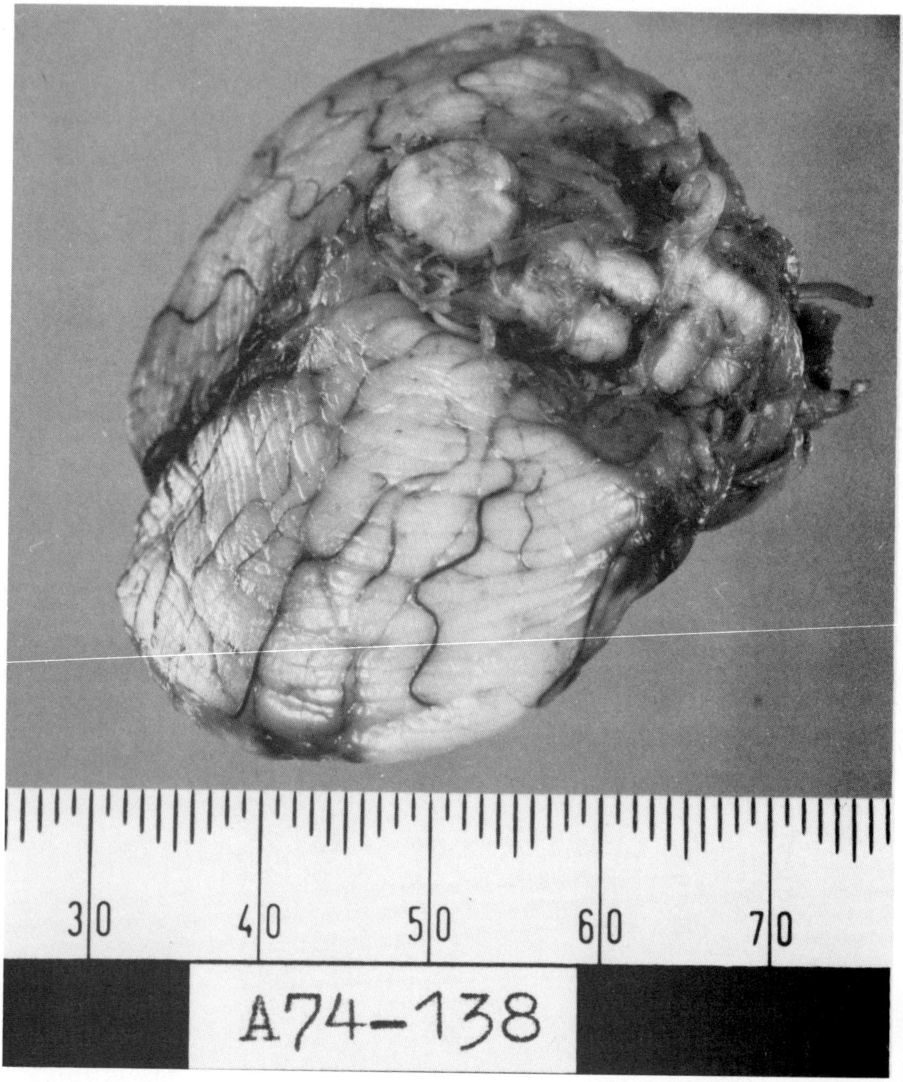

FIG. 7.4. Adult Chiari malformation. Tonsillar herniation is inconspicuous, but there is pronounced anterior angling of the herniated medulla oblongata due to impression from the basilar invagination of the odontoid process.

more complex malformations. Of greater interest are the instances in which the split in the spinal cord is the only change and which become symptomatic during growth of the individual. The problems arise from fixation of the spinal cord within the spinal canal, which continues to grow while the spinal cord "rides up." Early recognition and surgical intervention may be helpful in these cases. The best accepted pathogenetic theory was proposed by Bremer (1): he suggested that a primitive neurenteric canal persists beyond its usual stage and induces splitting of the cord. The frequent occurrence of malformations containing enteric epithelium or teratomas in the region related to malformation supports this theory. Diplomyelia, in turn, means duplication of the spinal cord. Dryden (2) proposed that several mechanisms may be involved, depending on the location of the lesion. In the part of the cord formed through the neural tube formation, two central canals may be formed through infolding of the neural folds, while in the end bud zone several lumina may persist during its neurulation. Since the cells that are to form the spinal cord all arise from the ventricular zone, the presence of two lumina can result in formation of two complete spinal cords. We have examined an unusual case of diplomyelia, in which two complete, side-by-side spinal cords were joined to two medullae in the posterior fossa. In addition, there were two infundibular recesses of the third ventricle, two pituitary stalks, and two complete pituitary glands. All of these structures are directly apposed to the notochord during early development, and it is likely that the malformation in this case resulted through induction from the notochord.

Agenesis of the cerebellar vermis is the last malformation to be included in the schisis group; it results in the so-called Dandy-Walker malformation. This term is used loosely to designate any form of hydrocephalus, involving primarily the 4th ventricle. This may be due to agenesis of the roof or to obstructive lesions such as atresias of the foramina of Luschka and Magendie, or even arachnoid cysts of the cisterna magna.

The second important step in the development of the central nervous system involves separation of the two cerebral hemispheres. The process begins around the 28th day, and the two vesicles are clearly developed by the 31st or 32nd day. Failure of separation results in various malformations, depending on the severity of the lesion. Olfactory tract and bulb aplasia is the finding most common to them. For this reason, the group is called arhinencephaly. More severe abnormalities are holoprosencephaly or unicameral brain; cyclopia is the most severe form. Failure of division is of considerable interest to the geneticists because the lesions are frequently associated with chromosomal abnormalities, although they also occur without evidence of genetic impairment. When these malformations are significant, they are usually not consistent with prolonged survival and therapeutic intervention.

At the same time the hemispheres begin to grow, the tissue between them at the anterior end of the neural tube—lamina terminalis—begins to proliferate and expand backward to eventually form the commissural system. The part particularly involved in formation of the corpus callosum—pars crassa—begins to form after the 38th day; any interference with its growth after this age results in partial or total agenesis of the corpus callosum. Agenesis by itself may not interfere with normal development of the central nervous system function, but it tends to occur in conjunction with a bewildering array of other malformations that can be severely incapacitating (7).

The last group of malformations is called disorders of migration. It consists of interference with gyration, which results in pachygyria or lysencephaly; arrest of migration of potential neurons, which results in heterotopias; and, finally, destruction of the neurons after they have reached the cortex and after formation of polymicrogyria. Most of the neurons that populate the cortex arrive there in two large migratory waves which begin after the end of the second month (8). All these malformations result from damage occurring after this point. It is becoming evident that such damage is usually caused by interference with oxygenation of the growing tissue, either through hypoxemia of the entire brain or through circulatory disturbances in various parts of the cerebral hemispheres. Consensus is developing that this type of malformation and its pathogenetic mechanisms approximate more closely the encephaloclastic type of lesions usually associated with perinatal problems; they should therefore not be classified with other malformations that result from the problems of induction, potency, and determination.

REFERENCES

1. Bremer, J. L. Dorsal intestinal fistula: Accessory neurenteric canal; diastematomyelia. Arch. Pathol., *54:* 132–138, 1952.
2. Dryden, R. J. Duplication of the spinal cord: A discussion of the possible.
3. Friede, R. L., and Roessmann, U. Chronic tonsillar herniation. An attempt at classifying chronic herniations at the *foramen magnum*. Acta Neuropathol. (Berl.), *34:* 219–235, 1976.
4. Jennings, M. T., Clarren, S. K., Kokich, V. G., and Alvord, E. C., Jr. Neuroanatomic examination of spina bifida aperta and Arnold-Chiari malformation in a 130-day human fetus. J. Neurol. Sci., *54:* 325–338, 1982.
5. Lemire, R. J. Variations in development of the caudal neural tube in human embryos (Horizons XIV to XXI). Teratology, *2:* 361–370, 1969.
6. Marin-Padilla, M. Morphogenesis of anencephaly and related malformations. Curr. Top. Pathol. *51:* 145–174, 1970.
7. Parrish, M. L., Roessmann, U., and Levinsohn, M. W. Agenesis of the corpus callosum: A study of the frequency of associated malformations. Ann. Neurol., *6:* 349–354, 1979.
8. Sidman, R. L., and Rakic, P. Neuronal migration with special reference to developing human brain: A review. Brain Res., *62:* 1–35, 1973.

CHAPTER

8

Neural Tube Defects: Clinical Correlations

RONALD J. LEMIRE, M.D.

The concept of neural tube defects (NTD) can be better understood if correlations with known neuroembryological processes are made. Scientific literature in recent years has tended to include many lesions within the term NTD, even though they may be unrelated when approached from the viewpoint of pathogenesis. Clinicians are then confronted with the task of engaging in many decisions with insufficient facts. A clear understanding of basic neuroembryology is key to addressing the lesions found in infants from the neurosurgical and neuropathological aspects. The purpose of this paper is to present the clinical correlations of defects in morphogenesis of the human neural tube. While it is impossible to cover the entire spectrum of neurodevelopmental defects, an attempt will be made to give a framework that the reader can utilize in other areas of interest.

NEURULATION DEFECTS VS. POSTNEURULATION DEFECTS

Neurulation Defects

Separation of NTD into those that arise during the process of neurulation from the postneurulation period is easier when viewed from either pathogenesis or clinical presentation. In humans the process of neurulation encompasses Stages 8 through 12 (Table 8.1), beginning with identification of the neural plate and ending with closure of the posterior neuropore (16, 20, 23). Malformations of the nervous system arising during this period are termed "neurulation defects," and they represent an important component of the spectrum of NTD. While the most severe neurulation defects are incompatible with life they are directly associated with one of the major congenital malformations confronting the neurosurgeon in newborns, the meningomyelocele. Correlation of these defects with the proposed time they arise is shown in Table 8.2.

CRANIORACHISCHISIS

Craniorachischisis (total dysraphism) is the result of nonclosure of the entire neuroaxis. This condition originates in humans during Stages 8

TABLE 8.1
Neurulation in Human Embryos

Stage	Event	CR length (mm)	Age (days)	Somites
8	Neural plate	1.0–1.5	17–19	
9	Neural folds	1.5–2.5	19–21	1–3
10	First fusion	2.0–3.5	22–23	4–12
11	Anterior neuropore closes	2.5–4.5	23–26	13–20
12	Posterior neuropore closes	3–5	26–30	21–19

TABLE 8.2
Timing of Neurulation Defects in Human Embryos

Defect	Events	Stage (s)
Craniorachischisis	Nonfusion of neural folds	8–10
Anencephaly	Nonclosure of anterior neuropore	11
Meningomyelocele	Nonclosure of posterior neuropore	12

through 10, and most such reported specimens undergo early spontaneous abortion. Occasionally, there is survival to term, but stillbirth invariably occurs. Numerous experimental animal models have been reported (12). It is remarkable that some of these specimens have normal appearance except for the head and spine, but numerous internal malformations are usually present.

ANENCEPHALY

When the rostral neuropore (or neural folds) fails to close in Stage 11, the condition of anencephaly occurs (17). Depending upon the extent of nonclosure this may involve the occipital-cervical region (anencephaly with rachischisis), the foramen magnum only (holoacrania), or just the membranous neurocranium (meroacrania). Classification is of little practical value, however, and frequently any dysraphic state involving the head is included under the term anencephaly.

MENINGOMYELOCELE

Meningomyelocele (myelomeningocele, myelocele) arises in Stage 12 of human development if the posterior neuropore fails to close. If the segmental nature of the embryo is correlated with the timing and level, then this probably takes place when the embryo has 25 somites (4 occipital, 7 cervical, 12 thoracic and 2 lumbar). While this count conveniently agrees with the usual site of meningomyelocele, the vertebral segmentation is, of course, much more complex.

Neurulation defects are amenable to prenatal diagnosis. Amniocentesis in the 15th and 16th week of pregnancy should be performed on any woman who has previously had a child with a neurulation defect. α-fetoprotein (AFP) and acetylcholinesterase (ACh) levels in the amniotic fluid are abnormally high at this time if an open neural tube defect is present. Ultrasound can then determine the nature of the defect, and therapeutic abortion can be offered in the event that anencephaly is present.

In contrast to other NTD, those that arise during neurulation do not have an association with known syndromes or other malformation complexes. There is a suggestion that anencephaly may be found occasionally with the holoprosencephaly spectrum (18), but this is unclear (Table 8.3). Epidemiological studies have not clarified the etiology of neurulation defects, although there is a strong association with low socioeconomic conditions (7). Recent work suggests dietary factors may be important, and confirmatory studies are in progress.

TABLE 8.3

Holoprosencephalic Facial Features Found in Human Anencephalics[a]

Facial Type	CNS Feature	Facial Features to Classify	No. of Reported Cases
Cyclotia	Cannot classify type of anencephaly	Median orbit; supraorbital proboscis; ears fused below eye; defects of maxilla	1
Cyclopia	Holocrania with rachischisis	Median orbit; supraorbital proboscis	9
	Cannot classify type of anencephaly		3
Ethmocephaly		Ocular hypotelorism; double proboscis attaches between the eyes	0
Ethmocephaly-like	Meroacrania	Ocular hypotelorism; microphthalmia; unusual nasal structure between eyes	1
Cebocephaly	Holocrania with rachischisis meroacrania	Ocular hypotelorism; single nostril	3
Premaxillary agenesis	Cannot classify type of anencephaly	Ocular hypotelorism; median cleft lip	1
Less severe facial dysmorphism	Meroacrania	Bilateral cleft lip and palate; bilateral iris colobomas	1

[a] Adapted from R. J. Lemire *et al.* (18).

Postneurulation Defects

The clinical presentation of NTD that arises after neurulation is easily recognized in most cases if the lesion is covered with skin. As with neurulation defects, the present conditions can be segregated as to whether they involve the craniovertebral axis, the cranium alone, or only the spinal canal.

INIENCEPHALY

Iniencephaly is a fatal malformation complex that involves the head and spine. It consists of severe spinal retroflexion, abnormal enlargement of the foramen magnum, and spina bifida to a considerable degree. When associated with an occipital encephalocele or myelocele, it is called iniencephaly apertus. Numerous accompanying defects can occur, including diaphragmatic hernia, and infants having the condition are usually stillborn. Consideration has been given to an overlap between this condition and Klippel-Feil syndrome (9). There are also suggested features which relate it to a category of neurulation defect called "anencephaly with spinal retroflexion" (Table 8.4). Perhaps more than any other condition, iniencephaly in its varied forms provides the greatest overlap between the open and closed neural tube lesions.

ENCEPHALOCELE

Encephaloceles represent one type of cranial postneurulation NTD. These skin-covered lesions have varied terminology (*e.g.*, meningoencephalocele, encephalocystocele, ventriculocele, encephalocystomeningocele, hydraencephalocele), depending on the neuropathological variations. They are further divided relative to locations such as occipital, parietal, or anterior. When the anterior encephalocele is visible, it is termed "sincipital" and, when not, it is termed "basal" (Table 8.5) (1, 24, 25).

In the United States up to 75% of encephaloceles occur in the occipital region, with the incidence varying between 1 per 2000 and 1 per 5000 live births. This is in contrast to its incidence other countries (*e.g.*, Southeast Asia) where anterior encephalocele is more common. The frequency of encephalocele does not reflect the number of cases referred for neurosurgical considerations. Many encephaloceles are associated with complex malformations which are associated with early death. The large size of some encephaloceles also is a factor in the decision to withhold aggressive treatment. Table 8.6 lists conditions that should be considered when evaluating a patient with an encephalocele and other anomalies (6). It is important that these syndromes be delineated prior to surgical intervention. In most cases where there is an isolated ence-

TABLE 8.4

Similarities between Iniencephaly, Klippel-Feil Syndrome, and Anencephaly (with Spinal Retroflexion)

Malformation	Iniencephaly (Clausus/Apertus)	Klippel-Feil Syndrome	Anencephaly (with Spinal Retroflexion)
General			
Female sex preponderance	+	+	+
Hydramnios	+	(±)	+
Common experimental teratogen	+	0	(+)
Neural			
Myeloschisis	+	(±)	+
Skeletal			
Retroflexion	+	(±)	+
Absent or short neck	+	+	+
Enlarged foramen magnum	+	(±)	(±)
Posterior cervical spina bifida	+	+	+
Anomalies of occipital bone	+	+	(±)
Hypoplasia of cervical vertebrae	+	+	+
Cephalorachidian space	+	(±)	0
Anterior spina bifida	+	0	(+)
Hemivertebrae	+	+	+
Rib anomalies	+	+	+
Enlarged upper extremities	+	(?)	+
Fusion of cervical vertebrae	+	+	+
Visceral			
Adrenal hypoplasia	(±)	(±)	+
Diaphragmatic hernia	+	0	+
Hypoplastic lungs	+	0	+

[a] Adapted from R. J. Lemire *et al.* (16).
[b] Parentheses indicate that condition is not commonly found, but has been reported nonetheless.

phalocele, the infant can undergo a proper period of stabilization anyway and resection performed in a reasoned manner.

SKIN-COVERED SACROCOCCYGEAL LESIONS

The final area of postneurulation NTD that will be discussed encompasses lesions found in the sacrococcygeal region. These also include some more lumbosacral in position but only those that arise after closure of the posterior neuropore in Stage 12 of human embryonic development. That there are approximately 50 different developmental malformations or embryonic tumors (Table 8.7) that arise in this region is not surprising. However, the clinical correlation of these lesions with the neuropathology is better appreciated if one has an understanding of the development of the caudal neural tube.

Following closure of the posterior neuropore in Stage 12, the neural tube continues development by a process different than neurulation. The exact nature of this development is poorly understood in humans, as relatively few descriptive studies have been done (4, 14, 15). The caudal cell mass is a large group of undifferentiated cells that occupies the area formerly marked by the primitive streak. These cells are regarded as totipotent (or pleuripotential), *i.e.*, they can be induced to form many different tissues. In some manner small vacuoles appear, and cells destined to become neural tube orient themselves around these vacuoles. Finally, there is a coalescence of these developing vacuoles into tubular structures which then connect with the rostral neural tube formed by neurulation. This process, termed "canalization" results in many abnormal appearing structures such as duplications, but it is apparently the manner in which the elongation continues into the tail of the embryo between Stages 13 and 20. Over the remainder of the embryonic and fetal periods, much of this area is transformed into the filum terminale by a

TABLE 8.5
Classification of Sincipital and Basal Encephaloceles[a]

	Presentation	Boundaries
Sincipital		
Frontoethmoidal		
Nasofrontal	Midline at root of nose	Cribriform plate of ethmoid Nasal process of frontal Frontal process of maxillary
Nasoethmoidal	One or both sides of nose	Ethmoid Frontal Nasal
Nasoorbital	Superior medial angle of orbital cavity; displaces eye laterally; may be bilateral	Lacrimal Frontal
Interfrontal		
Craniofacial cleft		
Basal		
Sphenoorbital	Enters orbit, causing exophthalmos	Superior orbital fissure
Sphenomaxillary	Pterygopalatine fossa	Superior orbital, then inferior orbital, fissure
Transethmoidal	Anterior nasal fossae	Defect in cribriform plate
Sphenoethmoidal	Posterior nasal fossae	Sphenoethmoidal suture
Sphenopharyngeal	Rhinopharynx; sphenoid sinus	Defect in sphenoid

[a] Adapted from G. Avanzini and G. Crivelli (1) and C. Suwanwela and N. Suwanwela (24).

process called "retrogressive differentiation" (13, 22). Within this latter structure, many ependymal rests can be found, some of which may be clinically significant.

It is reasonable to expect that the above formation of caudal neural tube can in itself result in a large number of malformations (19). In addition to the neural differentiation, the same group of undifferentiated cells are precursors for other structures such as vertebrae, metanephros, and various other tissues in the hindgut region. The marked overlap between tumors and malformations in this region is striking but reasonable when all of the inductive influences in differentiation are considered. Several lesions selected from Table 8.7 are presented to illustrate the diversity that can confront the neurosurgeon.

LUMBOSACRAL LIPOMAS

The spectrum of abnormal deposits of fatty tissue in the lumbosacrococcygeal region is unlimited. Depending on the location and attachments, they range from simple, subcutaneous lipomas to lipomas of the cauda equina, lipomeningoceles, and lipomyelomeningoceles (3, 8, 11). Small deposits of fat underlying an intact skin are often misleading, and many clinicians elect to "follow" their progress rather than to evaluate and refer to the neurosurgeon for resection. The most common lesion in our series involves a fibrous stalk traversing the lumbodorsal fascia and laminal defect to connect with an intraspinal lipoma. The latter can be extradural or intradural, the latter of which may attach to the conus medullaris or be entwined within the cauda equina. Neurological examination may be normal in the infant, but progressive and insidious deterioration can occur with time. This may be due to traction by a tethering effect or direct pressure on nerves as the fatty mass enlarges. Loss of innervation to bowel, bladder, and legs can follow.

Regardless of the size of the superficial lesion, CT scans of the region should be performed early (1–3 months), and in the event there is intraspinal involvement a decompression laminectomy and debulking of fat should be done. When there is involvement with nerve roots, microscopic dissection may be required. In spite of early aggressive therapy, 10–25% of cases still have neurological problems at a later date. This group of patients has a very low incidence of associated anomalies and rostral CNS malformations.

MYELOCYSTOCELE

Skin-covered cystic masses over the lower spine are found in association with cloacal exstrophy and less commonly with the other ventral body defects such as gastroschisis. Myelocystoceles have one or more

TABLE 8.6
Conditions with Encephaloceles

Site(s) of Encephalocele	Condition	Etiology	Associated Features
Occipital	Chemke syndrome	Autosomal recessive	Hydrocephaly, agyria, absent cortical lamination, cerebellar dysgenesis, retinal dysplasia, corneal opacities, cataracts
	Cryptophthalmos syndrome	Autosomal recessive	Extension of forehead skin covers one or both eyes, ear anomalies, notching of the nasal wings, syndactyly of hands and/or feet, genital anomalies
	Dyssegmental dwarfism	Autosomal recessive	Lethal dwarfism; short, broad, tubular bones with metaphyseal widening; accelerated carpal bone maturation; bowing of legs and forearms; short, broad pelvis with widely flared iliac wings; vertebral anomalies; small thorax; cleft palate; micrognathia
	Knobloch syndrome	Autosomal recessive (presumed)	Myopia, vitreoretinal degeneration, retinal detachment, meningocele
	Meckel Syndrome	Autosomal recessive	Polydactyly, polycystic kidneys, holoprosencephaly, microphthalmia, retinal dysplasia, cardiac anomalies, orofacial clefting, ambiguous genitalia, other abnormalities
	Pseudo-Meckel syndrome	t(3p+;)	Arhinencephaly, absent corpus callosum, Arnold-Chiari defect, cleft palate, congenital heart defects, accessory spleen, clubfoot, hammertoes
	von Voss syndrome		Agenesis of corpus callosum, hypoplastic olives and pyramids, phocomelia, urogenital anomalies, thrombocytopenia
	Warfarin syndrome	Warfarin during pregnancy	Nasal hypoplasia, bone stippling, limb shortening, optic atrophy, mental retardation, seizures, hydrocephaly

	Encephalocele-ectrodactyly		Ectrodactyly
	Encephalocele-hemifacial microsomia	Most cases sporadic; some familial	Unilateral dysplastic ear, with tags or pits; unilateral hypoplasia of mandibular ramus; ocular, skeletal, and cardiac defects, anomalies
	Encephalocele-iniencephaly; Klippel-Feil		Iniencephaly apertus, Klippel-Feil anomaly
Occipital frontal	Encephalocele-craniosynostosis		Craniosynostosis; association can occur alone or with other anomalies and syndromes
Occipital parietal	Encephalocele-Dandy-Walker; Arnold-Chiari		Dandy-Walker or Arnold-Chiari malformation
Occipital frontal	Encephalocele-meningomyelocele		Meningomyelocele
Multiple, predominantly anterior	Aberrant tissue band syndrome	Aberrant tissue bands	Constrictions and amputations of digits and limbs, irregular or asymmetric encephaloceles, microcephaly, microphthalmia, bizarre orofacial clefts
Frontal	Frontonasal dysplasia	Most cases sporadic; some familial	Ocular hypertelorism, anterior cranium bifidum occultum, widely set nostrils with lack of elevation of the nasal tip, notching of nostrils
Parietal Transsphenoidal Other	Encephalocele-absent corpus callosum		Absent corpus callosum; optic nerve abnormalities may occur with transsphenoid encephalocele; can occur with various syndromes including holoprosencephaly
Transsphenoidal	Encephalocele		Cleft lip, cleft palate, less commonly oblique facial cleft; common and bizarre orofacial clefts can occur with various syndromes
Transsphenoidal	Encephalocele-hypothalamic-pituitary dysfunction	Presumed embryonic secondary	Different patterns of hypothalamic-pituitary dysfunction; sometimes optic nerve abnormalities; ocular hypertelorism; cleft lip palate

[a] Adapted from M. M. Cohen *et al.* (6).

TABLE 8.7
Tumors and Malformations of the Sacrococcygeal Region

Tumors		Tumors *vs.* Malformations		Malformations and Anatomical Variations		Other	
Aneurysmal bone cyst		Cutaneous nevi	(4)	Atretic meningocele	(2)	Abscess	(2)
Chondroma		Cysts	(1)	Bone malformation other		Aneurysm	
Chondrosarcoma		Epidermal sinus with		than sacrum	(1)	Granuloma	
Chordoma		dermoid cyst	(2)	Conjoined twins			
Endodermal sinus	(1)[b]	Giant hairy nevus	(1)	Diastematomyelia	(5)		
Ependymoma		Hamartoma		Duplication of rectum	(1)		
Fibromatosis	(1)	Hemangioma		Epidermal sinus	(3)		
Fibrosarcoma		Hemangioendothelioma		Meningocele	(5)		
Ganglioneuroma	(1)	Lumbosacral lipoma	(49)	Myelocystocele	(11)		
Giant cell tumor of sacrum		Tail appendage	(4)	Neurenteric fistula			
Glomus tumor		Teratoma in meningo-		Pilonidal sinus	(8)		
Leiomyoma		myelocele		Prune perineum			
Liposarcoma				Sacral agenesis	(2)		
Lymphoma				Sacral anomaly	(5)		
Mesenchymoma				Sacral dimple	(6)		
Myxopapillary ependymoma	(1)			Tight filum terminale			
Neuroblastoma	(1)						
Neurofibroma							
Osteogenic sarcoma							
Paraganglioma							
Reticulum cell sarcoma	(1)						
Rhabdomyosarcoma							
Subcutaneous lipoma	(9)						
Teratoma	(17)						
Wilms' tumor in teratoma							
Totals	32		61		49		2

[a] Adapted from R. J. Lemire and J. B. Beckwith (19).
[b] Number in parentheses is number of tumor cases in this series.

cystic spaces which are in part lined by ependyma and seem to arise within the conus medullaris (2). They are best regarded as a massive localized hydromyelia, perhaps arising from the ventriculus terminalis. Neurological loss frequently accompanies myelocystocele, and rostral CNS anomalies can be a common feature. Unfortunately, only one experimental model (21) exists, and the pathogenesis remains obscure.

EPIDERMAL-DERMAL SINUS AND CYST

The presence of a sinus tract extending from the skin to a dermoid cyst within the spinal canal is another clinical problem confronting the neurosurgeon. These lesions are felt to arise when a tract of epidermal cells follow the neural tube as it separates from the skin. The predilection for lumbosacral and occipital-hindbrain sites is intriguing but unexplained. While cutaneous tracts are found within many caudal lesions, those that connect with dermoid cysts are usually characterized by a small dimple with a surrounding cutaneous hemangioma and possibly a small patch of hair. As with other lesions, a CT scan is helpful in identification of the intraspinal component. No association with syndromes or other CNS malformations is known.

MALFORMED LUMBOSACRAL VERTEBRAE

A variety of vertebral malformations arising from the caudal cell mass can be associated with neurological deficit. Historically these have been referred to the orthopedic surgeon but in some cases of caudal regression syndrome (found in infants of diabetic mothers) there are lumbosacral lipomas in addition to segmentation problems. These infants can have neuromuscular, bowel, and bladder deterioration and should be considered for diagnostic work-up and possible exploration of the lumbar canal. Sacral agenesis without lipoma is more common, and while neurological involvement may be present there is some question as to whether surgical exploration is beneficial.

DIASTEMATOMYELIA

This interesting problem has numerous presentations and associations (5, 10). One of the basic distinctions is whether or not there are separate dural sheaths surrounding each cord. Presumably this would be helpful in delineating whether the duplicated cords have arisen as a primary developmental phenomenon (if lower lumbosacral in position) in that the dura mater is formed by delaminating from the vertebral arch itself. In some cases the intervening septum is characterized as being fibrous, and in other situations a calcified spur separates the cords. Diastematomyelia is associated with other developmental malformations but does not play a major role, except for the neurological compromise that it produces. Diagnosis by anteroposterior radiographs can suggest the diagnosis, and CT scans confirm it when necessary.

SACROCOCCYGEAL TERATOMA

The final example of the numerous clinical lesions that arise out of the postneurulation caudal neural tube is the sacrococcygeal teratoma. This is one of the most fascinating lesions when viewed from the standpoint of its biological behavior. Most occur in females (as high as 9:1 sex ratio), and during the first 3 months after birth about 90% are benign. Many of those that are malignant have only a few foci of neoplastic cells. Unfortunately, if early resection is not accomplished, there is a propensity for malignant transformation such that after about 5–6 months of age, up to 30% can have malignant cells. These tumors are assumed to arise in the presacral region because of their attachment. However, they more commonly present as a cystic mass over the sacrococcygeal region by passing either caudal or lateral to the coccyx. When resected, it is essential that the coccyx be removed, or else there is a significant recurrence of a malignant tumor (even if the original lesion was benign). Reasons for this behavior are poorly understood but because some appear to be papillary adenocarcinomas and resemble choroid plexus, the role of the ependyma rests along the filum terminale (*e.g.*, the coccygeal medullary vestige) should be considered an etiological possibility.

SUMMARY

There are several approaches that can be applied to the analysis of malformations of the CNS. One practical way in making clinical correlations is to divide neural tube defects into those that arise during the period of neurulation and those that arise thereafter. This concept applies to cranial and spinal lesions and makes it possible to interpret clinical findings with embryological events. Malformations of the CNS that arise during the period of neurulation are not covered by skin and can be diagnosed prenatally by amniocentesis. Postneurulation CNS malformations are skin-covered and have differing patterns of associated malformation and etiologies. There is an overlap of the latter group with congenital tumors, and for the most part these malformations are not apt to be diagnosed prenatally.

ACKNOWLEDGMENT

The author is deeply appreciative of the preparation of the manuscript by Donna Neumann.

REFERENCES

1. Avanzini, G., and Crivelli, G. A case of spenopharyngeal encephalocele. Acta Neurochir., *22:* 205–212, 1970.

2. Ballantyne, J. W. *Manual of Antenatal Pathology and Hygiene. II. The Embryo.* New York, William Wood, 1905.
3. Barson, A. J. Symptomless intradural spinal lipomas in infancy. J. Pathol., *104:* 141–144, 1971.
4. Bolli P. Sekundäre Lumenbildungen im Neuralrohr und Ruckenmark menschlicher Embryonen. Acta Anat. (Basel) *64:* 48–81, 1966.
5. Cohen, J., and Sledge, C. G. Diastematomyelia. Am J. Dis. Child., *100:* 257–263, 1960.
6. Cohen, M. M., Lemire, R. J. Syndromes with cephaloceles. Teratology, *25:* 161–172, 1982.
7. Elwood, J. M., and Elwood, J. H. *Epidemiology of Anencephalus and Spina Bifida.* Oxford, Oxford University Press, 1980.
8. Emery, J. L., and Lendon, R. G. Lipomas of the cauda equina and other fatty tumors related to neurospinal dysraphism. Dev. Med. Child Neurol. (Suppl.) *20:* 62–70, 1969.
9. Gilmour, J. R. The essential identity of the Klippel-Feil syndrome and iniencephaly. J. Pathol. Bacteriol. *53:* 117–131, 1941.
10. James, C. C. M., Lassman, L. P. Diastematomyelia: A critical survey of 24 cases submitted to laminectomy. Arch. Dis. Child., *39:* 125–130, 1964.
11. James, C. C. M., Lassman, L. P. *Spina Bifida Occulta: Orthopaedic, Radiological and Neurosurgical Aspects.* London, Academic Press, 1981.
12. Kalter, H. *Teratology of the Central Nervous System.* Chicago, University of Chicago Press, 1968.
13. Kernohan J. W. The ventriculus terminalis: Its growth and development. J. Comp. Neurol., *38:* 107–125, 1925.
14. Kunitomo, K. The development and reduction of the tail bud and of the caudal end of the spinal cord. Contrib. Embryol., *8:* 161–198, 1918.
15. Lemire, R. J. Variations in development of the caudal neural tube in human embryos (Horizons XIV–XXI). Teratology, *2:* 361–370, 1969.
16. Lemire, R. J., Loeser, J. D., Leech, R. W., Alvord, E. C., Jr. *Normal and Abnormal Development of the Human Nervous System.* Hagerstown, Md., Harper & Row, 1975.
17. Lemire, R. J., Beckwith, J. B., Warkany, J. *Anencephaly.* New York, Raven Press, 1978.
18. Lemire, R. J., Cohen, M. M., Jr., Beckwith, J. B., Kokich, V. G., and Siebert, J. R. The facial features of holoprosencephaly in anencephalic human specimens. I. Historical review and associated malformations. Teratology, *23:* 297–303, 1981.
19. Lemire, R. J., and Beckwith, J. B. Pathogenesis of congenital tumors and malformations of the sacrococcygeal region. Teratology, *25:* 201–213, 1982.
20. O'Rahilly, R. Developmental Stages in Human Embryos. Part A. Embryos of the First Three Weeks (Stages 1 to 9). Washington, D.C., Carnegie Institute of Washington, 1973.
21. Shenefelt, R. E. Morphogenesis of malformations in hamsters caused by retinoic acid: Relation to dose and stage of treatment. Teratology, *5:* 103–118, 1972.
22. Streeter, G. L. Factors involved in the formation of the filum terminale. Am. J. Anat., *25:* 1–11, 1919.
23. Streeter, G. L. Developmental Horizons in Human Embryos. Age Groups XI–XXIII. Embryology Reprint, Vol. 2, Carnegie Inst. Wash., Washington, D.C., 1951.
24. Suwanwela, C., and Suwanwela, N. A morphological classification of sincipital encephalomeningoceles. J. Neurosurg., *36:* 201–211, 1972.
25. Warkany, J., Lemire, R. J., Cohen, M. M., Jr. *Mental Retardation and Congenital Malformations of the Central Nervous System.* Chicago, Year Book Mecical Publishers, 1981.

III

Posterior Fossa Tumors in Childhood

CHAPTER

9

Cerebellar Tumors in Children

FLOYD H. GILLES, M.D.

The child who develops the symptoms and signs of a cerebellar tumor carries a prognosis ranging over a wide spectrum of survival; for the two most common tumors he is either likely to survive or likely to die. The neurosurgeon needs to know at the time of the first operation those clinical, neuroradiologic, operative, and histologic features that will allow an intelligent assessment of outcome in order to rationally plan auxillary therapy and to counsel the family.

The *pathology* of a brain tumor, in its broadest sense, starts with the exposure of the child to the significant risk factors that lead to the proliferation of cells we call a tumor. While we glibly use the word "tumor" (implying a singular, local process of enlargement), nervous system neoplasms are often diffuse changes of many cells over a wide region. Once begun, the neoplastic process continues insidiously for an unknown period of time before neural dysfunction appears. Eventually, for cryptogenic reasons, the process makes itself known. When the neoplasm is located primarily in the cerebellum, the usual symptoms and signs and their evolution are all too well known to the neurosurgeon.

At some point the progressive impairment of neurologic function brings the child to the attention of the neurosurgeon. It is important to remember that the onset of clinical symptoms in the child does not necessarily mark the actual beginning of the neoplastic process, but merely the onset of the neurologic dysfunction induced by the process. It may even be that the rapid evolution of neurologic dysfunction may result from some secondary aspect of the tumor, *e.g.*, a cyst occluding outflow from the fourth ventricle. Thus, rapid evolution of neurologic impairment does not always herald the presence of a rapidly growing tumor.

The *pathology* of cerebellar tumors encompasses more than the histology of the tumor. It includes each aspect of the tumor: symptoms and signs indicate the first site or sites of breakdown of neural function; neuroradiologic findings provide one view of location, operative findings (including the border, cyst, location, secondary sites, etc.) a view of the biology, and histologic findings an entirely different view.

The *histology* of the tumor is often used exclusively in estimating the possibility of a good or bad outcome. However, each of the aspects of the pathology mentioned above contributes its facet to the ultimate judgment about potential outcome. Four decades ago Scherer (1) recognized the unfortunate tendency among pathologists to overlook other anatomic features or their clinical expression that constitutes pathology:

> Unfortunately, the slowly increasing custom of neglecting other aspects of gliomas in favor of cytological studies is accompanied by the tendency to violate or neglect facts in favor of preconceived ideas or systems based on the study of isolated aspects of glioma pathology.

The *pathology* of a brain tumor includes the evaluation of all evidence of the development of the tumor.

What is the value of a fragment of a tumor removed at the time of the first surgical prodedure? One often hears the lament that the outcome of the child cannot be evaluated on the basis of the first surgical specimen, as it does not include the entire tumor, that one needs the entire specimen at autopsy to make a statement as to prognosis. However, the histology of the tumor at the time of autopsy may have changed since the time of the operation, may have been modified by reparative reactions to the surgery, or may have been modified by the effects of radiotherapy or chemotherapy. In any case the child's prognosis is clear; he is dead, and information about his longevity cannot be extrapolated directly to living children without two additional pieces of information. To compare the histology of a tumor at autopsy with the histology of a biopsy taken at the time of the first surgical procedure for the purposes of estimating future outcome of a new child with a tumor, the original histology is needed as well as survival information about *all* children with similar tumors at the specific site, not just information about those children who are dead. That is, the clinician and pathologist will learn nothing about the likelihood of encountering those brain tumors that are not lethal. Thus, survival information garnered from autopsy series or from series in which the source of specimens (surgical or autopsy) is not indicated, is unlikely to provide information of prognostic value at the time of the first operation on a new child, at the time when a judgment must be made in order to decide about further intraoperative resection, or, immediately postoperatively, when a judgment must be made about the kind and amount of auxiliary therapy. Some have taken the position that (for certain sites, at least) all tumors are equally ominous and that the risks of a course of radiotherapy are less than those of operative intervention. However, the problem with this position is that it potentially unnecessarily exposes a group of children of unknown size to unneeded irradiation.

The histology of a brain tumor provides information about the nature of the cellular type or types undergoing proliferation, the degree of anaplasia, the nature of other processes in the tumor (*e.g.*, necrosis, endothelial reactions, leaky blood vessels, etc.), and the manner in which the tumor interacts with the tissue in which it is growing. The *prognostic pathology* of the neoplastic process in each specific child certainly includes all aspects of the histology just mentioned, but it also includes all of the clinical aspects previously mentioned. This is important to remember, as the clinician and pathologist may find important prognostic information in each of these other features as well as in the histology. Finally, the *prognostic pathology* of the child with a brain tumor includes not only the length of survival of the child and the responsiveness of the tumor to the various auxiliary therapies but also the quality of the postoperative life as well.

The remaining portions of this presentation will provide the reader with two varieties of specific information. The first will be about the frequency of each of the World Health Organization diagnoses in tumors whose major bulk lies within the cerebellum in children. The second will be about the other sites commonly involved at the time of operation upon what was thought to have been primarily a cerebellar tumor.

Some years ago a group of coinvestigators at 10 North American pediatric institutions organized the Childhood Brain Tumor Consortium with the hope that far better prognostic information could be provided the clinician at the time of the first operation. The combined resources of these institutions and a large number of neuropathologists, neuroepidemiologists, and biostatisticians were brought to bear upon the problems of prognosis. We used all of the children with brain and spinal cord tumors in the records of each institution without preselection. The population is approximately 3400 children with brain tumors. In addition to classifying these tumors into the categories of the World Health Organization (WHO) in a consistent fashion, a large amount of additional data was sought. Data about 290 clinical questions and about 150 histologic features were gathered for each child. Each child was followed until death, up to 5 years, or until lost to follow-up. At this time preliminary information is available about the kinds of tumors in the cerebellum in children, their locations within the cerebellum, and secondary sites recognized during the first hospitalization.

The slides of each child's brain tumor are being screened by multiple teams of experienced neuropathologists who work objectively, *i.e.*, without information about the child, the operative or clinical findings, or prior diagnoses. Prior to the slide review the 3400 cases in the study were randomized, and computer-generated slide reading lists were prepared for each team. To monitor intrateam observational variation, 25% of cases are randomly reinserted into the list for each team at places unknown to the team. To monitor interteam observational variation, 8% of cases are read by each team. One team is responsible for coding the slides of each case into one of the WHO categories. To study the large number of arrays of histologic features in brain tumors, the Consortium members prepared a master checklist of 150 histologic features. Each feature has a specific definition agreed upon prior to beginning the study. Four teams are responsible for coding the slides of each case for their histologic features without regard to or knowledge of the WHO diagnosis. A sixth team of neuropathologists is reviewing the records and slides of the 600 children in the original population who were autopsied. An individual trained to review clinical records collects the data from each clinical record with the help of a checklist of 290 questions, each specifically defined. At this time, all teams have completed their work on the slides of the first surgical sample of tumors whose bulk lay within the cerebellum and various analyses are in progress. The collection of the clinical information is complete. However, it is necessarily limited to what was recorded in each child's record, and no statement can be made for what was not recorded. That is, a negative for a sign or a symptom may mean that it was, in fact, not present or that it was not looked for or was not recorded. Specifically, the site information is a "least statement." That is, we recorded merely those sites noted by the neurosurgeon in his operative note, and therefore our information likely underestimates the true frequency of secondary sites (Table 9.1).

Thus, when these cerebellar tumors were classified by the World

TABLE 9.1

Kinds of Tumors at First Operation (1241 Children)[a]

	%
Medulloblastoma	33
Pilocytic astrocytoma	32
Ependymoma (grades i or ii)	7
Desmoplastic medulloblastoma	6
Astrocytoma	2
Fibrillary astrocytoma	2
Protoplasmic astrocytoma	2
Anaplastic astrocytoma, oligodendroglioma, anaplastic ependymoma, hemangioblastoma	1% each
Mixed oligodendroglioma and astrocytoma, papillary ependymoma, anaplastic plexus papilloma, pineoblastoma, gangliocytoma, ganglioglioma, neurilemmoma, meningioma, epidermoid, hemangiopericytoma, malignant lymphoma, and craniopharyngioma	<1% each
Unclassified	2%

[a] Preliminary data.

Health Organization Classification, it became apparent that the medulloblastoma (including the desmoplastic medulloblastoma) is the most frequently encountered tumor, followed closely by the pilocytic astrocytoma. However, if the astrocytomas are lumped together, then there is no difference in frequency, and the astrocytomas and medulloblastomas account for about three-fourths of the cerebellar tumors in children. The remaining quarter of cerebellar tumors includes a wide variety of tumors, each occurring in a small proportion, except for the ependymoma (grades i or ii), which appeared in 7% of cases.

Two questions remain to be asked for the three individual neoplastic processes encountered most commonly in the cerebellum in children, medulloblastoma (without the desmoplastic medulloblastoma), pilocytic astrocytoma, and ependymoma (grades i or ii). The first is that given the fact that the major bulk of these tumors was in the cerebellum, what other sites were noted as being simultaneously involved by tumor during the first hospitalization? The second question is related to the fact that the World Health Organization categories are, of necessity, summary categories (as are all classifications) based upon a set of *a priori* assumptions. The tumors classified under each of the names of the summary categories include a large amount of histologic information. Thus, the second question is twofold. How wide is the range of histologic features encompassed in each of the three diagnostic categories most commonly encountered and do any of the histologic features within each of these categories carry more specific prognostic information? At this time, I can provide information about primary and secondary sites, but not yet about the prognoses associated with the specific histologic features (Table 9.2).

At the time of the first hospitalization, the incidental notes in the clinical records of these children indicate that other sites were occupied by these tumors in a substantial number of cases. Since the cases accepted for study in the Childhood Brain Tumor Consortium were not preselected but included all cases contained in the records of each of the participating institutions, then a large proportion of children with these common posterior fossa tumors have multiple noncerebellar sites involved at the time of the first hospitalization.

The medulloblastoma was found in vermal and hemispheral locations in almost equal portions of cases, and the masses occupied both locations in some children. Secondary deposits or direct invasion of contiguous structures were recognized during the first hospitalization at one or more extracerebellar sites in 49% of children. Whether involvement at these other sites results entirely from direct extension or metastasis from the primary site or whether the high proportion of cases with secondary deposits already at the time of the first hospitalization supports a regional

TABLE 9.2

Sites Involved at the First Operation

Medulloblastoma	
Cerebellar sites	
Vermis	57.8[a]
Hemisphere	53.6
Fourth ventricle (roof)	19.8
Location not specified	13.8
Extracerebellar (In 49% of cases,[b] one or more other sites were also involved)	
Fourth ventricle (floor or wall)	28.9
Brainstem	23.0
Extramedullary	5.7
Cerebellopontine angle	1.8
Cervical spinal cord	5.5
Meninges	2.3
Third ventricle	1.3
Tentorium	3.1
Pilocytic astrocytoma	
Cerebellar	
Vermis	44.6[a]
Hemisphere	74.9
Fourth ventricle (roof)	8.7
Location not specified	13.6
Extracerebellar (In 33% of cases,[b] one or more other sites were also involved)	
Fourth ventricle (floor or wall)	16.2
Brainstem	18.0
Extramedullary	2.8
Cerebellopontine angle	3.3
Cervical spinal cord	2.8
Meninges	0.8
Third ventricle	1.5
Tentorium	11.3
Ependymoma	
Cerebellar	
Vermis	53.3[a]
Hemisphere	52.0
Fourth ventricle (roof)	14.7
Location not specified	17.3
Extracerebellar (In 87% of cases[b] or more, other sites were also involved)	
Fourth ventricle (floor and wall)	44.0
Brainstem	57.0
Extramedullary	42.7
Cerebellopontine angle	21.3
Cervical spinal cord	49.3
Meninges	5.3
Third ventricle	0
Tentorium	6.7

[a] % of cases.
[b] Tentorium not included.

or multicentric origin of the tumor cannot be decided. In either case the observation supports the well-known tendency of this neoplastic process to spread.

The pilocytic astrocytoma was predominately located in the cerebellar hemisphere but not exclusively. The surprising finding, though, was that involvement of one or more noncerebellar secondary sites were recognized at the time of the first hospitalization in one-third of cases. In most instances the secondary involvement was either the floor or wall of the fourth ventricle or one or more sites in the brainstem. While much of this spread could be direct extension, the multiple site involvement provides a little support for the notion that some of the neoplastic processes labeled pilocytic astrocytoma might reflect more widespread field changes in the posterior fossa, in both the brainstem and the cerebellum. In any case, it is clear that the morphologic statement that this a benign process pales in the light of the large proportion of cases already exhibiting brainstem involvement at the time of the first surgical procedure and must be brought to bear upon several decisions. Intraoperatively, knowledge that the tumor has extended into or involves the brainstem may influence the aggressiveness of the surgical attack upon the tumor. Postoperatively, this information will clearly influence further therapeutic decisions.

The ependymoma occupied vermal and hemispheral positions in equal portions of cases. However, most children with this kind of neoplastic process were recorded at the time of the first hospitalization as having one or more secondary noncerebellar deposits. Many of these were direct extensions of this neoplastic process into the floor or wall of the fourth ventricle or, in an even greater proportion of cases, at other sites in the brainstem. Furthermore, the cervical spinal cord was invaded in about half of these children. Once again I would raise the possibility that this widely spread early involvement of many structures in the posterior fossa really reflects a primary neoplastic change over a very wide field in the posterior fossa or tumor originating in multiple sites simultaneously. No matter how the speculation about the origin of this neoplastic process turns out, the intraoperative diagnosis of an ependymoma (grades i or ii) in the posterior fossa carries the implication of multiple site involvement, and it behooves the neurosurgeon to record this fact for the considerations of postoperative therapy. Life tables for children in the Childhood Brain Tumor Consortium have not yet been calculated. However, the primary diagnostic histologic criterion of ependymoma, the perivascular pseudorosette, was found in a previous study of cerebellar gliomas to have been associated with an ominous outlook (3), supporting the earlier study of Shuman *et al.* (2) concerning the malignancy of childhood ependymomas. We plan to see if the children included in the consortium with this histologic feature have a similar poor outlook.

Tumor intimately attached to or invading the tentorium provided some operative difficulty for the neurosurgeon in a surprising proportion of cases. For the medulloblastoma and the ependymoma the surgeon usually described the attachment as direct invasion. For the pilocytic astrocytoma the wall of the macrocyst was usually found to be particularly difficult to separate from the tentorium. In any case, tentorial attachments were not included among the secondary sites recorded above.

The neuropathologist, seemingly secure in the histologic and cytologic classification of brain tumors, can provide one view of prognosis. However, the clinician must not be trapped into the untenable position that his information about the location of the tumor and its secondary sites cannot be used in evaluation of the patient. Formal measures of the survival of these children are not complete but will be provided in the near future.

SUMMARY

All of the available classifications of brain tumors, including that provided by the World Health Organization, fail to take site into consideration when they provide estimates of prognosis. It seems from the preliminary information provided in this report that the common posterior fossa brain tumors frequently occupy extracerebellar sites already at the time of the first hospitalization, and that this information is likely to be helpful in planning further therapy.

ACKNOWLEDGMENTS

This study was conducted in the Department of Neurology-Neuropathology, Harvard Medical School, and the Department of Pathology (Neuropathology), Children's Hospital Medical Center, Boston, Mass. It was supported in part by Grant RO1-CA20462-06 from the National Cancer Institute.

REFERENCES

1. Scherer, H. J. The pathology of cerebral gliomas. J. Neurol. (Lond.), *3:* 147–177, 1940.
2. Shuman, R. M., Alvord, E. C., and Leech, R. W. The biology of childhood ependymomas. Arch. Neurol., *32:* 731–739, 1975.
3. Winston, K., Gilles, F. H., Leviton, A., and Fulcheiro, A. Cerebellar gliomas in children: Clinical considerations and a proposed classification. J. Natl. Cancer Inst. *58:* 833–838, 1977.

CHAPTER

10

Neuroradiology of Posterior Fossa Tumors in Children

CHARLES R. FITZ, M.D.

INTRODUCTION

The statistics for these tumors have been gathered from patients presenting at the Toronto Hospital for Sick Children (HSC) with previously untreated tumors over the past 6 years since the acquisition of a CT scanner by the hospital. The current survey of tumors (Table 10.1) shows a change which has some differences, as compared with the previous HSC series (3) and the large Vienna series (6). Cerebellar astrocytomas account for a smaller percentage, and brain stem tumors account for a higher number. This may reflect the ability of the CT scanner to better localize tumors. The percentage of medulloblastomas is higher than that of the previous HSC series but is approximately equal to the Vienna series.

Previous authors have ascribed certain definite characteristics to the CT appearance of posterior fossa tumors, so much so that there is a feeling among some radiologists and surgeons that one can predict tumor histology with nearly 100% accuracy on CT. As one grows more experienced, and sees more variations of each tumor, this confidence is somewhat tempered.

Using common sense, general principles, and specific observations, the large majority of tumors can correctly be identified, although some error will still be present.

TUMOR CHARACTERISTICS

Examination of easily identifiable characteristics is instructive in illustrating the occasional usefulness and frequent futility of labeling a single finding as diagnostic.

Calcification is often thought of as diagnostic of ependymoma. Naidich *et al.* (7) found 50% of their ependymomas calcified, and Swartz *et al.* (9) found 46% calcified. The present series has a 42% rate of calcification (Table 10.2), but because of the small number of ependymomas accounting for only 10% of posterior fossa tumors, the likelihood of a calcification

TABLE 10.1

Brain Stem Astrocytomas Divided into 16 Biopsied and 20 Unbiopsied Tumors

Posterior Fossa Tumors (Total: 124)		
Medulloblastoma	44	35%
Astrocytoma brain stem	16	29%
	20	
Astrocytoma cerebellum	22	18%
Ependymoma	12	10%
Miscellaneous	10	8%

TABLE 10.2

Calcification

	% Tumor	% Total
Ependymomas	42[a]	15
Medulloblastoma	23	39
Astrocytoma	27	23
Brain stem	6	8
Other	40	15

[a] Percent of tumors indicates the percent of tumors within the individual tumor groups that had calcifications. Percent of total indicates the proportion of calcified tumors represented by each individual tumor group.

being an ependymoma is only 15%. Because cerebellar astrocytoma with a 27% calcification incidence and medulloblastoma with a 23% calcification rate are far more common than ependymoma, a calcified posterior fossa tumor is more likely to be one of these. In fact, in this series, medulloblastoma accounted for 39% of calcified tumors. Swartz *et al.* (9) noted half their ependymomas had multiple punctate calcifications, and this author agrees that this finding, more than the calcification itself, is highly indicative of an ependymoma (Fig. 10.1).

Cyst formation is usually thought of as being characteristic of cerebellar astrocytomas. Indeed, it occurred in 64% of these tumors (Table 10.3). However, it was also present in 23% of medulloblastoma and 8% of ependymomas. The likelihood of a cystic tumor being an ependymoma in this series is only 4%, a medulloblastoma 33%, and a cerebellar astrocytoma 47%. Remarkably similar findings were obtained by Kingsley and Kendall (5). It does remain true that the cystic tumor with a single mural nodule, as noted by Naidich *et al.* (7), is very characteristic of astrocytoma.

INDIVIDUAL TUMORS

Ependymoma

In previously reported series, the precontrast density was quite variable. Swartz *et al.* (9) found that 80% were isodense. Naidich *et al.* (7)

found that 9% were isodense, and Kingsley and Kendall (5) found that none were isodense. It seems unlikely that the tumor in fact varied so greatly, and perhaps the differences are explained by technical differences in scanners and observer experience. The author's own series agrees closely with that of Swartz *et al.* (9), with 9 of 12 isodense before contrast enhancement (Table 10.4).

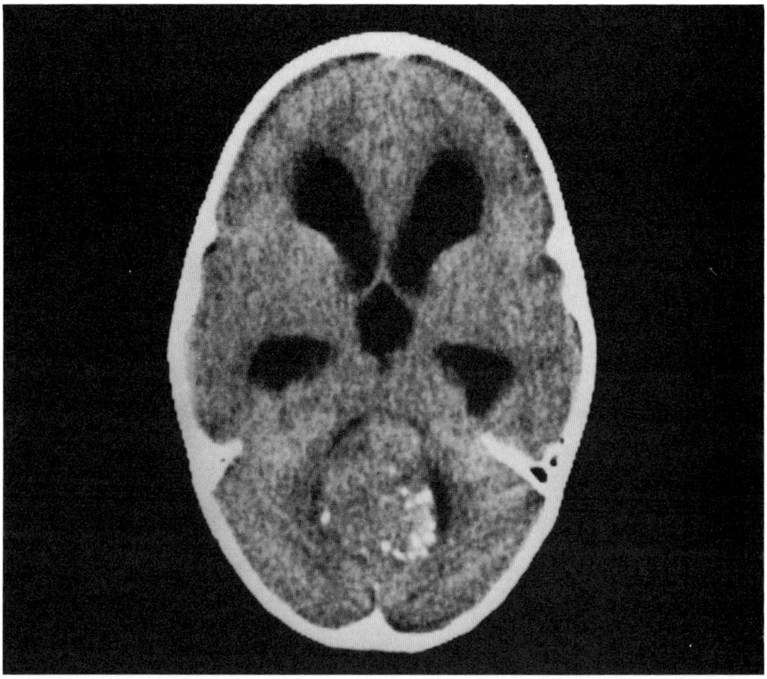

FIG. 10.1. Ependymoma. CT without intravenous contrast enhancement shows a moderate-sized isodense posterior fossa mass with multiple punctate calcifications, especially on the left. A thin rim of fourth ventricle can be seen surrounding the tumor, except in its most posterior aspect.

TABLE 10.3
Cyst

	% Tumor	% Total
Ependymomas	8[a]	4
Medulloblastoma	14	23
Astrocytoma cerebellum	64	54
Brain stem	14	19
Other	0	0

[a] Percent of tumor indicates the percent of each tumor type that was cystic. Percent of total is the proportion of cystic tumors represented by each individual tumor group.

TABLE 10.4

Ependymomas: Density

C-	↓	↓→	→	→↑	↑↓	↑
	-	25%	75%	-	-	-
C+	NONE	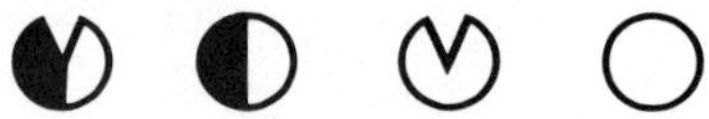				
	-	8%	33%	42%	17%	

[a] C– indicates tumor density before intravenous contrast. *Single downward arrow* indicates a uniformly hypodense tumor. The *downward* and *horizontal arrows* indicate a hypodense and isodense tumor, respectively. A single horizontal arrow indicates a homogeneously isodense tumor. The *horizontal* and *upward arrows* indicates a mixed isodense and hyperdense tumor. *Upward* and *downward arrows* indicate a tumor of mixed density varying from hyper to hypodense. A single *upward arrow* indicates a homogeneously hyperdense tumor. C+ indicates pattern following intravenous contrast. The *open black* and *white circles* signify mixed density enhancement through less than the entire tumor. The *closed black* and *white* circles signify a mixed enhancement of the entire tumor. The *white open* and *closed circles* indicate homogeneous enhancement of a portion or of the entire tumor. In both the pre- and postcontrast densities, they refer to the solid noncalcified portions of the tumor.

Although ependymomas are primarily intraventricular tumors, only 4 of the 12 were visibly surrounded by the fourth ventricle on CT (Fig. 10.1). A similar number of medulloblastomas also appeared to be within the fourth ventricle. The ability of an ependymoma to grow out of the lateral recess of the fourth ventricle and onto the lower medulla or upper cervical cord is an important CT finding (Fig. 10.2), both from a diagnostic and a therapeutic sense. This was present in 2 of the 12 ependymomas in this series and is best seen when the tumor is calcified.

All 12 tumors showed contrast enhancement (Table 10.4), which was frequently throughout the entire tumor. This observation is similar to that of a previously reported series, although Swartz *et al.* (9) found that 2 of 15 tumors showed no enhancement. Naidich *et al.* (7) noted that ependymomas are smaller than other posterior fossa tumors. The difference was not significant in this series, with a mean size of 4.7 cm across the greatest diameter *vs.* 4.8 cm for medulloblastomas and 5.3 cm for cerebellar astrocytomas. In fact more medulloblastomas (45%) were under 5 cm than were ependymomas (33%). However, no ependymoma was 6 cm or more in size, unlike astrocytomas and medulloblastomas.

Overall, the most prominent features of ependymoma are an isodense tumor in the midline, especially within the fourth ventricle and having multiple flecks of calcification. These unfortunately are not the most frequent findings. The type of contrast enhancement is of no particular diagnostic value.

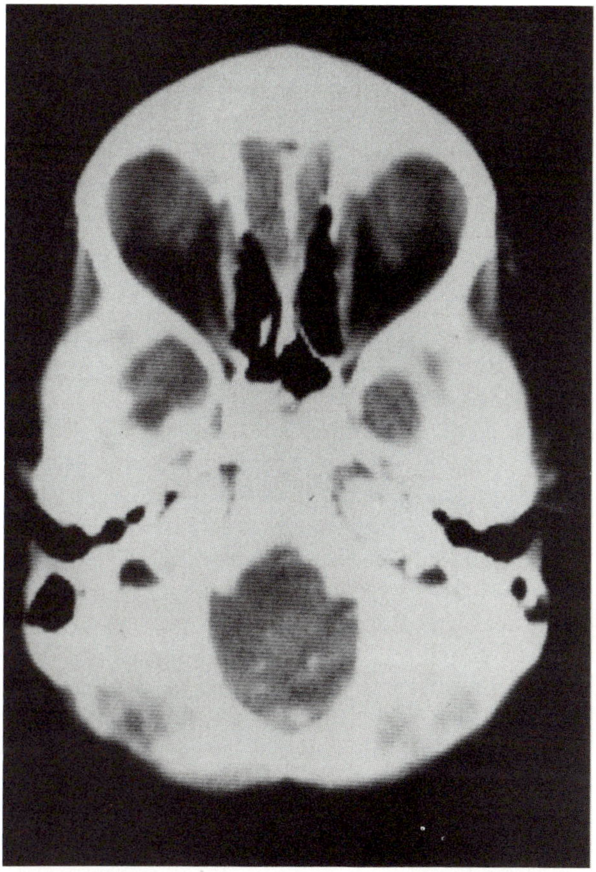

FIG. 10.2. Ependymoma. CT at the level of the foramen magnum without intravenous contrast shows multiple small punctate calcifications, indicating spread of this tumor out of the fourth ventricle and into the lower cisterna magna and upper cervical cord.

Medulloblastoma

This was the most common and most variable tumor in appearance. Like the ependymoma, none were of homogeneously low density (Table 10.5). This is a helpful fact when attempting to diagnose a small midline tumor. The tumor is often described as homogeneously hyperdense (13); however, this was the case in only 23% of the present series. This may be due to the better resolution of newer scanners. For example, 80% of the tumors examined on the GE 8800 were thought to be heterogeneous in density.

Contrast enhancement was variable. Two tumors (5%) had no enhancement. This observation has previously been documented by Zee *et*

TABLE 10.5

Medulloblastomas: Density[a]

C-	↓	↓→	→	→↑	↑↓	↑
	-	14%	21%	28%	14%	23%
C+	NONE					
	5%	12%	40%	10%	33%	

[a] See Table 10.4 for explanation of symbols.

al. (11), Woodrow *et al.* (10), and Gado *et al.* (2). Enhancement of the entire portion of the solid tumor was seen in 73%, and 33% were of a homogeneous quality. However, this observation is not especially helpful in an individual case, as ependymomas may enhance in a similar manner.

Of the 10 medulloblastomas having calcifications, 4 were large and dense on CT (Fig. 10.3). Not visible on skull x-ray, they were extensive, fine, gritty calcifications at operation. It appears that a large dense calcification on CT may be typical of medulloblastoma. This finding has previously been commented on by Swartz *et al.* (9).

Another relatively common finding was gross extension beyond the vermis and fourth ventricle. This was present in 10 tumors. Five of these were extensions to the cerebellopontine angle, and the others were into the midbrain and thalamus. Most of the large tumors with such extensions were of the desmoplastic variety and were solid. Zee *et al.* (11) also commented on these large tumors. This author believes that a large solid tumor extending to the cerebellopontine angle or into the midbrain or above is nearly always a medulloblastoma (Fig. 10.4).

Cystic medulloblastomas may closely resemble astrocytomas (Fig. 10.5). Cystic tumors that are in the midline and have small cysts with heterogeneous densities in the solid portion of the tumor are especially difficult to classify.

Brain Stem Tumor

This group includes tumors which were not histologically proven but had CT and clinical characteristics thought to be diagnostic of a tumor. For purposes of analysis, they are divided into those biopsy proven (16) and not biopsy-proven (20) (Table 10.6). Of those biopsied, no differences in density or contrast enhancement were present in six malignant or 10 benign tumors. This is unlike the description of Bilaniuk *et al.* (1), who

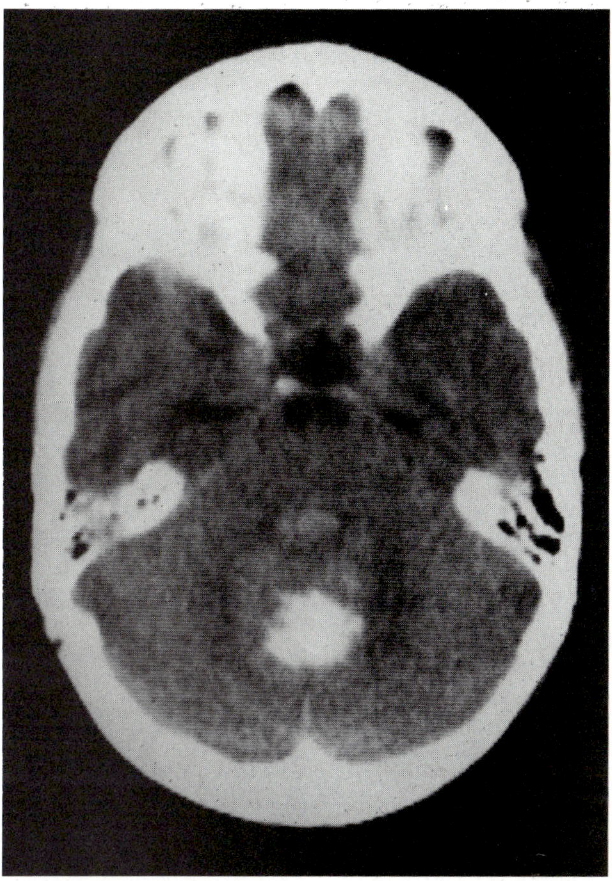

FIG. 10.3. Medulloblastoma. A large calcification is usually visible in this tumor, which has a mixed isodense and hyperdense appearance before contrast enhancement.

found the malignant tumors to be of low density and showing no enhancement.

None of the brain stem tumors were of homogeneous increased density, and only four had any element that was more than isodense. Nearly half (15) were uniformly hypodense. The most significant difference between the successfully biopsied tumors and those that were not was the lack of contrast enhancement that was present in 9 of the 20 nonbiopsied tumors *vs.* 1 of 16 of the proven astrocytomas.

This reflects the use of CT in picking a biopsy site, which is more likely to be positive in an area with contrast enhancement. It also reflects the fact that those tumors with contrast enhancement were more often

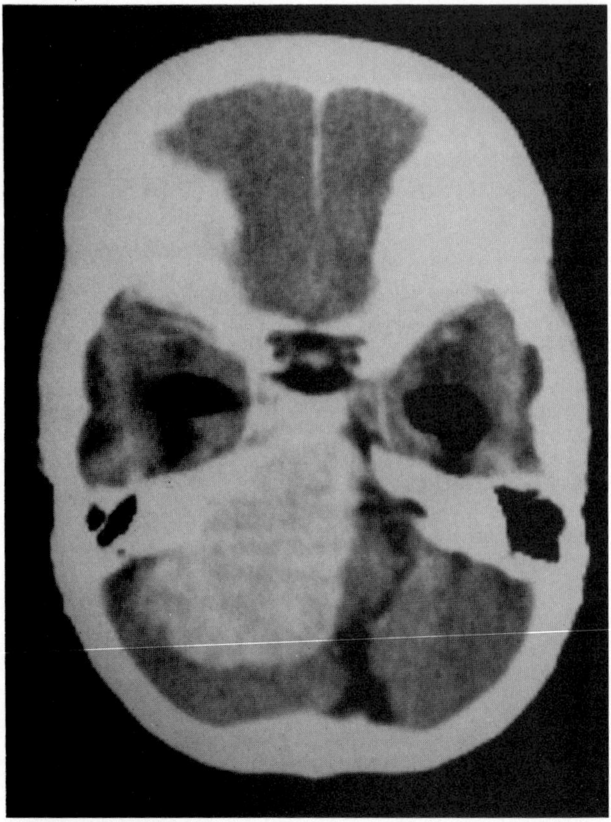

FIG. 10.4. Medulloblastoma. Huge desmoplastic medulloblastoma in a 1-year-old extends nearly the entire length of the petrous ridge. There is enhancement throughout the tumor, and it is relatively homogeneous, but foci of less dense enhancement can be seen.

exophytic into the fourth ventricle or laterally, as noted by Hoffman *et al.* (4). The biopsied tumors also had a much higher incidence of hydrocephalus, which though usually mild, was present in 77% of cases *vs.* 16% of the nonbiopsied tumors. While most of the tumors cause posterior displacement of the fourth ventricle as described by Bilaniuk *et al.* (1), 10% had an anterior displacement (Fig. 10.6).

The most significant features of brain stem tumor are the posterior displacement of the fourth ventricle, and a uniformly hypodense appearance before intravenous contrast, especially when combined with a lack of contrast enhancement. While contrast enhancement was very uncommonly as dense as in ependymomas of medulloblastomas, it was frequent and not specific enough to have any diagnostic features.

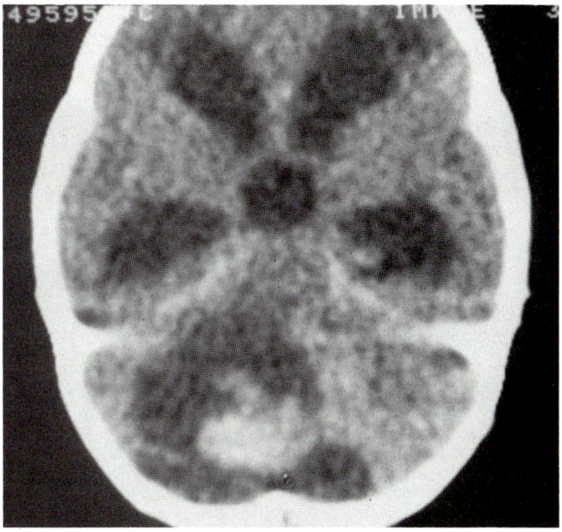

FIG. 10.5. Medulloblastoma. CT following intravenous contrast shows an enhancing nodule in a medulloblastoma that has a large cyst around it and is somewhat eccentric like a cerebellar astrocytoma.

TABLE 10.6

Brain Stem Tumors: Density

C-	↓	↓→	→	→↑	↑↓	↑
	42%	19%	28%	3%	8%	-
C+	NONE	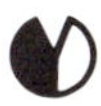	◐		○	☽
TOTAL	27.8%	13.8%	5.6%	30.5%	16.7%	5.6%
BIOPSY	6%	13%	13%	38%	31%	-
NO BIOPSY	45%	15%	-	25%	5%	10%

[a] No difference was noted between the biopsied and unbiopsied tumors before contrast enhancement, and this portion of the table is not divided. Because of some differences in contrast enhancement, the percentages are divided into the total and the individual tumors. Two of the unbiopsied tumors had only a crescentic enhancement, as indicated by the righthand symbol. No other tumors had this type of enhancement.

Cerebellar Astrocytoma

Like brain stem tumor, this tumor was homogeneously hypodense in a large minority (38%) of cases and was also never homogeneously hyperdense (Table 10.7). Contrast enhancement was quite variable. Naidich *et al.* (7) and Zimmerman *et al.* (12) noted the two cyst types that are

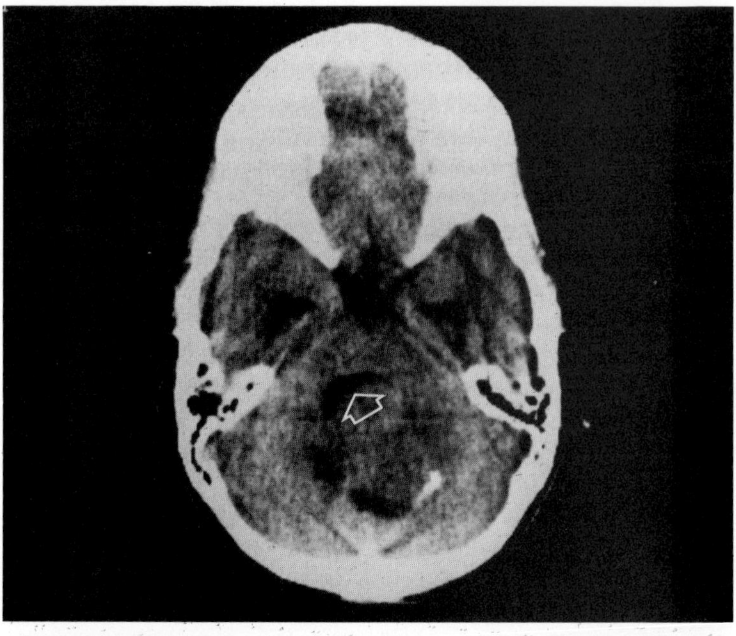

FIG. 10.6. Brain stem astrocytoma. CT before intravenous contrast shows a large grade III tumor with mixed low and isodense regions displacing the fourth ventricle (*arrow*) anteriorly. On the posterior edges of the tumor are two small surgically confirmed cysts, and to the left of these, a small calcification.

TABLE 10.7
Cerebellar Astrocytomas: Density[a]

C-	↓	↓→	→	→↑	↑↓	↑
	38%	24%	33%	5%	-	-
C+	NONE	◕	◐	Ⓥ		○
	5%	9%	27%	27%		32%

[a] See Table 10.4 for explanation of symbols.

commonly seen on CT. One is the cyst whose wall is thick and made up of tumor (Fig. 10.7), and the other which has a thin wall and a single small mural nodule (Fig. 10.8). These two types of cysts occurred in 41% of cases. The remaining cysts were smaller, being less than half the tumor volume.

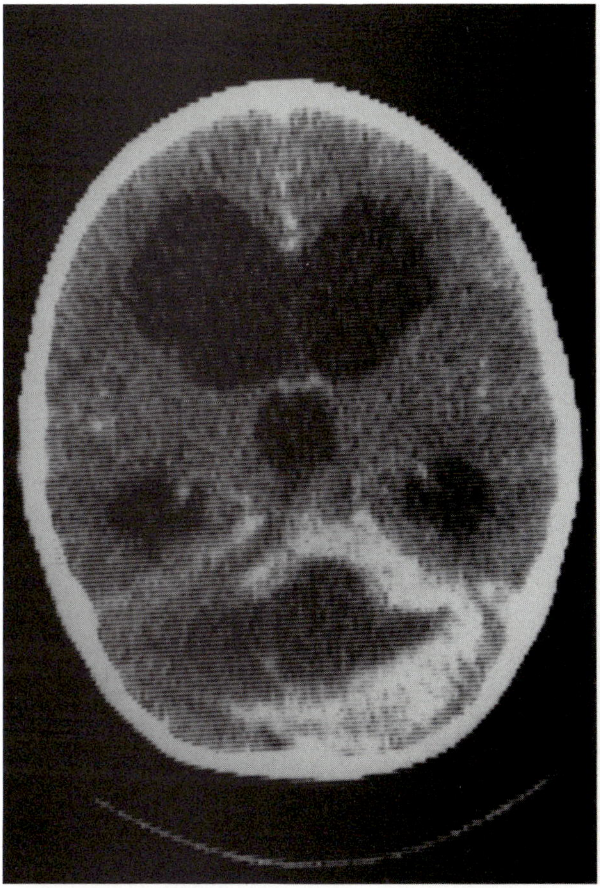

FIG. 10.7. Cerebellar astrocytoma. CT following intravenous contrast shows a large tumor with thick enhancing cyst wall through most of its circumference. Because the tumor is in both hemispheres, it is only minimally eccentric off the midline.

Cerebellar astrocytomas were slightly eccentric in 68% of cases, as can be seen in Figs. 10.7 and 10.8. The quality of the cyst and the location off the midline are important clues in the diagnosis of cerebellar astrocytoma, especially when it is not a hypodense tumor.

Miscellaneous Tumors

These included 1 hemangioblastoma with typical large cyst and small intensely enhancing nodule, as described by Seeger *et al.* (8). there were 5 acoustic neuromas. An important statistic of these is that four of the five had neurofibromatosis, and the fifth was 17 years old. One may infer

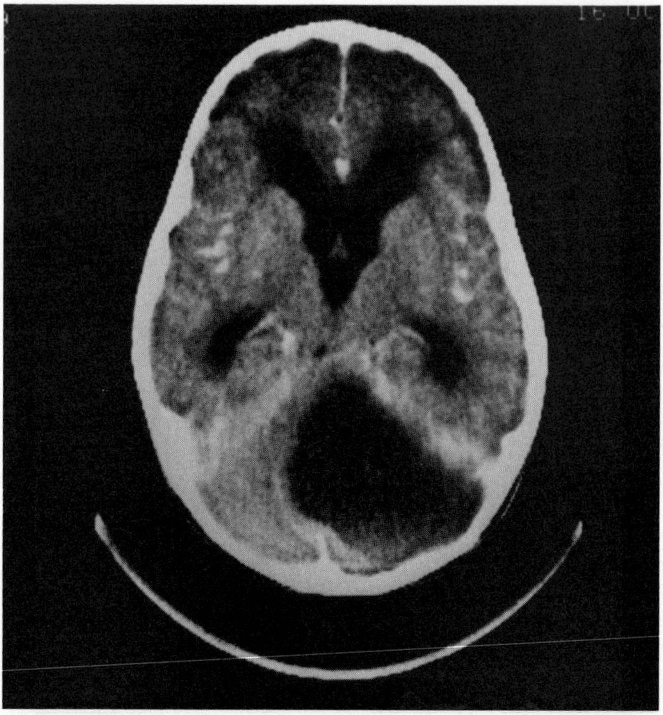

FIG. 10.8. Cerebellar astrocytoma. A cerebellar astrocytoma with a huge cyst and little or no enhancement of the cyst rim. The cyst is large enough to expand the occipital bone. The small mural nodule is not visible on this slice.

that a younger child with an angle mass does not have an acoustic neuroma unless neurofibromatosis is also present. The tumors themselves have CT characteristics like those of previously described adult tumors.

One cerebellar ganglioglioma, two mixed astrocytoma-oligodendriogliomas, and one astrocytoma-ependymoma were also found. The mixed ependymoma also had the multiple calfications typical of ependymoma. The mixed oligodendriogliomas had nonspecific calcification and no distinguishing features, as was also the case with the ganglioglioma, which was not calcified.

SUMMARY

In the examination of posterior fossa tumors, I believe that few findings are worthy of the term diagnostic. The small multiple focal calcifications of ependymomas are probably one such event, but it occurred in only 3 of the 124 tumors in this series. The large calcifications of medulloblastoma also seem to be close to a diagnostic sign, but this is also relatively uncommon. Extension to the midbrain or cerebellopontine angle in a large solid tumor is also fairly specific for medulloblastoma.

A homogeneously decreased density before intravenous contrast seems to hold up as a sign of an astrocytoma in both this series and previously reported cases. Large cysts of the type typical for astrocytoma are quite uncommon in nonastrocytomas, but they do occur. Small cysts or cysts of any size in tumors that are less than 4 cm in total diameter are nonspecific findings, as are solid or cystic tumors whose solid portions are of mixed density.

The relatively tumor-specific findings of the characteristic calcifications, low density and cysts of astrocytoma, and homogeneously hyperdense medulloblastomas account for approximately half of the tumors. Most of the remaining half can be accurately diagnosed by using combinations of size, location, and more general characteristics of density and contrast enhancement.

ACKNOWLEDGMENTS

The author wishes to thank Dr. E. B. Hendrick, Dr. H. J. Hoffman, and Dr. R. H. Humphreys, Division of Neurosurgery, Hospital for Sick Children, for the use of their clinical material, and Dr. L. Becker, Department of Pathology, Hospital for Sick Children, for the use of his pathological material.

REFERENCES

1. Bilaniuk, L. T., Zimmerman, R. A., Littman, P., Gallo, E., Rorke, L. B., Bruce, D. A., and Schut, L. Computed tomography of brain stem gliomas in children. Radiology, *134:* 89–95, 1980.
2. Gado, M., Huete, I., and Mikhael, M. Computerized tomography of infratentorial tumours. Semin. Roentgenol., *12:* 109–120, 1977.
3. Harwood-Nash, D. C., and Fitz, C. R. Neoplasms. In: *Neuroradiology of Infants and Children,* edited by D. C. Harwood-Nash, and C. R. Fitz. C. V. Mosby, St. Louis, 1976.
4. Hoffman, H. J., Becker, L., and Craven, M. A. A clinically and pathologically distinct group of benign brain stem gliomas. Neurosurgery, *7:* 243–248, 1980.
5. Kingsley, D. P. E., and Kendall, B. E. The CT scanner in posterior fossa tumours of childhood. Br. J. Radiol., *52:* 769–776, 1979.
6. Koos, W. T., and Miller, M. H. *Intracranial Tumours of Infants and Children.* C. V. Mosby, St. Louis, 1971.
7. Naidich, T. P., Lin, J. P., Leeds, N. E., Pudlowski, R. M., and Naidich, J. B. Primary tumours and other masses of the cerebellum and fourth ventricle: Differential diagnosis by computed tomography. Neuroradiology, *14:* 153–174, 1977.
8. Seeger, J. F., Burke, D. P., Knake, J. E., and Gabrielsen, T. O. Computed tomographic and angiographic evaluation of hemangioblastomas. Radiology, *138:* 65–73, 1981.
9. Swartz, J. D., Zimmerman, R. A., and Bilaniuk, L. T. Computed tomography of intracranial ependymomas. Radiology, *143:* 97–101, 1982.
10. Woodrow, P. K., Gajarawala, J., and Pinck, R. L. Computed tomographic documentation of a non-enhancing posterior fossa medulloblastoma: An uncommon presentation. CT *5:* 41–43, 1981.

11. Zee, C. S., Segall, H. D., Miller, C., Ahmadi, J., McComb, J. G., Han, J. S., and Park, S. H. Less common CT features of medulloblastoma. Radiology, *144:* 97–102, 1982.

12. Zimmerman, R. A., Bilaniuk, L. T., Bruno, L., and Rosenstock, J. Computed tomography of cerebellar astrocytoma. Am. J. Roentgenol., *130:* 929–933, 1978.

13. Zimmerman, R. A., Bilaniuk, L. T., and Pahlajani, H. Spectrum of medulloblastomas demonstrated by computed tomography. Radiology, *126:* 137–141, 1978.

CHAPTER

11

Posterior Fossa Tumors in Childhood: Radiation Treatment

DEREK JENKIN, M.B.

INTRODUCTION

Radiation treatment is an important component in the management of childhood posterior fossa tumors. In medulloblastoma and ependymoma radiation treatment follows as complete a resection as is possible and is required in all patients if a high cure rate is to be obtained. In brain stem gliomas, radiation treatment follows diagnosis, with or without exploration and biopsy, and is given to nearly all patients. Only a small fraction of patients with a posterior fossa astrocytoma receive postoperative irradiation, those with either a high grade solid tumor or gross tumor residual in a low grade tumor.

In all these situations, radiation is given with curative intent and increases substantially the cure rates obtained with resection alone, or in unresected patients it may offer the only prospect for cure.

The nature and results of irradiation will be considered separately for each of these tumor systems.

MEDULLOBLASTOMA

Medulloblastoma is a poorly differentiated tumor which occurs midline in the posterior fossa and usually involves the vermis. It is the classical example of a tumor which metastasizes via the cerebral spinal fluid pathway to seed at distal sites within the brain and the spinal cord. Systemic metastases, mainly in bone, are uncommon. Historically, cure was exceptional following even apparently complete resection and did not occur with lesser procedures. The first appreciable cure rate was reported by Patterson, some 30 years ago, when postoperative radiation was given not only to the posterior fossa but also to the whole craniospinal axis, that is, to include the whole brain and spinal cord down to the second sacral segment. This early report suggested that about one-half of patients would go on to long-term survival (8). It is now clear that absence of relapse in the first 5 years is associated in nearly all patients with cure of this neoplasm.

The importance of inclusion of the whole craniospinal axis in the volume irradiated was demonstrated by the early experience in Toronto (6). For some years postoperative radiation was given to the whole craniospinal axis, except for the frontal region of the brain. There were no survivors among 16 patients treated by this technique whereas following a change to whole craniospinal axis radiation the 5-year survival rate increased to approximately 50%. Comparable results were obtained at most large centers so that resection followed by craniospinal irradiation became the standard treatment for medulloblastoma for the last quarter of a century.

Factors which affect the outcome of postoperative craniospinal irradiation have been analyzed recently in the Toronto series of 122 patients with medulloblastoma who were referred to the Princess Margaret Hospital for irradiation 1958–1978 (1).

The overall 5-year survival rate for 89 patients treated with cobalt 60 since 1966 was 64%. The median dose given to the posterior fossa was 5000 rad and to the remainder of the craniospinal axis 3500 rad, utilizing 200-rad fractions 5 days/week. Increased survival was associated with an increased dose to the posterior fossa, thus in the range 5000–5100 rad ($N = 38$), the 5-year survival rate was 51%, as compared to 74% for doses in the range 5200–5350 rad ($N = 34$).

Survival was also related to the extent of resection of the primary tumor. Five-year survival rates were 64% for total resection, 56% for subtotal resection, and 33% for biopsy alone.

When these favorable factors were combined, we noted a subset of 15 patients who received a dose of 5200 rads or more to the posterior fossa following a gross total removal and who had a 5-year survival rate of 77% which remained constant for up to 10 years. The importance of the extent of the surgical resection has been confirmed in a recent large multicenter collaborative trial conducted by the International Society of Paediatric Oncology. Patients with medulloblastoma (a total of 287) were entered on trial between 1975 and 1979. Three-year survival rates for patients treated with resection and irradiation only were 27% for partial removal, 52% for subtotal removal, and 56% for total removal (3).

It is of interest that 5-year survival rates reported from major centers have been in the range of 30–40% until very recently (2), yet current multiinstitutional prospective trials suggest that resection and irradiation will give 50% 5-year survival rates. On the other hand, national or regional statistical studies suggest that overall 5-year survival rates of only about 20% are being obtained (4, 9).

It would seem likely that advances in surgical and radiation treatment have been occurring simultaneously in recent years and that superior results are being obtained at centers seeing large numbers of patients.

In the Toronto series the pattern of central nervous system relapse in 34 patients was posterior fossa, 26; spinal cord 5; and supratentorial brain 10 patients. Control of the posterior fossa tumor, therefore, remains the dominant problem. Control of the primary site may be improved by increasing the number of patients who undergo a complete resection and by increasing the radiation dose to the posterior fossa. Due to concern over possible late effects it has not been the practice in Toronto to use doses higher than 5250 rads and indeed in young children less than 3 years old not to exceed 4500 rad. These limits have been set by the fear of late effects, although there is no data to indicate that in younger children the tumor is more radiosensitive. By utilizing 4500 rad for small children, one accepts a lower tumor control rate, hoping that this will be balanced by decreased late effects. At the present time, control of the primary tumor is the limiting factor. Further improvement in local results can only come by the addition to current programs of new active agents or effective radiosensitizers. The low rate of spinal cord relapse in the Toronto series is noteworthy in that these patients did not undergo myelography unless there were overt symptoms of cord seeding or compression. Recent data indicate that the practice of screening myelography yields 15–20% of patients at diagnosis who have overt evidence of macroscopic seeding related to the spinal cord. Patients with overt cord compression at diagnosis do not usually survive. The implication is that elective irradiation of the spinal cord cures a number of patients who have gross deposits. It is not yet known whether the demonstration that an asymptomatic deposit is present will allow a change in radiation practice that will provide higher control rates at this site. Certainly, if such overt deposits were found, it would seem appropriate to boost the involved region to a dose of 4500–5000 rad. Likewise, computed tomography of the brain at diagnosis occasionally demonstrates meningeal or ventricular seeding. It is already clear that this is a bad prognostic sign, and again it is as yet unknown as to whether increasing the dose of radiation to the brain in these circumstances will give a higher survival rate, but in these circumstances it does seem appropriate to give the brain the maximum tolerable dose. One specific site of failure that may be due to inadequate radiation dose is the subfrontal region. Irradiation of the brain is normally undertaken by means of lateral opposed fields, and to shield the eyes it is inevitable that a small portion of the subfrontal brain, particularly in the midline, is also shielded. Thus, recurrence at this site may be due to inadequate radiation dose due to the eye shielding. In the Toronto series there were three examples of subfrontal relapse.

Overall, the current results obtained in large centers with resection and irradiation must be near the theoretical limit. Essentially, these results are obtained by maximizing both the resection and the irradiation.

A number of problems remain. In favorable patients, that is, in those with small midline tumors that can be totally resected, what is the optimal elective dose for the craniospinal axis? It is possible that doses lower than 3500 to 4000 rad may be as effective as these higher doses. This possibility needs to be put to a test in a clinical trial since obviously the optimal dose is the lowest dose that will produce a maximal therapeutic response. In all other patients there seems little room at present for reducing radiation dosage, and the emphasis is on finding other agents that will either be additive in their effect on tumor cell kill or will augment the radiation effect.

EPENDYMOMAS

Forty-six children with ependymoma were referred to the Princess Margaret Hospital, Toronto, for postoperative irradiation during the period from 1958 to 1977. In 28 of these patients the primary site was in the posterior fossa (supratentorial sites, 11 patients, and spinal cord, 7 patients) (7). Overall, the 5-year survival rate for this group of patients was 41%, but patients with posterior fossa tumors fared less well with 5-year rates of 28%, as compared to 42% for cerebral hemisphere sites and 86% for spinal cord involvement.

As with medulloblastoma the extent of resection appeared to be an important prognostic factor when all intracranial sites were considered. One of seven patients undergoing biopsy alone survived 5 years. This compared with 5-year survival rates of 33% for 24 patients undergoing partial excision and 42% for 6 undergoing complete excision.

Radiation dose to the primary site was a prognostic factor. The 5-year survival rates were 17% for less than 4500 rads ($N = 12$, 50% for 4500–4800 rad ($N = 7$), and 48% for greater than 4800 rads ($N = 16$).

The volume to be irradiated in ependymomas is controversial. Overall, approximately 12% of patients with ependymoma demonstrate, either at diagnosis or relapse, seeding by way of cerebral spinal fluid pathways (2). The risk appears somewhat higher for children with tumors in the posterior fossa and for high grade ependymomas. Thus, many radiation oncologists elect to treat grades III and IV ependymomas like medulloblastomas and utilize craniospinal irradiation, and they reserve local irradiation for grades I and II ependymomas only. However, since it is clear that even well-differentiated ependymomas occasionally metastasize, it has been the author's practice to treat all ependymomas with craniospinal irradiation, as for medulloblastoma. In the Toronto series, 6 of 18 children treated for posterior fossa ependymoma with craniospinal irradiation have survived, as compared to 1 of 8 treated by local irradiation. Comparable figures for supratentorial sites were 5 of 7, and 0 of 4, so that overall, 11 of 25 children treated with craniospinal irradiation have survived compared to 1 of 12 treated by local irradiation. However, the patients treated with local irradiation were from earlier years, when rather lower doses of radiation were utilized and other poor prognostic factors were associated with this particular subset.

In this series, utilizing all intracranial sites of origin, the pattern of relapse was known for 26 patients in whom the site of first relapse was the primary site in 21 and a distant CNS site in 5.

Summarizing, the common practice is to give craniospinal irradiation for high grade ependymomas and local irradiation for low grade ependymomas. It is the author's practice to treat ependymomas like medulloblastomas, regardless of grade. It is clear that the dose to the primary site should be that maximally tolerated: 5250 rad in 200-rad fractions for 5 days/week appears satisfactory and is associated with 5-year survival rates of about 50%.

BRAIN STEM GLIOMAS

Local radiation treatment of a brain stem glioma has been the standard practice for decades. Oftentimes, this is undertaken after neuroradiological investigation alone in view of the possible hazards associated with the exploration of tumors in the pons and medulla. The surgical procedure, when undertaken, is usually limited to a small biopsy. Unfortunately, about half of these tumors are high grade astrocytomas. Radiation treatment results are poor. In a recent literature review by Bloom (2), most 5-year survival results were in the range of 15–25% (2). Fifty-seven children treated at the Royal Marsden Hospital from 1952 to 1976 had a 17% 5-year survival rate which remained stationary at this level through 20 years. At the Princess Margaret Hospital from 1958 to 1975, 77 children were irradiated for a brain stem glioma, with an 18% 5-year survival rate. It would thus appear that a small fraction of these patients can be cured by irradiation and that this justifies the use of this treatment for all patients. However, while the majority obtain symptomatic improvement, relapse and death during the first 2 years is the common outcome. Again, the maximally tolerated radiation dose is required. Doses of 5250 rads in 200-rad fractions 5 days/week appear well tolerated in this moderate volume and are associated with cure of about 1 patient of every 5. There has been no significant change in radiation practice for children with brain stem gliomas during the last 2 decades.

The high early failure rate in this tumor and the small localized nature of the initial tumor should make this a good tumor model in which to demonstrate effects of radiation sensitizers or of additive cytotoxic agents but, to date, such trials have been disappointing, so that radiation alone remains the standard treatment, albeit an unsatisfactory one.

POSTERIOR FOSSA ASTROCYTOMAS

Since most children with cerebellar astrocytomas may be cured by resection alone, radiation treatment has a limited role restricted to those patients with gross residual tumor following attempted resection, either as a primary procedure or for local recurrence. When local irradiation is indicated, maximal tolerated doses should be used.

Even though only a small fraction of the most unfavorable cerebellar astrocytomas are irradiated, the outlook is still better than for astrocytomas in the cerebral hemispheres. Thus, the 5-year survival rates were 67% for irradiated cerebellar astrocytomas ($N = 34$), as compared with 30% for cerebral hemisphere astrocytomas ($N = 92$), for children irradiated from 1958 to 1975 at the Princess Margaret Hospital. After a partial excision of a low grade cerebellar astrocytoma, whether as a primary procedure or for recurrence, postoperative irradiation will decrease the subsequent rate of relapse by a factor of about two. Griffin *et al.* reported only a 36% relapse-free survival rate after partial resection alone, as compared to 82% after partial excision and postoperative irradiation (5).

Superior results will be obtained when the irradiated tumor is grade I or II and when there are cystic components, as compared to solid grade III or IV tumors.

The need for irradiation of a cerebellar astrocytoma in childhood is quite infrequent but should not be overlooked in these unfavorable situations.

REFERENCES

1. Berry, M. P., Jenkin, R. D. T., Keen, C. W., Nair, B. D., and Simpson, W. J. Radiation treatment for medulloblastoma. J. Neurosurg., *55:* 43–51, 1981.
2. Bloom, H. J. G. Intracranial tumors: Response and resistance to therapeutic endeavors, 1970–1980. Int J Radiation Oncol Biol Phys *8:* 1083–1113, 1982.
3. Bloom, H. J. G., Thornton, H., and Schweisguth, O. SIOP medulloblastoma and high grade ependymoma therapeutic clinical trial. Preliminary results. Int. Congr. Ser. *570:* 309–322, 1982.
4. Farwell, J. R., Dohrmann, G. J., and Flannery, J. T. Central nervous system tumours in children. Cancer, *40:* 3123–3132, 1977.
5. Griffin, T. W., Beaufaid, D., and Blasko, J. C. Cystic cerebellar astrocytomas in childhood. Cancer, *44:* 276–280, 1979.
6. Jenkin, R. D. T. Medulloblastoma in childhood. Radiation therapy. Canad Med Assoc J *100:* 1–3, 1969.
7. Jenkin, R. D. T. Childhood Ependymoma—Radiation treatment results. In: *Tumors of the Central Nervous System: Modern Radiotherapy in Multidisciplinary Management*, edited by Chang, C.H., and Housepian, E.M. pp 125–132. Masson, New York, 1982.
8. Patterson, E., and Farr, R. F. Cerebellar medulloblastoma: Treatment by irradiation of the whole central nervous system. Acta Radiol., *39:* 323–336, 1953.
9. Stewart, A. M., Lennox, E. L., and Sanders, B. M. Group characteristics of children with cerebral and spinal cord tumours. Br. J. Cancer, *28:* 568–574, 1973.

CHAPTER

12

Chemotherapy of Recurrent Pediatric Posterior Fossa Tumors

MICHAEL S. B. EDWARDS, M.D., VICTOR A. LEVIN, M.D., and CHARLES B. WILSON, M.D.

We will review our recent experience with chemotherapy of pediatric patients harboring recurrent posterior fossa tumors.

CEREBELLAR ASTROCYTOMAS

Cerebellar astrocytomas are slow growing tumors that often can be cured by surgery alone or with surgery and radiation therapy (20). We have used chemotherapy to treat 7 patients harboring this tumor (Table 12.1). Two patients with recurrent solid tumors have responded well to nitrosoureas and are alive at 100 and 275 weeks after treatment, respectively.

A third patient had a recurrent neoplastic cyst lined only with a thin layer of malignant cells that recurred after multiple operations, including aggressive resection and a cyst shunting procedure, and after irradiation. In an attempt to decrease fluid production within the cyst, we instilled P^{32} on two occasions, which alleviated symptoms of increased intracranial pressure. Based on the size of the cyst image on a radionuclide scan, the dose of P^{32} was calculated to deliver 10,000 rad to the cyst wall. Follow-up computerized tomographic (CT) scans (Figs. 12.1*A* and *B*) showed that the size of the cyst and ventricles had decreased. However, after 35 weeks, the disease recurred as a solid tumor that was resected.

Four other patients with recurrent solid tumors have been treated only by aggressive resection at a second procedure (Fig. 12.2*A* and *B*). All are alive and well without clinical or CT evidence of recurrence (56–204 weeks).

EPENDYMOMA

Using 1,3-bis (2-chloroethyl)-1-nitrosourea (BCNU) and, in two patients, vincristine and imidazole carboxamide, we have treated 6 children at the first appearance of recurrence of posterior fossa ependymomas (Table 12.2). Even though short-term responses were seen frequently and were often very dramatic (Fig. 12.3*A* and *B*), the overall results have

TABLE 12.1
Cerebellar Astrocytoma

	No. Tumors	Treatment	TTP(wks)
Solid recurrence	2	BCNU	100+/275+
Cystic recurrence	1	^{32}P	35R
Solid recurrence	4	Surgery	56+/204+

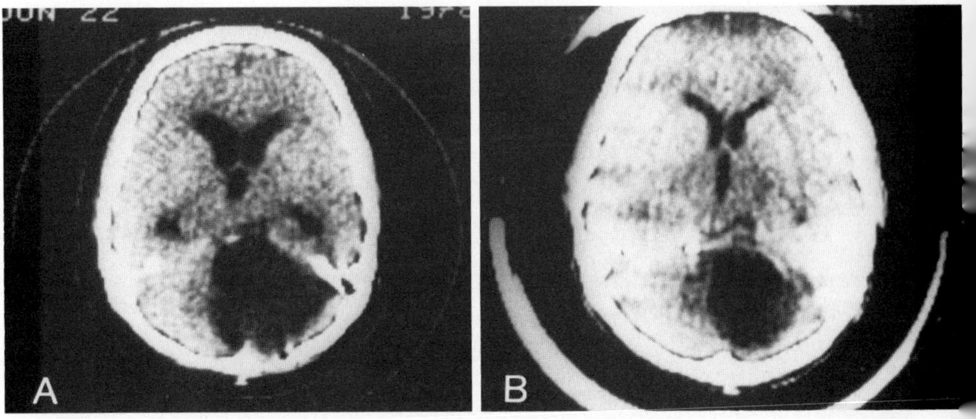

FIG. 12.1. (*A*) Axial contrast CT scan of recurrent cystic cerebellar astrocytoma (June 22, 1978). Note the presence of mild hydrocephalus. (*B*) Contrast axial CT scan after two injections of ^{32}P (October 12, 1978). The cyst has decreased in size, as has the ventricular system. Note rim of enhancement in cyst wall not present on previous scan.

been disappointing. Only one patient had a prolonged disease-free interval. We have performed multiple aggressive resections at the time of recurrence in two children (Figs. 12.3*A* and *B*); one child was reoperated 4 times during a 4-year period. Although it is technically possible to perform multiple resections, tumors recurred faster and were refractory to chemotherapeutic agents. In our hands, BCNU or 3-cyclohexyl-1-(2-chloroethyl)-1-nitrosourea (CCNU) have produced only short-term palliation. Aggressive reresection and chemotherapy may prove to be more effective than chemotherapy alone.

BRAIN STEM GLIOMAS

Our initial experience consisted of 30 children treated at the time of recurrence of brain stem glioma (Table 12.3). The most consistent responses were seen in patients who were treated with BCNU or CCNU, either singly or in combination with procarbazine and/or vincristine.

By 1981, we had treated 45 patients (8). We found no significant correlation between tumor pathology and median times to tumor progression or median survival. One of our 5-year survivors harbored a low

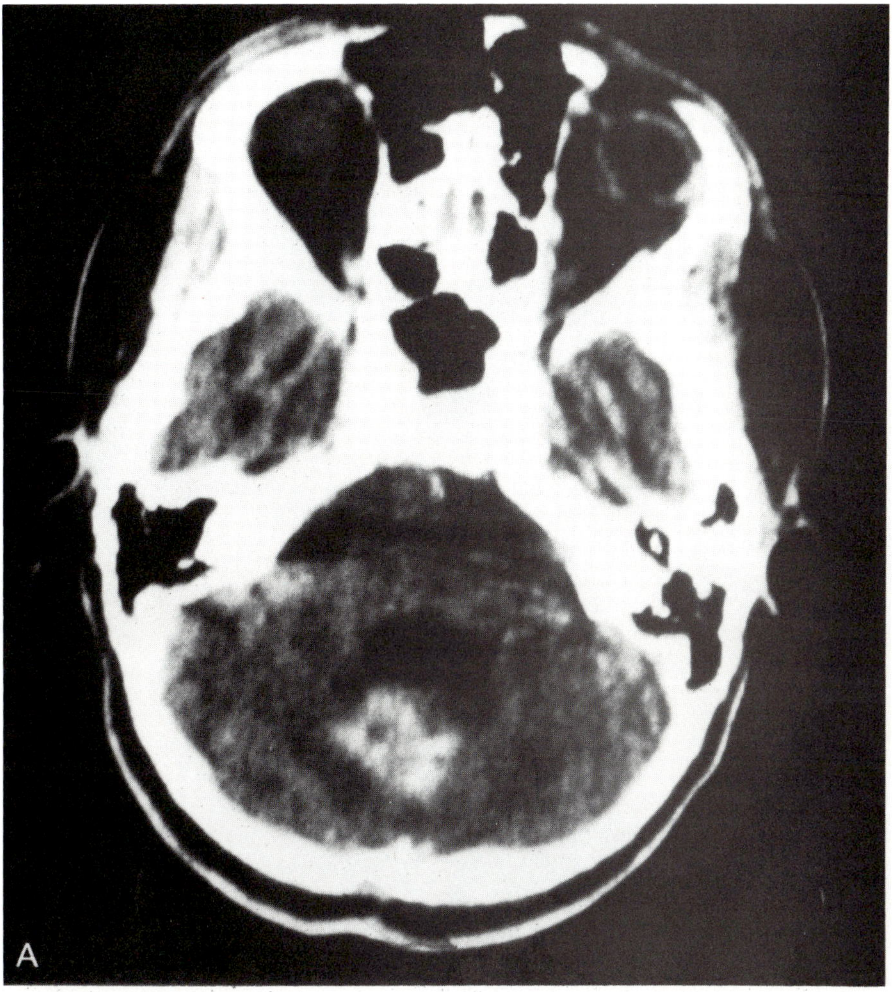

FIG. 12.2. (*A*) Axial contrast CT scan of 14-year-old female with a recurrent solid cerebellar astrocytoma.

grade glioma; however, after a 7-year disease-free interval, this patient died from a recurrent tumor.

We found no significant correlation between tumor location and median time to tumor progression or median survival. However, the largest number of long-term survivors were among patients whose tumors were confined to the midbrain at the time of initial diagnosis.

Patients treated with radiation therapy alone who received no further therapy at the time of tumor progression had significantly shorter median survival times (26 weeks) than patients treated with radiation therapy

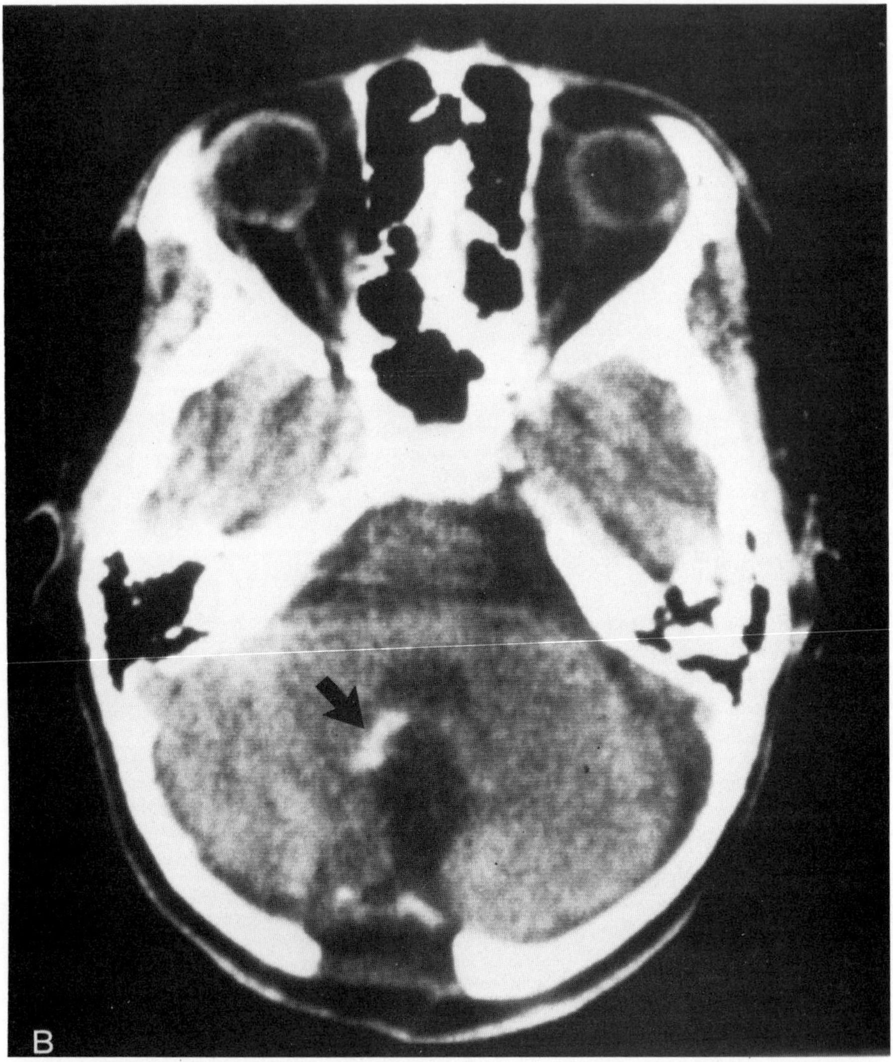

FIG. 12.2. (*B*) Axial contrast CT scan 2 years after resection of recurrent tumor (no other therapy was administered). There is a small area of residual contrast enhancement (*arrow*) that had not changed from the first postoperative CT scan.

alone initially and with chemotherapy at the time of tumor progression (56 weeks). These groups were not comparable, because patients who refused chemotherapy at the time of tumor progression generally had more severe neurologic deficits than those who received chemotherapy at the time of tumor progression. There was no significant difference in either median time to tumor progression (TTP) or median survival times (MST) between patients treated initially with adjuvant chemotherapy

TABLE 12.2
Recurrent Ependymoma

Patient No.	Site of Recurrence	Chemotherapy	Time to Progression (Wk)
1	Posterior fossa	BCNU	4
2	Fourth ventricle	BCNU	13
3	Fourth ventricle	BCNU	14
4	Fourth ventricle	BCNU	9 yr+[a]
5	Cerebellum	BCNU-procarbazine	10
6	Midline brainstem	BIC[b]	4

[a] + = continuing.
[b] Imidazole carboxamide (NSC-87196).

(TTP 31 weeks, MST 45 weeks) and those treated initially with radiation therapy alone followed by chemotherapy at the time of tumor progression (TTP 34 weeks; MST 56 weeks). However, there were more 5-year survivors in the latter group (Table 12.4).

BRAIN STEM GLIOMA (BTRC 8026-CSG 904P)

Because chemotherapy regimens used to treat brain stem gliomas were ineffective, we designed a protocol of aggressive chemotherapy that included irradiation before and concomitantly with drug therapy (Table 12.5). In animal models, 5-fluorouracil (5-FU) administered before CCNU had been shown to enhance CCNU cytotoxicity (16), and in humans hydroxyurea (HU) used in combination with radiation and BCNU was found to be more effective than BCNU and radiation against glioblastoma multiforme (12). Because of the normal vessel pattern in the brain stem, this region probably has a low blood flow, and tumor cells would presumably be hypoxic; because of this, misonidazole was used during radiation therapy in an attempt to improve response.

UCSF, Memorial Sloan Kettering Cancer Center, Children's Hospital of Los Angeles, and the Hospital for Sick Children of Toronto initiated this limited protocol in March 1980. Thirty patients were registered, 28 of whom were evaluable. Pathologic diagnoses are listed in Table 12.6. All patients received the full treatment, including a full course of radiation therapy.

As of September 1, 1982, the median time to tumor progression was 32 weeks (8 patients were free of disease), and the median survival was 48 weeks (13 patients still alive). In general, the therapy was well-tolerated, and there was minimal toxicity (Table 12.7).

MEDULLOBLASTOMA

In July of 1975 the Children's Cancer Study Group (CCSG-942) began a randomized prospective Phase III trial to determine the effect of

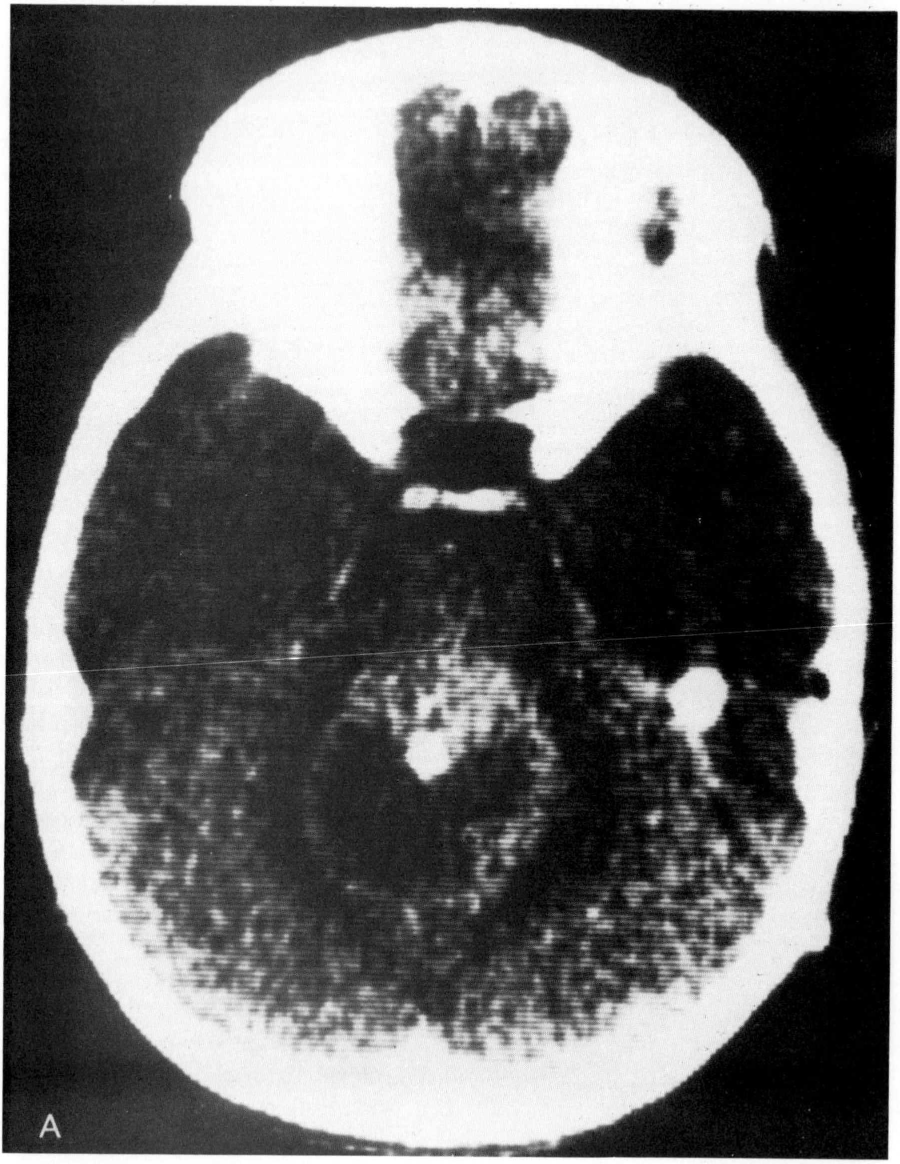

FIG. 12.3. (*A*) Axial contrast CT scan of 4-year-old male with a recurrent fourth ventricular ependymoma. A small dense area in the center of the mass is calcification.

adjuvant chemotherapy on the time to relapse and the survival rate of children with medulloblastoma. The protocol is summarized in Table 12.8. Children (228 of them) were entered into the study, which was closed in June 1981. Concurrently, a parallel study was conducted in

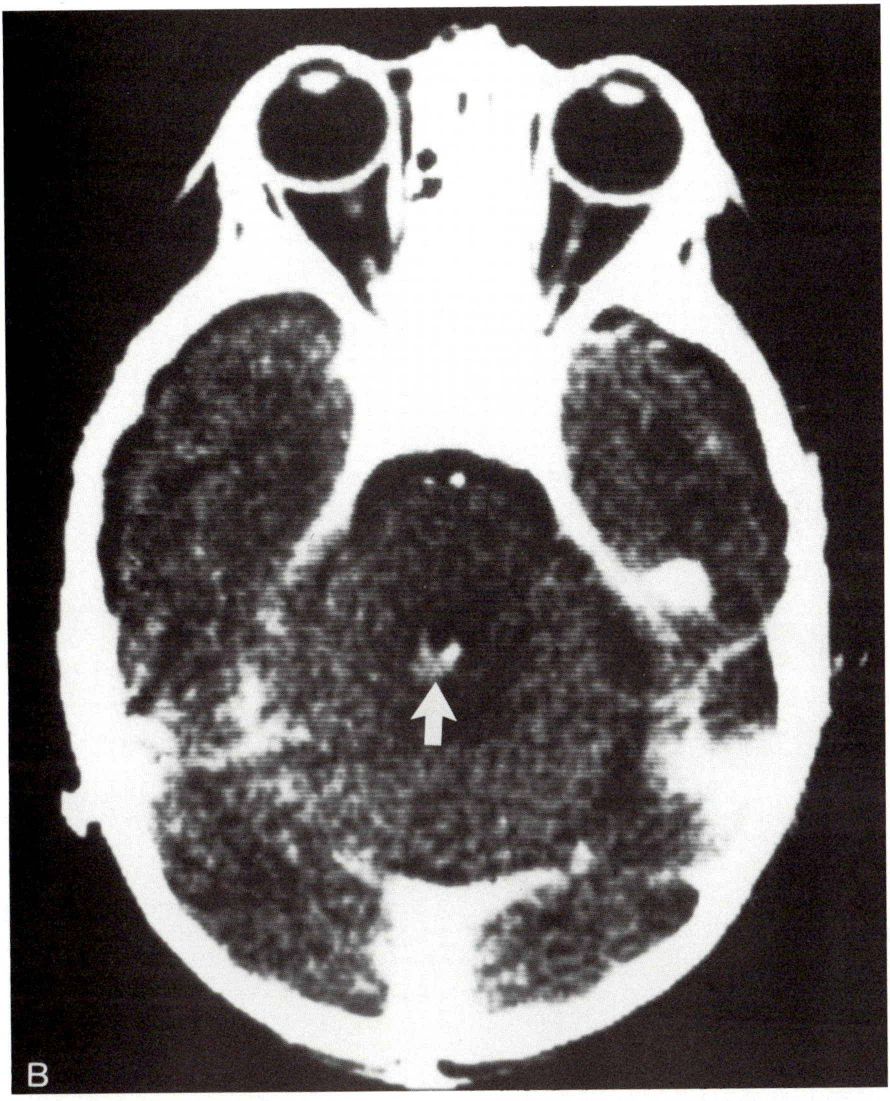

FIG. 12.3. (*B*) Axial contrast CT scan taken 24 hours after resection. There is a small residual area of calcification (*arrow*) but no enhancing tumor.

Europe by the International Society of Pediatric Oncology (SIOP). The major differences between the studies were the use of prednisone in the CCSG study and the inclusion of children under the age of 2 in the SIOP study.

For the 102 patients randomized to receive radiation therapy and concomitant chemotherapy, the CCGS 942 study demonstrated a 5-year

TABLE 12.3

Recurrent Brain Stem Glioma

No. of Patients	Chemotherapy for Recurrence	Time to Progression (Wk)	
		Individuals	Median
10	Procarbazine, CCNU, and vincristine	4,9,13,17,17,17, 19+,29,46,180+[a]	17
5	BCNU-procarbazine	6,9,9,9,11	9
5	CCNU	4,9,26,43,64	26
4	BCNU-vincristine	9,9,17,19	13
3	Procarbazine	4,9,17	9
2	Methotrexate	4,4	4
1	BCNU-5-FU	4	

[a] + = continuing.

TABLE 12.4

Efficacy of the Addition of Chemotherapy to Radiation Therapy for the Treatment of Brain Stem Glioma

N	Median TTP	Median Survival	% Survival	
	wk	wk	1 yr	5 yr
Radiation therapy				
5[a]	21[b]	26[+,c]	0	0
Radiation therapy with chemotherapy at progression				
24	34[a]	56*	65	9
Chemotherapy adjuvant to radiation therapy				
13	31[a]	45[⊕]	8	0

[a] Three additional patients received radiation therapy alone but, in them, tumors have not recurred.
[b] Values taken in pairs are not significantly different (Gehan analysis).
[c+] Significantly different; * $p = 0.02$;, [⊕], $p = 0.04$ (Gehan analysis).

TABLE 12.5

A Phase II Study of 5-FU and CCNU before Radiation Therapy with HU and Misonidazole for the Treatment of Primary Brain Stem Tumors (BTRC 8026/CCSG 904P)

Entry to Study

Days 1–3: 5-FU 1 (gm/sq m iv/day)
Day 7: CCNU (110 mg/sq m po)
Day 10[a] until end of irradiation:
RT: 170–180 rad/day (total dose, 5500 rad)
Hydroxyurea (HU): 275 mg/sq m q4 hr ×4 (8 a.m. on M-W-F)
Misonidazole: 0.5 gm/sq m daily 4 hr before each RT fraction

Progression of Disease

[a] Can be Days 10–14, depending on day of week of CCNU treatment.

recurrence-free survival (RFS) of 63% and a survival of 64%, as compared to the 104 patients receiving radiation alone, for whom RFS was 55% and survival was 56%. Measured in terms of survival, chemotherapy was of no benefit. Certain subsets of patients, especially those with advanced

TABLE 12.6

Patient Characteristics and Results of CCG 904P

Patients Entered—30 That Could Be Evaluated— Patients 28
Clinical diagnosis 14 Astrocytoma 9 Glioblastoma 2 Astrocytoma 3 (postmortem)
Radiation dose: 5000–5940 rad
September 1, 1980 TTP = 32 wk (8 disease free) MST = 48 wk (13 still alive)

TABLE 12.7

Toxicity Caused by CCG 904P Protocol

Steroid pancreatitis	1
Level 4 leukopenia	1
Level 4 nausea and vomiting	1
Myelosuppiression during radiation therapy[a]	4
Mild peripheral neuropathy	2

[a] Did not require discontinuation of chemotherapy.

TABLE 12.8

Childrens Cancer Study Group (CCSG-942)

Surgery and disease staging: Randomization to radiation therapy alone or radiation and chemotherapy
Radiation therapy (wk 1–8)
5000–5500 rad posterior fossa
3500–4000 rad whole brain and spinal cord
Vincristine (1.5 mg/sq m IV) on day 1 of each wk of radiation therapy
Rest (wk 8–12)
Chemotherapy (6-wk cycle)
Vincristine (1.5 mg/sq m IV) on day 1 of the first 3 wk of each cycle
CCNU (100 mg/sq m po) on day 1 of each cycle
Prednisone (40 mg/sq m/day po × 14) on day 1 of each cycle
Repeat chemotherapy every 6 wk for a total of 8 cycles

disease, appear to have a longer relapse-free survival. Although it appeared initially that gross total tumor resection enhanced relapse-free survival, as compared to biopsy and subtotal resection, the difference was not significant when survival was used as the end point. Toxicity and complications were minimal. The majority of patients recurred at the primary site despite adequate radiation therapy. The consequences of aggressive radiation therapy in long-term survivors are still under investigation.

RECURRENT MEDULLOBLASTOMA

Because it was known that 3 of 4 patients with recurrent medulloblastoma responded to procarbazine (10), a Phase II study of a 3-drug combination of procarbazine, CCNU, and vincristine (PCV) was tested and found to be as effective as BCNU against recurrent cerebral glioma (9) and against recurrent medulloblastoma. However, the initial protocol (PCV_1, Table 12.9) caused severe myelotoxicity that compromised therapy. Using animal models, we showed that oncolytic potency could be obtained using comparatively small doses of procarbazine and that when procarbazine was administered several days after CCNU, the combination was fully oncolytic but had decidedly less myelotoxicity than PCV_1 (11).

Based on these findings, the original protocol was revised and tested in 16 patients (PCV_2, Table 12.9). Ten of 16 patients responded, 5 of 16 stabilized, and 1 of 16 had rapid progression of tumor. The median time to tumor progression was 45 weeks; at 2 years, 25% of the patients were alive. The results of this study suggested that the PCV_2 combination has striking short-term effectiveness against recurrent medulloblastoma but that myelotoxicity secondary to previous craniospinal irradiation severely compromised therapy (4).

Usually, dianhydrogalactitol (DAG) and dibromodulcitol (DBD) have been given after PCV failure at a time of marked myelosuppression. DAG was used initially, but because of greater flexibility in dosing, DBD is the preferred hexitol epoxide. Even though treatment conditions were unfavorable because of previous craniospinal irradiation and systemic chemotherapy, DBD produced stabilization in 6 of 10 patients for as long as 53+ weeks (Table 12.10). Because of severe myelosupression during some of the courses of DBD, 3-day courses of HU and 6-mercaptopurine (6-

TABLE 12.9

PCV_1 and PCV_2 Patients with Medulloblastoma

Entry into study	
PCV_1	*PCV_2*
Day 1: CCNU (75 mg/sq m po)	Day 1: CCNU (75 mg/sq m po)
Day 1: Vincristine (1.4 mg/sq m iv)	Day 8: Vincristine (1.4 mg/sq m iv)
Days 1–14: Procarbazine (100 mg/sq m/day po)	Days 8–21: Procarbazine (100 mg/sq m/day po)
Day 8: Vincristine (1.4 mg/sq m iv)	Day 29: Vincristine (1.4 mg/sq m iv)
Wait 2 wk	
Courses to be repeated at 6-wk intervals	
Dose adjustments to be made for toxicity	
Progression of disease	
Other therapy at discretion of investigator	
Follow for survival	

TABLE 12.10
DBD and DAG for Recurrent Medulloblastoma

Patient	Age	Sex	Drug	Response
J.S.	5	M	DBD	53+S
M.G.	6	M	DBD	6S
C.T.	14	M	DBD	47S
J.A.	16	M	DAG/DBD	DAG(6+S), DBD(NR)
P.N.	7	M	DAG	28S
A.C.	18	M	DAG	13S
K.H.	6	F	DBD	10D
J.M.	4	M	DBD	NE[a]
L.B.	14	F	DAG	NE
L.K.	15	F	DAG	NE
H.L.	9	M	DHM	61S
J.S.	9	M	DHM	50+S

[a] *NE*, norepinephrine.

MP) were given to two patients in an attempt to achieve some antitumor activity without further compromising bone marrow reserves or exacerbating myelotoxicity. Both patients have shown stability of disease for greater than 50 weeks (Table 12.10). This approach appeared to have limited but definite short-term benefit.

As survival following recurrence of medulloblastoma increased because of more effective chemotherapy, the problem of leptomeningeal dissemination became more prominent. Intrathecal chemotherapy produces significantly higher cerebrospinal fluid (CSF) concentrations of certain drugs than can be attained with systemic administration. Thirteen children, 10 of whom were receiving systemic chemotherapy at the time they developed signs and symptoms of leptomeningeal dissemination, have been treated (7). The diagnosis was suspected clinically when fatigue, weight loss, anorexia, nausea, vomiting, or headaches developed, radiographically when a CT scan revealed enhancement of the ependyma, tentorium, or convexity, and/or when a radionuclide (RN) brain scan demonstrated ventricular and convexity labeling (resembling a CSF cisternogram), and/or when CSF polyamines and/or protein levels were elevated. In all 13 patients the diagnosis was confirmed by CSF cytology and myelography. The protocols used for intrathecal therapy are listed in Table 12.11.

The results of treatment are listed in Table 12.12. The most effective chemotherapeutic agent was methotrexate (MTX); however, it was also the most toxic and caused an encephalopathy in 2 of 5 patients. Intrathecal Ara-C also showed activity, but the responses were of extremely short duration. Our experience with thio-TEPA is too limited to make any statement regarding its effectiveness. The most effective regimen was

TABLE 12.11
Drug Administration Protocols

Induction therapy	
Ara-C	12 mg twice weekly for 4 wk or 20 mg on 3 successive days/wk for 4 wk
MTX	6.5 mg weekly for 4 wk
thio-TEPA	10 mg twice weekly for 4 wks
Maintenance therapy	
Ara-C, thio-TEPA, MTX: weekly for 4 wk, then once monthly	

TABLE 12.12
Results of Therapy

Ara-C	1 Complete response (13 wk)[a]
	4 Stable disease (9,10,26[a],35[a] wk)
	7 Nonresponders
MTX	2 Complete response (20,112 wk)
	3 Nonresponders
thio-TEPA	1 Complete response (4 wk)
	1 Stable disease (60 wk)

[a] Concomitant irradiation with misonidazole.
[b] Reirradiated with misonidazole.

craniospinal reirradiation (3000 rad) with misonidazole. To date, no evidence of radiation toxicity has been observed, but only 3 patients have survived for longer than 1 year after reirradiation.

Monitoring the progression of patients with medulloblastoma poses particular problems, especially for the early detection of spinal cord seeding. RN and CT scanning are of limited value, and myelography is not a routine monitoring procedure. We have monitored CSF polyamine levels to determine progression and response to therapy in patients with medulloblastoma (14, 15). The polyamines putrescine, spermidine, and spermine are small cationic molecules that are involved in many cellular functions (1, 3). These compounds are associated with nucleic acid metabolism, structure, and function and thus with cellular proliferation. Polyamine concentrations and activities of the polyamine biosynthetic enzymes increase during periods of cell proliferation (1, 3, 17); tumors usually have higher polyamine concentrations than their counterpart normal tissues.

CSF polyamine levels were determined sequentially in 32 patients harboring medulloblastoma. Over 210 lumbar CSF samples were analyzed. Polyamine levels were correlated with the clinical exam, CT scan, RN scan, CSF cytology, and myelography.

Polyamine levels were predictive of recurrence in 15 patients and increased before any clinical signs or neurodiagnostic test abnormalities indicative of recurrence were noted. Polyamine levels were elevated at the time of recurrence in 8 other patients; in 7 patients, stable or decreasing polyamines levels correlated with tumor stability or response to therapy. Neurodiagnostic tests showed evidence of recurrence in three patients in whom polyamine levels were not elevated (false negative); however, subsequent samples were elevated. No false positives (elevated levels in the absence of tumor progression or recurrence) have been noted to date. On our service, CSF polyamine levels are routinely monitored to determine response and/or progression. We are currently studying changes in CSF polyamine levels that occur during postoperative radiation therapy.

The effects of polyamines on cell growth might be used to advantage in a clinical setting. Polyamine production can be inhibited by specific inhibitors (18), such as DL-α-difluromethylornithine (DFMO), which is an enzyme-activated, irreversible inhibitor of ornithine decarboxylase, an enzyme that catalyzes the biosynthesis of putrescine, the first step in the polyamine pathway (4). In several animal tumor models, repeated administration of DFMO slows tumor growth and increases survival times (18, 19).

Methylglyoxal bisguanylhydrazone (MGBG) is a competitive inhibitor of the enzyme *S*-adenosylmethionine decarboxylase, which catalyzes the synthesis of spermidine from putrescine and spermine from spermidine (Fig. 12.4). MGBG appears to act selectively on polyamine synthesis and inhibits initiation of DNA synthesis, RNA synthesis, and mitochondrial respiration. We designed a protocol (BTRC 8221) to test the effects of the combination of DFMO and MGBG in depleting polyamines and

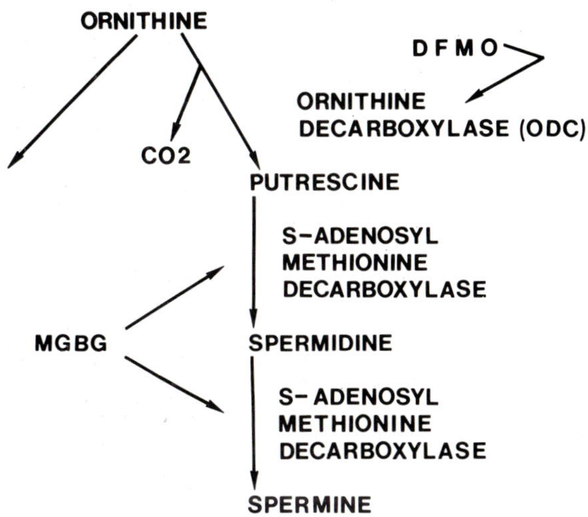

FIG. 12.4. Polyamine biosynthetic pathways.

stopping tumor growth in children with medulloblastoma (Table 12.13). Four children were treated on this protocol at the time of second and third recurrence (Table 12.14). The longest response was only 11 weeks despite a marked decrease in CSF polyamines in all 4 patients. Further testing of this protocol is under consideration.

We have reported our experience with 36 patients with recurrent medulloblastoma treated on various chemotherapy protocols after initial treatment failure (13). Patients were initially treated with PCV_3 and usually with one of the hexitol expoxides (DAG, DBD). If leptomeningeal seeding was noted, intrathecal therapy with Ara-C, MTX, or thio-TEPA was instituted. Frequently, systemic chemotherapy was limited by compromised bone marrow reserves secondary to previous craniospinal irradiation. When chemotherapy failed or myelosuppression prevented further drug therapy, reirradiation, with or without misonidazole, was performed. These therapies have extended postrecurrence median survival to 2 years; 25% of patients are alive at 2.9 years, and a few are currently disease free. Long-term follow-up will be necessary to determine whether these extended survival rates in fact represent cures.

Because previous therapies did not extend survival long enough, it was not necessary to evaluate the quality of life of long-term survivors. This group is now being studied. Intellectual deficits, probably secondary to whole brain irradiation, are seen in 30–60% of patients tested, and growth abnormalities have been noted in 40–65% of patients secondary to whole brain and spine irradiation (2). In an attempt to decrease these late complications and maintain survival we undertook a study of preradiation

TABLE 12.13
BTRC 8221: DFMO-MGBG Combination Therapy for Recurrent Adult and Childhood Gliomas

DFMO (1 gm/sq m) daily for 42 days
MGBG, (350 mg/sq m, iv) on days 14, 28 and 42
Cycle repeats after a 1-wk break

TABLE 12.14
BTRC Protocol 8221: DFMO-MGBG Patients

Medulloblastoma			Response (wk)
Patient	Sex	Age	
M.G.	M	8	8D
M.S.	M	7	11D
H.L.	M	12	6+D
G.K.	M	5	7D(Spinal metastases

TABLE 12.15
BTRC 7922—PHRT

Surgery (Day 1)
Procarbazine (100 mg/sq m/day) (Days 7–14)
Hydroxyurea (275 mg/sq m/q6h qod) (Days 14–56)
Radiation therapy (Days 14–56)
  Posterior fossa (5500 R) (Days 14–56)
  Whole brain (3500 R) (Days 28–56)
  Whole spinal cord (2500 R) (Days 28–56)

TABLE 12.16
BTRC Protocol 7922: Phase II Study of Chemotherapy with Procarbazine and Hydroxyurea before and during Irradiation for Medulloblastoma

Patients			Radiation Therapy			TTP (wk)[a]
Initials	Age	Sex	SC[b]	PF	WB	
N.J.	6	F	2500	5500	3500	175+R
M.G.	8	F	2520	5500	3520	98+R
K.A.	9	M	720	5500	3520	43R
R.L.	13	M	2520	5500	3500	90+R
C.U.	13	F	2500	5500	3500	98+R
F.S.	8	M	2500	5500	3500	184+S
A.M.	13	F	4480	5580	4860	163+S
S.C.	7	M	2500	5500	3500	37+S
C.K.	3	M	2580	5400	2520	26+S
M.S.	4	M	4480	5580	4860	61S
T.G.	11m	M		4665		22+R

[a] Median follow-up is 71 weeks.
[b] SC, spinal cord; PF, posterior fossa; WB, whole brain.

and/or concomitant radiation and chemotherapy with a decreased radiation dose to the whole brain and spinal axis in good risk medulloblastoma patients (BTRC 7922, Table 12.15).

Before initiation of therapy, all patients had CT scans performed to assess the extent of resection (gross total or aggressive subtotal (>90%)) and to rule out the presence of intracranial metastases. Complete myelography and CSF cytology were performed to rule out spread of tumor to the spine. If any disease was noted outside the posterior fossa, a boost was delivered to the lesion.

The results of treatment in 11 patients are listed in Table 12.16. A response to therapy was seen in 6 patients and stability of disease in the other 5 patients. The longest survival is 184 weeks posttreatment without evidence of recurrence. Median follow-up is 71 weeks, and the results, while preliminary, are very encouraging. Long-term follow-up will be necessary to determine the efficacy of this treatment.

CONCLUSIONS

Despite the fact that patients respond in some measure to drug therapy, cures of recurrent tumors are not obtained. Failures probably reflect *de novo* or acquired drug resistance or the intrinsic inability to deliver a high enough drug concentration to the tumor, either because of the blood-brain barrier or inadequate tumor blood flow. Before chemotherapy can be effective, new drugs and more information on appropriate drug scheduling, cellular drug resistance, and drug delivery will have to be obtained. Readers interested in a more extensive review of chemotherapy for central nervous system tumors should consult Refs. 5 and 6.

ACKNOWLEDGMENTS

Supported in part by Program Project Grant CA-13525 from the National Cancer Institute. We are deeply indebted to neurosurgeons in private practice and especially at the Kaiser-Permanente Medical Centers of the Greater Bay Area for referring patients to our Service. We thank Neil Buckley for editorial assistance.

REFERENCES

1. Campbell, R. A., Morris, D. R., Bartos, D., Daves, G. D., and Bartos, F. (Eds.). Adv. Polyamine Res., *1* and *2*: 1978.
2. Le medulloblastome. Societe de neuro-chirurgie de langue francaise XXXII. Congres Annuel (Strasbourg 16–18 Juin 1982) par M. Chou and G. Lena et coll. Neurochirurgie, 28 (Suppl 1): 229, 1982.
3. Cohen, S. S. *Introduction to the Polyamines.* Prentice-Hall, Englewood Cliffs, N.J., 1971.
4. Crafts, D. C., Levin, V. A., Edwards, M. S., Pischer, T. L., and Wilson, C. B. Chemotherapy of recurrent medulloblastoma with combined procarbazine, CCNU, and vincristine. J. Neurosurg., *49:* 589–592, 1978.
5. Edwards, M. S., Levin, V. A., and Wilson, C. B. Brain tumor chemotherapy: An evaluation of agents in current use for phase II and III trials. Cancer Treat. Rep., *64:* 1179–1205, 1980.
6. Edwards, M. S., Levin, V. A., and Wilson, C. B. Chemotherapy of pediatric posterior fossa tumors. Child's Brain, *7:* 252–260, 1980.
7. Edwards, M. S., Levin, V. A., Seager, M. L., and Wilson, C. B. Intrathecal chemotherapy for leptomeningeal dissemination of medulloblastoma. Child's Brain, *8:* 444–457, 1981.
8. Fulton, D. S., Levin, V. A., Wara, W. M., Edwards, M. S., and Wilson, C. B. Chemotherapy of pediatric brain-stem tumors. J. Neurosurg., *54:* 721–725, 1981.
9. Gutin, P. H., Wilson, C. B., Kumar, A. R. V., Boldrey, E. B., Levin, V. A., Powell, M., and Enot, K. J. Phase II study of procarbazine, CCNU, and vincristine combination chemotherapy in the treatment of malignant brain tumors. Cancer, *35:* 1398–1404, 1975.
10. Kumar, A. R. V., Renaudin, J., and Wilson, C. B. Procarbazine hydrochloride in the treatment of brain tumors. Phase 2 study. J. Neurosurg., *40:* 365–371, 1974.
11. Levin, V. A., and Wilson, C. B. Correlations between experimental chemotherapy in the murine glioma and effectiveness of clinical therapy regimens. Cancer Chemother. Pharmacol., *1:* 41–48, 1978.
12. Levin, V. A., Wilson, C. B., Davis, R. L., Wara, W. M., Pischer, T. L., and Irwin, R. L.

A phase III comparison study of BCNU, hydroxyurea, and irradiation for the treatment of primary malignant gliomas. J. Neurosurg., *51:* 526–532, 1979.

13. Levin, V. A., Vestnys, P. A., Edwards, M. S., Wara, W. M., Fulton, D. S., Barger, G., Seager, M. L., and Wilson, C. B. Improvement in survival produced by sequential therapies in the treatment of recurrent medulloblastoma. Cancer, in press, 1983.
14. Marton, L. J., Edwards, M. S., Levin, V. A., Lubich, W. P., and Wilson, C. B. Predictive value of cerebrospinal fluid polyamines in medulloblastoma. Cancer Res., *39:* 993–997, 1979.
15. Marton, L. J., Edwards, M. S., Levin, V. A., Lubich, W. P., and Wilson, C. B. CSF polyamines: A new and important means of monitoring patients with medulloblastoma. Cancer, *47:* 757–760, 1981.
16. Mulder, J. H., Smink, T., and Van Putten, L. M. Schedule dependent effectiveness of CCNU and 5-fluorouracil in experimental chemotherapy. Eur. J. Cancer, *13:* 1123–1131, 1971.
17. Nishioka, K., and Romsdahl, M. M. Elevation of putrescine and spermidine in sera of patients with solid tumors. Clin. Chim. Acta, *57:* 155–161, 1974.
18. Prakash, N. J., Schechter, P. J., Grove, J., and Koch-Weser, J. Effect of α-difluoromethylornithine, an enzyme activated, irreversible inhibitor of ornithine decarboxylase, on L1210 leukemia in mice. Cancer Res., *38:* 3059–3062, 1978.
19. Prakash, N. J., Schechter, P. J., Mamont, P. S., Grove, J. Koch-Weser, J., and Sjoerdsma, A. Inhibition of EMT6 tumor grown by interference with polyamine biosynthesis; Effects of α-difluoromethylornithine, an irreversible inhibitor of ornithine decarboxylase. Life Sci., *26:* 181–194, 1980.
20. Winston, K., Gilles, F. H., Leviton, A., and Fulchiero, A. Cerebellar gliomas in children. J. Natl. Cancer Inst. *58:* 833–838, 1977.

CHAPTER

13

Management of Medulloblastoma in Childhood

HAROLD J. HOFFMAN, M.D., F.R.C.S.(C),
E. BRUCE HENDRICK, M.D., F.R.C.S.(C), and
ROBIN P. HUMPHREYS, M.D., F.R.C.S.(C)

INTRODUCTION

In 1954, Ingraham and Matson (23) stated that the "treatment of medulloblastomas of the posterior fossa is certainly one of the darkest chapters in pediatric neurosurgery." They went on to state that no patient with this lesion had ever been cured and that it was unlikely that any would be cured with the therapeutic methods then available. In 1925, Bailley and Cushing (3) clearly established medulloblastomas as distinct tumors of the cerebellum occurring in childhood and for the first time gave those neoplasms the name by which they have been known ever since. By 1930, Cushing (11) reported his experience with 61 medulloblastomas. His operative mortality was 32%. Postoperative radiotherapy was either nonexistent or poorly given, and only 1 patient survived 3 years after surgery.

This state of pessimism in regard to these tumors persisted until the historical publication of Patterson and Farr (32) in 1953. At that time, they reported 27 patients with medulloblastomas treated in Manchester between 1941 and 1950. Following surgical verification of the tumor, their patients were all irradiated with 5000 rad to the posterior fossa and 3500 rad to the rest of the craniospinal axis. Using this mode of therapy, they reported a 3-year survival in 65% of their patients.

Since then, we have seen an increasingly aggressive approach to this once hopeless tumor which has led to a steadily increasing survival rate. In the recent report of Norris *et al.* (31), the survival rate had reached 84% at 4 years.

CLINICAL PRESENTATION

Medulloblastomas are a common tumor of childhood. At the Hospital for Sick Children in Toronto, they constitute 24% of posterior fossa tumors and 14% of all brain tumors seen in childhood (21). Medulloblastomas are characteristically a tumor of childhood. Choux and Lena (9), in their review of 1707 cases of medulloblastoma, found that 74.6% of these occurred in children under the age of 16. In 144 patients reviewed in our institution from 1950 to 1980, the age of presentation ranged from 7 weeks to 15 years, with only 3 patients less than 1 year of age at the time of presentation and with the peak age of occurrence at 7.

Although there have been claims that there has been a decrease in the number of medulloblastomas seen, we have found quite the reverse. Between 1950 and 1959, we saw 24 patients with medulloblastoma, between 1960 and 1969 44 patients, and during the decade between 1970 and 1980 76 patients.

Medulloblastomas tend to occur more frequently in boys than girls. Choux and Lena found that of 3785 patients with medulloblastoma, 62.9% were boys and 37.1% were girls (9). At the Hospital for Sick Children, a similar incidence was found. Of 144 patients, 92 (63.9%) were boys and 52 (36.1%) were girls.

Medulloblastomas are quickly growing tumors and typically present with a short history. Of the 144 patients reviewed at the Hospital for Sick Children, more than 3/4 of the patients gave a history of less than 3 weeks' duration. Choux and Lena (9) found that in 676 tumors in their review of childhood medulloblastomas, the average duration of symptoms prior to presentation was 2 months. Signs of increased intracranial pressure, including headache, vomiting, and papilledema, were the most frequent signs among all the patients reviewed by Choux and Lena, occurring in over 80% of the cases (9). In those patients presenting under 18 months of age, an increasing head size with a clinical diagnosis of hydrocephalus is a common form of presentation. Truncal ataxia in association with nystagmus is a common finding and can be found in more than half the patients with this tumor. When one sees truncal ataxia without nystagmus in association with raised intracranial pressure, one must shift one's diagnosis to the third ventricle and away from the posterior fossa. Rarely, a patient with medulloblastoma can present with an abrupt neurological deterioration due to spontaneous hemorrhage within the tumor. We saw this in 4 of our 144 patients.

Occasionally, a medulloblastoma may present within the first week of life as a congenital tumor (38). Yamashita *et al.* (41) presented a family in which medulloblastoma occurred in two brothers and reviewed the literature up to that time, finding six families with multiple siblings affected by medulloblastoma. In view of this association, they wondered whether hereditary factors played a role in this particular tumor. Rarely, medulloblastoma can be seen as part of an autosomal dominant syndrome which consists of multiple nevoid basal cell carcinomas, jaw cysts, and skeletal anomalies (18).

PATHOLOGY

Medulloblastomas are characteristically tumors of the cerebellar vermis. Choux and Lena, in their review of 2307 medulloblastomas, found that 65.5% were in the vermis, 13.6% in the paravermian region, and 19.59% out laterally in the hemisphere (9). Characteristically, medulloblastomas are solid tumors. However, reports of cystic varieties have occurred in as many as 2 to 20% of reported cases (9). Rarely, on CT scan, the cyst can be large with a mural nodule and can very closely mimic the appearance of a typical cerebellar astrocytoma (Fig. 13.1).

Chang *et al.* (7) developed an operative staging system for medulloblastomas which they reported in 1969.

T1— Tumors less than 3 cm in diameter and limited to the classic midline position in the vermis and roof of fourth ventricle and less frequently to one cerebellar hemisphere.

T2— Tumors more than 3 cm in diameter and invading one adjacent structure or partially filling the fourth ventricle.

T3A—Tumors further invading two adjacent structures or completely filling the fourth ventricle with extension into the aqueduct of Sylvius, foramen Magendie, or foramen of Luschka.

T3B—Tumors arising from the floor of the fourth ventricle or brainstem and filling the fourth ventricle.

T4— Tumors further spreading into the aqueduct of Sylvius to involve the third ventricle and midbrain or tumors extending to the upper cervical cord.

M0— No evidence of gross subarachnoid or hematogenous metastases.

M1— Microscopic tumor cells found in the CSF.

M2— Gross nodular seeding demonstrated in the cerebellar, cerebral subarachnoid space, or in third or lateral ventricles.

M3— Gross nodular seeding in spinal subarachnoid space.

M4— Systemic metastases.

Recently, the Children's Cancer Study Group, using these categories, found that the "M" rating plays a very definite role in recurrence-free survival. The "T" grading of course influences the extent of surgical resection, and the extent of surgical resection seems to have a very direct bearing on recurrence-free survival (37).

In 1964, Rubinstein and Northfield (35) described the desmoplastic medulloblastomas. These tumors characteristically occurred in adults, frequently were located laterally in the cerebellar hemisphere, and tended to carry a better prognosis than the classical medulloblastomas (8). Choux and Lena (9), in reviewing the pathology on 1361 medulloblastomas,

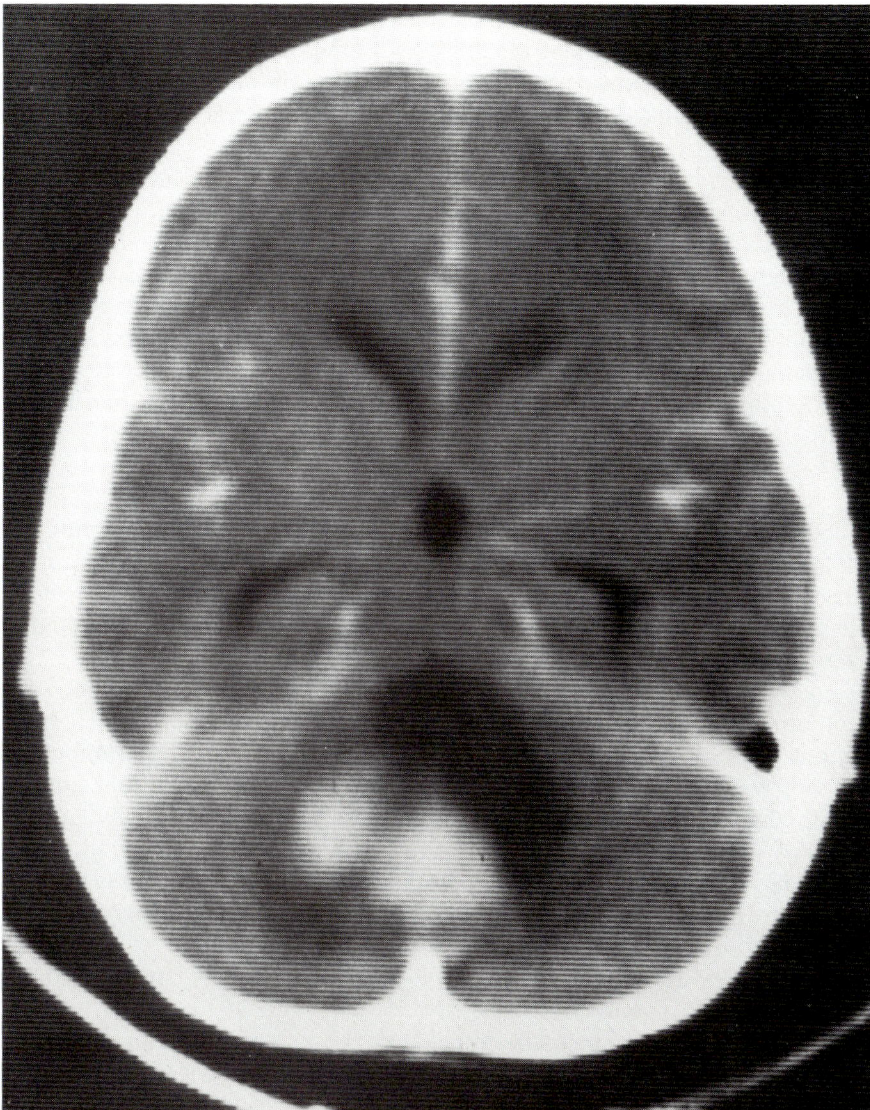

FIG. 13.1. CT scan of child with cystic medulloblastoma in posterior fossa displaying contrast-enhancing "mural nodule."

found that 1080 (79%) were classical, 236 (17%) were desmoplastic, and 45 (3%) were transitional. Of the 144 patients reviewed at the Hospital for Sick Children, 82% were classical, 15% were desmoplastic, and 3% were either pleomorphic or melanotic.

Our survival figures for the desmoplastic medulloblastomas were far worse than for the classical medulloblastomas. These poor results with the desmoplastic medulloblastomas may reflect the fact that all but 1 of our 21 patients with desmoplastic medulloblastomas were under 10 years of age.

In 1930, Percival Bailley (2) demonstrated that medulloblastomas tended to seed along CSF pathways. The knowledge of such seeding led Patterson and Farr (32) to report their revolutionary form of radiotherapy, which dramatically changed the survival rates of patients with this tumor. More recently, the presence of silent spinal cord metastases have been emphasized by Deutsch and Reigel (14). Rarely, the first sign of involvement in the patient with a medulloblastoma may be signs of spinal cord compression due to the metastatic deposits in the spine. We found this in 2 of our 144 patients.

SURGICAL MANAGEMENT OF MEDULLOBLASTOMAS

The early surgical experience with this tumor was disappointing. In 1930, when Cushing reported his experience with 61 medulloblastomas (11), his operative mortality was 32%. Because of this significant mortality rate, Cutler *et al.* (12) reported on the treatment of medulloblastoma with radiotherapy without the benefit of surgical biopsy. Sheline *et al.* (36) used a similar technique which they abandoned in 1949 because of their unhappiness with this mode of therapy. In 1947, Cone (4) began using a technique of twist drill biopsy of suspected cerebellar tumors. If the biopsy showed a medulloblastoma, no further surgery was undertaken, and the tumor was irradiated. When Berger and Elvidge (4) reviewed Cone's results, they found that open operation showed no great advantage over twist drill biopsy and radiation. However, the overall results were poor, with an average survival time in their patients of 3½ years. Furthermore, three of 24 cases (12.5%) died as a result of the biopsy. Mealey and Hall (28) reviewed their experience with 45 children with medulloblastomas treated between 1953 and 1973. About ⅓ had biopsy of the tumor. They concluded that the extent of tumor resection had no significant bearing on prognosis. Their operative mortality was 11%.

In 1969, Bloom *et al.* (6) reported the experience from the Royal Marsden Hospital and found that the survival rate among the patients who had had a complete excision of their tumor was better than among those who had had a partial removal or biopsy.

In recent years, there has been increasing evidence that the more radical the removal of the tumor, the better the long-term survival (6). Wilson (40) in 1970 stated very firmly that radical removal of a medulloblastoma carried a lower operative mortality, lower postoperative morbidity, and also an improved survival.

Recently, Raimondi and Tomita (34) found that the extent of surgical removal influenced survival in a dramatic fashion and that patients with a total resection had a 41.6% 5-year survival rate, as compared to a 30.2% 5-year survival rate for the patients who had a partial resection or biopsy.

In our review at the Hospital for Sick Children of 144 patients with medulloblastoma treated between 1950 and 1980, 129 patients have been included for survival studies. Thirty-one of these had a radical excision, 66 a subtotal excision, and 32 a partial excision or biopsy. The 5-year-survival rates were 59% for the radical excisions, 49% for the subtotal excisions, and 30% for the partial excisions or biopsies. There have been no operative deaths among 61 patients treated since 1973.

For over 20 years at the Hospital for Sick Children in Toronto, all surgical procedures on the posterior fossa have been carried out in the prone position (22). The arguments for the sitting position for posterior fossa surgery include the effectiveness of this position in draining blood and CSF away from the operative wound, as well as maintaining a lower venous pressure in the head. However, the sitting position has many pitfalls, including the risk of air embolism, systemic hypotension and the difficulty in maneuvering the patient into the sitting position.

On the other hand, the prone position is easily maintained. The table can be tilted to improve venous drainage, and the microscope can be easily used in the prone position. There is not the same tiring effects on the arms as there is when the patient is sitting. The risk of air embolism in the sitting position varies between 2 and 15% (25–27). Among 119 operative procedures in the prone position at HSC, there were only two suspected cases of air embolism (22). During the past 7 years, we have had no case of air embolism during posterior fossa surgery in the prone position.

Prior to surgery, the patient is started on dexamethasone in a dose of 4 mg every 6 hours for at least 24–48 hours prior to surgery. At the time of surgery, following anesthetic induction and placement of central lines, the head is carefully positioned without distortion in the prone position with the neck flexed at the occipital C1 junction. This is best done with the pin fixation headrest. The body is placed on a U-shaped bolster to leave the abdomen free (Fig. 13.2). Under the age of 2, because of fear of the pin fixation headrest penetrating the skull, the head is positioned on a U-shaped headrest, with care taken to protect the eyes.

With an indwelling urethral catheter in place, the patient is given mannitol (2 gm/kg). An occipital burr hole is rarely used, except in those patients with gross hydrocephalus in whom a preoperative shunt has not

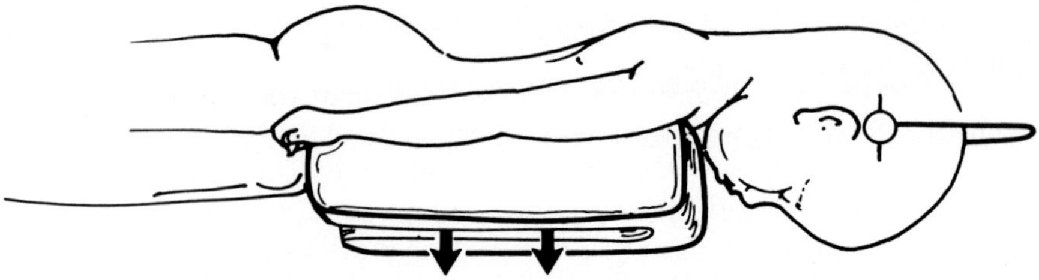

FIG. 13.2. Position of patient for posterior fossa craniotomy.

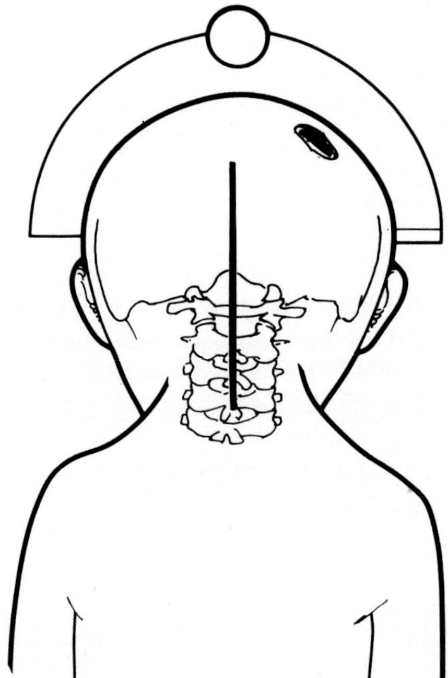

FIG. 13.3. Outline of skin incision utilized in posterior fossa craniotomy for medulloblastoma resection.

been placed. A midline skin incision is utilized from inion to the mid-cervical region (Fig. 13.3). Care must be taken once the skin is incised not to immediately insert a retractor since this may ruin anatomical landmarks and take one down a paramedian course into muscle with consequent brisk bleeding. No retractor is therefore inserted until the midline ligamentum nuchae have been incised down to the spinous processes. Once this is done, the skin and muscle are retracted. A horizontal incision is placed in the paraspinal muscle in the midoccipital region. This will be of help in the eventual suturing of the musculature. The muscle is then taken off the occipital bone. With sharp dissection, the periosteum is incised over the arch of C1. With an elevator, the periosteum is then lifted off the arch of C1 on either side, and then, using the index finger covered with gauze, the periosteum is stripped off the arch of C1. It is far safer to use the finger than sharp dissection or an instrument to carry out this dissection. With such dissection, one may inadvertently injure the vertebral artery.

With the power craniotome, a burr hole is placed on either side of the midline just below the inion. Bone is then rongeured between the burr holes, across the midline, and then downwards on either side towards the foramen magnum. Once this is done, the occipital bone is grasped with the rongeur and taken off the underlying dura, leaving the remaining attachment at the atlantooccipital membrane, which runs from the lip of the foramen magnum to the arch of C1 intact. This is sharply divided, and the occipital bone is removed. The arch of C1 is then removed.

The dura is now divided, running from a superolateral position inferiorly and thus creating a V-shaped incision in dura with the bottom of the V at the foramen magnum (Fig. 13.4). The occipital sinus is then coagulated or clipped, and the dura is then hinged upward by a ligature

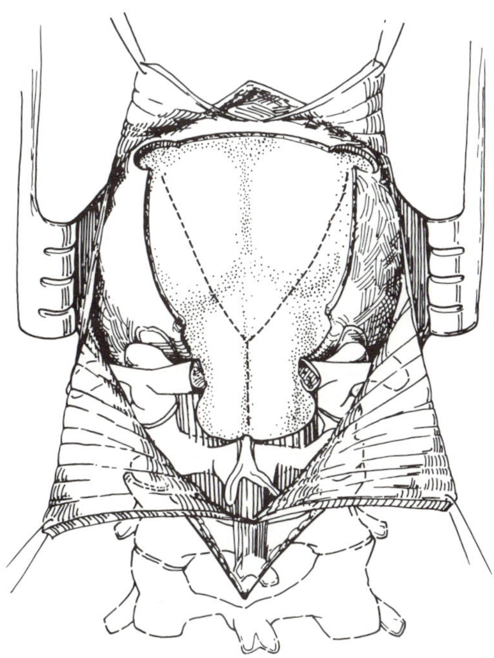

FIG. 13.4. Outline of dural incision utilized in posterior fossa craniotomy for tumor.

which is placed around the occipital sinus at its inferior extent. The dura is then divided over the cervical region and reflected laterally.

The cisterna magna is then opened, and frequently one can see medulloblastoma protruding between the two tonsils. On rare occasions, the tumor may have spread en plaque over the surface of the cerebellum, or the tumor may be located out laterally in one cerebellar hemisphere, distending it and mimicking the appearance of a cerebellar astrocytoma. Even more rarely, the tumor may be restricted to one cerebellopontine angle, lying in an extra-axial position. Commonly, however, the tumor occupies the vermis and protrudes into the fourth ventricle (Fig. 13.5).

Using bipolar cautery, the vessels over the surface of the inferior half of the vermis are coagulated and divided. A patty is slipped into the fourth ventricle between the floor of the fourth ventricle and the overlying tumor. The vermis is then split, exposing the tumor, which lies in the roof of the fourth ventricle (Fig. 13.6). The tumor is typically reddish grey in color. The microscope is usually brought in at this point; under magnification, the tumor is slowly removed. Frequently these tumors are very soft and friable, and ordinary suction may be sufficient for their removal. However, as the tumor enters the subarachnoid space, it picks up fibrous tissue, and certain areas can be quite firm. The cavitron becomes invaluable in removing the tumor in such instances. If the tumor fills the fourth ventricle, one can follow it into the fourth ventricle and up into the aqueduct, and eventually one can completely remove the tumor using biopsy forceps and the cavitron to dislodge fragments. Eventually, one should have a completely clean floor of fourth ventricle with no visible tumor. Occasionally, the medulloblastoma may invade the floor of the fourth ventricle, and of course here the tumor must be left adherent to the floor of the fourth ventricle for fear of disturbing vital signs. If one has to remove tumor from the floor of the fourth ventricle, it is wise to allow the patient to breathe spontaneously, so one can monitor both respiration and blood pressure and cardiac rate and know when he is disturbing these signs by manipulation of tumor in the floor of the fourth ventricle. If hydrocephalus and ventriculomegaly have been a problem, and one has cleared the fourth ventricle of tumor and exposed the aqueduct, then a Lapras catheter (Codman, Randolph, Mass.) is ideal for cannulating the fourth ventricle and allowing CSF access from the third ventricle into cisterna magna (Fig. 13.7 and 13.8).

Once the tumor is completely removed, if there is any venous ooze, Surgicel is applied to venous bleeders and then covered with Gelfoam, which will adhere to the Surgicel. This is then covered by a piece of rubber dam. Gentle pressure is then applied by instilling a piece of cotton, which has been soaked in 3% hydrogen peroxide for a period of 2 to 3

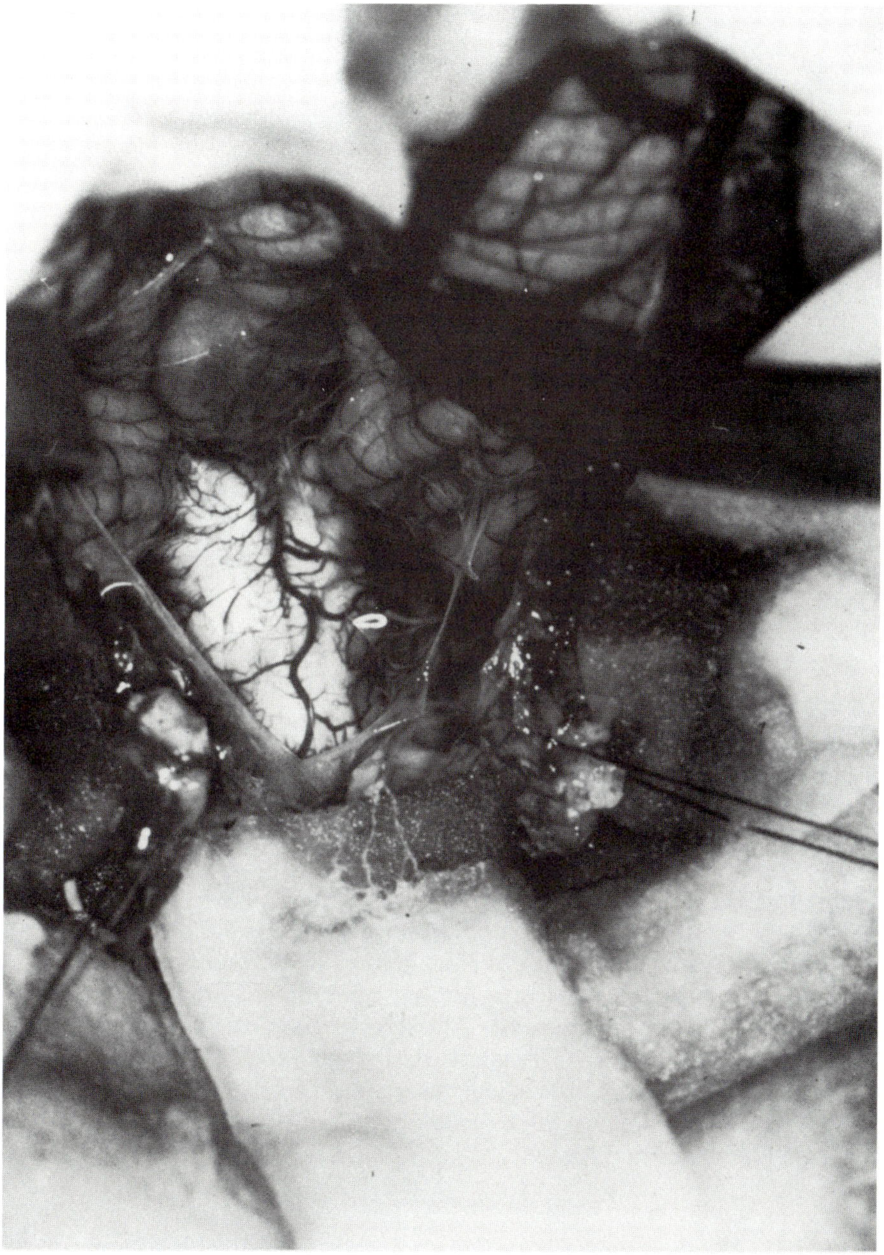

FIG. 13.5. Operative exposure of medulloblastoma protruding between cerebellar tonsils.

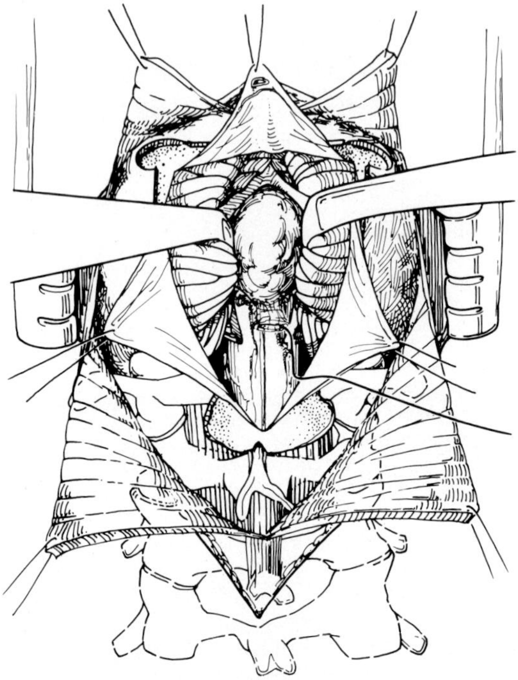

FIG. 13.6. Drawing of vermis split, which brings entire tumor into view.

minutes. The cotton and rubber dam are then irrigated out, leaving the Surgicel and Gelfoam adherent and thus providing a dry field.

Prior to dural closure, the venous pressure is raised by the anesthetist to make sure that there are no venous bleeders.

The dura is now replaced. Usually, there is not sufficient dura for adequate tight dural closure, so, in recent years, we have routinely made use of cadaver freeze-dried dura to produce a waterproof dural closure.

Postoperatively, the patient is closely monitored. If a Lapras catheter has been inserted, the patient is lumbar punctured 24 hours postoperatively and at intervals thereafter to ensure flow of CSF through the catheter. A postoperative CT scan is carried out 7 to 21 days after surgery to confirm the amount of surgical resection. Ten days to 2 weeks after surgery, a myelogram is done to rule out spinal metastases, and at that time, CSF is examined for cytology.

PRECRANIOTOMY SHUNTS

In 1963, Abraham and Chandy (1) pointed out the value of a precraniotomy shunt in the management of the patient with a posterior fossa tumor. In 1966, we were presented with two moribund patients with

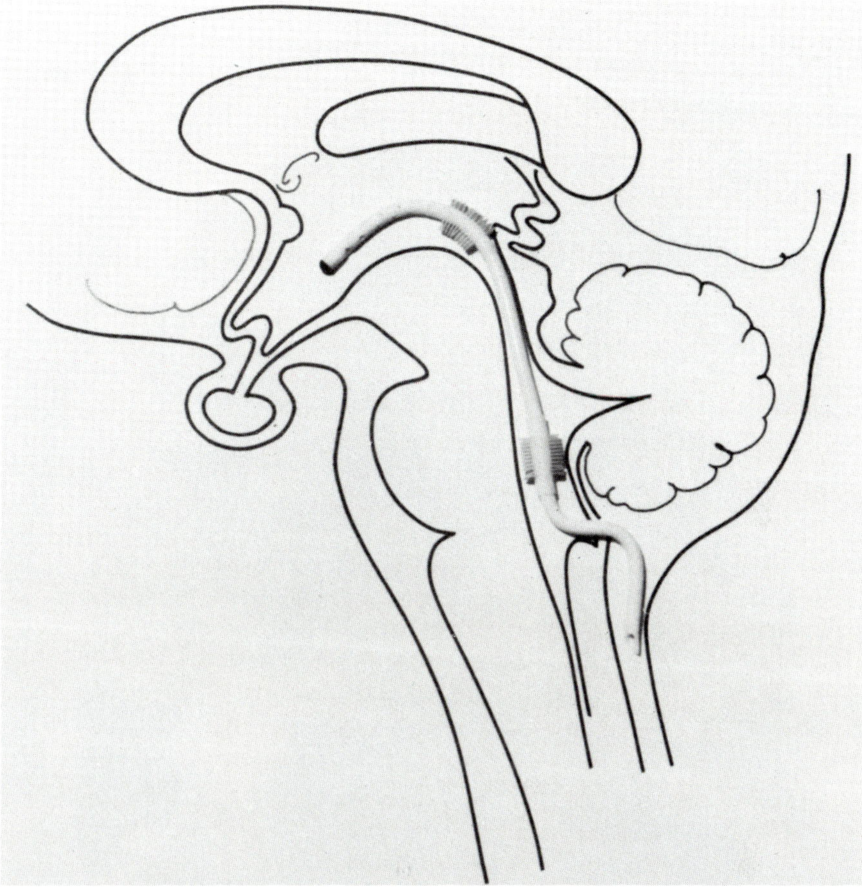

FIG. 13.7. Lapras catheter utilized for cannulating aqueduct of Sylvius.

posterior fossa tumors who were believed to be too ill to have a craniotomy. In order to improve their status, a ventriculoperitoneal shunt was inserted as an initial step. Both of these patients did surprisingly well, and it was at this point that we began inserting a ventriculoperitoneal shunt in all patients with a diagnosis of a posterior fossa tumor and significant hydrocephalus some 7 to 10 days before craniotomy (26). However, at that time prior to the advent of CT scanning, the common methods of investigating a child with a posterior fossa mass were ventriculography and angiography. These were both time consuming procedures necessitating general anesthesia in a child with raised intracranial pressure. If the child was ill prior to the investigative procedure, he was even more ill after the procedure. It was therefore elected at that time to

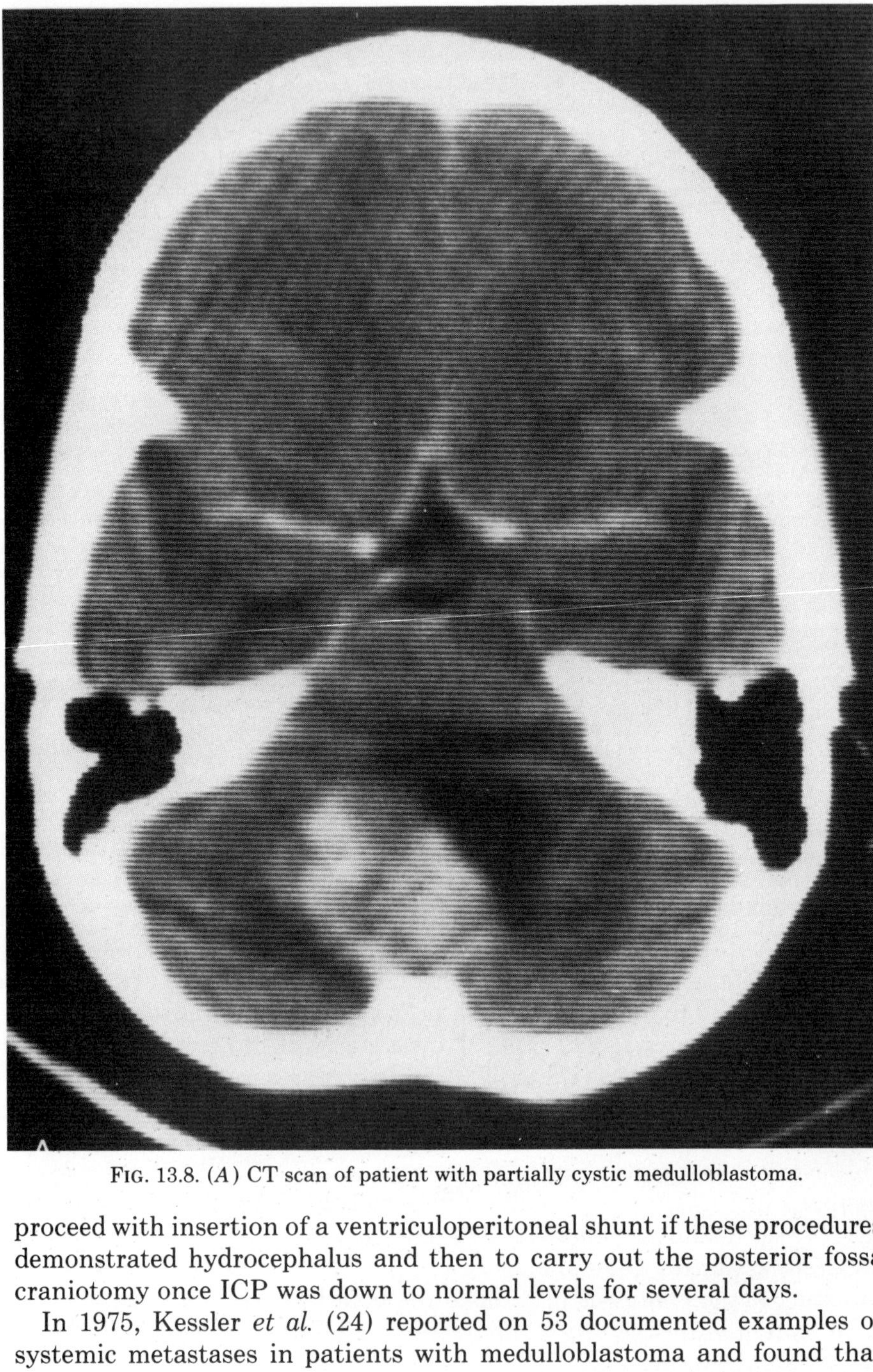

FIG. 13.8. (*A*) CT scan of patient with partially cystic medulloblastoma.

proceed with insertion of a ventriculoperitoneal shunt if these procedures demonstrated hydrocephalus and then to carry out the posterior fossa craniotomy once ICP was down to normal levels for several days.

In 1975, Kessler *et al.* (24) reported on 53 documented examples of systemic metastases in patients with medulloblastoma and found that

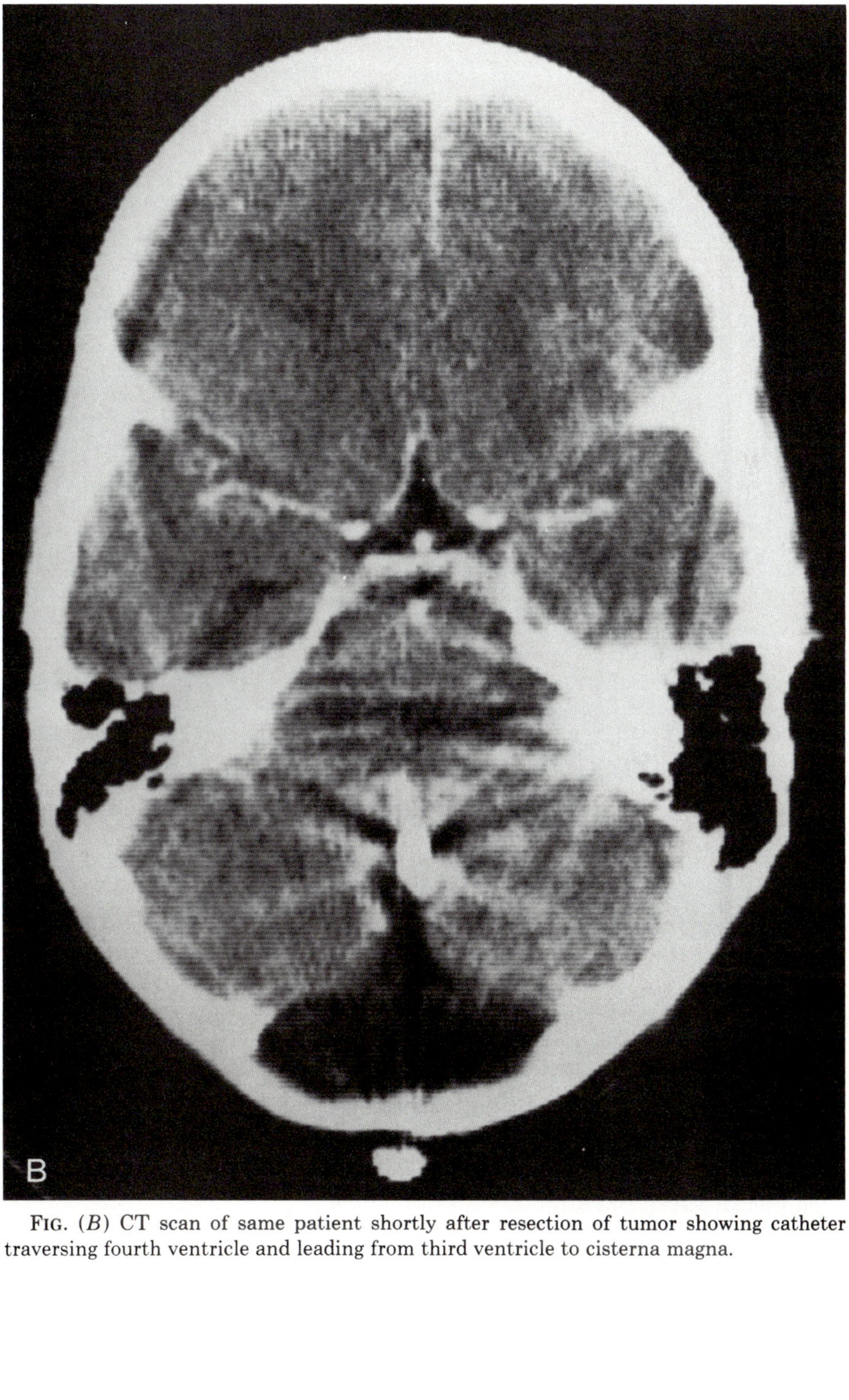

FIG. (*B*) CT scan of same patient shortly after resection of tumor showing catheter traversing fourth ventricle and leading from third ventricle to cisterna magna.

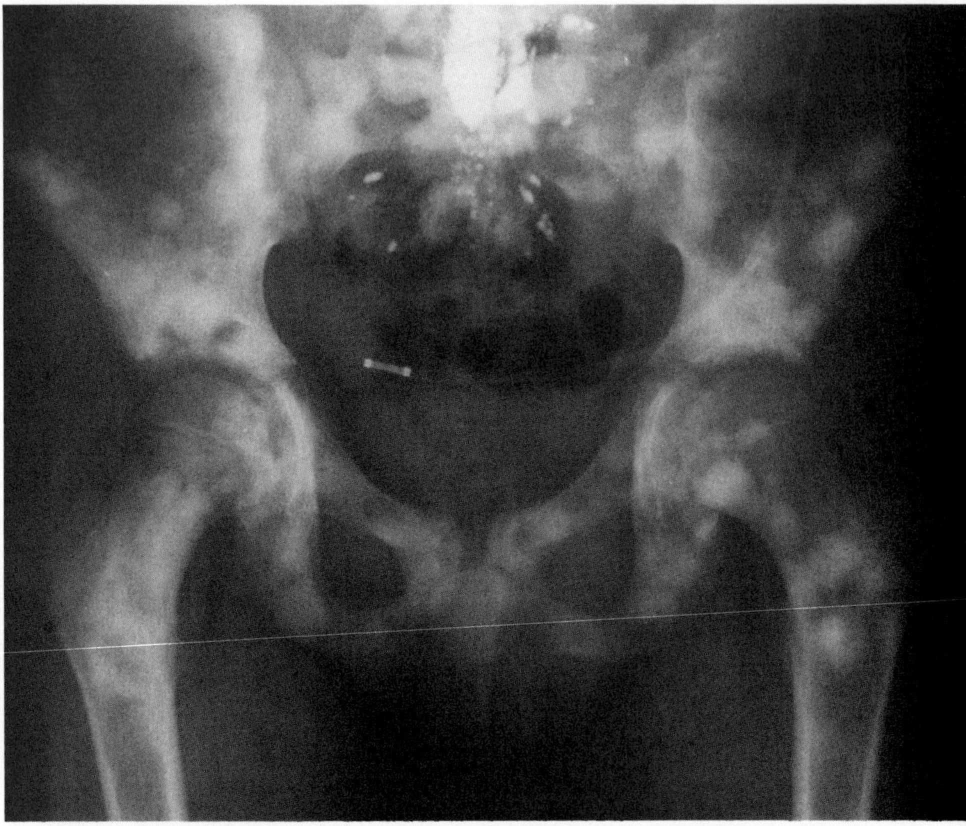

FIG. 13.9. Metastatic medulloblastoma in pelvis in child with unfiltered VP shunt.

eight of these patients had systemic CSF diversionary shunts. In our report of 1976 (2), we described 41 patients with medulloblastoma who had had a precraniotomy ventriculoperitoneal shunt, and six of these had systemic metastases, with four of this group having evidence of peritoneal spread, presumably on the basis of the VP shunts (Fig. 13.9).

As a result of this initial experience with systemic metastases through a ventriculoperitoneal shunt, we began using a 3-μm Millipore filter incorporated in the shunting system in patients with a suspect medulloblastoma. Between 1973 and 1980, 49 patients were treated on our service for medulloblastoma who had a preoperative ventriculoperitoneal shunt. In 24 of these patients, the shunts included a Millipore filter. Despite this, one of these patients did develop systemic metastases (4.2%). The systemic metastases could have been shunt related due to breakage of the fragile Millipore filter or on the basis of surgical manipulation and blood-borne metastases. On the other hand, 25 patients had unfiltered shunts, and five of these developed systemic metastases—an incidence of 20%. We found this to be a frightening statistic, since the presence of systemic metastases means the eventual death of the patient.

Since the availability of the CT scan, we have seen a steady decrease in the use of preoperative shunting in our patients for medulloblastoma. Between 1975 and 1980, the incidence of a preoperative shunting procedure in a patient in whom a preoperative CT scan was obtained was 75%. Between 1977 and 1980, the utilization had dropped to 60%, and at the present time, we rarely utilize a preoperative shunt in a patient with a suspected medulloblastoma.

However, when such a shunt becomes necessary, preoperatively or in the immediate postoperative period while tumor cells are free in the CSF, it is mandatory that a filtering device be inserted which can effectively block the spread of tumor cells into the peritoneal cavity. Millipore is fragile and can break and therefore may allow access of tumor cells. We are now using Versapor (Medical Device Division, Gelman Sciences Inc., Ann Arbor, Mich.), which is an acrylic, copolymer membrane, incorporating an integral nonwoven nylon substrate for support.

When one inserts a filtering device into a shunting system, we have found a 25% chance that the filter will eventually clog with fibrous tissue. At such a time, the patient may have completed his course of radiotherapy and the filtering device may no longer be necessary. Should the patient still require the shunt, it becomes necessary to reoperate on the patient and remove the filter. We now incorporate a bypass system into the filtering device so that if the filter should clog and if the shunting device remains necessary, we could percutaneously bypass the filter and thus open up the CSF diversionary device (Heyer-Schulte Corp., Santa Barbara, Calif).

CHEMOTHERAPY

Lassman *et al.* (25) reported on the value of vincristine in the management of intracranial gliomas in 1965. Since then, a variety of chemotherapeutic agents have been advocated for the management of recurrent medulloblastomas (15, 37). In January 1975, SIOP (Societe Internationale D'Oncologie Pediatrique) launched a study to determine the role of adjuvant chemotherapy in children with posterior fossa medulloblastomas (16). A randomized study was carried out in which half the children, in addition to their surgery and radiotherapy, received prophylactic chemotherapy consisting of vincristine and 1-(2-chloroethyl)-3-cyclohexyl-1-nitrosourea (CCNU).

In 1981, Julian Bloom (5) presented some of the data from the SIOP study. Chemotherapy for patients who had had a total resection of their tumor did not improve outcome. However, in patients who were at high risk, namely, patients who had only had a partial excision of their tumor or patients who were under 2 years of age, chemotherapy seemed to improve prognosis. The Children's Cancer Study Group conducted a similar randomized study and concluded that chemotherapy given prophylactically was not of benefit in improving prognosis (35).

RESULTS OF THERAPY FOR MEDULLOBLASTOMA

In 1955 Collins (10) formulated a rule in relation to Wilms' tumor that the period of risk for recurrence of a congenital tumor was equal to the time interval from the patient's conception to his age at diagnosis (expressed as patient's age plus 9 months). Bloom *et al.* (6) in 1969 applied this period of risk, initially formulated for Wilms' tumor, to patients with medulloblastoma and found that all recurrences in a series of 82 children with medulloblastoma had occurred within the period of risk as defined by Collins' rule. They concluded that once a child with medulloblastoma had passed this critical period without signs of recurrence, cure was likely.

Quest *et al.* (33), in 1978, in reporting on a series of medulloblastomas from Columbia University, found that Collins' rule seemed to hold true for their series of patients. In 1981 Dell *et al.* (13) in applying Collins' rule concluded that 10% of the patients satisfying Collins' rule would develop recurrences either of their primary tumor or of a malignant glioma. In our series of 144 patients with medulloblastoma, two have recurred beyond their period of risk.

Harisiadis and Chang (23), in reviewing the medulloblastoma treated in childhood at Columbia University, found that tumor staging was an accurate prognostic indicator of survival, with the T1 patients having a 75% 5-year survival rate, the T2 patients a 50.5% survival rate, the T3 patients a 32.3% survival rate, and the T4 patients not surviving.

The increasing survival seen in children with medulloblastoma has been accompanied by a growing concern for the long-term effects of radiotherapy on developing brain and spine. Hirsch *et al.* (19), in reviewing 57 children with medulloblastomas, found IQs below 70 in 31% of patients. About one-quarter of patients with medulloblastoma who have survived therapy in our series, have some degree of intellectual deterioration. Neuheuser *et al.* (30) has suggested that dosages in excess of 2000 R delivered to the spine will almost invariably cause growth retardation in children. Some 46.7% of our survivors exhibit a short stature. In some, this is due to impairment of growth hormone secretion, but in the majority it is due to the effect of radiation therapy on the growing spine. Almost one-fifth of our survivors have some degree of hormonal impairment affecting thyroid function, growth hormone secretion, or sex hormone secretion. Radiation can affect hearing by damaging the middle ear as well as the 8th nerve. Radiation necrosis can occur in brain and was

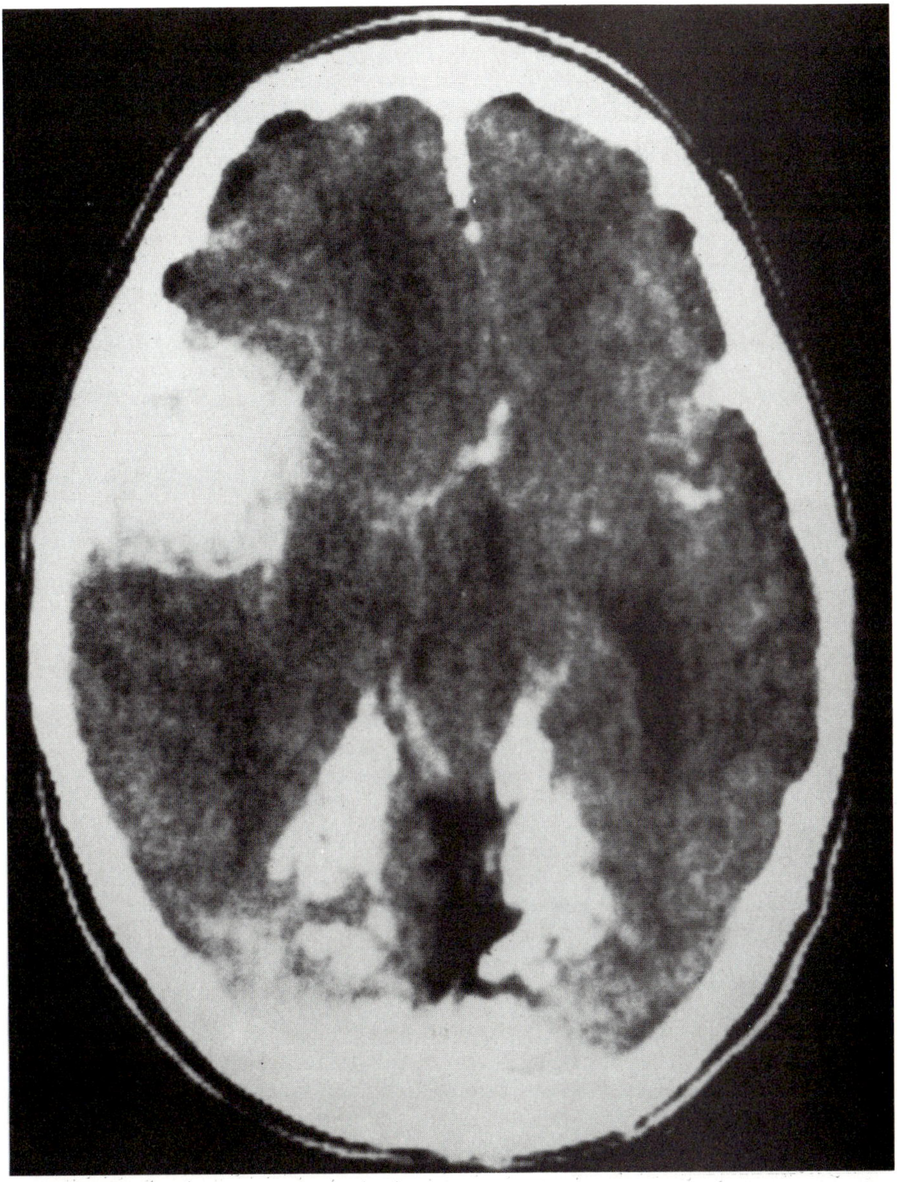

FIG. 13.10. CT scan of patient done 13 years after treatment of posterior fossa medulloblastoma and showing radiation-induced supratentorial meningioma as well as tentorial calcification.

seen in one of our patients. Radiation can induce tumors, and we have encountered one patient with a radiation-induced meningioma in our series (Fig. 13.10).

CONCLUSIONS

During the past 30 years, medulloblastomas have become curable tumors with more than 60% of the patients surviving. Our efforts now must be geared not only to improve upon these survival figures but also to improve the quality of life of the survivors.

REFERENCES

1. Abraham, J., and Chandy, J. Ventriculo-atrial shunt in the management of posterior fossa tumors. Preliminary report. J. Neurosurg., *20:* 252–253, 1963.
2. Bailley, P. Further notes on the cerebellar medulloblastomas. The effect of roentgen radiation. Am. J. Pathol., *6:* 126–136, 1930.
3. Bailley, P., and Cushing, H. Medulloblastoma cerebelli, common type of mid-cerebellar glioma of childhood. Arch. Neurol. Psychiatry, *14:* 192–224, 1925.
4. Berger, E. C., and Elvidge, A. R. Medulloblastoma and cerebellar sarcomas. A clinical survey. J. Neurosurg., *20:* 139–144, 1963.
5. Bloom, H. J. G. Presented at Second International Conference in Pediatric and Adolescent Hematology/Oncology, Niagara Falls, N.Y., August 31–September 2, 1981.
6. Bloom, H. J. G., Wallace, E. N. K., and Henk, J. M. The treatment and prognosis of medulloblastoma in children. Am. J. Roentgenol., *105:* 43–62, 1969.
7. Chang, C. H., Housepian, E. M., and Herbert, C. An operative staging system and a megavoltage radiotherapeutic technic for cerebellar medulloblastomas. Radiology, *93:* 1351–1359, 1969.
8. Chatty, E. M., and Earle, K. M. Medulloblastoma. A report of 201 cases with emphasis on the relationship of histologic variants to survival. Cancer, *28:* 977–983, 1971.
9. Choux, M., and Lena, G. Medulloblastoma. Neurochirurgie, *28*(Suppl. 1): 13–15, 26, 60, 66, 70, 81, 1982.
10. Collins, V. P. Wilms' tumor: Its behavior and prognosis. J. Louisiana State Med. Soc., *107:* 474–480, 1955.
11. Cushing, H. Experience with cerebellar medulloblastoma: A critical review. Acta Pathol. Microbiol. Scand., *7:* 1–86, 1930.
12. Cutler, E. C., Sosman, M. C., and Vaughan, W. W. The place of radiation in the treatment of cerebellar medulloblastomas. Report of twenty cases. Am. J. Roentgenol., *35:* 429–450, 1950.
13. Dell, S., Cohen, M., and Kushner, M. Period of risk hypothesis after prophylactic radiotherapy. Child's Brain, *8:* 372–381, 1981.
14. Deutsch, M., and Reigel, D. H. The value of myelography in the management of childhood medulloblastoma. Cancer, *45:* 2194–2197, 1980.
15. Edwards, M. S., Levin, V. A., Seager, M. L., and Wilson, C. B. Intrathecal chemotherapy for leptomeningeal dissemination of medulloblastoma. Child's Brain, *8:* 444–451, 1981.
16. Gerosa, M. A., di Stefano, E., Olivi, A., and Carteri, A. Multidisciplinary treatment of medulloblastoma: A 5-year experience with the SIOP trial. Child's Brain, *8:* 107–118, 1981.
17. Harisiadis, L., and Chang, C. H. Medulloblastoma in children: A correlation between staging and results of treatment. Int. J. Radiation Oncol. Biol. Phys., *2:* 833–841, 1977.
18. Hawkins, J. C., Hoffman, H. J., and Becker, L. E. Multiple nevoid basal-cell carcinoma syndrome (Gorlin's syndrome) possible confusion with metastatic medulloblastoma. J. Neurosurg., *50:* 100–102, 1979.

19. Hirsch, J. F., Renier, D., Czermichow, P., Beneviste, L., and Pierre-Kahn, A. Medulloblastoma in childhood survival and functional results. Acta Neurochir., *48:* 1–15, 1979.
20. Hoffman, H. J., Hendrick, E. B., and Humphreys, R. P. Metastasis via ventriculoperitoneal shunt in patients with medulloblastoma. J. Neurosurg., *44:* 562–566, 1976.
21. Humphreys, R. P. Posterior fossa brain tumors in children. Neurol. Surg., *5:* 2733–2758, 1982.
22. Humphreys, R. P., Creighton, R. E., Hendrick, E. B., and Hoffman, H. J. Advantages of the prone position for neurosurgical procedures on the upper cervical spine and posterior cranial fossa in children. Child's Brain, *1:* 325–336, 1975.
23. Ingraham, F. D., and Matson, D. D. Neurosurgery of infancy and childhood. Charles C Thomas, Springfield, Ill., 1954.
24. Kessler, L. A., Dugan, P., and Concannon, J. P. Systemic metastases of medulloblastoma promoted by shunting. Surg. Neurol., *3:* 147–152, 1975.
25. Lassman, L. P., Pearce, G. W., and Garg, J. Sensitivity of intracranial gliomas to vincristine sulphate. Lancet, *2:* 296, 1965.
26. Leivers, D., Spilsbury, R. A., and Young, J. V. Air embolism during neurosurgery in the sitting position. Two case reports. Br. J. Anaesth., *43:* 84–90, 1971.
27. Marshall, B. M. Air embolism in neurosurgical anaesthesia. Its diagnosis and treatment. Can. Anaesth. Soc. J., *12:* 255–261, 1965.
28. Mealey, J., and Hall, P. V. Medulloblastoma in children. Survival and treatment. J. Neurosurg., *46:* 56–64, 1977.
29. Michenfelder, J. D., and Terry, H. R. Current practices and trends in neuroanesthesia. Clin. Neurosurg., *13:* 252–264, 1966.
30. Neuheuser, E. B. D., Witlenborg, M. H., Berman, C. Z., and Cohen, J. Irradiation effects of roentgen therapy on the growing spine. Radiology, *59:* 637–650, 1952.
31. Norris, D. G., Bruce, D. A., Byrd, R. L., Schut, L., Littman, P., Bilaniuk, L., Zimmerman, R. A., and Capp, R. Improved relapse-free survival in medulloblastoma utilizing modern techniques. Neurosurgery, *9:* 661–664, 1981.
32. Patterson, E., and Farr, R. F. Cerebellar medulloblastoma: Treatment by irradiation of the whole central nervous system. Acta Radiol., *39:* 323–336, 1953.
33. Quest, D. O., Busman, R., Antunes, J. L., and Housepian, E. M. Period of risk for recurrence in medulloblastoma. J. Neurosurg., *48:* 159–163, 1978.
34. Raimondi, A. J., and Tomita, T. Medulloblastoma in childhood. Comparative results of partial and total resection. Child's Brain, *5:* 310–328, 1979.
35. Rubinstein, L. J., and Northfield, D. W. C. The medulloblastoma and the so-called arachnoidal cerebellar sarcoma. A critical examination of a nosological problem. Brain, *87:* 379–412, 1964.
36. Sheline, G. E., Phillips, T. L., and Baldrey, E. The therapy of unbiopsied brain tumors. Am. J. Roentgenol., *93:* 664–670, 1965.
37. Sposto, R. Reports to CCG-921 and CCG-923 studies committees, Children's Cancer Study Group, 1982.
38. Taboada, D. F., Froufe, A., Alonso, A., Alvarez, J., Muro, D., and Vila, M.: Congenital medulloblastoma. Report of two cases. Pediatr. Radiol., *9:* 5–10, 1980.
39. Thomas, P. R. M., Duffner, P. K., Cohen, M., Sinks, L., Tebbi, C., and Freeman, A. Multimodality therapy for medulloblastoma. Cancer, *46:* 666–669, 1980.
40. Wilson, C. B. Medulloblastoma. Current views regarding the tumor and its treatment. Oncology, *24:* 273–290, 1970.
41. Yamashita, J., Handa, H., and Toyama, M. Medulloblastoma in two brothers. Surg. Neurol., *4:* 225–227, 1975.

CHAPTER

14

Prognosis and Long-term Follow-up in Patients with Medulloblastoma

MAURICE CHOUX, M.D., G. LENA, M.D., and J. HASSOUN, M.D.

INTRODUCTION

A French monograph on medulloblastoma has been recently published by our group (24). It is the first general publication on this subject since that of Crue (26) in 1958.

Our report (24) was based on a review of 113 series grouping 6026 cases; 4636 cases from 85 series were taken from the literature, and 1388 cases from 28 series were not yet published. Our own material included 112 cases, but only 84 of them were selected for study.

Considering that most of the statistical data concerned a limited number of cases (only 19 series of 113 include more than 100 cases), we tried, with inclusion of material from the literature, to check the general trends of incidence, age, and sex proportion.

In 19 large series of intracranial tumors of all ages (43,578 cases), medulloblastomas represented 1630 cases (3.74%). In 48 series of intracranial tumors in children (14,317 cases), medulloblastomas represented 2609 cases (18.22%). Despite what is mentioned in some publications, the incidence of medulloblastoma is increasing slightly in the majority of centers.

In 24 series (1707 cases) of medulloblastomas, 74.6% are pediatric cases (1273). The age distribution in 2049 pediatric cases of the literature shows a "plateau" of major incidence between the ages of 3 and 8, with a peak occurrence at 6 years of age. Medulloblastomas in infants represent 10.5% of the cases. Nineteen congenital medulloblastomas have been described in the literature. Few cases are reported within the first year of life (4% of the cases). In adulthood, medulloblastomas are rare after the age of 40 and exceptional after 50 (13 cases).

Medulloblastomas are more common in males (62.9%) among 3766 cases. In children, the sex incidence shows a similar male predominance at different ages (62.6% in infant, 58% between the ages of 11 and 15). Desmoplastic medulloblastomas are encountered in male patients in 61.5% of the cases.

Familial medulloblastomas are rare. Seven confirmed cases and 6 probable cases were found in the literature. Personally, we have published the familial cases of two sisters operated on for medulloblastoma and one brother who died with posterior fossa symptoms from an unknown cause. Medulloblastomas in twins are exceptional, and 4 cases only have been published (Leavitt (55), Cushing (30), and Grienpentrog and Pauly (41).

In this paper, we have chosen to discuss four controversial problems: the pathological entity of the medulloblastoma from our own material, the survival rate and what is the expectancy of cured tumor, the factors influencing the prognosis, and the quality of survival. We do not pretend to bring firm answers to each of these questions, but we felt that the study of the major papers on medulloblastomas since 1930 permitted us to point out some questions and possible answers in regard to this fascinating lesion.

MORPHOLOGICAL STUDY

Material and Methods

Fifty-five cases of cerebellar medulloblastomas in 41 children and 14 adults were histologically studied on biopsy samples in all the cases and on autopsy specimens in 6 cases. In 47 cases, the tumor was located in the vermis. In 7 cases, it was laterally located, and in one case, the tumor was diffuse. Hematoxylin-eosin, Gomori's method for reticulin, and Bodian's method for neurofibrils were utilized to stain the tissue in all cases. Immunocytochemical reactions for GFAP were done in 28 cases according to Sternberger's method. Electron microscopy was done in 36 cases (Fig. 14.1).

Results

The morphological classification followed that proposed by Rubinstein and Northfield in 1964 (83). Four groups of tumors were described. Twenty-eight cases of classical medulloblastomas showed a uniform and dense cellular pattern (Fig. 14.1*A*), with typical Wright rosettes in 10 cases. Fourteen cases corresponded to the definition of desmoplastic medulloblastoma with an extensive production of reticulin in the stroma. Ten cases associated both previous types (mixed medulloblastomas). In 3 cases, the medulloblastoma cells formed diffuse meningeal or molecular infiltrates without any limited tumor mass (medulloblastomas "en plaque").

There was no relationship between the age of the patient and the histological pattern. However, a desmoplastic reaction was always present when the tumor was laterally located in the cerebellar hemispheres.

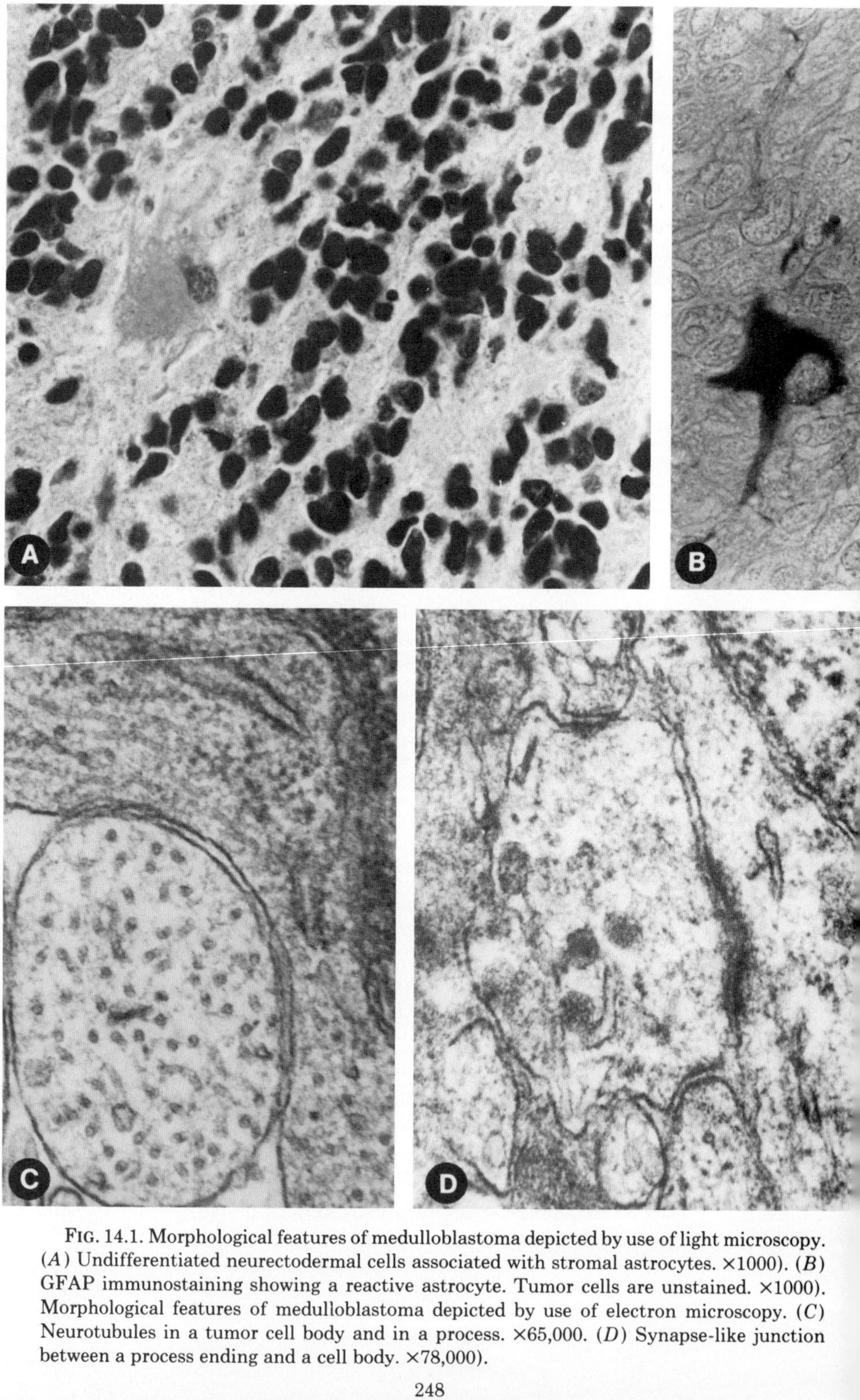

FIG. 14.1. Morphological features of medulloblastoma depicted by use of light microscopy. (*A*) Undifferentiated neurectodermal cells associated with stromal astrocytes. ×1000). (*B*) GFAP immunostaining showing a reactive astrocyte. Tumor cells are unstained. ×1000). Morphological features of medulloblastoma depicted by use of electron microscopy. (*C*) Neurotubules in a tumor cell body and in a process. ×65,000. (*D*) Synapse-like junction between a process ending and a cell body. ×78,000).

The differential diagnosis of medulloblastomas with other anaplastic primitive neurectodermal tumors of the cerebellum (such as malignant astrocytomas, ependymomas, and oligodendrogliomas) was problematic only in some cases. GFAP immunostaining and electron microscopy were very helpful in these cases.

GFAP immunostaining revealed more or less numerous positive astrocytes in 19 cases from the 28 tumors tested (Fig. 14.1*B*). It was never possible to assert that tumor cells were stained. The positive cells corresponding to astrocytes were easily recognizable with hematoxylin-eosin staining.

Electron microscopy performed in 36 cases revealed one tumor cell type. Organelles were rare, except for neurotubules, which were especially numerous in the cell processes (Fig. 14.1*C*). Dense core vesicles evoking a neurosecretory activity were observed in 4 cases, synapse-like junctions in 2 cases (Fig. 14.1*D*). Glial process cells were more frequent at the periphery of the tumor and in the infiltrated lamellae. Microfilaments were rather exceptional in the tumor cells themselves.

No supratentorial or extraneural metastases were morphologically studied in this present series. A supratentorial extension of the tumor was observed in 4 autopsy cases. Tumor metastases to spinal cord were analyzed in 7 cases.

The morphological conclusions from this study enhanced, if need be, the concept of an undifferentiated tumor with a pleomorphic architectural pattern but showed a unique neurectodermal cell type by electron microscopy. No proper definite astrocytic differentiation was obvious, either on ultrastructural specimens or on immunocytochemical reactions. Thus, the present study did not favor the widely accepted notion of a spontaneous astrocytic maturation of the neoplastic cells. It is possible that such a static approach does not allow any conclusion about this point. At the opposite extreme, an incomplete neuronal differentiation was suggested in a few cases by electron microscopy and was reminiscent of the so-called neuroblastomas of the cerebellum. The cytological uniformity of the various subtypes of medulloblastomas (tumors of children or adults, median or lateral tumors, classical, desmoplastic, and mixed forms) constitutes sufficient proof of a unique and unequivocal tumoral concept. The pleomorphism of the stroma reaction, well-known in other types of human tumors, cannot argue for different cerebellar tumors of different histogenesis.

SURVIVAL

We have indicated in Table 14.1 the survival rates at 1, 2, 3, 4, 5 and 20 years in 67 series of medulloblastoma from the literature.

TABLE 14.1

Survival in 67 Series of the Literature

Authors		No. of Cases	1 Yr (%)	2 Yr (%)	3 Yr (%)	4 Yr (%)	5 Yr (%)	7 Yr (%)	10 Yr (%)	More than 10 Yr
Cushing (30)	1930	61			1.6		1.6			
Spitz *et al.* (93)	1947	67 E			0					
		21 A[a]			62		19			
Ingraham *et al.* (48)	1948	56			13		5		3.6	
Keith *et al.* (51)	1949	84					0			
Ringertz and Tola (81)	1950	107		14	7		3			
Grant and Sayers (40)	1951	50					6		4	1 Case
Bodian and Lawson (15)	1953	36			0					
Paterson and Farr (73)	1953	Totally children			65		40			
					54		29			
Richmond (80)	1953	25			50		43			
Lampe and McIntyre (53)	1954				35		31			
Hoffmann *et al.*	1961	72	40	26	23.6	23	7			
Paterson (72)	1961	31			54		40			
Smith *et al.* (92)	1961	38			33		28		21.6	6 Cases
Tice (97)	1962	21			30		30	23		2 Cases
Liebner *et al.* (56)	1964	19			32		13			
Bouchard (17)	1966	37			35		28		17	
Simpson *et al.* (91)	1968						40		25	
Aron (2)	1969	24					35		26	
Borejko and Hartel-Ulkowska (16)	1970				33		20			
Chang *et al.* (22)	1969	30	87	70	60	55	50			
Bloom *et al.* (13)	1969	82			39		38		31	
Jenkin (49)	1969	47			62		53		26	1 Case
MacFarland *et al.* (57)	1969	26			48		38		14	10%
Faust *et al.* (36)	1970				50		38			
Hope-Stone (47)	1970	35					75		50	
Massaroti *et al.* (60)	1970	76 C	41.3	13	8.7		6			
		39 A	53.6	32	28.6		7			
Miles and Bhandhari (63)	1970	29	33		14		10		3	
Nöel and Methot (67)	1970	37	75		57		46			

TABLE 14.1 *Continued*

Aron (3)	1971	14					46		35	2 Cases
Chatty and Earle (23)	1971	105	44		22		12		6	3 Deaths
										4 Cases
Scherpereel (86)	1974	100	59	38	28		21		3	2 Cases
Bloom (11)	1975	45[b]	69	38	33	33	33	24	24	
		43[c]	79	38	37		33	23	13.4	
Brain Tumor Registry (in Japan)	1975	71	58.4	38.9	27	24.3	24.3			
Onoyama *et al.* (70)	1975	20	50	40	30	25	20			
Mealey and Hall (62)	1977	32	80	55	47	45	41		22	
Harisiadis and Chang (44)	1977	58			60		40.4		31	
Nuchel and Andersen (69)	1978	44	64	45	36	36	33		20	
Quest *et al.* (76)										
Hirsch *et al.* (46)	1979	57	75	63	61	58.5	54			
Paillas *et al.* (71)	1979	17	70		47	30	23			1
Raimondi and Tomita (78)	1979	34	79.4	54.6	42.9	26.9	23.1		4.5	
Scuccimara *et al.* (87)	1979	119	36.1		16.7		13.4	6.6	5	
Tokars *et al.* (98)	1979				88		73			
Nakamura *et al.* (64)	1980				19		13			
Gerosa *et al.* (37)	1980	29	89.6	72.5	41.3	31	13.8	6.9		
Saladino (85)	1980	17 C	47	29.5	23.5	23.5	23.5	11.7	5.8	1
		11 A	36.4	27.3	27.3	27.3	27.3	27.3	27.3	3
Wilson and Gutin (102)	1980						30		25	
Amacher (24)	1981	20	88	87.5	80		71.4			
Berry *et al.* (9)	1981	122					56		43	
Berchet (7)	1981	74	55	41	28	23.5	23.5		7	3 Cases
HSC (24)	1981	144	89	79	60	52	47	42	42	
Mazza *et al.* (61)	1981	47	67		43		27			
Migliavacca (24)	1981	51	88	78	70	68.6	68.6			
Pauri-Boatto (24)	1981				33.3		14.3			
Santini (24)	1981				60		49			
Chin and Maruyama (25)	1981	20	90	70	56	45	45	40		
SIOP (14)	1982	287	88	72	62	56	51			
Choux and Lena	1982	60 C	61	50	41	41	37	37	37	
		22 A	73	63	52	45	32	21	17	

[a] *A*, adult; *C*, child. [b] 1950–1958. [c] 1959–1970.

What Is the Evolution of the Results from 1930 to 1981?

PERIOD FROM 1930 TO 1953

The statistics are essentially surgical, and survival at 5 years is exceptional (between 0 and 5%). The survival rate is higher in adults. During this period, survival at 10 years was observed only by Ingraham *et al.* (48) (2 cases) and Grant and Sayers (40) (2 cases). Lampe and McIntyre (53), in reviewing the literature from 1925 to 1945, found only 22 survivors at 3 years. Cuneo and Rand (29) state precisely that 21 of 22 children less than 13 years old were dead within the first 2 years after surgery.

THE PERIOD FROM 1953 TO 1960

Since the publication of Richmond (80) and Paterson and Farr (73), which stressed the advantages of global radiotherapy, the results improved to between 30 and 60% for 3-year survival and between 15 and 40% for 5-year survival. Bodian and Lawson (15), in the same year, do not mention any survivors at 3 years (but only 6 of the 23 survivors of surgery underwent radiotherapy). In a study of 93 cases, Christensen and Alo (27) found only 8 survivors, who ranged in age from 15 months to 9 years (again only a small number of patients had undergone radiotherapy).

THE PERIOD FROM 1960 TO 1969

By this time, the series were increasing in number, and surgical treatment and radiotherapy had improved greatly. The 3-year survival rate was always above 30%, the 5-year survival rate above 20%. Ten-year survivors were now mentioned (reaching 15 to 20%). Smith *et al.* (92) were the first to mention 6 survivors after 10 years in a group of 29 cases, of whom 3 were alive at 13, 15, and 17 years of age.

THE YEAR 1969

In 1969, Aron (3), Chang *et al.* (22), Jenkin (49), McFarland *et al.* (57), and Bloom *et al.* (13) published their series. All stressed the technique of radiotherapy. For the first time, the survival rate at 3 years reached 60%, and survival at 5 years varied between 40 and 50%; survivors at 10 years were now common.

THE PERIOD FROM 1970 TO 1981

Total radiotherapy advantages have been confirmed since the studies of Bouchard (17) and Hope-Stone (47). Medulloblastomas series were more frequent and better studied. Results included the complementary effect of chemotherapy.

In reviewing the evolution of these results, we were surprised to see that the survival rate from 1969 to 1975 had not changed significantly. However, since the period from 1975 to 1976, the 5-year survival has improved markedly to reach 60% in some series.

What Is the Survival Rate Now at the Different Survival Periods (Fig. 14.2)?

The 1-year survival rate varies now between 60 and 90% (in recent series, it is situated between 80 and 90%). This outcome is related to the decrease in operative mortality. The 1-year survival rate was at 63.4% for Bouchard in 1966 (17) and at 87% for Chang *et al.* (22) in 1969. These figures change significantly whether the operative mortality was considered or not.

The 3-year survival rate varies between 40 and 60% (it was 62% in the 1981 SIOP study). Before 1970, the survival rate was 54% for Paterson (72), 60% for Chang *et al.* (22), and 62% for Jenkin (49).

The 5-year survival rate is not substantially different from the results at 3 years: 10 to 15%. In 38 series, the 5-year survival rate is less than 30% 16 times, between 30 and 40% 7 times, between 40 and 50% 8 times, and more than 50% 7 times. The highest survival rates are mentioned in the series coming from departments of radiotherapy. Thirty series out of 38 mention a 5-year survival rate of less than 50%. However, when we take into consideration the number of cases in each series, we can find the mean 5-year survival rate at 43%. Six series mention a survival rate of less than 20%. However, in these series, the number of cases is small, and several observations include old data.

It is interesting to note that in groups of patients treated since 1975, the 5-year survival rate is beyond 50%, approaching 60%.

The 10-year survival rate is mentioned in 22 series (of 38) since 1970. Figures were then variable. Eight series mention a survival rate of less than 10%; 8 other series have rates ranging between 20 and 30%. Only 3 series note survival at 10 years of more than 40%.

By taking into consideration the size of each series and its data, we can evaluate presently the 10-year survival rate at about 22%. We note that in series before 1970, it was 21% for Smith *et al.* (92), 17% for Bouchard (17), 25% for Simpson *et al.* (91), 26% for Aron (2), and 26% for Bloom *et al.* (13). If we exclude the series of Berry *et al.* (9) at 43% and the series of the Toronto HSC in 1981 at 42%, we can state that the survival rate at 10 years has remained unchanged since 1960.

In most statistics, *survival rates beyond 10 years* are mentioned but are generally not great in number, ranging between 1 and 6 cases in each series. Some prolonged survivals have been described despite many tumor recurrences. We can mention 3 characteristic cases.

Stolzenberg *et al.* (95) described a case with a 14-year evolution: the

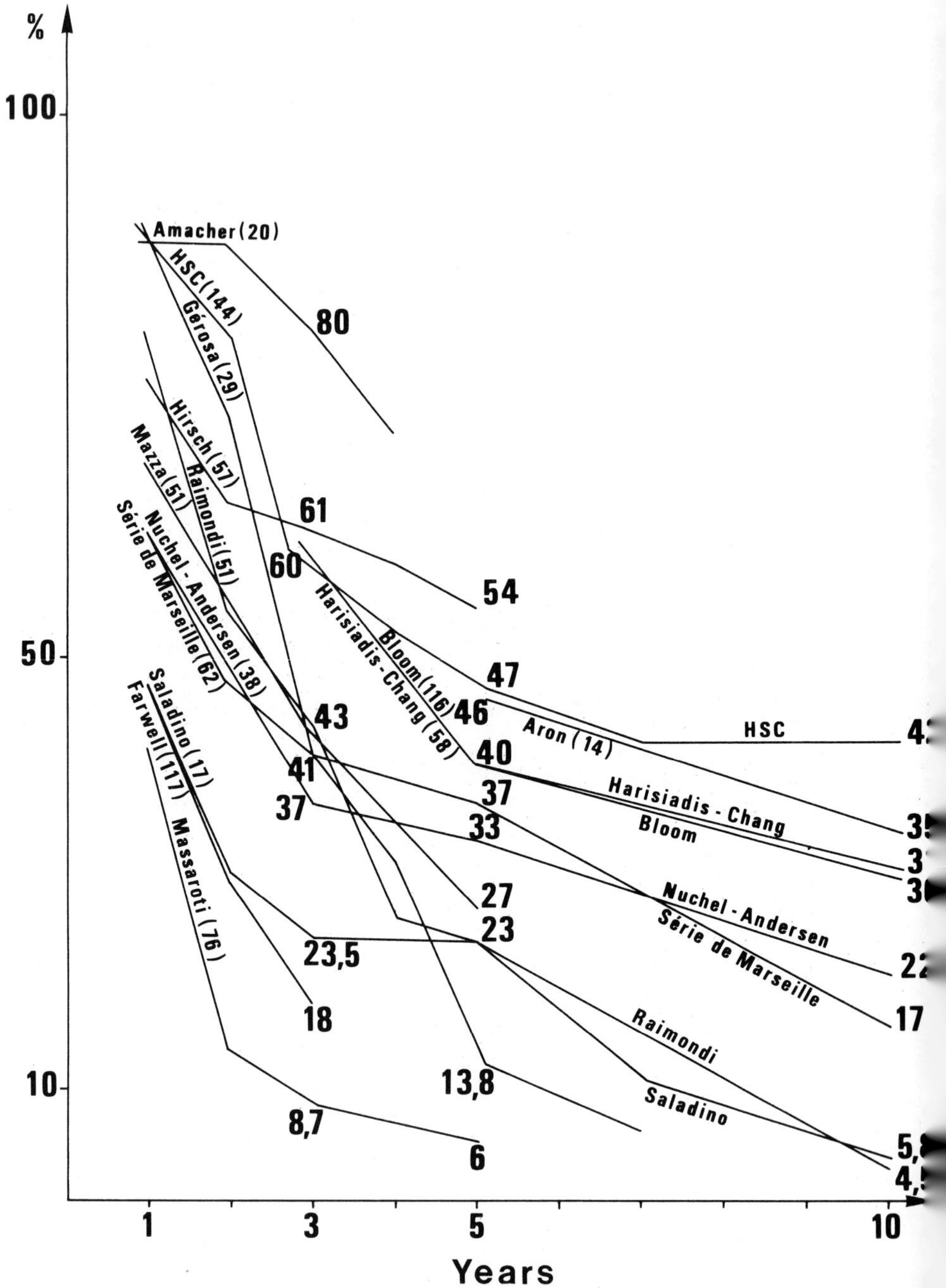

FIG. 14.2. Survival in 11 pediatric series of medulloblastoma.

patient was operated on at the age of 15, had spinal metastases 10 years after surgery and radiotherapy, had spinal metastases again 1 year later (surgery and radiotherapy), and went through final evolution with bone metastases.

Debnam and Staple (33) described a case in 1973 with an 18-year evolution: a child was operated on at the age of 7, had local recurrence 3 years later (surgery and radiotherapy), had diffuse bone metastases 3 years later (treated by chemotherapy), and had recurrence again 3 years later.

The Toronto HSC case (1981) involved an evolution of 18 years: the child was operated on when he was 5 years old, had recurrence 9 years later (radiotherapy and chemotherapy), then had spinal metastasis after 7 years (radiotherapy), and is still alive after 2 years.

The calculation of the *mean survival* gives no precise idea of survival duration. We must consider the age of the patient, the operative mortality, and the type of treatment. The mean survival is now about 25 months at any age on the basis of data from current series.

Now it is possible to mention cured cases of medulloblastoma. These cases are few in number, but their incidence will increase certainly in the coming years. Considering series in which the initial treatment is well managed, the expected cured medulloblastomas can be estimated to range between 18 and 24%.

FACTORS OF PROGNOSIS

The factors which influence the survival rate and the quality of that survival rate are multiple. Some are common to all intracranial tumors (age, sex, clinical symptoms, tumoral localization). Some are specific to the medulloblastoma (histological type, extent of removal, radiotherapy, and chemotherapy).

We intend to discuss all 8 of these factors.

Survival and Age

Medulloblastoma is a pediatric tumor but is not always present at birth; it develops from pre-existing cellular islets at any age. Consequently, it should be logical to affirm that an early medulloblastoma is more evolutive and has a poor prognosis. The same can be said for craniopharyngioma.

Some authors confirm classical data on a better prognosis of medulloblastoma in the adult (Spitz *et al.* (93), Rubinstein and Northfield (83), and Miles and Bhandari (63)). The 5-year survival rate is given in Table 14.2.

The better prognosis of medulloblastoma in the adult is classically

TABLE 14.2
Five-Year Survival by Age

Authors	Yr	5-Yr Survival Rate	
		Children (%)	Adults (%)
Ringertz and Tola (81)	1950	0	9
Aron (2)	1969	29	39
Chatty and Earle (23)	1971	1	16
Quest *et al.* (76)	1978	28	38

explained by a slower evolution, a predominant cerebellar localization, and the frequency of the desmoplastic variety.

However, many authors do not find significant differences in the survival rate in children and in adults; Cushing (30), Alekseeva (1), Berger and Elvidge (8), and Miles and Bhandari (63) are among that number. For Nöel and Méthot (67), the 5-year survival rate is similar in children (22%) and in adults (18%). For Berry *et al.* (9) and Chin and Maruyama (25), there are no differences.

In our series also, the 5-year survival rate in children is 37% and in adults 32%.

If the classical longer survival in the adult is not constant in the literature, the poor prognosis in young children is found in all series, especially in children under 2 years of age.

The reasons are usually the large size of the lesion, a frequently poor clinical status, a particular quick evolution of the tumor at this age, and the dramatic consequences of radiotherapy. The operative mortality is also higher in infants.

The 5-year survival rate is different in children younger than and older than 5 years of age; for Berry *et al.* (9) it was 48% *vs.* 60%, and in the Toronto series, it was 41% *vs.* 51%). In our pediatric series, the 5-year survival rate is 17% in infants and 59% in older children.

In conclusion:

1. Medulloblastoma in the adult does not have a significantly better prognosis than in children.
2. Medulloblastoma in infancy has a very poor prognosis in all the series.
3. Medulloblastoma in children under 5 years old results in a lower 5-year survival rate than in older children.
4. The 10-year survival rate is somewhat higher in children than in adults.

Survival and Sex

Classically, medulloblastoma in the female results in a longer survival rate, as confirmed by Paterson (72), MacFarland *et al.* (57), and Chin and Maruyama (25).

In 4 pediatric series, the 5-year survival rate data show females with longer survival than males.

However, others do not mention significant differences between the two sexes, such as Smith *et al.* (92), Sherpereel (66), Mealey and Hall (62), and Berry *et al.* (9).

Moreover, some authors find a longer survival in males (Table 14.3).

In the adult, long-term survival seems better in females than in males.

In conclusion:

1. Childhood medulloblastoma has not a significantly better prognosis in females.
2. In children long-term survival is often higher in boys.
3. In the adult long-term survival is higher in females.

Survival and Clinical Symptoms

We have correlated the survival rate with the duration of symptoms and the presence of hydrocephalus in 46 cases of our series (Table 14.4).

DELAY OF SYMPTOMS

There is no direct correlation between duration of symptoms before operation and survival, if we consider a duration of less than 3 months, which represents the majority of the cases. If the duration of symptoms is longer than 5 months, the 5-year survival rate increases.

We did not find any correlation between the duration of symptoms and the presence of a tumoral dissemination at the time of surgery.

TABLE 14.3
Five-Year Survival by Sex

Authors	Yr	Boys (%)	Girls
Bloom *et al.* (13)	1969	29	45
Harisiadis and Chang (44)	1977	13	33
Nuchel and Andersen (69)	1978	44	56
Raimondi (77)	1979	35	44
HSC (24)	1981	42	28
SIOP (24)	1981	37	29
Choux and Lena (24)	1982	52	47

TABLE 14.4
Survival and Clinical Symptoms

Duration of Symptoms	No. of Cases	Alive at 3 Yr (%)	Alive at 5 Yr (%)
Before 1 mo	14	64	28.5
1–2 mo	13	61.5	30.7
3–5 mo	13	69	15.3
After 5 mo	7	42.8	42.8

HYDROCEPHALUS

The presence of hydrocephalus influences the short-term survival but not the long-term survival. On the other hand, we think that postoperative hydrocephalus can influence significantly the quality of survival. In our series, the rate of late hydrocephalus is very low (1 of 36 cases), probably because we use routinely preoperative drainage.

Five-year survival is mentioned in three series where correlation was made between shunting procedure and survival. No significant difference was found (Table 14.5).

Survival and Aspect of the Tumors

Three tumoral factors can influence the prognosis: the character of the tumor, the localization, and the extent of the disease.

CHARACTER OF THE TUMOR

If the presence of a cyst in tumor (10 to 20% of the cases) does not influence the survival, spontaneous tumor bleeding (3 to 5% of the cases) explains some examples of acute presentation.

The volume of the tumor is important to consider, especially in children under 3 years of age. The commonly large size of the tumor in infants explains the high operative mortality at this age.

After 3 years, we did not find any differences in the survival rate, whether the tumor is less or more than 3 cm in size. This point is important to be noted since the great majority of medulloblastomas are more than 5 cm in size. Considering the first two categories of the operative staging proposed by Chang *et al.* (22), we obtained the results shown in Table 14.6 in 4 series.

TABLE 14.5

Correlation between Shunting and Survival

Authors		5-Yr Survival Rates	
		With Shunting (%)	Without Shunting (%)
HSC at Toronto (24)	1981	40	49
Berry *et al.* (9)	1981	59	54
Choux (24)	1982	27	40

TABLE 14.6

Correlation between Size of Tumor and Survival

Authors	Yr	T_1 (Less than 3 cm) (%)	T_2 (More than 3 cm) (%)
Harisiadis and Chang (44)	1977	8.4	33
Pindaro (24)	1981	10	34
Berchet (7)	1981	1.4	21.4
Choux (24)	1982	14	28

LOCALIZATION OF THE TUMOR

We have studied the localization of the tumor in 37 series in the literature (2307 cases of medulloblastomas), and we found the following proportion: median 1511 (65.5%); paramedian 314 (13.6%); and hemispheric 452 (19.6%).

In the adult, the hemispheric location represents 55% of the cases *vs.* 9.3% in children.

Generally, in the literature hemispheric localization goes with a better prognosis than midline localization. The reason is that the latter is more frequently attached to the brain stem (Table 14.7).

In our series, we did not observe such a difference. The midline tumors are often larger but less infiltrative and easier to remove.

However, the point that seems to us the most important is the continued localization to the vermis and to the hemisphere. In two series in which this point has been considered, we see that correlations with the survival rate are notable.

ADHESIONS TO THE BRAIN STEM

In 790 cases of the literature, we found involvement of the brain stem in 257 cases (33.4%). In 4 series, the 3- and 5-year survival rates were not significantly modified, except in the Toronto series (Table 14.8).

The 10-year survival rate seems to correlate better with the brain stem involvement.

TABLE 14.7

Correlation between Location of Tumor and Survival

		5-Yr Survival Rate (%)	10-Yr Survival Rate (%)
HSC at Toronto (24)	1981		
	Vermis	60	48
	Vermis and hemisphere	39	38
Choux (24)	1982		
	Vermis	42	33
	Vermis and Hemisphere	29	18

TABLE 14.8

Five-Year Survival and Involvement of Brain Stem

		Brain Stem Involvement	
		Present (%)	Absent (%)
Bloom (10)	1971	32	36
HSC Toronto (24)	1981	35	54
SIOP (14)	1981	40	48
Choux (24)	1982	34	39

Finally, the extension to the brain stem is one of the main factors of prognosis because the brain stem is often deeply invaded at the time of surgery. Furthermore, local recurrences appear generally at the level of the floor of the fourth ventricle, especially where such invasion existed.

Survival and Tumor Type

Many authors have tried to correlate the survival rate with the histologic aspects of the tumor. Generally, medulloblastoma in adults is described as having a better prognosis because the desmoplastic type is considered more frequent in adulthood.

A large group of authors do not find any significant difference in the prognosis of classical or desmoplastic types; Cutler *et al.* (31), Spitz *et al.* (93), Kernohan and Sayer (52), Smith *et al.* (92), Miles and Bhandari (63), and Russell and Rubinstein (84) are among them. In our personal series, we did not find differences in the survival rate in the two histologic types. Particularly in the 14 cases of desmoplastic medulloblastoma, the survival rate was no longer for either children or adults.

A second group of authors mention correlation between the tumor type and the survival. The great majority of these authors point out a better prognosis in desmoplastic medulloblastomas; Berger and Elvidge (8), Dexter and Howell (34), Chatty and Earle (23), and Marty-Double and Barneon (59) are among them.

In the pediatric series of the Toronto HSC (1981) (24), the 5-year survival rate was longer in the classical type (50%) than in desmoplastic type (37%).

Histological differentiation of the tumor into neuroblastic or astrocytic components does not change significantly the survival rate. In conclusion, due to the small number of cases in the majority of the series, it is difficult to confirm that a tumor type provides for a different survival:

In children, the desmoplastic medulloblastoma does not have a better prognosis.

In the adult, a better prognosis of desmoplastic medulloblastoma exists in many series but is not of great significance.

In long-term survivors, the desmoplastic tumors are more frequently found.

Survival and Importance of Removal

Even if a simple biopsy procedure or a partial excision of the tumor may go with a satisfactory survival rate in a few series, we must point out that total removal yields the best long-term survival. However, in many series, it is difficult to appreciate exactly what is described as a partial or a subtotal removal.

A few authors do not find any relationship between the survival rate and the extent of removal; Miles and Bhandari (63), Mealey and Hall (62), De la Torre *et al.* (99), and Venes *et al.* (101) are among them. Most authors think that complete removal provides the longest survival; Christensen and Alo (27), Bloom *et al.* (13), Wilson (103), Massarotti *et al.* (60), Hirsch *et al.* (46), Succimara *et al.* (87), McIntosh (58), Raimondi (77), Thomas *et al.* (96), Berry *et al.* (9), Mazza *et al.* (61), Norris *et al.* (68), Choux (24), are among them.

In some studies (9, 14, 44) there are no significant differences of survival after subtotal or total removal.

In 3 pediatric series the 5-year survival rate is shown in Table 14.9.

It is interesting to note that the operative mortality is no higher after total removal; the postoperative period is often simpler, and the morbidity is frequently lower.

In conclusion:

1. In medulloblastoma, surgical abstention or simple biopsy cannot be maintained as therapeutic methods.
2. Total removal gives the best short- and long-term survival.
3. Total removal gives longer survival in children than in adults.

Survival and Radiotherapy

The importance of a postoperative radiotherapy is stressed in all the series. Very few 8-month survivors are seen without radiotherapy. The mean survival with surgery alone is 7 months (4) 5.6 months (31), 2.4 months (15), and 13 months (8). Pichler *et al.* (75) mentions that 37 of 38 patients treated by surgery alone died. Only 1 was alive 14 years after diagnosis. Irradiation is indicated in all the cases, but the extension and the modalities of irradiation are also important.

IRRADIATION OF THE POSTERIOR FOSSA

This radiotherapy must be systematic and total. Recurrences appeared in the posterior fossa (67.3%), and in the case of spinal or supratentorial recurrence there is generally an associated local recurrence. Consequently, the quality of irradiation of the posterior fossa is the most important factor for prognosis.

In 4 recent series in which the importance of irradiation is correlated

TABLE 14.9

Correlation between Removal of Tumor and Survival

Authors	Yr	Total Removal (%)	Partial Removal (%)	Subtotal (%)	Total (%)
Raimondi (77)	1979		12.5		40
SIOP (14)	1981	27		47	49
Choux (24)	1982	18		27	43

with the 5-year survival, we see that a minimum of 5000 rad must be given and that more than 5300 rads are not necessary. In the literature, results are not significantly improved with doses of more than 5500 rads (Table 14.10).

The results are not notably modified when radiotherapy is delayed after surgery. Berry *et al.* (9) do not find a different prognosis when postoperative radiotherapy is started before or after 10 days. In our series, 11 patients were irradiated for more than 20 days after surgery. The prognosis was not worse in these cases.

IRRADIATION OF SPINE

The spine represents the second most important location of recurrence. Spinal recurrences are encountered in 17% of the cases in 32 series in the literature. We have seen in our series and in many series of the literature that spinal extension of the tumor is present at the moment of the diagnosis, even without any symptomatology. We are convinced that irradiation of the spine must be systematic and total. When spinal radiotherapy is not carried out, the survival rate is drastically lower in all the series, and spinal recurrence is common (20, 61). For Jenkin (49), there is no 5-year survival rate after local irradiation alone, and for Hope-Stone (46), the 5-year survival rate is 6%. Landberg *et al.* (54) find differences in the 10-year survival rate when irradiation is restricted only to the posterior fossa (5%), posterior fossa and spinal region (25%), or complete craniospinal irradiation (35%).

TABLE 14.10

Correlation between Radiation and Survival Rates

	Five-Yr Survival Rate (%)
Harisiadis and Chang (44)	
4500–4700 rads	33
4700–5200 rads	45
>5200 rads	48.25
Cumberlin *et al.* (28)	
4500 rads	25
4500–5000 rads	10
>5000 rads	50
Chin and Maruyama (25)	
4500 rads	0
5000 rads	8
5000–5500 rads	7
Berry *et al.* (9)	
Less than 5000 rads	50
5000–5100 rads	51
5200–5350 rads	74
More than 5350 rads	71

Concerning the doses of spinal irradiation, the survival rate is not improved by more than 2500 rads. This conclusion is important since the consequences on spinal growth can be subsequently diminished without increasing the number of spinal recurrences. In cases of spinal localization, detected at the time of surgery, the doses should be increased at the level of the lesion.

IRRADIATION OF SUPRATENTORIAL COMPARTMENT

In 22 series of the literature (1152 medulloblastomas), we have found 98 supratentorial metastases (8.68%). This frequency is substantially higher in pediatric series (24, 44, 61).

It is important to note that in 3 series the existence of supratentorial recurrences is directly related to the absence of supratentorial irradiation: for Landberg *et al.* (54), 5 of 6; for Mazza *et al.* (61), 6 of 7; and for Choux (24), 3 of 4.

Another point of interest is the frequency of the subfrontal location of metastases. In 90 cases in the literature in which the location of supratentorial recurrences was mentioned, the following sites were noted: frontal (50%) and multiple (27%, with a majority of frontal lesions (9, 43, 50). It is well-known that the subfrontal region receives a lower dose of irradiation.

The problems raised by supratentorial irradiation are the neurological, intellectual, and endocrinal consequences of this irradiation. These complications must be compared with the risk of supratentorial metastases.

The doses generally used in the literature are around 3000 to 4000 rad. We have noted that the incidence of recurrence is not significantly higher with doses exceeding 3500 rad. Consequently, we suggest irradiating the supratentorial compartment in children with 3000–3500 rad, taking particular care of the frontoethmoidal region.

Considering the consequences of irradiation in young children, we do not irradiate routinely the supratentorial compartment in infants with medulloblastoma, except in those with high risk (tumoral extension at the moment of the operation, positive myelography, and positive CSF).

In conclusion:

1. The necessity of extensive postoperative irradiation is imperative.
2. The most important point is irradiation of the posterior fossa carefully and totally, with doses ranging between 5000 and 5300 rad.
3. Spinal irradiation is necessary in all the cases, with doses not exceeding 2500 rad.
4. Supratentorial irradiation must be seriously considered in young children, in relation to the consequences of radiother-

apy at this age and the incidence of supratentorial recurrences.

Survival and Chemotherapy

Chemotherapy as initial treatment does not significantly change the prognosis of the patient with medulloblastoma. Chemotherapy seems to delay recurrences but does not prevent them. However, high risk patients (extensive lesion at the time of operation, brain stem invasion, partial removal, positive myelography, and positive CSF) can benefit from chemotherapy. In 2 series in which survival is considered in the case of brain stem extension of the tumor, it is clear that the 5-year survival rate is drastically higher when chemotherapy has been associated with radiotherapy (Table 14.11).

The survey of the major recent trials and studies permits similar conclusions about the effects of chemotherapy in the initial treatment of medulloblastoma.

PILOT STUDY OF THE ROYAL MARSDEN HOSPITAL (1975)

Vincristine—CCNU—Methotrexate. Fourteen children treated between 1970 and 1973 with surgery, radiotherapy, and chemotherapy are compared with 88 children treated between 1950 and 1970 with radiotherapy alone. In this study, the results of chemotherapy are encouraging but not decisive, and a cooperative multicentric study is proposed.

SIOP THERAPEUTIC CLINICAL TRIAL

Preliminary results (1975–1981) on the use of **vincristine** and **CCNU** were presented by H. J. G. Bloom at the SIOP Meeting in Marseille.

Some 287 medulloblastomas from 44 centers are included in this study. The 5-year survival rate is 42% in the control group and 52% in the group receiving chemotherapy, but the differences are not significant. The conclusion of the authors is: that the present adjuvant chemotherapy program does not appear to benefit all children with medulloblastoma, but it appears to achieve significantly better results in certain high risk

TABLE 14.11

Correlation between Chemotherapy and Survival

	Survival Rates (%)	2 Yr (%)	3 Yr (%)	5 Yr (%)
SIOP (14) (90 patients)	RT[a] + CT (46 patients)	64	60	60
	RT (44 patients)	36	36	0
Choux (24) (32 patients)	RT + CT (18 patients)	56	56	51
	RT (14 patients)	48	41	16

[a] RT, radiation therapy; CT, chemotherapy.

cases (in patients in whom tumor excision has been incomplete, in those with involvement of the brain stem, and in children under age 2).

CHILDREN'S CANCER STUDY GROUP (CCSG)

Vincristine—CCNU—Prednisone. The preliminary results of this study were presented by Evans at the SIOP Meeting in Budapest in 1980.

Ninety-one children with medulloblastoma are included in this study. Forty-four received adjuvant chemotherapy. In the two groups, the 2-year survival rate is the same, about 60%. Berry *et al.* (9) looked at 48 patients treated with the same protocol and found the same results: the 3-year survival rate is the same, 60%, in the two groups.

STUDY OF THE SOUTH WEST ONCOLOGY GROUP (SWOG)

Vincristine—Methotrexate—Hydrocortisone. This study was presented by J. Van Eys in 1981. Among 34 patients, 16 received adjuvant chemotherapy. The results do not mention any significant differences in the two groups studied.

TWO STUDIES USING A "SANDWICH" PROTOCOL

These studies included chemotherapy between surgery and radiotherapy.

Voute presented in 1981, at the SIOP meeting in Marseille, France, a protocol with vincristine, prednisone, and methotrexate that was started in 1979. Chemotherapy is given after surgery and again after radiotherapy.

Neidhart, at the same meeting, presented the preliminary results of the West Berlin pilot study and the West German cooperative trial (using procarbazine, CCNU, methotrexate, and the citrovorum factor). Forty patients with medulloblastoma had been registered for this study by July 31, 1981. The preliminary results are encouraging, but it is too early to affirm the definite effects of chemotherapy.

In these two pilot studies, the number of patients is too small, the duration of the trials too short to allow a significant conclusion.

THE STUDY OF MAZZA *ET AL.* (61)

Mazza *et al.* (61) presented a randomized trial in 47 children. Ten received adjuvant chemotherapy with CCNU. The 5-year survival rate is almost the same in the two groups: 35% with radiotherapy alone and 30% with adjuvant chemotherapy.

THE SIOP PROTOCOL AT MARSEILLE

In Marseille, 38 children have been entered in the SIOP protocol since 1977. The first group of 21 cases treated with radiotherapy alone and the second group of 17 cases received adjuvant chemotherapy. The 3-year-survival rate is 68% in the first group and 57% in the second group. The 5-year survival rate is exactly the same in the two groups, 57%.

A NEW PROTOCOL FROM THE PEDIATRIC ONCOLOGY GROUP (POG)

The Pediatric Oncology Group (PIOG) is using a MOPP protocol that has just been started.

In conclusion, as of 1982, chemotherapy as an initial treatment has not significantly modified the survival rate of medulloblastoma in children and in adults. Chemotherapy has demonstrated its benefit in high risk patients and especially in patients with recurrence. In these patients, when addition of radiotherapy is impossible, chemotherapy can in some cases delay significantly the eventual mortality. We remember the case of a 6-year-old boy presenting with a medulloblastoma treated by surgery and radiotherapy. Two years later, he developed spinal recurrence and 2 supratentorial tumors. Chemotherapy (with oncovin and CCNU) was given, and 3 months later the frontal lesion disappeared, and the occipital lesion decreased in size. The boy had a comfortable survival of 20 months.

In the literature, we collected 113 recurrent cases in which chemotherapy was used. Ninety-four presented a positive response. In our department at the present time, we do not prescribe routinely and systematically initial chemotherapy. We restrict its use for recurrence only.

QUALITY OF SURVIVAL

While most statistics, since 1975, have demonstrated a significant improvement in the survival rate, many publications have been devoted to the problems of the delayed ill-effects of the treatment of medulloblastoma. It is surprising that the quality of the survival has rarely been mentioned and has never been evaluated in the majority of publications until recent years. According to the literature, problems arise when late sequelae of medulloblastoma are not evaluated with the same criteria in all series being studied.

Many classifications or scales have been used to characterize the results. We can mention the Karnofsy scale, the four grades of Bouchard (17) and Bloom et al (13), the complex evaluation of Rosenblum *et al.* (82), the evaluation of Bamford *et al.* (6) and, more recently, the "composite quality of survival scale" (CQS) proposed by Spunberg *et al.* (94). This last classification takes into consideration all the factors which participate in the quality of life: physical status, neurological status, intellectual status, endocrine disorders, psychological factors, and school or professional life. Without considering all of these 6 factors we have only a partial view of the consequences of the treatment of medulloblastoma. This explains the differences existing in the results in most statistics on this tumor. Of interest is the fact that the best results are found in series originating from departments of radiotherapy. Jenkin (49) described 24 of 30 patients with a normal life. Bloom (10) states that 70 to 75% of survivors have an active and useful life. On the contrary, Hirsch *et al.* (46) mentions intellectual problems in 82% of the survivors. Broadbent *et al.* (19) in 8 patients describes 8 examples of ataxias and 5 patients with growth deficiency. These few examples stress the necessity to assess the results in the series and to require a precise testing of the sequelae.

Neurological Sequelae

These are the most common, even if they are scarcely mentioned. The tumor itself, hydrocephalus, surgery, and radiotherapy are the main causes of these neurological symptoms.

The frequency of the neurological sequelae is difficult to appreciate. In 17 series grouping 358 cases, such sequelae are found in 188 cases that represent 52.5% of the cases. In 34% of the cases, the neurological deficit was severe. The authors who looked for them found a proportion of 60 to 70% of neurological sequelae. Gutjar *et al.* (42) in a series of 12 cases did not find any normal neurological examinations, and in 42% of the cases the sequelae were extreme.

In our series, we have studied the neurological status in 48 patients. Only 21 patients (43%) presented a normal examination. Seven patients (14.5%) had severe neurological deficits.

Three groups of sequelae can be distinguished: cerebellar, cranial nerve, and visual.

Cerebellar signs are almost constant in the postoperative period. They improve in many cases, but even if symptoms can decrease over a long period of time, mild cerebellar signs remain present in the great majority of cases, especially in ataxia, clumsiness of a hand, and nystagmus.

Cranial nerve palsy is generally the consequence of surgery. Oculomotor and facial nerves are the most frequently involved.

Visual impairment is not rare, particularly a diminution of a visual acuity due to a long period of increased intracranial pressure. Shunting does not always prevent this complication.

Epilepsy has been described in many series and does not necessarily represent recurrence.

Residual normal pressure hydrocephalus might be a factor of importance in secondary neurological symptomatology. Preoperative shunting diminishes markedly the risk of secondary hydrocephalus. In our series, of 26 cases with preoperative shunting, only one had residual hydrocephalus on CT scan.

Intellectual Sequelae

For a long time ignored, the intellectual deficit after irradiation of medulloblastoma is now recognized and, in a few cases, has been tested. In 22 series with 291 survivors, intellectual deficit is mentioned in 32.6% of the cases. When children are tested, the incidence is significantly higher (Table 14.12).

In our personal series, IQ testing was performed in 24 survivors. The age at time of surgery was less than 2 years in 2 cases, between 3 and 5 years in 3 cases, between 6 and 10 years in 14 cases, and between 11 and 15 years in 5 cases. Children were tested 2 to 4 years after irradiation.

Verbal IQ score was normal in 15 patients (62.5%) while only 9 patients (37.5%) had normal performance IQ score. The existence of cerebellar dysfunction in these patients can explain the lower score in performance.

The IQ testing has been evaluated in 5 series. The results are shown in Table 14.13.

School attendance has been studied in several series. We must remember that in the normal population, only 80% attended normal school (Table 14.14).

Many factors can influence the existence of an intellectual deficit.

TABLE 14.12

Correlation between Irradiation of Medulloblastoma and Intellectual Deficit in Children

Hirsch *et al.* (46)	1979	88.4
Raimondi and Tomita (79)	1979	63
HSC at Toronto (24)	1981	43
Berchet (7)	1981	50
Choux (24)	1982	62.5

TABLE 14.13

Correlation between Irradiation of the Medulloblastoma and IQ

Authors	No. of Patients	Verbal IQ Score (%)		
		70	70–90	90
Hirsch *et al.* (46)	26	31	58	11
Berchet (7)	12	25	25	50
Choux (24)	24	12.5	25	62.5
		70	70–85	90
Raimondi and Tomita (79)	11	45	27.5	27.5
HSC at Toronto (24) (1981)	16	12.5	19	68.5
Authors	**No. of Patients**	**Performance IQ Score (%)**		
		70	70–85	85
Raimondi and Tomita (79)	11	63		33
HSC at Toronto (24) (1981)	16	56		44
		70	70–90	90
Choux (1982) (24)	24	12.5	50	37.5

Some of them can be easily recognized: age, hydrocephalus, radiotherapy, and aspects of the tumors. Others are less easily appreciated: psychological factors and social and familial environment.

The effects of radiotherapy in the pediatric age are well-known, especially in young patients. The quantity of irradiation, as well as the time distribution of irradiation, influence brain damage.

To appreciate the consequences of radiotherapy, we have compared the intellectual level in 2 groups of children who have been treated, one for a cerebellar astrocytoma (without radiotherapy) and one for a medulloblastoma (with radiotherapy). Our results (Table 14.15) are compared with those of Hirsch *et al* (46) and Raimondi and Tomita (79).

It is evident that children who have been irradiated present a lower

TABLE 14.14

School Attendance of Children after Irradiation of Medulloblastoma

Authors	Yr	Cases	Cases Attending Normal School
Jenkin (49)	1969	30	24 (80)[a]
Bloom *et al.* (12)	1969	12	5 (41.6)
Harisiadis and Chang (44)	1977	11	7 (63.6)
Hirsch *et al.* (46)	1979	16	4 (25)
Raimondi and Tomita (79)	1979	16	4 (25)
Gerosa *et al.* (38)	1981	28	20 (71.4)
Gutjahr *et al.*(42)	1981	10	1 (10)
Choux (24)	1982	26	16 (61.5)

[a] Numbers in parentheses are percentage.

TABLE 14.15

Effects of Radiotherapy on Intellect of Two Groups of Treated Children

Authors	No. of Cases	IQ (%)		
		70	70–90	90
Hirsch *et al.* (46)				
Medulloblastoma	26	31	58	11
Astrocytoma	31	19	19	62
Authors	**No. of Cases**	**IQ (%)**		
		70	70–85	85
Raimondi and Tomita (79)				
Medulloblastoma	11	45	27	27
Astrocytoma	6	0	16	83
Authors	**No. of Cases**	**IQ (%)**		
		70	70–90	90
Choux (24)				
Medullobastoma	24	12.5	50	37.5
Astrocytoma	15	6.6	20	73.33

intellectual level. It is interesting to note that children with cerebellar astrocytoma do have an intellectual deficit (6.6 to 19%), which can be the consequence of a psychological trauma (due to the hospitalization, the familial reaction, *etc.*).

The age of patient is important since the most important intellectual deficits are encountered in infants. Spunberg *et al.* (94), in 36 irradiated infants, found only 23% of them with a normal intellectual level. In our personal series, the proportion of intellectually normal patients is lower in children under 4 years (38%), as compared to 62.5% at all ages.

Residual hydrocephalus can explain the intellectual deficit in some cases. Hirsch *et al.* (46) did not find a significant correlation between the size of the ventricle and the IQ score.

Endocrine Sequelae

The endocrine status of patients treated by radiotherapy for medulloblastoma has been rarely reported before 1975. Now, many papers, mainly originating from endocrine departments, have been documented in the literature.

The first description of growth deficiency in a child with medulloblastoma is that of Cushing (30), who described a girl with a diminution of 10 cm in height, as compared with her twin sister.

The majority of publications on medulloblastoma until 1979 neglected this complication (13, 17, 92).

Jenkin (49) describes a moderate growth deficiency in nearly all the cases.

Aron (2) mentions the case of a 6-year-old girl who presented at 16 years with short stature, amenorrhea, and hypothyroidism.

Harisiadis and Chang (44) describe a short stature in the majority of 11 survivors.

Cumberlin *et al.* (28) in a study of 33 children, describe 2 examples of growth failure, 2 and 3 years after treatment.

Raimondi and Tomita (78) describe the endocrine status in 13 patients; two have kyphoscoliosis with short stature (but laminectomy was performed) and two have a diminution of growth hormone and delayed puberty.

Hirsch *et al.* (46), in 29 patients, mention endocrine sequelae in more than 50% of the cases; 17 (58.6%) present with a short stature, 19 (65.5%) have an important diminution of growth hormone, and 17 (58.6%) have a thyroid dysfunction.

Chin and Maruyama (25) state that growth deficiency is common, and they recommend a systematic endocrine evaluation.

Gerosa *et al.* (38) mention endocrine deficits in a significant number of their 62 survivors. Five patients developed hypothyroidism, GH deficiency was detected in 5 patients, and 1 patient had a GH deficiency as well as hypothyroidism.

In our personal series, the endocrine status has been documented clinically in 40 children, hormonally in 16. A short stature was clinically evident in 24 children. Three children of 16 presented with moderate hyperthyroidism. No patient had symptomatic diabetes insipidus. In prepubertal patients, delayed puberty was noted in one girl, and in postpubertal patients, gonadotrophic function was clinically and hormonally normal.

In the endocrinologic literature, the consequence of radiotherapy in brain tumor is now well-known. In these papers, many of the patients had a medulloblastoma. It is interesting to point out the higher incidence of endocrine dysfunction in endocrinologic series.

Shalet *et al.* (88, 90) mention the importance of endocrine sequelae in irradiated children:

1975: In 16 patients (9 with medulloblastoma), they found GH deficiency in 68% of the cases.
1976: In 9 patients (4 with medulloblastoma), GH deficiency was present 6 times.
1977: In 20 patients (8 with medulloblastoma), GH deficiency was present in 9 patients.

Perry-Keene *et al.* (74) in 8 patients (1 with medulloblastoma) found 3 examples of panhypopituitarism and 5 cases of isolated GH deficiency.

Czernichow and Rappaport (32) studied clinically and hormonally the endocrine status in 30 children with medulloblastoma. Twenty-seven were tested. GH deficiency was present in 15 cases (it was total in 11 cases and partial in 4). Thyroid function was mildly affected, and cortisol levels were normal.

All these publications stress the importance of growth deficiency in irradiated patients. In series in which GH was assayed, the incidence of growth deficiency is established between 60 to 70% (6, 32, 74, 90). In our personal series, growth hormone deficiency was confirmed in 72% of the cases and was clinically evident in 60% of the cases.

The causes of growth deficiency after irradiation can be due to the effect of radiotherapy on vertebral bodies, especially between the ages of 6 and 12. With more than 2500 rad, the consequences on spinal growth are increasingly significant. We see the need to reduce the doses of spinal irradiation since we have demonstrated that those doses of more than 2500 rads are not necessary to prevent spinal recurrences. The other cause of growth deficiency is hypothalamic irradiation during the supratentorial radiotherapy and thyroid irradiation during the cervical spine

TABLE 14.16

Results of Survey Showing Survivors and Survivors Living Normal Lives

Authors		Survivors	Survivors in Normal Condition
Smith *et al.* (92)	1961	11	5 (45.5)[a]
McIntosh (58)	1969	17	5 (29.4)
Jenkin (49)	1969	30	24 (80.5)
Hope-Stone (47)	1970	7	6 (85.7)
Noël and Methot (67)	1970	10	2 (20)
Harisiadis and Chang (44)	1977	11	6 (54)
Mealey and Hall (62)	1977	9	6 (66)
Nuchel and Andersen (69)	1978	13	3 (23)
Raimondi (77)	1979	13	5 (38)
Berry *et al.* (9)	1981	68	41 (60)
Gerosa *et al.* (81)	1981	28	5 (17.8)
Broadbent *et al.* (19)	1981	8	5 (62)
Choux (24)	1982	48	16 (33.3)

[a] Numbers in parentheses are percentages.

radiotherapy. It is clear that irradiation of posterior fossa and spine exclusively reduces the risk of growth deficiency. The endocrine consequences of supratentorial irradiation in children must be carefully considered before making the decision to irradiate the supratentorial compartment.

The survey of the consequences of the treatment of medulloblastoma points out the necessity of establishing a strict therapeutic protocol adapted to each case and considering all the factors of prognosis.

The different treatments must have the same goal: healthy and long survival. Now the length of survival alone, cannot be the main purpose in medulloblastoma. We cannot ignore the quality of the survival, when we see the incidence of survivors living normal lives (Table 14.16).

REFERENCES

1. Alekseeva V. S. Medulloblastomes de la fosse postérieure chez l'adulte. Vopr. Neurochir., *6:* 30–33, 1959.
2. Aron B. S. Twenty-years experience with radiation therapy of medulloblastoma Am. J. Roentgenol., *105:* 37–42, 1969.
3. Aron B. S. Medulloblastoma in children. Am. J. Dis. Child., *121:* 315–317, 1971.
4. Bailey P. and Cushing A. Medulloblastoma cerebelli: a common type of mid-cerebellar glioma of childhood Arch. Neurol. Psychiatry, *14:* 192–224, 1925.
5. Bamberg M., Schmitt, G., Quast, U., Bongartz, E. B., Nau, H. E., Bayindir, C., and Reinhardt, V. Therapie et pronostic du medulloblastome: progrès à l'aide de techniques d'irradiations nouvelles. Strahlentherapie, *156:* 1–17, 1980.
6. Bamford F. N., Morris-Jones, P., Pearson, D., Ribeiro, G. G., Shalet, S. M., Beardwell C. G., Residual disabilities in children treated for intracranial space occupying lesions. Cancer, *37:* 1149–1151, 1976.
7. Berchet, T. Médulloblastome de l'enfant et de l'adulte. A propos de 74 observations. Ph.D. Thesis, Nancy, France, 1981.

8. Berger, E. C., and Elvidge, A. R. Medulloblastomas and cerebellar sarcomas. A clinical survey J. Neurosurg., *20:* 139–144, 1963.
9. Berry, M. P., Jenkin, R. D. T., Keen, C. W., Nair, B. D. and Simpson, W. J. Radiation treatment for medulloblastoma. A 21-year review. J. Neurosurg., *55:* 43–51, 1981.
10. Bloom, H. I. G. Concepts in the natural history and treatment of medulloblastoma in children: Increasing survival rates and possible risks with current radiotherapy techniques CRC Crit. Rev. Radiol. Sci., *2:* 89–143, 1971.
11. Bloom, H. J. G. Combined modality therapy for intracranial tumours. Cancer, *35:* 111–120, 1975.
12. Bloom, H. I. G. Recent concepts in the conservative treatment of intracranial tumours in children. Acta Neurochir., *50:* (1–2): 103–116, 1975.
13. Bloom, H. I. G., Wallace, E. N. K., and Henk, J. M. The treatment and prognosis of medulloblastoma in children. A study of 82 verified cases. Am. J. Roentgenol. Radium Ther. Nucl. Med., *105:* 43–62, 1969.
14. Bloom, H. J. G., Thornton, H., and Schweiguth, O. S.I.O.P. medulloblastoma and high grade ependymoma therapeutic clinical trial: Preliminary results (1975–1981). In: *Pediatric Oncology*, pp. 309–322. Excerpta Medical, Amsterdam, 1982.
15. Bodian, M., and Lawson, D. The intracranial neoplastic disease of childhood: A description of their material history based on a clinical pathological study of 129 cases. Br. J. Surg., *40:* 368–392, 1953.
16. Borejko, J., and Hartel-Ulkowska, N. Medulloblastoma in the records of a radiotherapy clinic in the years 1955–1969. Pol. Przegl. Radiol., *34:* 395–401, 1970.
17. Bouchard, J. Radiation Therapy of Tumors and Diseases of the Nervous System, pp. 104–128. Philadelphia, Lea & Febiger, 1966.
18. Bouchard, J., and Peirce, C. B. Radiation therapy in management of neoplasm of central nervous system, with special note in regard to children: Twenty years experience 1939–1958. Am. J. Roentgenol., *84:* 610–628, 1960.
19. Broadbert, V. A., Barnes, N. D., and Wheeler, T. K. Medulloblastoma in childhood: Long-term results of treatment. Cancer, *48:* 26–30, 1981.
20. Brown, R. C., Gunderson, L., and Plenk, H. P. Medulloblastoma. A review of the L.D.S. Hospital experience. Cancer, *40:* 56–60, 1977.
21. Carteri, A., Scuccimarra, A., Giordano, R. Giovanelli, M., Gaini, S. M., and Villani, R. Histological aspects of medulloblastomas in infancy and their correlations with survival. J. Neurol. Sci., *1:* 29–33, 1978.
22. Chang, C. H., Housepian, E. M., and Herbert, C. Jr. An operative staging system and a megavoltage radiotherapeutic technic for cerebellar medulloblastomas. Radiology *93:* 1351–1359, 1969.
23. Chatty, E., and Earle, K. M. Medulloblastoma. A report of 201 cases with emphasis on the relationship of histologic variants to survival. Cancer, *28:* 977–983, 1971.
24. Choux, M., and Lena, G. Medulloblastoma. Neurochirurgie *28* (Suppl.): 1–229, 1982.
25. Chin, H. W., and Maruyama, Y. Results of radiation treatment of cerebellar medulloblastoma. Inst. J. Radiat. Oncol., *7:* 737–742, 1981.
26. Crue, B. L. Medulloblastoma. Charles C Thomas, Springfield, Ill. 1958.
27. Christensen, E. and Alo, E. Medulloblastomas. Acta Physicatr. Neurol. Scand. *108* (Suppl.): 87–100, 1956.
28. Cumberlin, R. L., Lu, K. H., Wara, W. M. Sheline, G. E., and Wilson G. B. Medulloblastoma. Treatment results and effect on normal tissues. Cancer, *43:* 1014–1020, 1979.
29. Cuneo, H. M., and Rand, C. W. Brain tumours of childhood. Charles C Thomas, Springfield, Ill., 1952.
30. Cushing, H. Experiences with the cerebellar medulloblastomas. A critical review. Acta Pathol. Microbiol. Scand., *7:* 1–86, 1930.

31. Cutler, E. C., Sosman, M. C., and Vaughan W. W. The place of radiation in the treatment of cerebellar medulloblastomas. Report of twenty cases. Am. J. Roentgenol. *35:* 429–450, 1936.

32. Czernichow, P., and Rappaport, R. Sequelles endocriniennes après irradiations pour tumeurs de la tête et du cou. J. Parisiennes: 171–183, 1978.

33. Debnam, J. W., and Staple, T. W. Osseous metastasis from cerebellar medulloblastoma. Radiology, *107:* 363–365, 1973.

34. Dexter, D., and Howell, D. A. Medulloblastomas and arachnoidal sarcomas. Brain, *88:* 367–374, 1965.

35. Evans, A. E., Anderson, J., Chang, C., Jenkin, R. D. T., Kramer S., Schoenfeld, D., and Wilson, C. Adjuvant chemotherapy for medulloblastoma and ependymoma: Multi-disciplinary aspects of brain tumor therapy, p. 275. Elsevier-North Holland Biomedical Press, Amsterdam, 1979.

36. Faust, D. S., Tatem, R., Brady, L. W., Olsen, A. K., Osterholm, J. L., Kasem, I., and Mancall, E. L. Radiation therapy in the management of medulloblastomas. Neurology *20:* 519–522, 1970.

37. Gerosa, M., Di Stefano, E., Carli, M., and Iraci, G. Combined treatment of pediatric medulloblastoma. A review of an integrated program (two-arm chemotherapy trial). Child's Brain, *6:* 262–273, 1980.

38. Gerosa, M., Di Stefano, E., Olivi, A., and Carter A. Multidisciplinary treatment of medulloblastoma: 5 year experience with the SIOP trial. Child's Brain *8:* 107–118, 1981.

39. Goldberg, M. B., Sheline, G. E., and Mallamud, N. Malignant intracranial neoplasms, following radiation therapy for acromegaly. Radiology, *80:* 465–470, 1963.

40. Grant, F. C., and Sayers, M. P. Notes on series of brain tumors. Trans. Am. Neurol. Assoc.: 102–106, 1951.

41. Griepentrog, F., and Pauly, H. Intra und extrakranielle frühmanifeste Medulloblastome bei erbglichen Zwillingen. Zentralbl. Neurochir., *17:* 129, 1957.

42. Gutjahr P., Dieterich E., and Walther B. Spätstatus Langzeitüberlebender nach infratentoriellen Tumoren im Kindersalter. Acta Neuropediatr., *2:* 94–104, 1981.

43. Hardy, D. G., Hope-Stone, H. F., McKenzie, C. G., and Scholtz, C. L. Recurrence of medulloblastoma after homogeneous field radiotherapy. Report of three cases. J. Neurosurg., *49:* 434–440, 1978.

44. Harisiadis, L., and Chang C. H. Medulloblastoma in children: A correlation between staging and results of treatment. Int. J. Radiol. Oncol. Biol. Phys., *2:* 833–841, 1977.

45. Hoffmann G. R., Thiry S., Achslogh J., Brihaye J., Dereymaeker A. Etude statistique de 202 cas de tumeur de la fosse postérieure de l'enfance. Neurochirurgie, *7:* 97–107, 1961.

46. Hirsch, J. F., Renier, D., Czernichow, P., Benveniste, L., and Pierre-Kahn, A. Medulloblastoma in childhood. Survival and functional results. 1979.

47. Hope-Stone, H. F. Results of treatment of medulloblastomas. J. Neurosurg., *32:* 83–88, 1970.

48. Ingraham, F. D., Bailey, O. T., and Barker, W. F. Medulloblastoma cerebelli: Diagnosis treatment and survivals, with a report of fifty six cases. N. Engl. J. Med., *238:* 171–174, 1948.

49. Jenkin, R. D. T. Medulloblastoma in childhood: Radiotherapy Can. Med. Assoc., J., *100:* 51–53, 1969.

50. Jereb, B., Sundaresan, N., Horten, B., Reid, A., and Galicich J. A. Supratentorial recurrences in medulloblastoma. Cancer, *47:* 806–809, 1981.

51. Keith, H. M., Kraig, W., and Kernohan, J. W. Brain Tumors in children. Pediatrics, *3:* 839–843, 1949.

52. Kernohan, J. W., and Sayer, G. P. Tumours of the Central Nervous System. Atlas of tumor pathology. Section X., Fascicle 35 Publication of the Armed Forces Institute of Pathology, Washington, D.C., 1950.
53. Lampe, I., and McIntyre R. S. Radiation therapy of medulloblastoma. Am. J. Roentgenol., *71:* 659–668, 1954.
54. Landberg, T. F., Lindgren, M. L., and Cavallin-Stahl E. K. Improvements in the radiotherapy of medulloblastoma, 1946–1975. Cancer, *45:* 670–678, 1980.
55. Leavitt, F. H. Cerebellar tumors occurring in identical twins. Arch. Neurol. Psychiatry, *19:* 617–622, 1928.
56. Liebner, E. J., Pretto, J. I., Hochhauser, M., and Kassaraba, W. Tumors of the posterior fossa in childhood and adolescence. Their diagnostic and radiotherapeutic patterns. Radiology, *82:* 193–201, 1964.
57. McFarland, D. R., Horwitz, H., Saenger, E. L., Bahr, G. K. Medulloblastoma. A review of prognosis and survival. Br. J. Radiol., *42:* 198–214, 1969.
58. McIntosh, N. Medulloblastoma. A changing prognosis? Arch. Dis. Child., *53:* 200–203, 1979.
59. Marty-Double, C., and Barneon, G. Le médulloblastome de l'adulte (à propos dune série de 22 cas). Ann. Anat. Pathol., *19:* 189–210, 1974.
60. Massarotti, M., Paoletti, P., Gaini, S. M., and Bollatti, A. Resultats à distance du traitement du médulloblastome. Analyse de 115 cas opérés. Minerva Neurochir., *14:* 92–99, 1970.
61. Mazza, C., Pasqualin, A., Da Pian, R., and Donati, E. Treatment of medulloblastoma in children: Long-term results following surgery, radiothérapy, and chemotherapy. Acta Neurochir., *57:* 163–175, 1981.
62. Mealey, J., and Hall, P. V. Medulloblastoma in children: Survival and treatment. J. Neurosurg., *46:* 56–64, 1977.
63. Miles, J., and Bhandari, Y. S. Cerebellar medulloblastoma in adults: Review of 18 cases. J. Neurosurg. Psychiatry, *33:* 208–211, 1970.
64. Nakamura, S., Harada Y., and Tabuchi, K. Medulloblastoma in childhood. Nerv. Syst. Child., *5:* 91–97, 1980.
65. Neidhart., *Pediatric Oncology*, pp. 323–327. Excepta Medica, Amsterdam, 1982.
66. Neidhardt, M. K., Hanefeld F., Henze, G., Langermann, H. J., Riehm, H. Treatment of medulloblastoma with postoperative chemotherapy before neuroaxis irradiation: An interim progress report on the West Berlin Pilot study and the West German cooperative trial.
67. Noël, J., and Méthot, Y. La radiotherapie du medulloblastome: Dix ans d'expérience. U. Méd. Can., *99:* 1848–1851, 1970.
68. Norris D. G., Bruce, D. A., Byrd, R. L., Schut, L., Littman, P., Bilaniuk, L., Zimmerman, R. and Capp, R. Improved relapse-free survival in medulloblastoma utilizing modern techniques. Neurosurgery, *9:* 661–664, 1981.
69. Nuchel, B., and Andersen, A. P. Medulloblastomas: Treatment and results. Acta Radiol. Ther. Phys. Biol., *17:* 305–311, 1978.
70. Onoyama, Y., Abe, M., Takahashi, M., Yabumoto, F., and Sakamoto, T. Radiation therapy of brain tumor in children. Radiology, *115:* 687–693, 1975.
71. Paillas J. E., Hassoun J., Torres Garcia P., Michotey P., Vialet G. Les medulloblastomes de l'adulte. Etude clinique, anatomique et thérapeutique de dix-sept observations. Arch. Anat. Cytol. Pathol., *27:* 78–84, 1979.
72. Paterson, E. Distant metastases from medulloblastoma of the cerebellum. Brain, *84:* 301 and 309, 1961.
73. Paterson E., and Farr R. F. Medulloblastoma: Treatment by irradiation of the whole central nervous system. Acta Radiol., *39:* 323–336, 1953.

74. Perry-Keene, D. A., Connelly, J. F., Young, R. A. Wettenhal, H. N. B., and Martin F. I. R. Hypothalamic hypopituitarism following external radiotherapy for tumors distant from the adeno-hypophysis. Clin. Endocrinol. *5:* 373–380, 1976.

75. Pichler, E., Kogelnik, H. D., Reinartz G., Karcher, K. H. Zaunbauer, F., Jurgensen, O. A., Koos, W., Kundi M. Therapeutic results achieved during the past 15 years in cases of medulloblastomas. Strahlentherapie, *157:* 508–513, 1981.

76. Quest, D. O., Brishan R., Antunes J. L., and Housepian, E. M. Period of risk for recurrence in medulloblastoma. J. Neurosurg., *48:* 159–163, 1978.

77. Raimondi, A. J. Medulloblastoma in childhood: Comparative results of partial and total resection. Child's Brain *5:* 310–328, 1979.

78. Raimondi, A. J., and Tomita, T. Medulloblastoma in childhood. Acta Neurochir., *50:* 127–138, 1979.

79. Raimondi, A. J., and Tomita, T. The disadvantages of prophylactic whole C. N. S. post-operative radiation therapy for medulloblastoma. In: Multidisciplinary Aspects of Brain Tumor Therapy, pp 209–218. Elsevier-North Holland Bio-medical Preps, Amsterdam, 1979.

80. Richmond, J. J. Radiotherapy of intracranial tumors in children. J. Fac. Radiol. (Lond.), *4:* 180, 1953.

81. Ringertz, N., and Tola, J. H. Medulloblastoma. J. Neuropathol. Exp. Neurol., *9:* 354–372, 1950.

82. Rosenblum, M. L., Reynolds, A. F., Smith, K. A. Rumack, B. H., and Walker, M. D. Chloroethyl cyclohexyl nitrosurea (CCNU) in the treatment of malignant brain tumour. J. Neurosurg., *39:* 306–314, 1973.

83. Rubinstein, L. J., and Northfield, D. W. The medulloblastoma and the so-called arachnoidal cerebellar sarcoma. Brain, *87:* 379–412, 1964.

84. Russel, D. S., and Rubinstein, L. J. Pathology of Tumours of the Nervous System. E. Arnold, London, 1959, 1971, and 1977.

85. Saladino, J. Les médulloblastomes et leurs traitements. Ph.D. Thesis, Lausanne, Switzerland, 1980.

86. Scherpereel. Des médulloblastomes. A propos de 100 dossiers. Thèse Médecine, Lille, France, 1974.

87. Scuccimarra, A., Carteri, A., Giordano, R., Crotti, F. M., Tomei, G., and Zavanone, M. L. Medulloblastoma in children: Review of 119 cases. J. Neurosurg. Sci., *23:* 37–46, 1979.

88. Shalet, S. M., Beardwell, C. G., Mac Farlane, I. A., Morris-Jones, P. H., and Pearson D. Endocrine morbidity in adults treated with cerebral irradiations for brain tumours during childhood. Acta Endocrinol. *84:* 673–680, 1977.

89. Shalet, S. M., Beardwell, C. G., Morris-Jones, P., Bamford, F. N., Ribeiro, G. G., and Pearson, D. Growth hormone deficiency in children with brain tumours. Cancer, *37:* 1144–1148, 1976.

90. Shalet, S. M., Morris-Jones P. H., Beardwell C. G., and Pearson D. Pituitary function after treatment of intracranial tumours in children. Lancet, *1:* 104–107, 1975.

91. Simpson, D. A., Carter, R. F., and Ducrow, W. Intracranial tumours in infancy. Dev. Med. Child. Neurol. *10:* 190–199, 1968.

92. Smith, R. A., Lampe, I., and Kahn, E. A. The prognosis of medulloblastoma in children. J. Neurosurg., *18:* 91–97, 1961.

93. Spitz E. B., Shenkin H. A., and Grant, F. C. Medulloblastoma in adults. Arch. Neurol. Psychiatry, *57:* 417–422, 1947.

94. Spunberg, J. J., Chang, C. H., Goldman, M., Auricchio, E., and Bell, J. J. Quality of long-term survival following irradiation for intracranial tumors in children under the age of two. Int. J. Radiat. Oncol., *7:* 727–736, 1981.

95. Stolzenberg, J., Fischer, . J., and Kligerman, M. M. Extradural metastasis in medulloblastoma 10 years after treatment. Am. J. Roentgenol., *108:* 71–74, 1970.
96. Thomas, P. R., Duffner, P. K., Cohen, M. E., Sinks, L. F., Tebbi, C., and Freeman, A. I. Multimodality therapy for medulloblastoma. Cancer, *45:* 666–669, 1980.
97. Tice, G. M. Traitement et pronostic du medulloblastome. J.A.M.A., *182:* 629–631, 1962.
98. Tokars, R. P., Sutton, H. G., and Griem, M. L. Cerebellar medulloblastoma. Results of a new method of radiation treatment. Cancer, *43:* 129–136, 1979.
99. De La Torre, A., Sacchetti, A., Polo, E., Aramburo, P., and Otero, J. Medulloblastoma: A proposito de trece cases. Med. Clin. (Barcelona), *74:* 342–346, 1980.
100. Van Eys, J., Chen, T., Moore, T., Cheek, W., Sexauer, C., and Starling K. Adjuvant chemotherapy for medulloblastoma and ependymoma using IV vincristine intrathecal methotrexate and intrathecal hydrocortisone. A Southwest Oncology Group Study. Can. Treat. Rep., *65:* (7–8): 681–684, 1981.
101. Venes, J. L., McIntosh, S., O'Brien, R. T., and Schwartz, A. D. Chemotherapy as an adjuvant in the initial management of cerebellar medulloblastomas. A preliminary report. J. Neurosurg., *50:* 721–724, 1979.
102. Wilson, C. B., and Gutin, P. H. Therapy of malignant brain tumors: An update on progress. Texas Med., *76:* 40–43, 1980.
103. Wilson, C. B. Medulloblastoma. Current views regarding the tumor and its treatment. Oncology, *24:* 273–290, 1970.

CHAPTER

15

The Value of Precraniotomy Shunts in Children with Posterior Fossa Tumors

A. LELAND ALBRIGHT, M.D.

Almost all neurosurgeons who treat children with posterior fossa tumors agree on two points. First, the condition of a child before posterior fossa craniotomy correlates with the condition afterward; children alert before craniotomy are more likely to be alert afterward, and moribund children are more likely to be moribund. Second, children who are obtunded because of hydrocephalus from posterior fossa tumors improve remarkably after insertion of internal or external CSF shunts. There is, however, wide disagreement about the role of CSF shunts for children with hydrocephalus from posterior fossa tumors. The reason for this lies partly in the history of the neurosurgical treatment of these children.

Before 1960, children with cerebellar tumors were seriously ill by the time their tumors were correctly diagnosed. Most children were dehydrated and had lost weight because of recurrent vomiting. Twenty to thirty percent were lethargic and bradycardic because of increased intracranial pressure. Visual impairment was evident at the time of diagnosis in 43% of Cushing's patients with medulloblastomas and 52% of those with astrocytomas. Cushing said, "It is the hydrocephalus that is responsible for the most serious of all complications from the standpoint of the useful life after a successful operation: namely, blindness" (5). The tumors were usually diagnosed by ventriculography, and further clinical deterioration often occurred. By the time of craniotomy, many children were restless or opisthotonic. Cushing and neurosurgeons since then realized that substantial hydrocephalus complicated the care of these children, and they treated the hydrocephalus by ventricular taps at the time of craniotomy. The taps decompressed the ventricles rapidly, but subdural hematomas or effusions sometimes resulted. The operative mortality was 40–50%. Children who survived the craniotomy often worsened dramatically during the first week after operation because of increased intracranial pressure. For these children, hydrocephalus was a serious component of their illness, and its treatment was of major importance.

In 1941, Ingraham and Campbell (11) began inserting external CSF shunts—external ventricular drains— to treat the hydrocephalus associated with posterior fossa tumors. Their system and the drainage systems of Dott and others during the next 15 years were not the sterile preassembled systems of today but rather were usually valveless tubes that drained into sterile gauze or into an air-vented drainage bottle. The systems often became disconnected. They drained too much CSF and caused supratentorial subdural hematomas, or too little fluid, depending on the height of the water column. Ten to twenty percent became infected if they were used longer than 72 hours. The drains treated the hydrocephalus but with considerable morbidity.

In 1960, the operative mortality for posterior fossa tumors was still about 40%, due in large part to the effects of hydrocephalus. German (7) wrote in Clinical Neurosurgery in 1961, "I am sure our lives would be more tranquil if we were able to operate on slack brains". By that time, internal CSF shunts were acceptably dependable and were an obvious option to treat the hydrocephalus associated with posterior fossa tumors. In 1963, Abraham and Chandy (1) reported 13 patients in whom ventriculoatrial shunts were inserted 3–15 days before removal of posterior fossa tumors. They observed the numerous changes after shunt insertion that have been reported many times since then: headache and vomiting ceased, vision improved, false localizing signs disappeared, and many of the classic signs of cerebral dysfunction, such as incoordination and ataxia, also disappeared. Diagnostic studies were obtained with less risk. At the time of craniotomy, the posterior fossa was slack, and no ventricular taps were necessary. The postoperative course was smooth, without the usual deterioration on the second or third day. There was only one operative death, a child with congenital cyanotic heart disease. This development was a striking improvement in the care of these children.

Three years later, Hekmatpanah and Mullan (8) verified Abraham and Chandy's observations. They inserted ventriculocaval shunts into 15 children with suspected posterior fossa tumors and observed similar clinical improvement. They had no operative mortality, and the postoperative convalescences were short. They attributed the improvement to recovery of normal function in vital brain stem centers and to an improvement in the children's general condition. Similar observations were reported in 1965 by Taptas *et al.* (19) and in 1967 by Raimondi *et al.* (16).

In 1973 Jane *et al.* (12) reported other advantages of precraniotomy shunts. First, tumors were easier to localize because neurodiagnostic procedures could be performed more deliberately in the absence of intracranial hypertension. Second, valves in the shunt system lessened the risk of upward herniation that occurred occasionally with valveless systems. Third, neurosurgeons were not obligated to reopen CSF pathways if the tumor removal was unduly hazardous. The precraniotomy shunts results in better patient care but, as Jane *et al.* noted, their report was not a controlled trial that proved the superiority of shunts. They noted that factors such as patient condition, slackness of the posterior fossa, and more adequate tumor localization were difficult to quantify.

None of the articles to that time had compared children with untreated hydrocephalus from posterior fossa tumors with children treated by internal or external shunts before tumor removal. In 1977, this author and D. H. Reigel reported 86 children with hydrocephalus secondary to posterior fossa tumors treated at Children's Hospital of Pittsburgh between 1965 and 1975 (2). Only 20% of the children were in good condition at the time of admission; 70% were in fair condition and 10% were in poor condition. The hydrocephalus was treated by a precraniotomy VP shunt in 27 and was untreated before craniotomy in 47. Children in the two groups were in comparable condition at the time of admission. The operative morbidity was significantly less in the group with shunts than in those without a shunt, and the operative mortality was less for those with shunts (3.7%) than for those without (12.8%), although the difference was not statistically different. The remaining 12 children were not comparable to the others; their condition on admission was worse, and they were treated with external shunts.

Thus, the majority of articles since 1960 indicate that CSF shunts benefit children who are ill from hydrocephalus of posterior fossa tumors. They improve the condition of the child before craniotomy, normalize the posterior fossa pressure for craniotomy, improve the postoperative course and, most importantly, decrease the operative mortality.

After the benefits of precraniotomy shunts were evident, some neurosurgeons began inserting shunts into virtually all children with posterior fossa tumors, regardless of the severity of the hydrocephalus. Other neurosurgeons remained skeptical of the value of shunts and never used them.

Raimondi has been perhaps the strongest advocate of shunts for children with posterior fossa tumors. In his experience from 1967 to 1979, he observed papilledema at the time of diagnosis in 70% of 117 children with cerebellar and fourth ventricular tumors and thought this was a strong indication for a precraniotomy shunt (17). Hydrocephalus was documented in 94% of his patients, and internal shunts were inserted in 86%. Craniotomies were delayed an average of 8 days until papilledema subsided. After craniotomy, permanent internal shunts were required in 19 of 53 patients (36%) with medulloblastomas and in 25 of 42 patients (60%) with cerebellar astrocytomas.

The four major arguments against precraniotomy shunts have been: (a) the risk of upward herniation after shunt insertion (6, 10); (b) the possibility of transshunt metastases (10); (c) the belief that corticosteroids restore patency to obstructed CSF pathways (6); and (d) the belief that most children do not need a permanent shunt after tumor removal (3).

Upward herniation refers to herniation of the anterior vermis or tumor in the vermis through the tentorial incisura, compressing the dorsal brain stem. This usually occurs within a few hours after decompressing severe hydrocephalus in children with large anterior vermis tumors and causes progressive obtundation. The neurologic deterioration is usually, although not always, reversed by shunt occlusion or by tumor removal. Fortunately, upward herniation is infrequent; it occurred in an average of 3.4% of patients with precraniotomy shunts in a compilation of series (3 of 103 (17); 9 of 96 (10); 0 of 60 (Mark O'Brien, personal communication); and 2 of 68 (author's experience)). CT scans occasionally demonstrate upward herniation of vermis or tumor before shunt insertion, and these children are probably at increased risk of further herniation. Mild upward herniation compresses the quadrigeminal cistern, moderate herniation obliterates the posterior angle of the peritectal CSF diamond, and severe herniation flattens the posterior aspect of the third ventricle (14). In children with hydrocephalus and these CT findings, CSF must be removed slowly. Intratumoral hemorrhages occur rarely after insertion of internal or external shunts and may be temporally, rather than causally, related to the shunt operation but may be due to increased blood flow to the tumor (20).

A second objection to precraniotomy shunts has been the possibility of transshunt metastases. This is a concern primarily for medulloblastomas, which frequently metastasize along CSF pathways and are the most common brain tumor to metastasize outside the central nervous system (13). The relationship between shunts and systemic metastases can be evaluated either (a) by determining whether most patients with systemic metastases have had shunts, or (b) by comparing the frequency of metastases in patients with and without shunts.

Kleinman *et al.* (13) reviewed 686 medulloblastoma patients and found that 33 (4.8%) developed systemic metastases at some time in their illness. They also reviewed all of the cases of medulloblastoma with systemic metastases reported before 1981 (103 cases). They found that 80% of the patients had no CSF shunt at any time during their illness. The incidence of visceral metastases was not increased in patients with CSF shunts, although pulmonary metastases occurred more often in patients with ventriculoatrial shunts (31%) than in those without (9%).

The seminal question in this issue is whether the low (4.8%) incidence of systemic metastases is increased by a CSF shunt. We do not know. To definitively answer that question, we would need to know the incidence of systemic metastases in children with comparable tumor excisions, half with shunts and half without, followed prospectively. The extent of tumor resections must be comparable because children with residual medulloblastoma after craniotomy would be more likely to develop local or systemic metastases. This question will probably never be answered with statistically significant data, because we would need 700 children with and 700 without shunts to detect a doubling (from 5 to 10%) of systemic metastases, with a 95% confidence level (Floyd Taylor, Sc.D., personal communication).

Berry *et al.* (4) recently analyzed the survival of patients with medulloblastomas with and without shunts. They reviewed 122 patients who received radiotherapy at the Princess Margaret Hospital in Toronto between 1958 and 1978. The 5-year survival for 71 patients with a precraniotomy shunt was 59%, and for the 51 patients without a shunt, it was 54%. Of the 52 patients who relapsed, 18 had systemic metastases at the time of relapse. Fifteen of the 18 had been treated with a shunt. Unfortunately, the extent of tumor removal was not reported for children with or without shunts. Total removals were performed in only 36% of the patients, and it is possible that the shunts were inserted more frequently into children with incomplete tumor resections; metastases would be more likely in these children.

The rarity of transshunt metastases can be explained by the fact that although medulloblastomas metastasize frequently down the spinal axis and occasionally cephalad into the extracerebral subarachnoid space, they rarely seed into the lateral ventricle; cytology of ventricular CSF is rarely positive for medulloblastoma cells.

A third objection to precraniotomy shunts has been that they are unnecessary because corticosteroids allegedly restore patency to obstructed CSF pathways (6). This hypothesis has not been substantiated by data. Many posterior fossa tumors are associated with peritumoral edema that may compress both the brain stem and the cerebral aqueduct. The improvement often seen after giving corticosteroids is more likely due to a reduction in peritumoral edema than to reopening of CSF pathways. In our experience, ventriculomegaly has not improved after corticosteroids.

A fourth and perhaps the most cogent argument against precraniotomy shunts is that most children do not need a permanent internal shunt after removal of posterior fossa tumors. Shunts are inserted before craniotomy into 31–86% of children with posterior fossa tumors. The percentage of children who need a permanent CSF shunt after craniotomy is unknown and has varied from 15% (3) to 72% (17), but most authors (9, 15) indicate that 20–40% of children continue to need a shunt; this is in keeping with our experience. In the experience of Papo *et al.* (15), children with cerebellar hemispheric tumors are less likely (14%) to need permanent shunts than children with midline cerebellar tumors (29%).

As the arguments for and against precraniotomy shunts continue, the significance of the debate is lessening because a change is occurring in the patient population. Children are apparently being diagnosed earlier, before they are obtunded from hydrocephalus. I reviewed the charts of 57 children with posterior fossa tumors at the Children's Hospital of Pittsburgh from 1975 to 1982. The children's conditions at the time of admission were analyzed. The children were rated in good condition if they were alert with or without papilledema and with or without such cerebellar signs as dysmetria and ataxia. They were rated in fair condition if they were irritable, lethargic, or combative, or if they were dehydrated or unable to walk. They were rated in poor condition if they were obtunded or had decerebrate posturing, bradypnea, or bradycardia. Although this rating system is subjective and retrospective, it is comparable to the grading system reported previously (2). Hydrocephalus was present to some extent in 45 of 57 (79%) of the children, and shunts were inserted in 41 of 45, although some of the shunts may have been optional.

By this classification, 62% of the children were in good condition at the time of admission, 33% in fair, and only 5% in poor condition. This is a substantial improvement from the situation which we found between 1965 and 1975 (2) (20% good, 70% fair, and 10% poor) and is probably due to earlier diagnosis by CT scans. Therapy of the hydrocephalus should have been considered for the 38% of patients who were not in good condition.

For approximately the last 5 years the quality of the external shunts available has improved, so that they are a reasonable alternative to internal shunts, if not the procedure of choice (15, 18). Papo *et al.* (15) reported that the overall mortality of 62 children with precraniotomy external CSF shunts was only 6%. This also is substantial improvement in the mortality of previous years. Twenty-five percent of their patients needed permanent internal shunts.

The risks of external shunts are infection and excessive CSF drainage. The risk of infection with current external drainage systems is equilavent to that of internal shunts. To reduce the risk of infection, long ventricular catheters inserted into dilated frontal horns should be drawn subcutaneously for several centimeters before exiting, a technique similar to that used by general surgeons inserting Broviac catheters. Most current systems contain sterile reservoirs to permit daily CSF cultures, and some contain valves to regulate CSF flow into the collection bags. The reported incidence of subdural hematomas related to excessive drainage has declined precipitously.

Because 75% of children with medulloblastomas have hydrocephalus at the time of diagnosis, the small risk of transshunt metastases deserves careful consideration. Children with presumed medulloblastomas who need treatment of hydrocephalus should probably have an external shunt. If the hydrocephalus persists after craniotomy, as it will in 30–40% of the cases, an internal shunt will be required. Whether a Millipore filter in the shunt decreases the low incidence of shunt-related metastases is debatable; statistically significant data have not yet been published (10).

In summary, almost all of the published data indicate that precraniotomy shunts benefit the children who are ill from hydrocephalus of posterior fossa tumors by improving their condition before operation and by reducing operative morbidity and mortality. In the United States, children with cerebellar tumors are apparently being diagnosed earlier, and the need for treatment of hydrocephalus with internal or external shunts before craniotomy is diminishing. Advances in technology have made external shunts comparable to internal shunts in risks and benefits for children who need treatment of hydrocephalus before craniotomy.

REFERENCES

1. Abraham, J., and Chandy, J. Ventriculo-atrial shunt in the management of posterior-fossa tumours. Preliminary report. J. Neurosurg., *20:* 252–253, 1963.
2. Albright, L., and Reigel, D. H. Management of hydrocephalus secondary to posterior fossa tumors. J. Neurosurg., *46:* 52–55, 1977.
3. Amacher, A. L., and Hovind, L. Intracranial tumefactions in children. Surgical mortality. Child's Brain, *5:* 518–529, 1979.
4. Berry, M. P., Jenkin, D. T., Keen, C. W., Nair, B. D., and Simpson, W. J. Radiation treatment for medulloblastoma. A 21-year review. J. Neurosurg., *55:* 43–51, 1981.
5. Cushing, H. Experiences with the cerebellar astrocytomas: a critical review of seventy-six cases. Surg. Gynecol. Obstet., *52:* 129–204, 1931.
6. Epstein, F., and Rajagopalan, M. Pediatric posterior fossa tumors: Hazards of the "preoperative" shunt. Neurosurgery, *3:* 348–350, 1978.
7. German, W. J. The gliomas: A follow-up study. Clin. Neurosurg., *7:* 1–19, 1961.
8. Hekmatpanah, J., and Mullan, S. Ventriculo-caval shunt in the management of posterior fossa tumors. J. Neurosurg., *26:* 609–613, 1966.
9. Hemmer, R., Haensel-Friedrich, G., and Friedrich, H. The value of preoperative shunts in posterior fossa tumors. Mod. Probl. Paediatr., *18:* 48–50, 1977.
10. Hoffman, J. J., Hendrick, E. B., and Humphreys, R. P. Metastases via ventriculoperitoneal shunt in patients with medulloblastomas. J. Neurosurg., *44:* 562–566, 1976.
11. Ingraham, F. D., and Campbell, J. B. An apparatus for closed drainage of the ventricular system. Ann. Surg., *114:* 1096–1098, 1941.
12. Jane, J. A., Kaufman, B., Nulsen, F., Yashon, D., and Young, H. The role of angiography and ventriculovenous shunting in the treatment of posterior fossa tumors. Acta Neurochir., *28:* 13–28, 1973.
13. Kleinman, G. M., Hochberg, F. H., and Richardson, E. P., Jr. Systemic metastases from medulloblastoma: Report of 2 cases and review of the literature. Cancer, *48:* 2296–2309, 81.
14. Osborn, A. G., Heaston, D. K., and Wing, S. W. Diagnosis of ascending transtentorial herniation by cranial computed tomography. Am. J. Roentgenol., *130:* 755–760, 1978.

15. Papo, I., Caruselli, G., and Luongo, A. External ventricular drainage in the management of posterior fossa tumors in children and adolescents. Neurosurgery, *10:* 13–15, 1982.
16. Raimondi, A. J., and Tomita, T. Hydrocephalus and infratentorial tumors—Incidence, clinical picture and treatment. J. Neurosurg., *55:* 174–182, 1981.
17. Raimondi, A. J., Yashon, D., Matsumoto, S., and Reyes, C. A. Increased intracranial pressure without lateralizing signs: The midline syndrome. Neurochirurgia, *10:* 197–209, 1967.
18. Richard, K. E., Heller, R., and Frowein, R. A. Internal shunt or preoperative pressure-controlled ventricular fluid drainage in children and juveniles with infratentorial tumours (abstr). Acta Neurochir., *62:* 132, 1982.
19. Taptas, J. N., Apostolov, A., and Kordioli, N. La dérivation ventriculoatriale dans le traitement chirurgical des lésions de la fosse postériure. Presse Medicale, *73:* 15–16, 1965.
20. Vaquero, J., Cabezudo, J. M., DeSola, R. G., and Nombela, L. Intratumoral hemorrhage in posterior fossa tumors after ventricular drainage. Report of two cases. J. Neurosurg., *54:* 406–408, 1981.

CHAPTER

16

Disadvantages of the Preoperative Shunt In Posterior Fossa Tumors

ROBERT L. McLAURIN, M.D.

The value of placement of a ventricular shunt prior to definitive surgery in patients with posterior fossa tumors was first recognized by Abraham and Chandy in 1963 (1). Neurosurgeons who dealt with pediatric problems recognized the contribution derived from relief of intracranial hypertension in such patients, and the procedure was adopted by many centers. During the ensuing period of time, however, there has occurred considerable discussion about the advantages and disadvantages of routine shunting, and it certainly seems that this forum is an appropriate one in which to reconsider this matter. The present author has not adopted the practice of routine precraniotomy shunting, and the following reasons are presented to justify this position.

The basis for the opinion that shunts should not be done routinely consists of two considerations: (a) the problems and potential risks resulting from the shunt placement, and (b) the lack of any demonstrated benefit consequent to its use. The negative effects of shunting can, in turn, be broken down into those due to the shunt itself and those which may be specifically due to the presence of a posterior fossa tumor in a shunted patient. The first consideration, therefore, will be directed toward the potential complications of the shunt.

As every neurosurgeon knows, shunting, however valuable and lifesaving it may be under conditions involving CSF obstruction, is not a benign procedure. Indeed, the history of the evolution of ventricular shunting is largely a history of efforts to prevent its complications. The most frequent complication is malfunction of the shunt and, while the incident of this problem is probably very infrequent during the first week or so after placement, it nevertheless cannot be totally ignored. Moreover, experience with shunting of other forms of hydrocephalus has taught that shunt dependence can be created simply by the presence of a shunt, perhaps due to aqueductal occlusion which was not present before shunting. That this is not a theoretical consideration only is evidenced by the case reported by Hekmatpanah and Mullan: a child 3½ years of age underwent removal of an ependymoma after shunting and returned 1 year later with neurologic deterioration secondary to shunt malfunction (4).

The problem of shunt infection, likewise, cannot be disregarded. Although infection is no longer the problem that it was a decade ago, it still occurs in approximately 3–5% of shunts. Such more rare complications such as perforation of a viscus, seizures, and surface hematomas due to craniocerebral disproportion need be mentioned only for completion's sake.

More important than the complications of the shunt itself are those problems that may arise from the coexistence of a shunt and a posterior fossa neoplasm. Epstein and Murali (3) have clearly documented one such problem: upward herniation and hemorrhage into the tumor. The authors presented the histories of three patients who demonstrated neurologic deterioration following placement of peritoneal shunts. In two of these cases the patient did not awaken from the anesthetic used for the shunting procedure, and repeat CT scans showed hemorrhage into the tumor. The third patient had deterioration over several days after shunting, despite decreased ventricular size, and upward herniation was demonstrated surgically. Jane *et al.* (6) also have described upward herniation after shunting and have demonstrated by pneumoencephalography the high position of the fourth ventricle, which subsequently returned to normal after tumor excision. The three patients of Epstein and Murali (3) occurred among 30 patients with posterior fossa tumors who were shunted, an incidence of 10%. Hoffman *et al.* (5) reported six instances of upward herniation in 126 cases of shunted infratentorial tumors.

The second major complication of shunting the ventricular systems of patients with tumors concerns the occurrence of metastases of medulloblastomas into the peritoneal cavity or vascular stream. This was first described by Makeever and King (7) in 1966 but later was emphasized by a report of the experience of Hoffman *et al.* (5). Between 1966 and 1974 the latter observers had shunted 96 of 126 patients with posterior fossa gliomas, of which 41 were medulloblastomas. Four of these patients died as a result of systemic metastases, with no evidence of local recurrence clinically or at autopsy. The peritoneal surfaces were covered by medulloblastoma, and the tumor had also spread systemically to the bone marrow in each patient. The authors incidentally noted that the survival curve for patients with medulloblastoma treated by shunting, including these four patients, was not as good as the survival cure for patients treated prior to the use of shunting. For this reason the authors devised a Millipore filter to be used when shunting patients with gliomas. As expected, however, the filters have also contributed to the malfunction of these shunts. It remains clear, nevertheless, that metastasis through a shunt is a very real risk, especially with medulloblastomas, and that justification for shunting should be strongly based on demonstrable benefit despite this risk. The fact that the majority of extracranial metastases of brain tumors occur only after craniotomy (or shunt) indicates that local mechanical barriers are of greater importance than the inability of the tumor to occur in a new environment.

This brings us to a consideration of whether there is, in fact, any positive value derived from preoperative shunting. This question was addressed by the American Society of Pediatric Neurosurgery, and some data has been collected to attempt to resolve the matter (8). The data were obtained from several pediatric neurosurgical centers, some of which made a routine practice of precraniotomy shunting and others who did not.

Thirty-nine cases were submitted, with 15 having been shunted and 24 having been operated without shunts. That the two cohorts were similar in clinical presentation is shown in Table 16.1. Among the shunted patients, 13 of 15 (87%) were alert preoperatively while among the nonshunted population 17 of 24 (71%) were recorded as alert; thus, the shunted population was somewhat more neurologically intact on admission. Another index of the severity of involvement was noted in the presence of papilledema in approximately 75% of each population.

The ventricular size, as noted on CT scan, was determined in each patient. It was recorded as a ratio (percentage) of the maximum width of the ventricles to the skull at that level. Table 16.2 reveals that 3 of 14 shunted patients and 5 of 23 nonshunted patients had a ratio greater than 50%. Again, therefore, it must be concluded that the two populations were similar.

Probably the most significant index of whether shunting was beneficial in the management of posterior fossa tumors was derived from an

TABLE 16.1

Clinical Presentation of Preoperatively Shunted and Nonshunted Patients

Conscious Level Preoperatively	Shunted		Nonshunted	
	No.	%	No.	%
Alert	13	86.7	17	70.8
Lethargic	2	13.3	6	25.0
Obtunded	0	0.0	0	0.0
Stuporous	0	0.0	0	0.0
Comatose	0	0.0	1	4.2
Total	15	100.0	24	100.0
Missing cases	0		0	
Response %	100.0%		100.0%	

TABLE 16.2

Ventricular Size of Preoperatively Shunted and Nonshunted Patients

Ventricular Size Preoperatively by CT Scan	Shunted		Nonshunted	
	No.	%	No.	%
15	1	7.1		
17			1	4.2
19			1	4.2
20			3	12.5
25			3	12.5
30	3	21.4	3	12.5
31			2	8.3
40			1	4.2
42	1	7.1		
43			1	4.2
50	6	42.9	3	12.5
55			1	4.2
57	1	7.1		
60			1	4.2
66	1	7.1	2	8.3
75	1	7.1	1	4.2
80			1	4.2
Total	14	100.0	24	100.0
Missing cases	1		0	
Response %	93.3%		100.0%	

evaluation of the duration of hospitalization. The shunted patients had a median precraniotomy hospitalization of 9 days (Table 16.3) while the nonshunted patients showed a median of less than 5 days (Table 16.3). The median period of postcraniotomy hospitalization for shunted patients was 18 days (Table 16.4), and for nonshunted patients it was 14 days (Table 16.4). The total difference in median period of hospitalization was, therefore, 8 days with the nonshunted patients hospitalized for 1 week less than the shunted population. There was no difference in the postoperative conditions at 30 days since all but one patient was fully alert.

It appears inescapably apparent from this small survey that there is no demonstrable value to precraniotomy shunting and that it simply subjects the child to another operative procedure and several extra days of hospitalization.

Other items of significance concern the need for postcraniotomy shunts. In the 15 patients who underwent preoperative shunting, 7 had their shunts removed postoperatively. Moreover, of 23 patients recorded without precraniotomy shunting, only 4 required postcraniotomy shunts. The argument that a significant percentage of patients will need shunts after tumor removal does not appear substantiated.

TABLE 16.3

Precraniotomy Hospitalization of Shunted vs. Nonshunted Patients

Precraniotomy Hospitalization (days)	Shunted		Nonshunted	
	No.	%	No.	%
1			2	8.3
2			2	8.3
3	1	6.7	3	12.5
4	2	13.3	3	12.5
5			5	20.8
6	1	6.7	2	8.3
7	1	6.7	1	4.2
8	1	6.7		
9	2	13.3		
10	4	26.7	4	16.7
11	2	13.3		
13			1	4.2
14	1	6.7		
47			1	4.2
Total	15	100.0	24	100.0
Missing cases	0		0	
Response %	100.0%		100.0%	

TABLE 16.4

Postcraniotomy Hospitalization for Shunted vs. Nonshunted Patients

Postcraniotomy Hospitalization (days)	Shunted		Nonshunted	
	No.	%	No.	%
7			3	12.5
8			2	8.3
10	1	6.7	4	16.7
11	1	6.7	1	4.2
13	1	6.7	1	4.2
14	2	13.3	1	4.2
15			2	8.3
16	1	6.7	1	4.2
17	1	6.7		
18	1	6.7	1	4.2
20	1	6.7	1	4.2
21			3	12.5
23	1	6.7		
28			1	4.2
34	1	6.7		
44	1	6.7		
45	2	13.3		
49	1	6.7		
78			1	4.2
92			1	4.2
99			1	4.2
Total	15	100.0	24	100.0
Missing cases	0		0	
Response %	100.0%		100.0%	

DISCUSSION

The use of a precraniotomy shunt appears presently to be anachronistic. Prior to the advent of steroid therapy, CT scan, and unidirectional external ventricular drainage (EVD), shunting unquestionably improved the child's preoperative state and facilitated surgery. Albright and Reigel (2) reviewed their experiences over an 11-year period between 1965 and 1976. They compared three groups of patients: 47 had no shunt or EVD, 12 had preoperative EVD, and 27 had preoperative shunts. Of 47 patients without preoperative decompression, 21 had no evidence of intracranial hypertension at surgery, and in 3 patients there was difficulty tapping the ventricles. It would appear, then, that the authors would have to agree that preoperative shunting would have been of no value in half of those patients. It is also noteworthy, although not well explained, that the highest mortality was in the group prepared for surgery by EVD.

The introduction of CT scan has, in our opinion, reduced considerably the preoperative morbidity of children with posterior fossa tumors. This factor, accompanied by the increased availability of pediatric neurologists and neurosurgeons, has allowed earlier diagnosis before the patient has reached a stage of brain stem, metabolic, and nutritional failure. Recent experience in one clinic has demonstrated that it is rare for the patient hospitalized for posterior fossa tumor removal not to demonstrate dramatic, and fairly complete, relief of symptoms from the use of steroids.

An alternative to the placement of a shunt in those patients who may not respond to steroids is external ventricular drainage. Papo *et al.* (9) have recently made a very strong case for EVD in the management of posterior fossa tumors in children (9). The authors reviewed a series of 62 patients, 58 of whom did not have preoperative shunting. They presented their results in relation to operative mortality and the need for late shunting. The early operative mortality was 3.2%, and one later complication was due to infection relating to the EVD. The infection rate in the series, therefore, was 1.6%.

The need for later shunting occurred in 14 patients (25%). The authors analyzed these patients and noted that the need for later shunting was considerably higher in those patients with midline tumors of the cerebellum than in those with hemispheric tumors. Moreover, the need for permanent shunt occurred 4 times as often in children less than 10 years of age as in those more than 10 years old.

Observations on the 39 patients surveyed by the American Society of Pediatric Neurosurgery showed that 3 of 5 nonshunted patients who had EVD inserted had it removed at the time of surgery, and the remaining 2 patients had theirs removed within 4 days postoperatively. Thus, it appears that prolonged use of EVD is not necessary in most instances.

The use of EVD seems to have considerable advantage over preliminary shunting in the management of acute intracranial hypertension. It is possible to control the intracranial pressure more precisely and to reduce it in a more progressive and gradual manner, thereby reducing the likelihood of complications of rapid decompression. Moreover, the procedure of placement of EVD is obviously a much simpler procedure than placement of a shunt.

REFERENCES

1. Abraham, J., and Chandy, J. Ventriculo-atrial shunt in the management of posterior-fossa tumours. Preliminary report. J. Neurosurg., *20:* 252–253, 1963.
2. Albright, L., and Reigel, D. H. Management of hydrocephalus secondary to posterior fossa tumors. J. Neurosurg., *46:* 52–55, 1977.
3. Epstein, F., and Murali, R. Pediatric Posterior Fossa Tumors: Hazards of the "Preoperative" Shunt. Neurosurgery, *3*(3)*:* 348–350, 1978.
4. Hekmatpanah, J., and Mullan, S. Ventriculo-caval shunt in the management of posterior fossa tumors. J. Neurosurg., *26:* 609–613, 1967.
5. Hoffman, H. J., Hendrick, E. B., and Humphreys, R. P. Metastasis via ventriculoperitoneal shunt in patients with medulloblastoma. J. Neurosurg., *44:* 562–566, 1976.
6. Jane, J. A., Kaufman, B., *et al.* The role of angiography and ventriculovenous shunting in the treatment of posterior fossa tumors. Acta Neurochir., *28:* 13–27, 1973.
7. Makeever, L. C., and King, J. D. Medulloblastoma with extracranial metastasis through a ventriculovenous shunt. Report of a case and review of the literature. Am. J. Clin. Pathol., *46:* 245–249, 1966.
8. McLone, D. G., Personal communication, 1982.
9. Papo, I., Catuselli, G., and Luongo, A. External ventricular drainage in the management of posterior fossa tumors in children and adolescents. Neurosurgery, *10:* 13–15, 1982.

IV

Spinal Dysraphism

CHAPTER

17

The Embryology of Spinal Dysraphism

BARRY N. FRENCH, M.D., F.R.C.S.(C), F.A.C.S.

INTRODUCTION

Neurosurgeons are confronted by embryological development gone awry, especially frequently in the various forms of spinal dysraphism listed in Tables 17.1 and 17.2. The open forms, or spina bifida aperta, display abnormal embryogenesis throughout the central nervous system whereas the less frequent closed forms, or occult dysraphism, involve predominantly the spine, spinal cord, and cauda equina. A host of theories have been proposed to explain the disordered development, but each theory must be assessed against a background of what is truly known, in contrast to only theorized, about normal embryogenesis. The purposes of this chapter are three: to review the normal processes occurring in the development of the central nervous system; to describe the morphology of the various forms of open and closed spinal dysraphism; and to review the many theories of their causation.

EMBRYOLOGICAL TERMINOLOGY

A neurosurgeon who reads the embryological literature meets an unfamiliar terminology used to describe the age of the developing conceptus (29). Embryologists divide the intrauterine period of development into the embryonic and the fetal periods. The embryonic period consumes approximately the first 52 days, laying down the basic tissues and forming the primitive organs and organ systems. The fetal period continues for the next 7 months of gestation and involves the sophisticated development of the primitive tissues and organs sketched in the embryonic period. The embryologist, rather than stating the gestational age of development in days or months, will generally use the terms horizon or stage for the embryonic period or record the crown-rump (CR) length of the embryo (Fig. 17.1*A* and *B*). The CR length is used well into the fetal period but in the later fetal period the crown-heel (CH) measurement is generally recorded (Fig. 17.1*C*).

Streeter (50) divided the embryonic period into a timetable of 23 "horizons" designated by Roman numerals, with each horizon described

TABLE 17.1
Classification of Spinal Dysraphism

Spina bifida aperta
Myeloschisis
Myelomeningocele
Hemimyelomeningocele
Hydrosyringomyelomeningocele
Spinal meningocele
Arnold-Chiari malformation

TABLE 17.2
Classification of Spinal Dysraphism

Occult spinal dysraphism
Spinal dermal sinus
Tethered cord syndrome
Lumbosacral lipoma
Lipomyelomeningocele
Diastematomyelia
Neurenteric cyst
Combined anterior and posterior spina bifida

by specific morphological features of the organ systems. O'Rahilly detailed the earlier phases and elected to use the term "stage" in preference to "horizon", and used Arabic numbers to designate each stage. The end of the embryonic period was arbitrarily defined by Streeter as the appearance of marrow formation in the humerus generally correlating with a CR length of 30 mm and a gestational age ranging from 50 to 62 days. The horizon or stage method of dating the development of the embryonic period is preferred because embryos of similar morphological development may have a marked variability in gestational age or length due to simple difficulties in measurement, anatomically incomplete embryos, or inaccurate menstrual cycle data.

The essential elements in both the open and closed forms of spinal dysraphism occur in the embryonic period, with developments in the fetal period modifying and complicating their eventual anatomical and clinical appearances. This chapter will deal predominantly with the abnormalities of the embryonic period.

NORMAL EMBRYOLOGY OF THE CENTRAL NERVOUS SYSTEM

Coordination of Development

The cellular migrations that occur in the embryonic period are well described; however, the mechanisms that coordinate developmental processes such as the interaction between different tissues, the migrations of cell populations, the regulated proliferation of cells, and the control of cellular death are poorly understood. Certain tissues in early embryonic

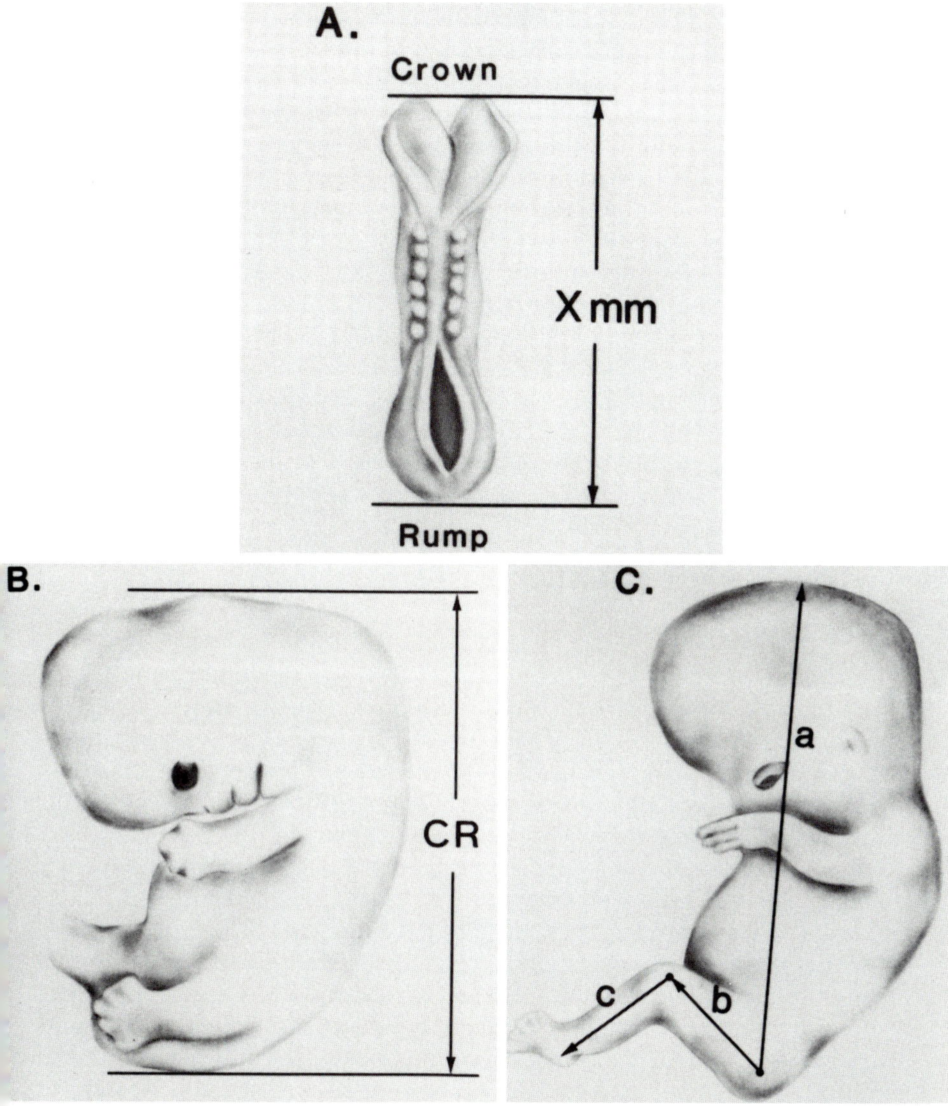

FIG. 17.1. Measurements of the length of an embryo or fetus used by the embryologist. (*A*) Crown-rump (*CR*) length (*X* millimeters) of a Stage 10 embryo with six pairs of somites. (*B*) CR length of an older embryo. (*C*) Crown-heel (CH) length of the fetus is the sum of a + b + c. Estimations of gestational age by length are complicated by anatomically incomplete or deformed embryos.

development influence adjacent tissues and are called inductors or organizers. Human inducers are unknown but in the avian embryo, the primitive streak, the notochord, and the paraxial mesoderm act as primary organizers of the central nervous system (CNS) (35). For instance, primitive streak tissue transplanted to another area of the embryonic disc will influence the formation of a neural plate; similarly, transplanted notochordal tissue will cause a localized neural tube to form. The chemical mediators that control induction are poorly understood in the experimental situation and not at all in human development. Indeed, once the major primary inductors have outlined the CNS, a series of secondary inductions occurs as, for example, in the development of the optic vesicle which ultimately forms the eye.

Abnormalities of these complex and poorly understood areas of embryology may contribute to many of the CNS anomalies that confront the neurosurgeon. Thus, while simple or easily understood mechanical explanations for complicated embryological anomalies may be attractive, such explanations should always be weighed against the essential complexities of embryological development. The development of certain structures during normal embryogenesis of the nervous system has to be discussed in series whereas, in reality, the formation of these structures is in parallel.

Formation of the Embryonic Disc

THE BILAMINAR EMBRYO

The first 2 weeks of development after fertilization (embryonic stages 1–5) consist of implantation of the conceptus into the uterine wall and development of a bilaminar, or two-layered, embryo. The union of sperm and egg creates the single-celled zygote and subsequent repeated divisions form the 12- to 16-cell morula which enters the uterus. A cavitation within the morula creates two cellular groups, the outer trophoblast which contributes to the formation of the placenta and a group of centrally located cells, the internal cell mass, which gives rise to the embryo. During stage 5 at 7–12 days of development, this structure, now called the blastocyst, implants into the uterine wall. With further development the internal cell mass separates from the overlying trophoblast to create a slit-like amniotic cavity which progressively enlarges and ultimately contains the embryo. Simultaneously, the internal cell mass becomes the flattened and circular embryonic disc with 2 cell layers, the so-called bilaminar embryo (Fig. 17.2). The outer layer adjacent to the amniotic cavity is the epiblast which gives rise to all or nearly all of the cells of the embryo. The inner layer adjacent to the primary yolk sac is the hypoblast, which is actually displaced laterally and does not contribute to the embryonic cellular development.

During stage 6, at 13–15 days of development, the hypoblastic cells near the future rostral end of the embryo form a thickened circular area

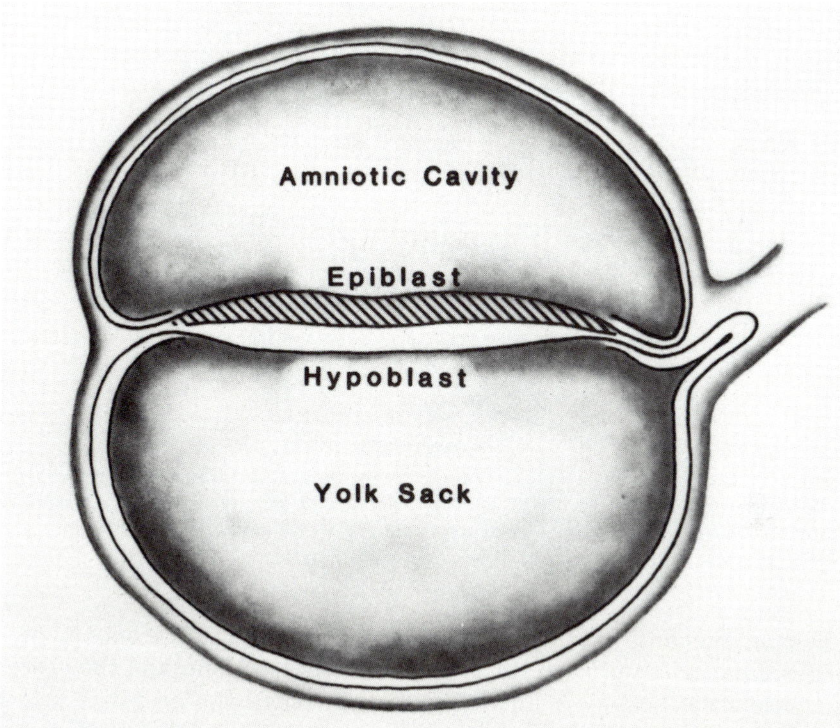

FIG. 17.2. Diagrammatic longitudinal section through the bilaminar embryonic disc within the blastocyst. The epiblast is adjacent to the amniotic cavity and the hypoblast to the yolk sac. The two cavities are separated by the embryonic disc.

called the prochordal plate at the future site of the mouth (Fig. 17.3). The prochordal plate is important not only because it is an organizer of the head region but also because the outer and inner layers of the bilaminar embryo are fused at this site. The interposition of mesoderm is prevented in later development, and the cephalic growth of the future notochord is limited by this fusion of tissue layers.

THE TRILAMINAR EMBRYO

Gastrulation is the process which converts the embryo from two layers to three by interposition of a mesoblastic layer between the epiblast and the hypoblast. In actual fact, some cells of the mesoblastic layer invade and displace the early hypoblastic cells. Thus, the epiblast is the eventual source of all three layers of the trilaminar embryo—the outer embryonic ectoderm, the middle intraembryonic mesoderm, and the inner embryonic entoderm.

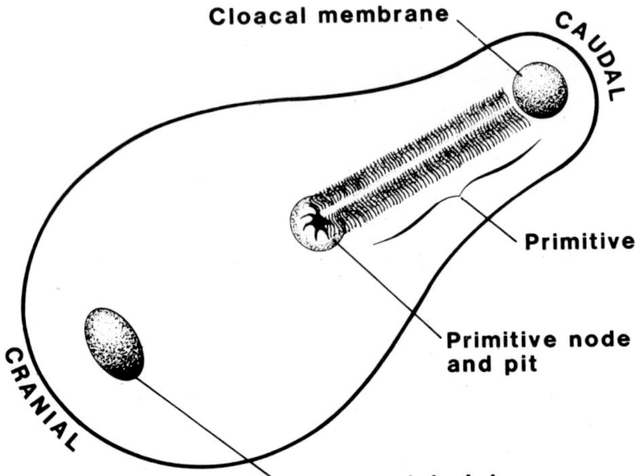

FIG. 17.3. Embryonic stage 6 (13–15 days) showing the cranial and caudal areas of fusion of the two-layered embryo at the prochordal plate (future mouth) and cloacal membrane (future anal area), respectively. These areas limit the rostral and caudal conversion of the embryo from 2 to 3 layers during the process of gastrulation.

During the end of stage 6, usually at 15 days of development, a longitudinal orientation of the embryo becomes evident, and the process of gastrulation begins. A linear thickening, called the primitive streak, appears in the epiblast in the midline of the caudal aspect of the embryonic disc (Fig. 17.3). The primitive streak is the site and source of the majority of migrating cells that form the middle and inner layers of the embryo. The interval between the primitive streak caudally and the prochordal plate rostrally mark the future posterior midline of the embryo. At the caudal end of the primitive streak is an area of fusion of the two cell layers similar to the rostral prochordal plate. This site is the circular cloacal membrane, which is the future location of the anus and urogenital structures.

Cellular proliferation increases the length of the primitive streak, and a thickening forms at its rostral end called variously the primitive knot or node or Hensen's node (Fig. 17.3). Simultaneously, a longitudinal central depression called the primitive groove develops along the streak and deepens somewhat at the rostral node level to form the primitive pit. Cells from the epiblast move into the primitive streak and groove, separate from the epiblast, and migrate rostrally between the epiblast and hypoblast to form the mesoblast, thus creating the earliest stage of the trilaminar embryo (Fig. 17.4). The epiblast (ectoderm) is destined to form the CNS (neuroectoderm) and the epidermis (cutaneous ectoderm);

the mesoblast (mesoderm) forms the skeleton, striated and smooth muscles, connective tissues, blood vessels, blood cells, and bone marrow, and the reproductive and excretory organs. The hypoblast (entoderm) is the source of the epithelial linings of the respiratory and digestive tracts and glandular cells of the liver and pancreas.

The primitive streak is the source of intraembryonic mesoderm until approximately the 4th week of development, and then it rapidly regresses in size and importance. During its functional lifetime, the embryo increases in length 5-fold, predominantly by the complex development of the embryo rostral to the primitive streak. The primitive streak occupies the sacrococcygeal area by this time and normally disappears in later development. Occasionally, cells persist and produce a tumor called a sacrococcygeal teratoma, which may contain a variety of tissue types which reflect the pleuripotential nature of primitive streak cells. These tumors present at birth and must be differentiated by the neurosurgeon from a sacral meningocele or a form of occult spinal dysraphism because the management is quite different (20).

DEVELOPMENT OF THE NOTOCHORD

During embryonic stage 7, at days 16 and 17 of development, some of the mesoblastic cells migrate in the midline rostral to Hensen's node between the ectoderm and entoderm all the way to the prochordal plate

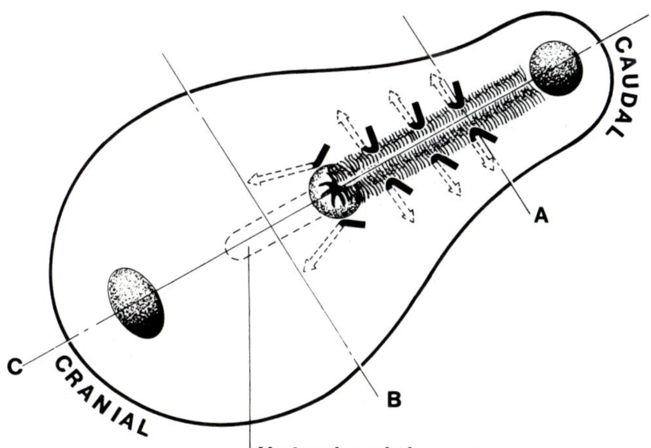

FIG. 17.4. Embryonic stage 7 (16 to 17 days) showing the cells of the epiblast moving into the primitive groove to form the mesoblast laterally and cranially. Cells passing rostrally in the midline between epiblast and hypoblast from Hensen's node form the notochordal process around which the future vertebral column will organize.

to create the rod-like notochordal process around which the skull base and vertebral column ultimately form (Fig. 17.4). The intraembryonic mesoderm that is originating simultaneously from the primitive streak cannot cross the midline but extends to the left or right sides of the midline and will eventually condense alongside the midline notochordal process. The development of the notochord itself extends through several of the later embryonic stages in concert with developments of the overlying neuroectoderm to be discussed later.

Initially, the notochordal process is a solid core of cells until an extension of the primitive pit at Hensen's node burrows into the notochordal process, converting it into a hollow cylinder of cells surrounding a central cavity called the notochordal canal (Fig. 17.5*A–C*). A complex

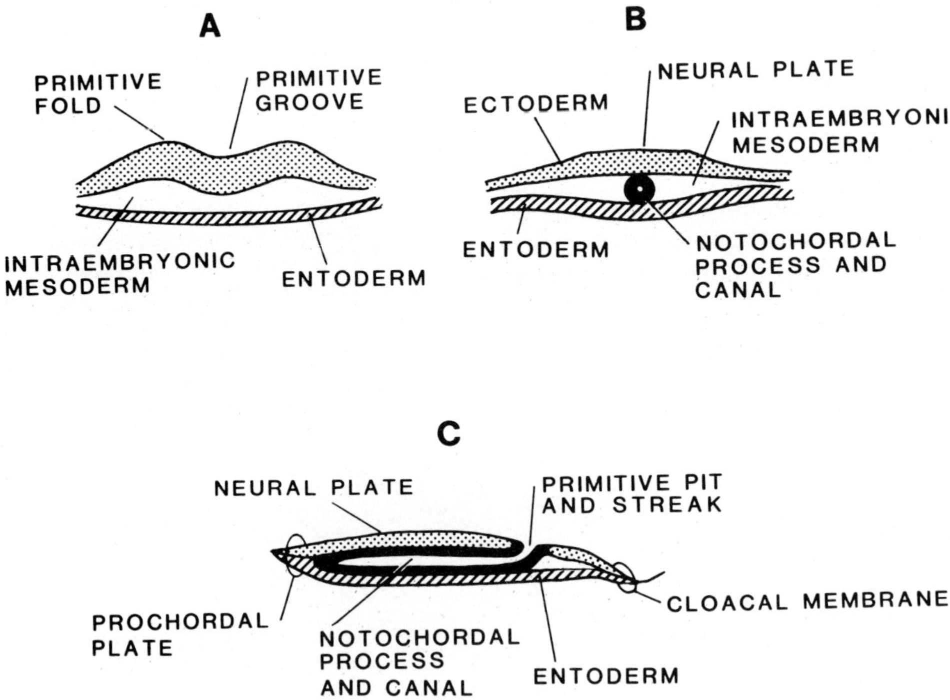

FIG. 17.5. Cross-sections through the embryonic disc sketched in Figure 17.4 at *A*, *B*, and *C*. (*A*) Section through the primitive streak showing the elevated primitive folds and central groove and the middle layer, the intraembryonic mesoderm, created during gastrulation. (*B*) Section through the notochordal process showing the central notochordal canal and early induction of the overlying ectoderm to form the neural plate. The notochordal process is in contact with both the ectoderm and the entoderm. (*C*) Longitudinal section reveals the hollow notochordal process now extending up to the rostral area of fusion in the bilaminar embryo, the prochordal plate.

series of steps now occurs to form the notochord itself, and several embryological anomalies of importance to the neurosurgeon are attributed to aberrations in this sequence. The hollow notochordal process fuses to the adjacent entoderm ventrally, and the two cellular layers degenerate along the length of the fusion (Fig. 17.6*A* and *B*). The notochordal canal then opens into the yolk sac, and the cells of the notochordal process form a longitudinally grooved notochordal plate in the roof of the yolk sac. This process is called intercalation of the notochord into the entoderm. At the caudal end of the notochordal plate, where the primitive pit first extended into the notochordal process as the notochordal canal, a communication called the neurenteric canal now extends directly through the dorsoventral thickness of the embryo. Temporarily, the amniotic cavity is in communication with the yolk sac.

Subsequently, the cranial end of the notochordal plate infolds to form a solid cord of cells called the notochord, and the process of infolding or excalation of the notochord proceeds to the Hensen node level (Fig. 17.7*A–C*). As the notochord reforms, the entoderm once again becomes a continuous layer ventrally, and the neurenteric canal ceases to exist. The notochord is the structure around which the mesoderm condenses to form the vertebral column, with the only remnants of the notochord in the adult represented by the nucleus pulposis of the intervertebral disc. However, in the early stages the notochord induces the overlying ectoderm to form the neural plate from which the CNS forms.

The processes of intercalation and excalation of the notochord from

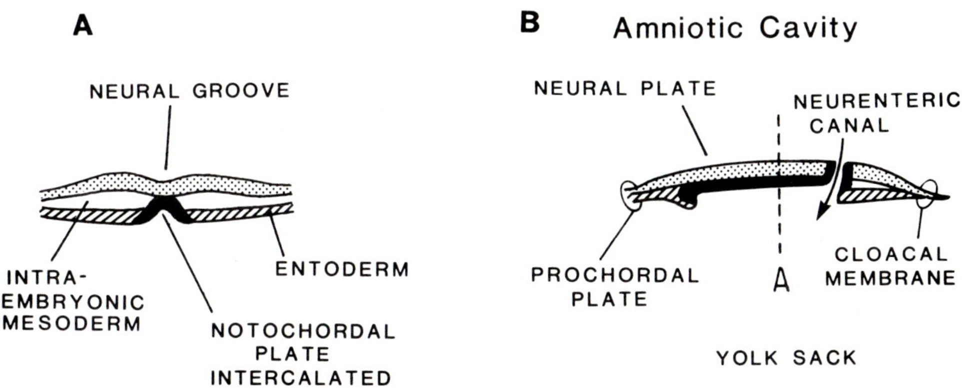

FIG. 17.6. Embryonic stage 7 (16–17 days). (*A*) Intercalation of notochordal process into the yolk sac roof has occurred along its entire length shown in cross-section. (*B*) Longitudinal section along the intercalated notochordal process shows that the amniotic cavity is in communication with the yolk sac through the neurenteric canal at the site of Hensen's node.

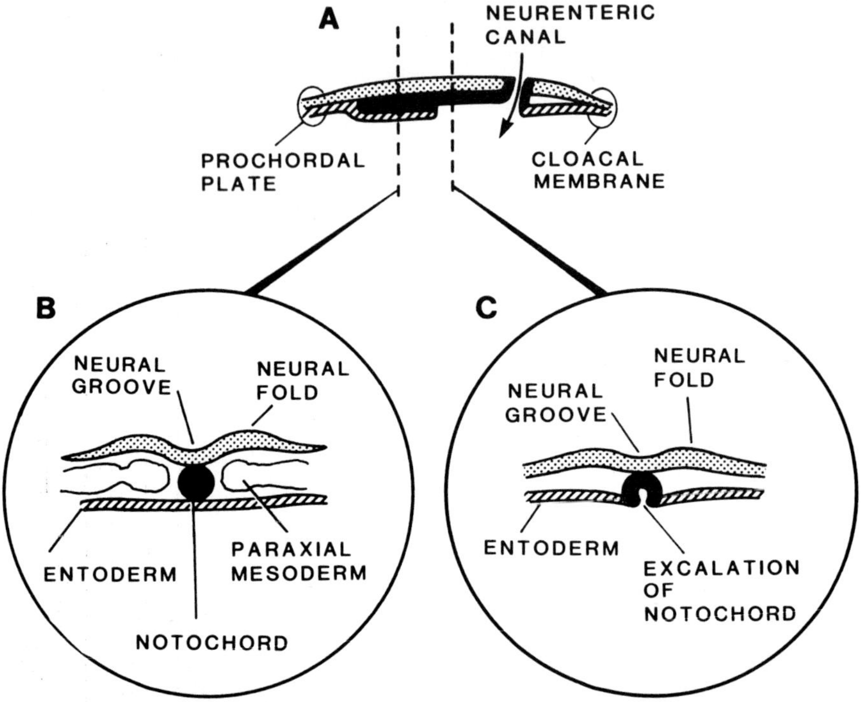

FIG. 17.7. (*A*) A longitudinal section shows that excalation of the notochordal plate begins rostrally. As the notochord tissue fuses, the entoderm becomes a continuous layer ventrally. (*B*) Cross-section shows that the notochord is now a solid cylinder of cells. (*C*) Cross-section shows that the process of excalation is by an infolding of the notochordal process which draws the entoderm towards the midline. The neurenteric canal is obliterated at the end of the process of excalation. By this stage the neural plate is beginning to form the heaped-up lateral edges, the neural folds, and a longitudinal central depression, the neural groove.

the entoderm are the likely stages at which three of the forms of occult spinal dysraphism may develop: the neurenteric cyst, diastematomyelia with septum, and combined anterior and posterior spina bifida. All of these anomalies may result from aberrations in notochord-entoderm-neurenteric canal-neural tube development (6–8, 20, 34, 48).

Formation of the Neural Tube

The neural tube is the primordium of the entire CNS and forms by a process called neurulation during embryonic stages 8–12 at gestational ages from 18 to 27 days. It is during these developmental stages or soon afterwards that the most severe and most frequent open forms of cranial and spinal dysraphism occur. In the later stages of embryonic development, the processes by which the caudal neural tube (canalization) and the filum terminale and cauda equina (regression) form take place. Aberrations during these processes contribute to some of the types of occult spinal dysraphism such as lumbosacral lipoma, lipomyelomeningocele, and the tethered cord syndrome.

NEURULATION

The ectoderm which overlies the notochordal process rostral to Hensen's node begins to thicken in response to the notochordal tissue and the adjacent mesoderm to form the neural plate. A longitudinal central depression called the neural groove develops along the neural plate as the edges of the plate heap up to form the neural folds (Fig. 17.8*A*). The neural folds in the cephalic region are always larger and anticipate the location of the future brain. The middorsal region of the embryo, which corresponds to the area of the future upper cervical spinal cord, is relatively precocious. The earliest developmental advances occur here and precede similar progress in the neural plate and adjacent tissues in the caudal regions.

While the notochord and the neural plate are developing, the paraxial mesoderm on either side of the notochord is thickening to form bilateral paramedian longitudinal mesodermal rods. Condensations of cells occur within the mesodermal rods to create the paired segments of mesoderm called somites which first develop during stage 9 (days 20 and 21) at the future level of the occipital bone just short of the rostral end of the notochord. Subsequent pairs form in a rostral-caudal sequence until about 30 to 35 pairs are formed by day 30. The maximum number of somite pairs is debatable but as many as 42–44 pairs may be formed as follows: occipital 4, cervical 8, thoracic 12, lumbar 5, sacral 5, and sacrococcygeal 8–10. The first occipital and caudal 5–7 coccygeal pairs regress (35).

At stage 10 (days 22–23), the neural groove deepens, and the neural folds meet in the dorsal midline to first form the neural tube (Fig. 17.8*B*, *C*, and *D*). First closure occurs at the level of the third or fourth somites and then extends cephalically and caudally simultaneously. By the end of stage 10 the neural tube has formed from the otic plate region of the rhombencephalon through the future cervical spinal cord to the level of the 12th somite which is the caudal-most somite formed in stage 10. Hereafter, caudal neural tube closure keeps pace with the level of the most distal somite formed in each embryonic stage (Fig. 17.9).

The ectoderm that is continuous lateral to the neural folds is destined to form the epidermis. As the folds close in the midline, the cutaneous

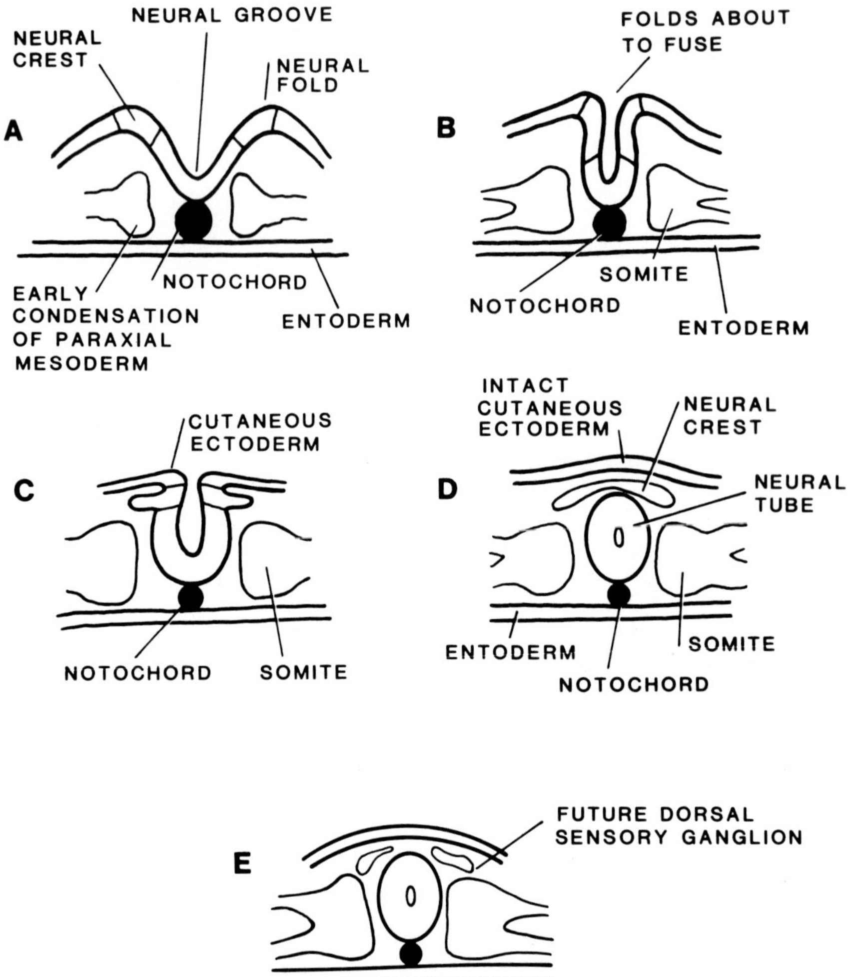

FIG. 17.8. Embryonic stages 8–12 (18–27 days) in cross-section show the process of neurulation which transforms the neural plate into a neural tube buried beneath the continuous layer of cutaneous ectoderm (*A–E*). The paraxial mesoderm condenses to form paired segmental blocks called somites from which the vertebral bodies will form. If the embryo were sectioned along its length in the early stages of neurulation, all of these steps could be seen in one embryo, with the advanced step *E* in the cervicomedullary area.

ectoderm is similarly drawn medially and fuses along the midline (Fig. 17.8*C* and *D*). Shortly thereafter, the cutaneous ectoderm separates from the neural tube and, ultimately, mesoderm interposes itself to form dermal appendages, muscle and skeletal structures. Abnormal persistent adhesion of the cutaneous ectoderm to the neural tube has been impli-

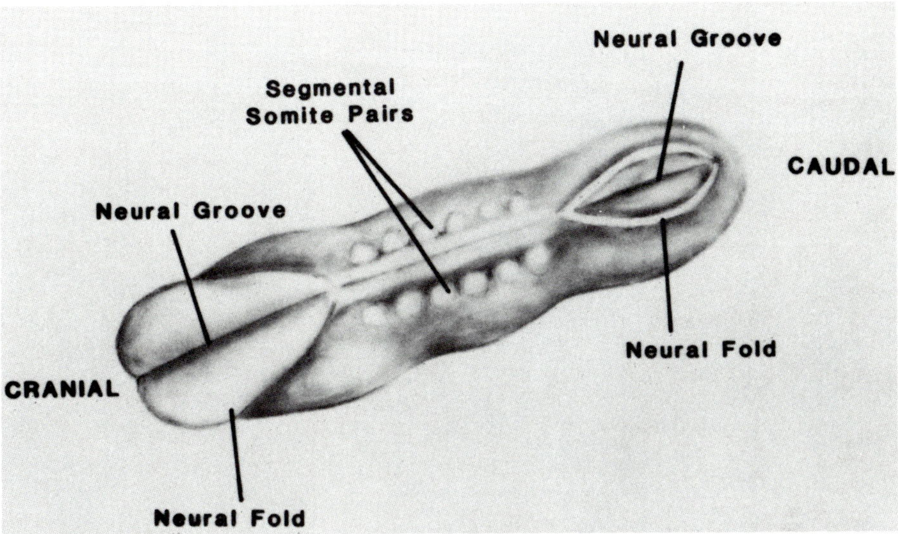

FIG. 17.9. Embryonic stage 10 (days 22–23) in dorsolateral view, showing the closed neural tube and 6 somite pairs and open neural groove cranially and caudally. Thus, cross-sections at various levels at this stage could show all stages of neurulation seen in Figure 17.8. Neural tube closure caudally keeps pace with somite formation from stage 11 on. Caudal to the posterior neuropore is the undifferentiated caudal cell mass of the primitive streak, extending into the future tail fold.

cated in the creation of congenital dermal sinuses and the intraspinal inclusion tumors of the epidermoid and dermoid varieties.

During stage 11 (days 24 and 25) the future thoracic spinal cord forms caudally while cephalically the neural tube completes its closure at the rostral opening, the anterior neuropore, at the level of the future lamina terminalis. Finally, during stage 12 (days 26 and 27), the caudal aspect of the neural tube closes at the level of the posterior neuropore which is at the level of the spinal cord segments L1 or L2 with a range of error of two segments above or below (T11 to L4) (29). In other words, the process of neurulation only accounts for the lumbar spinal cord segments, and the more caudal cord develops by a different process called canalization. Cutaneous ectoderm completely covers the neural tube by the end of neurulation.

CANALIZATION OF THE TAILBUD

The process of formation of the neural tube caudal to that formed by neurulation occupies embryonic stages 13 through 20 (days 28 to 48) (22, 29). Caudal to the posterior neuropore is the undifferentiated caudal cell mass of the primitive streak extending into the tail fold (Fig. 17.10).

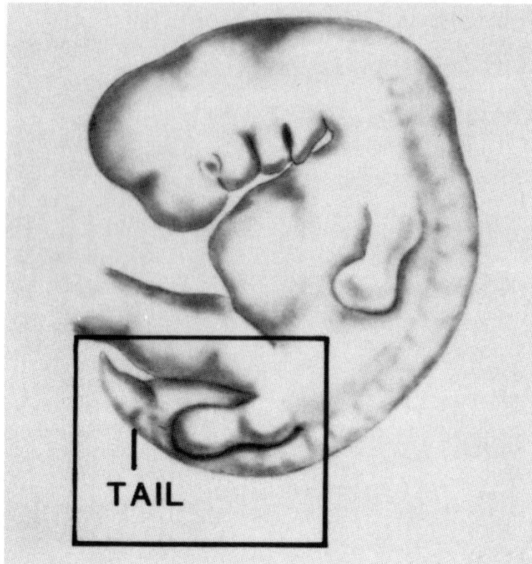

FIG. 17.10. Embryonic stage 15 (34–36 days), showing formation of the tail process within which neural tube formation is by the process of canalization.

Under an intact covering of cutaneous ectoderm, the caudal cell mass develops vacuoles around which the cells assume a neural appearance. Subsequently, the vacuoles coalesce to form the neural tube, which then fuses with the rostral neural tube formed by neurulation (Fig. 17.11*A*–*C*). The ventriculus terminalis, which marks the level of the future conus medullaris, becomes identifiable during stages 18–20 (days 43–48). The process of canalization is less precise than that of neurulation, with abnormalities such as central canal forking or duplication in the region of the conus medullaris, ventriculus terminalis, and filum terminale quite common (27, 28, 31). Forms of occult spinal dysraphism such as the lumbosacral lipoma and lipomyelomeningocele likely have their origin during the process of canalization of the tail bud.

REGRESSION

The processes by which the filum terminale and cauda equina are formed from that portion of the neural tube formed by canalization and by which the conus medullaris eventually comes to lie at its adult level opposite the L1-L2 intervertebral disc space is termed regression or retrogressive differentiation (26, 50). These processes begin as early as embryonic stages 18–20 (days 43–48) and extend throughout the fetal period and on into the the early postnatal period (Fig. 17.12). The ventriculus terminalis is a localized dilatation of the central canal in the conus medullaris and can be identified in stages 18–20, at which time it

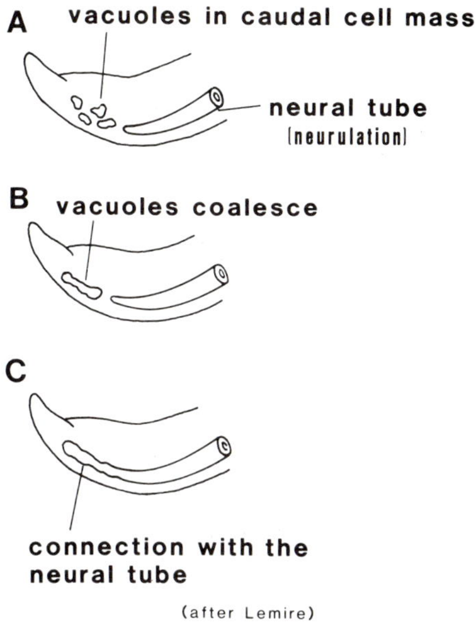

FIG. 17.11. Process of canalization of the tail bud may form the neural tube caudal to the midlumbar area between days 28 and 48 by vacuolization (*A*), coalescence (*B*) and fusion of the distal neural tube to the proximal neural tube formed by neurulation (*C*). (Reproduced with permission from R. J. Lemire *et al.* (29).)

lies opposite the level of the developing 32nd vertebra or coccygeal two level. In other words, in the early developmental stages, the spinal cord and the vertebral body levels correspond segment for segment. As the process of regression begins, an epidermal cell rest known as the coccygeal medullary vestige remains at the level of the tip of the coccygeal vertebral segments. Between this and the ventriculus terminalis, the caudal neural tube regresses and forms the fibrous band called the filum terminale, first identifiable during embryonic stage 23 (day 52). After approximately 9 weeks of development, the ventriculus terminalis "ascends" within the spinal canal by the simultaneous occurrences of regression and of disproportionate growth of the vertebral column relative to the neural tube. Rapid ascent occurs between 9 and 18 weeks of development, at which time the conus may have reached the L4 vertebral body level (Fig. 17.13). Thereafter, ascent slows such that the conus is at the L3 vertebral level by birth and at the adult level by as early as 2 months postnatal development (2). Of course, the spinal nerve roots, which early on in development exit directly opposite their segmental spinal cord level of origin, become elongated as the conus "ascends," thus creating the cauda equina.

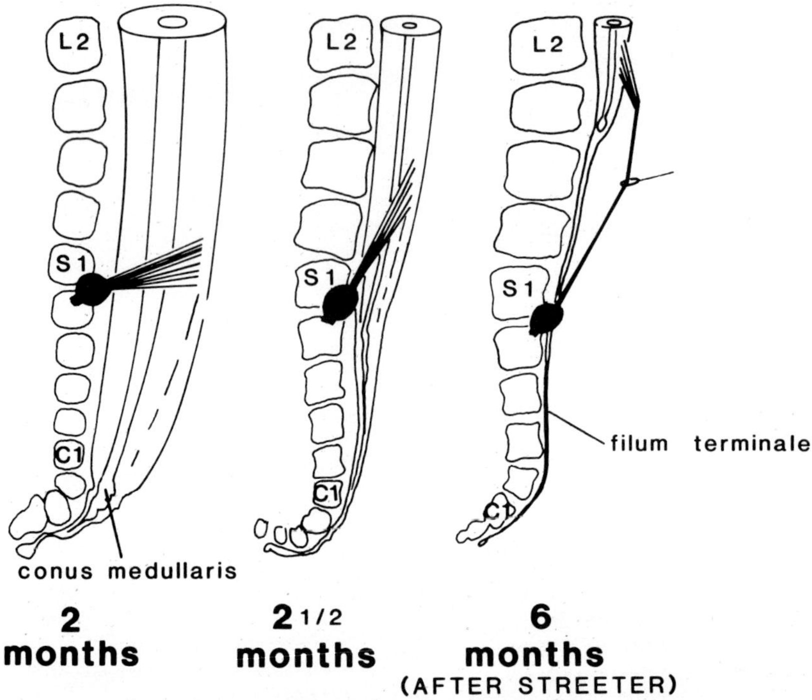

FIG. 17.12. The relationship of the caudal neural tube and the vertebral column during the 8th–25th weeks of development shows the conus medullaris "ascending" by a combination of regression and disproportionate elongation of the vertebral column. The cauda equina and filum terminale are formed as a result (Adapted from G. L. Streeter (50).)

Abnormalities of the process of regression may account for the form of occult spinal dysraphism known as the tethered cord syndrome due to a thick filum terminale or to bands and adhesions. Also, any of the processes which prevent the normal separation of neuroectodermal structures from those structures derived from the mesoderm or cutaneous ectoderm may prevent or impair ascent of the conus and so may tether the developing spinal cord at an abnormally low level early in development.

Formation of the Brain with Particular Reference to the Cerebellum

The reader is referred to specialized texts concerning the complex develoment of the brain, but a cursory review of the early development of the cephalic neural tube and cerebellum is important to an understanding of the so-called Arnold-Chiari malformation (ACM) occurring in association with the open forms of spinal dysraphism (29, 35).

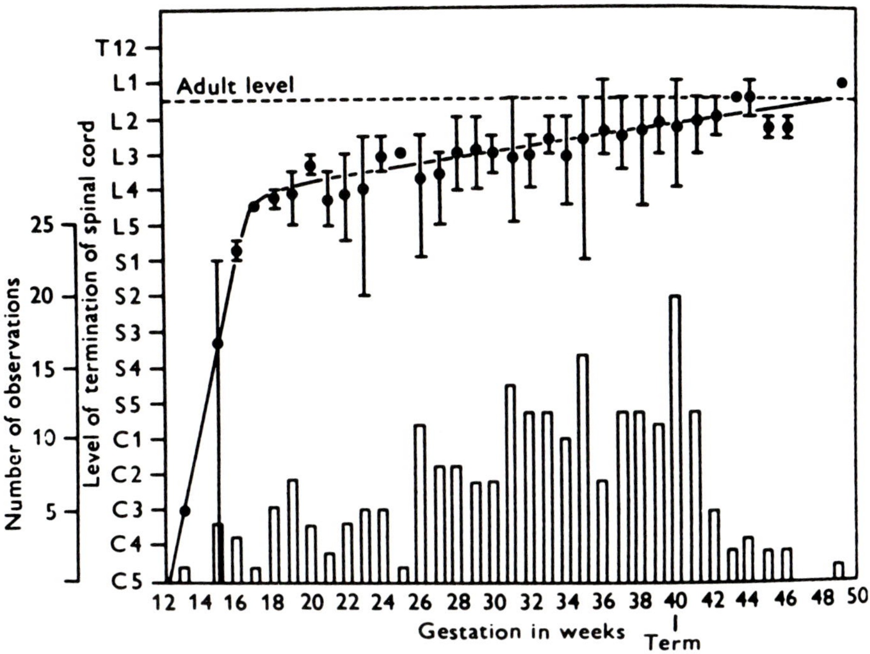

FIG. 17.13. The vertebral level of the conus medullaris in the human rapidly "ascends" between 12 and 18 weeks of development and more slowly thereafter. The conus reaches the adult level of L1–L2 2 months after birth on the average. (Reproduced with permission from A. J. Barson (2).)

EARLY FORMATION OF THE BRAIN

By embryonic stage 10 (days 22 and 23), the cephalic neural folds develop two constrictions which divide the area into the prosencephalon (forebrain), mesencephalon (midbrain), and rhombencephalon (hindbrain). The divisions become more prominent as the anterior neuropore closes at approximately day 25. In embryonic stage 12 (days 26 and 27) the major brain segments are clearly demarcated and the ventricular cavities are continuous with the central canal of the spinal cord. The embryo begins to develop a convex dosal curve to assume the eventual shape of the letter "C" by a process of flexion. The first to form is the cephalic flexure between the prosencephalon and mesencephalon, and in the following stage, the cervical flexure forms between the rhombencephalon and the spinal cord. In that same stage the ventral rhombencephalon bulges at the site of the developing pontine flexure which is convex ventrally in contrast to the two prior flexures.

EARLY FORMATION OF THE CEREBELLUM

The ventrally convex pontine flexure of the rhombencephon is established at the future level of the trigeminal nerve during embryonic stages 13–16 (days 28–39). The pons and cerebellum form from the apex and rostral limb of the flexed rhombencephon while the caudal limb forms the medulla oblongata. The pontine flexure likely forms because of some intrinsic differential growth within the rhombencephon and is quite different in formation from the earlier two flexures. Somewhat akin to bending a hollow rubber tube acutely, the concave dorsal surface buckles laterally, carrying the alar plates laterally with it and making the lumen of the rhombencephaon the widest portion of the neural tube. The cavity destined to become the fourth ventricle becomes rhomboidal or diamond-shaped due to the buckling. Also, the rhombic roof is attenuated and transversely creased during the buckling phenomenon. Within this transverse crease, called the plica choroidea, the choroid plexus eventually forms with the lateral edges of the crease corresponding to the foramina of Luschka. The cerebellum will develop rostral to the transverse crease with a portion of the rhombic roof called the area membranacea superior (AMS) separating the developing cerebellum from the developing choroid plexus. The AMS eventually forms the posterior medullary velum. The rostral rhombic roof is more active histologically than the inert-looking caudal rhombic roof or area membranacea inferior (AMI). The caudal roof extends from the plica to the cervical spinal cord and eventually attenuates to form the midline foramen of Magendie.

The cells in the laterally lying alar plates rostral to the AMI proliferate extensively during stages 15–17 (days 34–42) to form the thickened paired rhombic lips that are the precursors of the cerebellum and which ultimately fuse in the midline at approximately 8 weeks of development. The most primitive portions of the cerebellum, the flocculus and nodulus, form the earliest at the level of the vestibular nuclei. The cerebellum lies within the cavity of the rhombencephalon (the fourth ventricle) during the first 2 months of development, but during the 3rd month at a CR length of 40–90 mm, it enlarges rapidly and begins to bulge extraventricularly. The early linear structure of the cerebellum, viewed in a sagittal plane alters as the central portions undergo rapid proliferation and the cerebellum mushrooms dorsally. The relative inactivity of the roof of the IVth ventricle ventral to the rapidly enlarging cerebellar vermian lobules causes the roof to buckle in a fashion similar to that of a kernel of popcorn exploding and inverting a part of its shell (29). As a result, the nodulus of the vermis, the posterior medullary velum, and the adjacent choroid plexus become tucked in and hidden from view under and between the cerebellar tonsils by approximately 3½ months of development. The inactive portion of the rhombic roof caudal to the choroid plexus, the AMI, which forms the foramen of Magendie also becomes hidden from view by the cerebellar tonsils.

FORMATION OF THE CHOROID PLEXUS AND CEREBROSPINAL FLUID FLOW

Choroid plexus first appears in the fourth ventricle during embryonic stage 18 (days 43 and 44), in the lateral ventricles during stage 19 (days 45 and 46), and in the third ventricle in stage 21 (days 48.5 and 49). The relationship of the developing choroid plexus and the perforation of the rhombic roof to form the foramen of Magendie are important to a critical evaluation of the hydrodynamic theory of Gardner (21). The rhombencephalic roof protrudes from the dorsal surface of the embryo and becomes attenuated during stages 13 and 14. However, the caudal rhombencephalic roof or the AMI, does not perforate to form the foramen of Magendie until approximately stage 20 (days 47 and 48) or even until 8 or 9 weeks of development (10, 39). In this same stage the choroid plexus cells develop the appearance of secretory epithelium and first produce extraventricular CSF which helps to open up the loose meshwork of mesenchymal cells surrounding the brain to create the subarachnoid space. The opening up process begins in the cisterna magna and spreads to other basal areas and then over the hemispheres and spinal cord. Which comes first, perforation or CSF formation, is the crux of the argument. Brocklehurst's histological studies of the roof of the fourth ventricle suggest that perforation of the caudal roof is due to active differentiation occurring prior to the ability of the choroid plexus to form CSF rather than a bursting of the roof in response to an increase in the intraventricular CSF pressure (10).

The central canal of the spinal cord is obliterated normally after birth by the cellular proliferation within the cord, and thus the ventricular system terminates at the obex. The disturbed embryology of the caudal cerebellum in the ACM frequently alters this normal course of events such that the central canal remains patent and enlarged to the point of symptomatic hydromyelia developing on occasion.

Formation of the Vertebrae

The vertebral unit is composed of a vertebral body and posterior elements (pedicles, transverse processes, laminae, and spinous process) and is separated from the other units by the intervertebral discs. Cells originating from the medial portion of the somites form the vertebral units in three stages: a period of membrane formation from stages 11 to 16 (days 22–39), the period of cartilage formation from stages 17 to 23 and on into the early fetal period (days 40–64); and the period of bone formation which overlaps the later portions of the period of cartilage formation and carries on throughout the fetal period to well beyond birth. The notochord is an important influence on the formation of the vertebral bodies, and the neural tube appears to direct formation of the posterior elements (4).

PERIOD OF MEMBRANE FORMATION

The notochord, which is in contact with the neuroectoderm above and the entoderm below in stages 10 and 11 (days 22–25), is flanked by the somites. Each somite is divided into a medial half, the sclerotome, which ultimately forms the vertebral structures and a lateral half, the myotome, which develops into the supporting musculature. Cells from the sclerotome portion migrate medially to form a perichordal tube after the notochord separates from the neural tube and the entoderm. This process occurs first in the cervical segments and then proceeds rostrally and caudally. The vertebral bodies will ultimately form from the perichordal tube of mesoderm, and other sclerotomic cells migrate dorsally to eventually surround the neural tube to form the posterior elements.

PERIOD OF CARTILAGE FORMATION

The vertebral body which does form is not from the segmental somites at its level; rather, the segmental arrangement is altered. The sclerotome cells which condense around the notochord to outline a vertebral body originate from adjacent sclerotome pairs. Cells from the caudal half of the sclerotome above condense with cells from the rostral half of the sclerotome below. Thus, each vertebral body is composed of portions of 4 somites. Later on the intervening sclerotome cells form the anulus fibrosis of the intervertebral disc, and the notochord persists as the nucleus pulposus. The notochord within the future vertebral body regresses.

Chondrification begins in the vertebral body first and later in a separate center in each neural arch. The centra and arches are chondrified by 47 days of development, but the arches are incomplete dorsal to the neural tube. Arch closure is progressive, and by 64 days the arches are complete in the thoracic and upper lumbar regions but remain open in the upper cervical and lower lumbar areas. These are common sites for failure to close completely, leaving a simple spina bifida.

PERIOD OF BONE FORMATION

Endochondral ossification centers develop in the centra and in each of the neural arch processes and the costal processes. The neural arch processes extend dorsally and medially to form the laminae, and with fusion and further dorsal prolongation, the spinous process is formed. The ventral extension of each arch fuses with the vertebral body; the lateral extension forms the transverse process with which the rib articulates. The shafts of the ribs are formed by extension of their primary ossification centers. Thus, any process that interferes with development and growth of the vertebral unit may be associated with malformations such as aplasia or fusion of one or more ribs, hemivertebrae, fused vertebrae, or anterior or posterior spina bifida.

The formation of the sacrococcygeal vertebrae deserves special attention. As already mentioned, a maximum of 42–44 somite pairs may be formed, with the caudal 7 to 8 pairs formed in the embryonic tail. The neural tube extends to the level of the most distal somite pair and even beyond, into the tip of the so-called nonvertebrated tail which does not contain somites. The period of regression which must involve the caudal neural tube also involves these terminal somites. The sacrum is formed at somite levels 25 through 29, and the coccygeal segments usually consume the 30th to 35th pairs, and all the remaining somite pairs have regressed by the end of stage 17 (42 days).

Formation of the Skull

The skull, or neurocranium, is subdivided into two sections. The skull base (occipital, sphenoid, ethmoid, and petrous temporal bones), which is formed by endochondral ossification, and the cranial vault, which is formed by the membranous process. The latter process does not involve a cartilaginous phase. A brief review of the formation of the skull base is pertinent to one of the theories for the origin of the ACM proposed by the Marin-Padillas (33).

The notochord separates from the neural tube in the cervical and cranial areas during stage 12 (days 26–27) and subsequent prechordal and parachordal mesodermal condensations form nearly all of the major bones of the skull base. The rostral tip of the notochord marks the junction between the occipital bone and the sphenoid bone. The first chondrification begins during stage 17 (40–44 days) in the basiocciput and the body of the sphenoid.

The occipital bone has four endochondral ossification centers which create the clivus, the occipital arch around the foramen magnum, and the supraoccipital part of the occipital bone, which is that portion below the inion and the superior nuchal line. The occipital bone above the superior nuchal line is termed the interparietal occipital bone, and it is formed by the membranous process, as are all of the bones of the cranial vault. These two portions of the occipital bone unite in approximately the 3rd month.

The other three bones of the skull base are: the sphenoid bone; the ethmoid bone, including the crista galli, cribriform plate, ethmoidal labyrinth, and the cartilaginous nasal septum; and the petrous portion of the temporal bone. The endochondral skull base appears to have its own intrinsic growth potential and, in contrast to the passive intramembranous bone of the cranial vault, is subject to abnormal osseous development independent of the influence of the overlying neural structures. This is particularly true of the bones around the foramen magnum which are malformed in occipitoatlantal fusion, platybasia, and basilar impression.

SPINA BIFIDA APERTA AND THE ARNOLD-CHIARI MALFORMATION

Spina Bifida Aperta

The subtypes of spina bifida aperta (SBA) listed in Table 17.1 refer to those open forms of spinal dysraphism most familiar to neurosurgeons (20). The anatomy of the open defect fits well with a process disordering the normal development already described. At the open area the neural malformation is exposed on the surface and, obviously, the other tissue layers that were to close in the midline over neural tissue are separated. The skin is deficient but is in continuity with the edge of the neural plaque through an intervening layer of modified epithelium and arachnoid called the zona epitheliosa. The dura is splayed widely open with its lateral margins ballooned over the edges of the spina bifida. It lies gently adherent to the underlying fascia covering the paraspinous muscles and fuses laterally to the edge of the skin defect. The spina bifida varies in its extent, depending on whether the posterior elements of the T12-L1 level are normally formed. If T12 and L1 are involved, the entire lumbar and sacral spine is also bifid, regardless of the level of the neurocutaneous lesion; if the T12 and L1 posterior elements are normal, the posterior spina bifida may be localized to the lumbar or to the sacral spine and correlates closely with the level of the neurocutaneous malformation (3). As a consequence of the time during embryological development that the neural defect forms, the spinal cord is always abnormally low in myelomeningocele and is tethered to a degree to the surrounding tissues.

The subtypes show fascinating clinical and pathological variations which should be explained by any theory of abnormal embryology (16).

In myeloschisis the neural tube at the site of the defect is totally open with no evidence for the central canal having been formed. It is commonly found at the thoracolumbar junction and is associated with a posterior spina bifida of the entire lumbar and sacral spines.

In myelomeningocele and hemimyelomeningocele, a central canal has been formed, although it may be partially open to a variable degree on the dorsal surface of the neural plaque. These forms seem to be more commonly found in the lumbar and sacral regions in contrast to a myeloschisis. The hemimyelomeningocele is a special variation which involves a diastematomyelia with septum. One hemicord is found in its own bony spinal canal and, usually, the ipsilateral lower limb has a better level of function than the limb supplied by the adjacent hemicord, which is exposed on the surface as a "hemimyelomeningocele."

The hydrosyringomyelomeningocele is a rare form usually found in the cervical or thoracic areas and often misinterpreted as a meningocele because the patient's neurological function is usually normal. The malformation appears to be a herniation of a dilated central canal and dysplastic neural tissue between the dorsal columns of a fused spinal cord through a localized posterior spina bifida. The dysplastic neural tissue in the wall of the sac differentiates this lesion from a benign meningocele.

Spinal meningocele is unfortunately rare. This form, by definition, means the patient is neurologically normal, and it usually involves only an outpouching of the meninges, with a normally formed spinal cord located safely within the spinal canal. This is not to say that nerve roots cannot be adherent to the neck of the meningeal sac and cannot be endangered by cavalier dissection or that the spinal cord is not tethered abnormally low by intraspinal anomalies, but at least at birth, the neural structures function normally. Also, the incidence of the ACM and of hydrocephalus is much less than in the complex forms.

Any theory offered to explain the formation of these forms of SBA should also explain frequently found associated malformations such as the ACM (to be discussed in more detail later), diastematomyelia (without septum) found above the plaque in approximately one-quarter of cases, and hydrosyringomyelia of the proximal cord in 43% of cases. Other minor malformations are frequently found as well (20).

The Arnold-Chiari Malformation

Whether the eponym "Arnold-Chiari" is applied properly to this malformation in an historical sense has been debated. The term has been used in the clinical setting for years, although some authors refer to this malformation occurring in 90% of all infants with SBA as the Chiari Type II anomaly (13, 20). In any event the essence of the anomaly is a caudal displacement of a prolongation of the inferior cerebellar vermis and IVth ventricle into the upper cervical spinal canal, an associated caudal displacement or prolongation of the cervicomedullary junction often kinked dorsally over the upper cervical spinal cord, a cephalad course of the upper cervical nerve roots, and the frequent occurrence of hydrosyringomyelia and hydrocephalus as well as other anatomical variations listed in Table 17.3 (20). However, in infants with SBA, there is

TABLE 17.3

Anomalies Associated with the Arnold-Chiari Malformation

Structure	Anomaly
Cerebellum	Caudal displacement of vermis and fourth ventricle; cerebellum smaller than normal
Brain stem	Caudal displacement of pons, medulla, and cervicomedullary junction with kink; displaced basilar and vertebral arteries; stretching of lower cranial nerves
Cervical and lower spinal cord	Compression of upper segments; hydromyelia or hydrosyringomyelia
Midbrain	Tectal "beak"; aqueduct stenosis or forking
Cerebral hemisphere and third ventricle	Polymicrogyria; cortical heterotopia; enlarged massa intermedia; Meynert's commissure; hydrocephalus
Meninges	Hypoplasia of falx cerebri; low set tentorium with enlarged incisura; low set and large venous sinuses in dura of foramen magnum; thickened, obliterative leptomeninges at level of foramen magnum
Skull and cervical spine	Craniolacunia; enlarged foramen magnum; small posterior fossa, scalloped petrous bone; enlarged upper cervical spinal canal

a gradation of the severity of the anatomical abnormalities that is described well by Emery and MacKenzie (18), but the degree of severity does not correlate directly with the anatomical level of the spinal lesion. A number of the more minor degrees of ACM occur with the caudal lumbar or sacral myelomeningocele. The influence of the hydrodynamic effects of hydrocephalus may modify some of the features of the malformation, including the degree of caudal displacement of the brain stem and cerebellum, the molding of the collicular plate, the shape and size of the aqueduct, the presence of the cerebellar "tower," and the development of hydrosyringomyelia.

Embryological Timing of Development of SBA and ACM

The anatomical and pathological variations in SBA and ACM imply that the causative multifactorial teratogenic events may occur at any time from near the end of neurulation at 28 days to some period after neurulation to cause the less complex anomalies such as the spinal meningocele. In general, the earlier the event occurs during the development of the nervous system, the higher the neuroanatomical level of the spinal lesion and the more severe are the associated anomalies. For example, an insult occurring just prior to or just after closure of the posterior neuropore at 28 days is likely to cause a myeloschisis at the thoracolumbar junction, a posterior spina bifida of the entire lumbosacral and sacral spines and, likely, a more severe degree of the ACM and other brain anomalies. This latter assumption has yet to be pathologically proven, although clinical experience suggests the higher the spinal lesion, the greater is the incidence of hydrocephalus and the lower the intellectual achievements. In contrast, an insult occurring after closure of the posterior neuropore is associated with a lower lumbar or sacral myelomeningocele in which the spinal cord has developed through the neural tube stage by neurulation or by canalization, the posterior spina bifida may be localized, and the spinal cord may be formed normally below the level of the open lesion in occasional cases. Clinical experience indicates that the frequency of hydrocephalus and ACM is less in the lower lesions and that intellectual development may be normal. Indeed, in spinal meningocele, the neural tube development is virtually normal, and the meningeal, posterior elements, and skin are the main participants in the lesion.

The pathological material studied in SBA would suggest that the spinal lesion may develop just before or just after neurulation and may create a myeloschisis at a higher level, or it may involve the lower regions of the spine where the neural tube has formed, either by neurulation or canalization, and where myelomeningocele is created. Such a lower lesion could form early in the 2nd month of development if these observations are valid.

The embryological timing of the occurrence of the ACM is not clear. The terms prolongation and displacement and herniation are used interchangeably to describe the caudal location of the cerebellar vermis and brain stem, as compared to those of normal individuals. Prolongation implies that the structures are abnormally lengthened and are, thereby, in an abnormal location; displacement or herniation implies some active process forcing the structures into their abnormal location. Both factors, a primary embryological malformation and a secondary active displacement may, in fact, play a part in the evolution of the malformation. For example, the choroid plexus of the fourth ventricle is frequently found external to the ventricle and matted over the cervicomedullary junction; the anatomical divisions of the vermis are straightened out over the upper cervical cord area, rather than being "tucked-up" within the fourth ventricle; the brain stem does appear to be truly elongated. These anatomical variations could have their origin in the failure of the pontine flexure to form normally during 28–39 days of gestation leading to an elongated brain stem. The normal growth of the midportion of the cerebellum during the 3rd month ultimately leads to the caudal vermis and choroid plexus tucking in under the cerebellar tonsils. A failure of this process could lead to the persistent extraventricular position of the vermis and choroid plexus seen pathologically. Once this anatomical malformation is created, the normal processes of CSF circulation may be disturbed, leading to an embryological hydrocephalus and direction of the fourth ventricular CSF outflow into the central canal since formation of the foramen of Magendie is impaired. A persistent hydromyelia could follow. The hydrocephalus could also cause an increase in the extent of prolongation or herniation of the cerebellar tissues into the upper cervical spine and push the tentorium further inferiorly to decrease the size of the posterior fossa. In other words, a primary embryological malformation could, in itself, lead to secondary hydrodynamic factors important in increasing the severity of the anatomical malformation. The earlier in gestation the causative event acts, the more likely these normal embryological steps are to be disturbed and lead to a higher, anatomically more primitive spinal lesion and an increase in the occurrence of associated malformations. The later in gestation the event occurs, the more likely these critical steps are to be initiated normally, resulting in a lower, more developmentally advanced spinal lesion and a less frequent occurrence and lesser severity of the associated malformations.

THEORIES OF ABNORMAL EMBRYOGENESIS OF SPINA BIFIDA APERTA AND THE ARNOLD-CHIARI MALFORMATION

Unfortunately, no single theory proposed to date satisfactorily explains all of the pathological variations witnessed clinically in SBA or ACM. The theories that have been offered do discuss the mechanisms for the malformations but do not stipulate the cause that initiates that mechanism. This is understandable since the etiology of SBA is multifactorial with both genetic and environmental interactions involved (51). The theories fall into four general groups with one additional theory reserved for the ACM: (a) developmental arrest; (b) the overgrowth hypothesis; (c) the hydrodynamic theory; (d) the theory of neuroschisis; and (e) the outmoded traction theory suggested as a cause of the ACM. Woven into all these theories is the question of whether the spinal defect develops before the neural tube closes or after it has closed and becomes covered with cutaneous ectoderm. The fact that the cutaneous ectoderm is in continuity with the exposed neuroectoderm has been used as proof that the neural tube never closed; however, experimental work suggests that a closed neural tube covered by cutaneous ectoderm can reopen and develop continuity with the edges of the split cutaneous ectoderm (47). The presence of a central canal in many human specimens indicates that neurulation did occur before the neural plaque became exposed, and thus reopening of fused cutaneous ectoderm to expose the neurulated cord must occur in many forms (16). In addition, the sacral myelomeningocele involves spinal cord created by canalization under intact cutaneous ectoderm. Thus, opening of this intact ectoderm layer must occur in the lower lesions.

The Theory of Developmental Arrest

This theory proposes that myeloschisis is a simple failure of the neural plate to close due to an arrest of normal development with subsequent secondary changes in the surrounding tissue (56). However, not all open lesions are in the form of a myeloschisis, and the theory does not explain adequately the neurulated types. Indeed, the occurrence of open lesions at levels of the spinal cord formed by canalization under intact cutaneous ectoderm is not addressed. Such lesions must involve breakdown of the cutaneous layer to expose the neural tissue. Developmental arrest of the brain stem was invoked as a cause of the ACM by Daniel and Strich (15) in 1958 and was expanded later by other authors (17, 44, 45). If the pontine flexure which develops at the level of the pons at stages 13–16 (days 28 to 39) were to fail to form, then the pons and medulla would be abnormally elongated. With straightening of the cervical flexure during the 2nd month, the elongated brain stem could bulge dorsally over the upper cervical cord which is fixed by the dentate ligaments and could thus create the "kink." Failure of the vermis of the cerebellum and the adjacent choroid plexus to become tucked up within the fourth ventricle as a result of the rapid development of the central cerebellum during the 3rd month would create the elongated tail of the caudal vermis and the matted choroid plexus found over the cervicomedullary junction. The caudal displacement of the cerebellum and brain stem cause the foramen magnum to be enlarged and the posterior fossa to be small and permits the tentorium to migrate to an abnormally low position.

While the theory of developmental arrest has been expanded to explain the malformations of the ACM complex, it is deficient in describing all the subtypes of the open spinal lesions, the associated spinal cord anomalies, and the associated cerebral anomalies.

A new theory has been offered by Marin-Padilla and Marin-Padilla (33) in 1981. The explanation for the spinal lesion has yet to be presented in as detailed a fashion as for the ACM, but it does involve the same basic mechanism. A primary mesodermal deficiency is the cause of all of the neural developmental abnormalities.

Their theory for the ACM is an extension from observations in pregnant hamsters treated with vitamin A. A primary paraxial mesodermal insufficiency results in underdevelopment of the occipital bone, particularly the basal portion. As a result, the posterior fossa is short and small and is therefore inadequate to contain the developing cerebellum and brain stem. Also, the skull base is flattened, compared to that of a normal person. The overall consequence is that the cerebellum must grow towards the foramen magnum, the pontine flexure is reduced, and the angle of the cervical flexure is increased. The mesodermal abnormality might affect an embryo before, during, or after closure of the neural folds and thus might explain all varieties of cranial and spinal dysraphism, open and closed. No experimental embryo had displacement of the cerebellum below the foramen magnum because that displacement is attributed to the postnatal growth of the cerebellum or possibly to the development of hydrocephalus.

Several problems exist in applying this experimental model to the human situation as the Marin-Padillas do. The model demonstrates a tendency towards but not the full expression of the ACM; which malformation comes first, neural or mesodermal envelope, is not proven; the ACM has been shown to exist in human embryos as early as at 16–18 weeks of development with and without hydrocephalus (1, 9, 36); and the cerebellum has been shown to be smaller than normal at all postnatal ages in the ACM, suggesting the small posterior fossa may be a secondary phenomenon (53).

The Overgrowth Hypothesis

This theory suggests that an overgrowth of the neural plate prior to neurulation everts the neural folds and prevents their fusion. Thus, an open neural tube lesion in the form of a myeloschisis is created. The theory was proposed in 1881 by Lebedeff from observations in chick embryos and was adopted by Cleland in 1883 to explain some forms of SBA in humans (14). More recently the theory has been associated with observations in human embryos by Patten (41, 42), by Lemire and coworkers (30), and by Osaka *et al.* (36). Debate exists as to whether overgrowth is the primary cause of, or is a secondary reaction to, either the failure of fusion or a reopening of a fused neural tube.

The same objection holds for this theory as for the theory of arrested development. The occurrence of open lesions at levels of the cord formed by canalization under intact cutaneous ectoderm and the occurrence of lesions with a central canal indicating neurulation are not addressed. Such lesions must involve an opening up of the cutaneous layer to expose the neural tube, which may or may not then open as a myeloschisis or remain partially or totally closed.

In 1957 Barry *et al.* (1) reported an increase in the volume of the cerebellum and brain stem in two human fetuses of 17 weeks and 18 weeks of development with evidence for the ACM (1). They noted that the posterior fossa was abnormally small and the tentorium was inferiorly situated. The overgrowth of the cerebral hemispheres was believed responsible for the diminution in the volume of the posterior fossa. They proposed that the too large cerebellum and brain stem in a too small container led to a caudal herniation and kinking. Hydrocephalus was present in only one of the specimens. Thus, overgrowth of the cerebellum and brain stem, along with overgrowth of the cerebrum, was invoked as a cause for the ACM. The fact that the cerebellum is smaller than normal in later life in children with SBA was attributed rather vaguely to changes in differential growth in the second half of gestation.

No other authors studying the problem have assessed the posterior fossa structures as overgrown and certainly not the cerebral hemispheres (9, 19). The cerebellum in infants with the ACM weighs uniformly less than normal at all ages (53). Thus, the overgrowth theory can be abandoned as an explanation for the ACM.

The Hydrodynamic Theory

Although the hydrodynamic theory is associated with W. J. Gardner, many authors have espoused earlier but less expansive theories or alternative hydrodynamic mechanisms (11, 12, 18, 21, 52). Gardner's monograph, *The Dysraphic States*, published in 1973, details the historical development of the hydrodynamic theories through Morgagni and Chiari and his own concept that all dysraphic states can be explained by a series of mechanical steps consequent to the inadequate escape of fluid from the neural tube during the embryonic period or from the subarachnoid space during later development (21). The essential features of the theory depend to a great deal upon the developmental chronology of the rhombencephalic roof, through which communication with the primitive subarachnoid space first occurs. As already mentioned, the rhombencephalic roof is divided by a transverse fissure, the plica choroidea, in which the future choroid plexus develops into a superior and an inferior portion. The AMS develops between the cerebellum above and the plica choroidea below and is destined to thicken to form the posterior medullary velum. The AMI forms between the plica choroidea above and the obex region below and later perforates to form the foramen of Magendie. Initially, the attenuated roof of the rhombencephalon begins to bulge as early as days 28 to 34 soon after the closure of the posterior neuropore presumably due to the accumulation of a proteinaceous material within the neural tube, even before the formation of CSF. After formation of the choroid plexus in the IVth ventricle during days 43 and 44 of development a so-called physiological hydrocephalus and hydromyelia develop, according to Gardner, and the semipermeable membrane of the AMS is the first route of escape for fluid into the primitive subarachnoid space. With subsequent development the AMS thickens, the AMI opens to form the foramen of Magendie, and a defined anatomical communication is created between the IVth ventricle and the subarachnoid space. Early reports suggested that patency is achieved at 12–16 weeks of development but Brockelhurst (9) and Padget (39) have observed open foramina in human embryos as early as 8 or 9 weeks of development. Gardner suggests that either too rapid an accumulation of fluid or too little an escape through the rhombencephalic roof can cause an overdistension of the neural tube to a degree that a rupture can occur at some site. An extensive rupture at the cranial end of the neural tube can cause anencephalus; a rupture at the lower end causes a myeloschisis. Various stages and complexities of rupture can create virtually any of the open or occult dysraphic malformations.

According to Gardner, the ACM forms due to an unequal competition between the pulsating choroid plexus in the IVth ventricle against that of the lateral ventricles. He applies two mechanical theories. The Bering effect attributes the ventricular CSF pulse wave to the arterial pulsation within the choroid plexus; the law of Laplace finds the distending tension (T) in a cylindrical vessel of any given pressure (P) directly proportional to the radius (R) or $T = P \times R$. The choroid plexus of the IVth ventricle forms first at 6 weeks of development but is rapidly exceeded in size by that in the lateral ventricles a few days later. The Bering effect is more pronounced in the lateral ventricles and results in the cerebral hemispheres gradually encroaching posteriorly to cause the migration of the tentorium to its final resting place. In the event of a caudal neural tube rupture for reasons just explained, the Bering effect of the small IVth ventricle choroid plexus is completely dissipated, and the Bering effect of the lateral ventricles is relatively enhanced, producing a marked posterior migration of the tentorium. As a result the posterior fossa is small, and the hindbrain and cerebellum are forced or herniated out of the posterior fossa into the upper cervical spinal canal. The subsequent impairment of CSF circulation by this herniation leads to the hydrocephalus above with further compression on the midbrain perhaps leading to aqueductal stenosis and the usual midbrain tectal malformation.

Gardner's theory has been criticized on several points. Those who believe that myeloschisis forms due to a failure of the neural tube to close dismiss it out of hand. Others point to the fact that fetal myeloschisis has been found even before evidence of choroid plexus formation and have not found embryonic hydrocephalus in young embryos with myeloschisis (1, 30, 36). If CSF production is required to produce the overdistension necessary for rupture of the neural tube, then the theory is deficient. However, Gardner believes that excessive proteinaceous fluid found within the neural tube before choroid plexus formation is sufficient to rupture the tube. Anencephalus or craniorrachischisis are extensive lesions, and one would suspect that the initial point of rupture would decompress the distending forces within the neural tube and limit the extent of the lesion. Even more basic is the belief that the roof plate of the rhombencephalon is burst by the secretory pressure of the CSF in a physiologically distended neural tube. Brocklehurst (10) suggests that a sequential developmental process of the roof plate results in the foramen opening, rather than a mechanistic blowout.

These criticisms of Gardner's theory as the cause of SBA and the ACM should not be interpreted to mean that hydrodynamic mechanisms are not important to the pathological evolution or the clinical manifestations of spinal dysraphism. It is quite clear that active hydrocephalus can contribute to the clinical presentation of the ACM or to hydrosyringomyelia (20).

The Theory of Neuroschisis

Dorcas Padget (37–39) developed a theory of spinal dysraphism that postulates a reopening of the closed neural tube based on observations in monkey and human embryos. A cleft develops in the dorsal midline of the closed neural tube, permitting the proteinaceous material within to escape into the surrounding mesoderm and to elevate the overlying cutaneous ectoderm. Padget likened the elevation to a dermatological blister and named the embryonic lesion a neuroschistic bleb. The future of the bleb varies from total healing to creation of an adhesion between cutaneous and neuroectoderm (congenital dermal sinus) or to rupture through the cutaneous ectoderm to create an open spinal lesion. The edges of the cutaneous ectoderm become fused secondarily to the everted edges of the neural plate, thus converting the lesion into an appearance of the "never closed" neural tube lesion, which fits in with the prevailing theory of a nonclosure. Bleb formation can occur at any level of the neural tube and at any site around the circumference, thus explaining some of the ventral lesions as well as forms of cranial dysraphism.

Padget also explained the ACM as a sequela of the neural cleft, which allows fluid to escape from the neural tube. Embryonic microcephaly results, and the cerebellar primordia prematurely approximate and fuse in a posterior fossa already small. Subsequent development of the cerebellum in the too small posterior fossa leads to herniation into the upper cervical spinal canal. Hydrocephalus follows this obstruction at the IVth ventricular level or is due to aqueduct stenosis caused by the folding and fusion at the level of the midbrain due to microcephaly. Support for the theory of primary embryonic microcephaly with secondary hydrocephalus is provided by the frequent clinical observation that infants with myelomeningocele may have a normal head circumference and marked hydrocephalus. The head becomes microcephalic after successful shunting.

Objections to this theory are few, as it is a relatively recent proposal.

Osaka *et al.* (36) observed neuroschistic lesions in both normal embryos and those with myeloschisis but could not relate the lesions to neural tube defects. They suggested that the neuroschistic lesion could even be an artifact of handling (36).

The Traction Theory in the ACM

The traction theory was described by Penfield and Coburn (46) and suggested that the fixation of the spinal cord to the skin at a low level prevented upward migration of the spinal cord during early development. Thus, the cerebellum and brain stem were pulled down into the cervical spinal canal as the vertebral column elongates.

Objections to the theory are incontrovertible (20). The traction force caused by the fixation of the spinal cord low in the spinal canal is dissipated within five segments above the fixation; the spinal cord is tethered low in the spinal canal in occult spinal dysraphism, and yet the ACM is not found; the dorsal aspect of the pons, medulla, and upper cervical cord is displaced more than the ventral portions, which would not be the case in traction from below; the anatomy of the dorsal kink can only be explained by the structures being displaced from above rather than pulled down from below; the Arnold-Chiari malformation is absent in some cases of low lumbar or sacral myelomeningoceles in which traction forces might be expected to be maximal and has been reported in a case with a normal lower spine and spinal cord; the malformation may be seen in embryos before the spinal cord ascends to a great degree; experimental tethering of the spinal cord in animals has failed to produce the malformation (1, 12, 17–20, 22, 36, 43). Thus, the traction theory is an outdated historical theory that should not be invoked as an explanation for the occurrence of the ACM.

OCCULT SPINAL DYSRAPHISM

Classification

Occult spinal dysraphism, or spina bifida occulta as it has been termed by James and Lassman (24), is an entity composed of a variety of malformations of embryological development varying from the very simple to the very complex (20). The major subtypes are listed in Table 17.2. Spinal dermal sinus and the neurenteric cyst have special clinical features, whereas the other types generally present with one or more features of a cutaneous malformation, a neuromusculoskeletal syndrome, sphincter disturbance, spinal curvature and, occasionally, back or leg pain. The infant may have a neurological deficit at birth or may be normal and, in either case, a new deficit or progression of an existing one may occur in the first or second decade. Spinal dermal sinus exhibits the special presentation of meningitis in the very young and spinal cord or cauda equina compression by tumor in the older child. The neurenteric cyst may present with an associated congenital thoracic cyst or an enteric duplication with vertebral body defects and a compressive intraspinal lesion at the cervicodorsal level. A brief description of the clinical and pathological abnormalities in each type is appropriate before discussing the abnormal embryology that might contribute to the lesions.

A congenital spinal dermal sinus is an epithelium-lined tract that may occur anywhere along the posterior midline of the body along the spine. It forms a potential communication between the skin surface and the deeper tissues. The tract may end in the subcutaneous tissues, on the bone, in the epidural or subdural space, or in the neural tissues, with the intraspinal extension often expanding into a dermoid or epidermoid inclusion tumor. The posterior elements may be normal radiologically, although usually a minor degree of posterior spina bifida is present. The vertebral bodies are virtually always normal. If the tract attaches to the neural elements and the normal degree of ascent of the conus has occurred during early development, then the cutaneous opening may be lower than the ultimate termination of the tract on the spinal cord by two or three segments. On occasion, the tract itself may act a a tethering agent to prevent the normal extent of upward migration, resulting in a low-lying conus medullaris.

The tethered cord syndrome can be defined as an abnormally low conus medullaris tethered by one or more forms of intradural abnormalities such as a short, thickened filum terminale, fibrous bands or adhesions, or a totally intradural lipoma fixing the neural elements to the caudal dural sac. The pathological feature that distinguishes this from congenital dermal sinus, lumbosacral lipoma, and lipomyelomeningocele is the lack of continuity between the visible cutaneous lesion, if there is any, and the intradural pathology. Important clinical features are the fact that cutaneous manifestations are present in only approximately 50% of the patients, and scoliosis is as frequent an occurrence as in diastematomyelia with septum. Posterior spina bifida is usually present, but the vertebral bodies are usually normal. The syndrome has been known by a variety of terms over the years such as the tethered conus, tight filum terminale, filum terminale syndrome, and the meningocele manque (20).

The forms lumbosacral lipoma and lipomyelomeningocele are quite related, with the latter a more complex lesion. The pathological hallmark is a subcutaneous lipoma overlying the lumbar or sacral region that extends through a defect in the fascia and posterior elements to merge with the neural elements, which are invariably tethered low in the spinal canal. The feature that merits differentiating the two lesions is that, in the simpler form, the neural elements are within the spinal canal; in the complex lipomyelomeningocele, the spinal cord rises out of the spinal canal to enter the subcutaneous lipoma. Thus, the complex lesion is somewhat akin to the open forms where the neural tissues are exposed at skin level; hence, the term "lipomyelomeningocele." In addition a meningocele component may be present in the lipomatous mass itself. The bony anomalies are more complex with lipomas than in the dermal sinus or tethered cord syndrome. Frequently, the vertebral bodies are malformed by scalloping of their posterior margins, the interpedicular distance is more likely to be widened and hemivertebrae or hypoplasia of the iliac wing may occur. An important factor in treatment is that compression of the neural elements may be a cause of a neurological deficit as well as tethering. The compression may be due to the intraspinal fat itself, usually by the portion extending under intact posterior elements or in the lipomyelomeningocele; the last intact neural arch may compress the exiting spinal cord at the point of its angulation around the arch.

Diastematomyelia is a fascinating pathological entity already mentioned as a part of SBA, especially in the spinal cord proximal to the neural plaque. In that setting there is usually no structural element between the hemicords, and the hemicords are located in a single dural sac. The infrequent form of hemimyelomeningocele is an exception, however. In occult spinal dysraphism, the division of the spinal cord into two more or less equal halves is usually associated with a midline septum of fibrous tissue, cartilage, or bone separating the hemicords, each of which are located in a separate dural sac. The conus medullaris is usually low in the spinal canal, with the transfixing septum located between T7 and T12 in 25% of cases and between L1 and L4 in 67% (20). Scoliosis is a frequent clinical manifestation that is no doubt related to the spinal anomalies that are more complex than seen in the other forms of occult dysraphism just discussed. Vertebral body anomalies occur frequently, especially in those patients with scoliosis, and posterior spina bifida is virtually always present near the level of the septum.

The neurenteric cyst occurs in an intramedullary or intradural extramedullary location ventral to the spinal cord in the cervicodorsal region of the spine. The usual presenting syndrome is a nonspecific spinal cord compression. As will be discussed later, the embryological origin of these lesions seems to be related to entoderm development. As a result, an associated intrathoracic or intraabdominal cyst can occur, and the vertebral bodies are virtually always malformed. In rare cases a transvertebral communication between the intraspinal cyst and the cyst anterior to the spine may be found. The posterior elements are virtually always normal, and no cutaneous manifestations are seen.

Finally, the very rare combined anterior and posterior spina bifida is mentioned only to give evidence of the potential validity of some of the theories of abnormal embryology. These rare instances of a longitudinal division of the vertebral bodies anteriorly forming a cleft and a posterior spina bifida at the same level usually occur in the cervicodorsal or lumbar areas of the spine. The higher lesions are associated with severe anomalies in other organ systems and are of pathological interest only. The lower lesions have been reported rarely in living children and usually involve prolapse of intestinal duplications through the anterior and posterior vertebral defects to the back. The neural elements are either open and exposed as a myeloschisis or they are closed. In the latter case a diastematomyelia ringing the enteric structure is seen, and the enteric duplication may appear as a skin-covered swelling which can mimick a meningocele or lipoma. Rarely, the enteric duplication may open onto the back and drain meconium.

Pathogenesis of the Clinical Presentation

The pathogenesis of the clinical presentation in occult spinal dysraphism is usually the product of one or more factors such as true myelodysplasia, traction, compression and, rarely, inflammation in congenital dermal sinus complicated by meningitis. True myelodysplasia, that is, an embryological malformation of the neural structures, may be seen in all of the types but is a source of neurological deficit at birth more often in lipomyelomeningocele, lumbosacral lipoma, and diastematomyelia. The source of neurological deficits after birth, whether new or progressive, is usually the result of compression or the traction phenomenon. Compression occurs more frequently in the lipomatous malformations by the lipoma itself or is caused by the vertebral arch in lipomyelomeningocele or, rarely, by the septum in diastematomyelia. Traction occurs in any situation wherein the neural elements are fixed at a lower than normal level in early embryological development when the spinal cord and spine are symmetrical in length. The normal ascent of the conus medullaris during regression of the tail bud is prevented, and the spinal cord is stretched. Although the stretching or tethering itself may not create a neurological deficit, the day-to-day repetitive incremental trauma of stretching occurring during normal spinal movements in active children can produce neurologic deficits. Ischemia of the stretched caudal spinal cord appears to play a part in the neurological dysfunction, and Yamada *et al.* (57) show that release of the tether can improve oxidative metabolism within the caudal cord.

THEORIES OF ABNORMAL EMBRYOGENESIS OF OCCULT SPINAL DYSRAPHISM

Occult spinal dysraphism in its many subtypes would appear to form in the earliest embryonic stages, as evidenced by the intimate cutaneous-neural (congenital dermal sinus) and enteric-neural (neurenteric cyst) communications, abnormal neurulation (diastematomyelia), and abnormal canalization and regression of the tail bud (tethered cord syndrome, lumbosacral lipoma, lipomyelomeningocele) (Table 17.4). The theories offered to explain these malformations involve five basic mechanisms: (a) abnormal separation of tissue layers: (b) abnormal neurulation; (c) abnormal formation of the notochord; (d) abnormal formation of the neurenteric canal; and (e) abnormal canalization and regression of the tail bud. Except for the latter mechanism, they are variations on a theme and are mutually interactive with the main dispute, focusing on which feature is the primary cause. The theories are more easily discussed by separating the malformations into three groups: (a) congenital dermal sinus; (b) tethered cord syndrome, lumbosacral lipoma, and lipomyelomeningocele; and (c) diastematomyelia, neurenteric cyst, and combined anterior and posterior spina bifida.

Congenital Dermal Sinus

The spinal dermal sinus can occur at any level of the spine and is rarely, if ever, associated with complicated vertebral abnormalities unless it is related to one of the more complex forms of occult dysraphism such as diastematomyelia with septum. The more common simple forms likely represent adhesion between the neural tube and cutaneous ectoderm at the time when separation of these layers should occur just after neurulation or canalization of the tail bud. (Figure 17.14) The mechanism was popularized by Walker and Bucy (55) in 1934. The misplaced ectodermal cells can then develop into the inclusion epidermoid or dermoid tumor. Since the communication may be small, the mesoderm can condense in

TABLE 17.4

Time of Onset of Spinal Dysraphism during Normal Embryogenesis

Entity	Gestational Age (days)
Neurenteric cyst Diastematomyelia with septum Combined spina bifida	16–17
Congenital dermal sinus	22–48
Myeloschisis	26–27 or 28+
Myelomeningocele Lumbosacral lipoma Lipomyelomeningocele	28–48
Tethered cord syndrome Spinal meningocele	43–fetal period

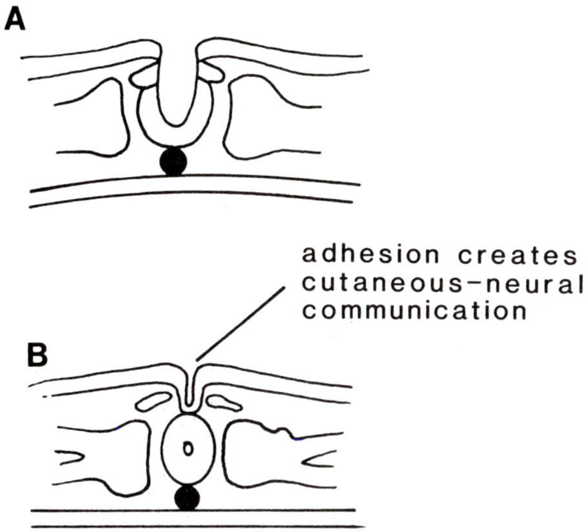

FIG. 17.14. (*A*) As the neural folds approximate, the cutaneous ectoderm ventrally fuses and then separates from the closed neural tube. (*B*) If separation fails to occur, a sinus of cutaneous ectoderm may remain attached to the neural structures, but the mesodermal condensations from virtually unimpaired and bony malformations are minimal.

a virtually normal fashion and result in only a minor degree of posterior spina bifida.

Padget (37) proposed the neuroschisis theory as a cause of congenital dermal sinus. The neuroschistic bleb that forms between the neural tube and the cutaneous ectoderm largely heals, leaving the neural tube to develop normally but creating an adhesion between skin and cord and, thus, the sinus.

Spinal dermal sinus has also been related to the more complex anterior form, in theory at least, and will be discussed shortly.

Tethered Cord Syndrome, Lumbosacral Lipoma, and Lipomyelomeningocele

These malformations which involve the caudal spinal cord are very likely related to some abnormality of canalization of the caudal cell mass, regression of the neural tube, and ascent of the conus medullaris. Abnormal canalization during 28–48 days of development would likely cause the lumbosacral lipoma and lipomyelomeningocele while abnormal regression, starting as early 43–48 days of development and continuing to the postnatal period, would be related to the tethered cord syndrome. Few theories of causation have been advanced, and none has been advanced in great detail.

Since canalization occurs in the caudal cell mass of pleuripotential cells under intact cutaneous ectoderm, it is not unrealistic to believe some cells of mesodermal nature destined to form fat tissue could be misplaced in conjunction with those cells destined to form the neural tube. Subsequent development of both tissues result in a dorsal subcutaneous lipoma fused to the caudal spinal cord in varying degrees of intimacy. In the complex lipomyelomeningocele, the spinal cord is drawn out of the confines of the spinal canal, the fusion is intimate, and the potential for primary myelodysplasia with congenital neurological deficit is high. The simpler lipoma fuses with the spinal cord within the canal and produces no functional impairment of neural development. In both instances, the lipoma transgresses several tissue planes extending from the subcutaneous plane through fascia, bone, dura, and arachnoid-pia. Tethering of the cord low in the spinal canal results, and ascent of the conus is prevented, setting the stage for postnatal neurological deficit from traction.

In the tethered cord syndrome the process of canalization has usually occurred normally, but regression is abnormal, leading to various abnormalities such as lipoma of the filum terminale, and abnormally thick and short filum terminale or a variety of bands and adhesions between neural structures and the dura. These intradural tethering lesions impair ascent of the conus medullaris and have the same potential for later postnatal neurological deficit.

These mechanisms would not explain spinal cord lipomas at the higher levels of the spine unassociated with spina bifida or cutaneous anomalies. The embryological abnormality should involve a misplacement of pleuripotential cells that ultimately form fat, possibly during the migration of those cells from the caudal cell mass which condenses alongside the notochord and under the neural plate prior to neurulation.

Diastematomyelia, Neurenteric Cyst, and Combined Anterior and Posterior Spina Bifida

These forms of occult spinal dysraphism involve the higher levels of the spine and are often associated with malformation of the vertebral bodies. In neurenteric cysts and combined spina bifida, the enteric structures may also be abnormal and may even communicate, to a variable degree, through the anterior spina bifida with the spinal canal and spinal cord. The primary abnormality must involve either the neural tissue itself, the mesoderm, the notochord, or the entoderm, and since all are abnormal to some degree, each has been implicated in one or more theories. Some theories are expansive and describe all three malformations whereas others are limited to a description of only one malformation.

ABNORMAL SEPARATION OF TISSUE LAYERS

Beardmore and Wiglesworth (5) and McLetchie *et al.* (34) reviewed the development of the theories regarding abnormal fusion of tissue layers as it relates to the neurenteric cyst. A primary adhesion could develop between the ectoderm and entoderm in the midline prior to the formation of the notochord, perhaps akin to the type of fusion that marks the future mouth and anus (Fig. 17.15*A*). Subsequently, the notochord cells extending rostrally split around the adhesion, forming a split notochord (Fig. 17.15*B*). Further development of the tissues and persistence of the adhesion results in an entoderm to neuroectoderm band. Evidence that adhesions can occur in this area is supported by Patten's (40) observation of an area of fusion between the notochord and neural tube in an embryo of 6 weeks development. This abnormal communication has a variable potential in its ultimate expression, depending upon the degree of healing. The adhesion impairs the formation of the vertebral bodies around the split notochord and can lead to hemivertebrae or midline cleft formation. An enteric-neural fistula, an enteric diverticulum with abnormal vertebral body formation or a localized cyst can form anterior to the spine or intraspinally, or both could occur (Fig. 17.15*E*). Abnormal adhesions can develop between the notochord and entoderm during the process of intercalation and excalation of the notochord from the yolk sac, but the neural malformations are not explained on this basis alone (54). This theory was not extended to explain diastematomyelia or combined spina bifida as some later authors have done with similar theories.

ABNORMAL NEURULATION

Abnormalities of neurulation have been involved to explain diastematomyelia with septum for many years. In 1940 Herren and Edwards (23) suggested that diastematomyelia was due to a "twinning" in which the neural folds turned inward excessively and fused with the neural plate rather than with one another. Subsequently, two neural tubes formed, and the mesoderm migrated between the neural tubes to form the separate dural envelopes and the septum. They offered no explanation for the behavior of the neural folds themselves. In the same year, Lichtenstein (32) suggested that the mesoderm created the midline septum primarily and split the neural plate with subsequent secondary formation of the separate neural tubes. Several authors have indicated mechanisms for the abnormal neurulation as a primary phenomenon. Kapsenberg and Van Lookeren Campagne (25), in 1949, suggested that overgrowth of the neuroectoderm as had been observed in SBA by Patten (41) might explain diastematomyelia. Since the overgrown neural folds and plate cannot bend sufficiently to meet in the midline, each fold fuses with the plate

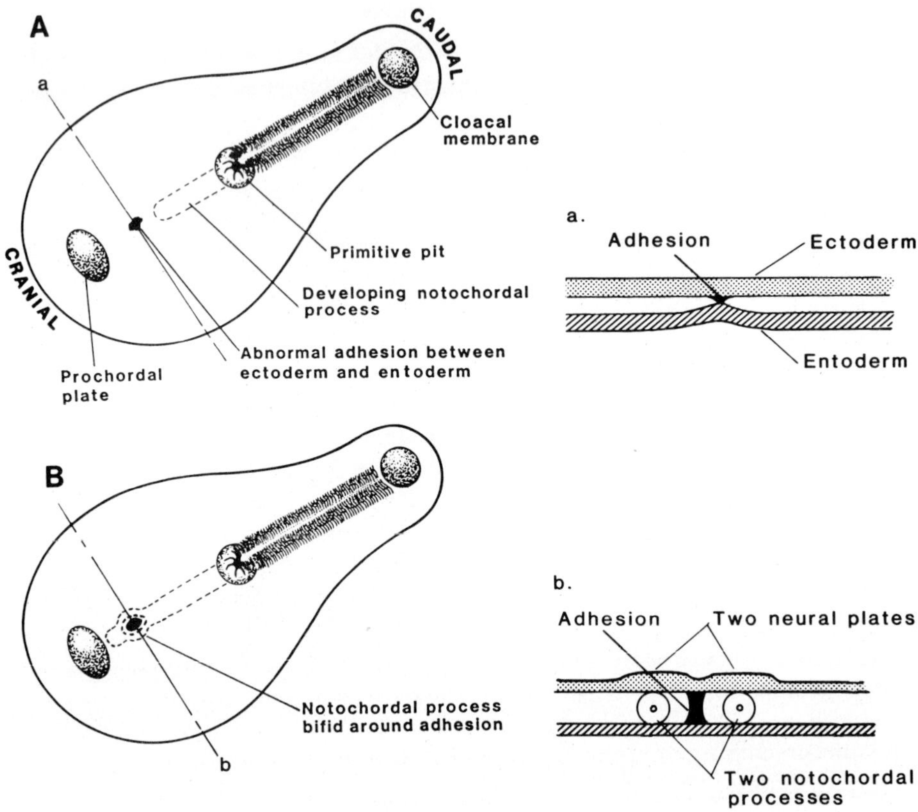

FIG. 17.15. (*A*) An adhesion between the ectoderm and entoderm of the two-layered embryo cranial to the developing notochordal process is shown in cross-section (*a*). (*B*) The notochordal process is forced to divide around the adhesion creating two notochordal processes which ultimately can induce two neural plates as shown in *b*. A diastematomyelia could occur. (*C*) An enterocutaneous fistula, as in combined anterior and posterior spina bifida, penetrates the cleft through the vertebral bodies, diastematomyelia, and posterior elements. (*D*) Healing of the anterior and posterior portions of the fistula could lead to diastematomyelia with septum, which is usually accompanied by posterior element and vertebral body abnormalities. (*E*) Healing of the posterior and midportions of the fistula could lead to neurenteric cyst with an intraspinal cyst, vertebral body defect of variable severity, and variable enteric anomalies.

on its own side, thus forming two separate neural tubes. Padget (37) suggested the theory of neuroschisis could explain the malformation if neuroschistic blebs formed simultaneously dorsally and ventrally to the neural tube and each half tube then creates a separate neural tube. Gardner (21) postulated that hydrodynamic overdistension of the embryonic neural tube ruptures the roof and floor plates simultaneously with two neural tubes forming as a result. In each case the mesoderm fills in

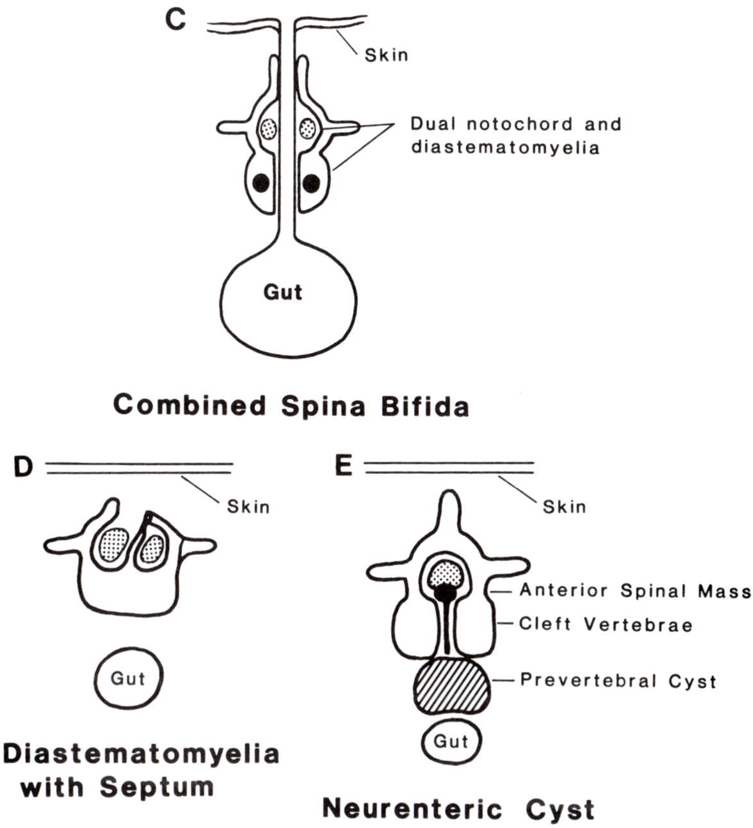

FIG. 17.15-C–E

the space between the neural tubes secondarily to form the separate dural sheaths and septum. None of the theories, except for Gardner's, explain the mechanism for the vertebral body anomalies. The primary role of the neural tube in the creation of this malformation does not fit comfortably with that of the notochord and mesoderm functioning as important inductors of neural tube formation. Gardner's theory is alone in suggesting that overdistension of the neural tube may also cause the notochord to split to create a neuroectoderm-entoderm communication and thus explain the neurenteric cyst.

ABNORMAL FORMATION OF THE NOTOCHORD

Abnormal formation of the notochord is an attractive theory for these malformations if the notochord truly has an important role in inducing the formation of the neural tube and is the framework for vertebral body development. In 1943 Saunders (48) described a primary split in the notochord as being responsible for combined spina bifida but did not expand the description to other forms of occult spinal dysraphism. In 1960 Bentley and Smith (7) and Smith (49) separately reviewed the split notochord syndrome and believed that diastematomyelia, neurenteric cyst, combined spina bifida, and congenital dermal sinus could all be explained. A primary split develops in the notochord at a variable level and extent for reasons not stated, and thus a gap opens in the dorsal tissue between the two parts of the notochord. The spinal cord develops in two halves. Through this gap the entoderm herniates and adheres to the cutaneous ectoderm covering the dorsal embryo. If the hernia ruptures, a fistula from amniotic sac to yolk sac will exist, passing between the two halves of the notochord and spinal cord (Fig. 17.15*C*). The extent of the healing process will determine what type of lesion remains. If the entire hernial sac remains, true combined spina bifida occurs; if only the very dorsal portion persists and the remainder heals, a congenital dermal sinus may result; if the dorsal and ventral portions heal, a diastematomyelia may form (Fig. 17.15*D*); if only the ventral portion remains, a form of neurenteric cyst may develop (Fig. 17.15*E*).

The notochord theory is attractive because it explains all the types of occult spinal dysraphism, except for those due to abnormal canalization and regression of the caudal tail bud. However, congenital dermal sinuses are located frequently below the level of the spinal cord formed by neurulation, and spinal cord malformations or vertebral body malformations are rare, suggesting that the simpler theories of cutaneous ectodermal-neuroectodermal adhesion are a more likely explanation than persistence of the posterior remnant of a fistula between the yolk sac and the amniotic cavity.

ABNORMAL FORMATION OF THE NEURENTERIC CANAL

The neurenteric canal is the passageway that temporarily penetrates the caudal embryo to join the dorsal amniotic sac with the ventral yolk sac during the formation of the notochord at stage 8 (days 18 and 19). It ceases to exist as the process of excalation of the notochord from the yolk sac is completed and the entoderm becomes a continuous layer once again. The dorsal opening of the canal is at the level of Hensen's node, and at this early stage no somites have yet formed. Two theories involving abnormal development of the neurenteric canal have been offered as explanations for combined spina bifida, diastematomyelia with septum, neurenteric cyst, and for congenital dermal sinus.

In 1923, Bell (6) reviewed the early concepts that abnormal persistence of the neurenteric canal could give rise to anterior spina bifida at any level of the spine and thereby create lesions of the neurenteric cyst variety. Even at this time some authors discredited this notion as a cause of any abnormalities in the cervicothoracic area since the neurenteric canal is believed to be located at the caudal end of the embryo. However, those authors favoring the theory applied, to the human situation, the embryological development noted in amphibian embryos in which the neurenteric canal migrates craniocaudally. In that case, arrest of closure at different times could cause lesions at any level of the vertebral column. Bremer (8), writing in 1952, agreed that the final resting place for Hensen's node, through which the neurenteric canal was located, was the coccygeal tip. Thus, any abnormal enteric-neural communications proximal to the coccyx must be due to "... an ectopic or an accessory canal." Subsequent herniation of the entodermal layer through the gap creates the fistula, dividing the vertebral bodies and the spinal cord. Healing to a varying degree may create any of the types of occult dysraphism, as discussed for the split notochord syndrome (Fig. 17.15*C–E*).

The differences between the split notochord syndrome, described by Bentley and Smith in 1960, and the accessory neurenteric canal theory, described by Bremer in 1952 are minor, with the former suggesting that the notochord is at fault and the latter suggesting an "extra" neurenteric canal as responsible. Bremer's theory is less attractive because the mechanism for the so-called "accessory neurenteric canal" is difficult to describe embryologically. The true neurenteric canal is created during the complicated process of notochord formation at the caudal end of the embryo, and it never divides the neural plate or the notochord longitudinally; the accessory canal must divide both and thus fails its comparison to the true canal, except in the communication of the amniotic cavity and yolk sac.

SUMMARY

The theories of abnormal embryogenesis suggested as explanations for the various forms of SBA and occult spinal dysraphism appear in some instances too all encompassing, as in Gardner's hydrodynamic theory or Padget's neuroschisis theory, or too limited, as in the theory of arrested development proposed by Daniel and Strich for the ACM, or just too speculative in many cases. The observation of a completed defect does not allow one to venture backwards in development to a specific time and cause with any accuracy. Perhaps several different causes striking different tissues at different times can set up a series of aberrations that lead to morphologically similar mature anomalies. The ability of developmental processes to heal themselves, as shown experimentally, may obscure the true mechanism and timing of occurrence although the final morphological expression may be dramatic. Since the study of human embryogenesis in the experimental laboratory is ethically unacceptable although technically feasible, the elucidation of the mechanisms of these neural defects will be long in coming.

ACKNOWLEDGMENTS

The author would like to thank Hal Pullum and George Newton for their artistic talents, as displayed in their preparation of the illustrations.

REFERENCES

1. Barry, A., Patten, B. M., and Stewart, B. H. Possible factors in the development of the Arnold-Chiari malformation. J. Neurosurg., *14:* 285–301, 1957.
2. Barson, A. J. The vertebral level of termination of the spinal cord during normal and abnormal development. J. Anat., *106:* 489–497, 1970.
3. Barson, A. J. Spina bifida: The significance of the level and extent of the defect to the morphogenesis. Dev. Med. Child Neurol., *12:* 129–144, 1970.
4. Barson, A. J. Differentiation, growth and disorders of development of the vertebrospinal axis. In: *Scientific Foundations of Paediatrics*, edited by J. A. Davis and J. Dobbins, pp. 577–586. London, William Heinemann Medical Books, 1974.
5. Beardmore, H. E., and Wiglesworth, F. W. Vertebral anomalies and alimentary duplications. Pediatr. Clin. North Am., *5:* 457–474, 1958.
6. Bell, H. H. Anterior spina bifida and its relation to a persistence of the neurenteric canal. J. Nerv. Ment. Dis., *57:* 445–462, 1923.
7. Bentley, J. F. R., and Smith, J. R. Developmental posterior enteric remnants and spinal malformations: The split notochord syndrome. Arch. Dis. Child., *35:* 76–86, 1960.
8. Bremer, J. L. Dorsal intestinal fistula: Accessory neurenteric canal; diastematomyelia. Arch. Pathol., *54:* 132–138, 1952.
9. Brocklehurst, G. A quantitative study of a spina bifida foetus. J. Pathol., *99:* 205–211, 1969.
10. Brocklehurst, G. The development of the human cerebrospinal fluid pathway with particular reference to the roof of the fourth ventricle. J. Anat., *105:* 467–475, 1969.
11. Brocklehurst, G. *Spina Bifida for the Clinician*, pp. 1–195. London, William Heinemann Medical Books, 1976.
12. Cameron, A. H. The Arnold-Chiari and other neuro-anatomical malformations associated with spina bifida. J. Pathol. Bacteriol., *73:* 195–211, 1957.
13. Carmel, P. W., and Markesbery, W. R. Early descriptions of the Arnold-Chiari malformation: The contribution of John Cleland. J. Neurosurg., *37:* 543–547, 1972.
14. Cleland, J. Contribution to the study of spina bifida, encephalocele and anencephalus. J. Anat. Physiol., *17:* 257–292, 1883.
15. Daniel, P. M., and Strich, S. J. Some observations on the congenital deformity of the central nervous system known as the Arnold-Chiari malformation. J. Neuropathol. Exp. Neurol., *17:* 255–266, 1958.
16. Emery, J. L., and Lendon, R. G. The local cord lesion in neurospinal dysraphism (meningomyelocele). J. Pathol., *110:* 83–96, 1973.
17. Emery, J. L., and Levick, R. K. The movement of the brain stem and vessels around the brain stem in children with hydrocephalus and the Arnold-Chiari deformity. Dev. Med. Child Neurol., *11*(Suppl.)*:* 49–60, 1966.
18. Emery, J. L., and MacKenzie, N. Medullo-cervical dislocation deformity (Chiari II deformity) related to neurospinal dysraphism (meningomyelocele). Brain, *96:* 155–162, 1973.

19. Emery, J. L., and Naik, D. Spinal cord segment lengths in children with meningomyelocele and the "Cleland-Arnold-Chiari" deformity. Br. J. Radiol., *41:* 287–290, 1968.
20. French, B. N. Midline fusion defects and defects of formation. In *Neurological Surgery*, Ed. 2, edited by J. R. Youmans, pp. 1236–1380. Philadelphia, W. B. Saunders Co., 1982.
21. Gardner, W. J. *The Dysraphic States from Syringomyelia to Anencephaly*, pp. 1–201. Excerpta Medica, Amsterdam, 1973.
22. Goldstein, F., and Kepes, J. J. The role of traction in the development of the Arnold-Chiari malformation: An experimental study. J. Neuropathol. Exp. Neurol., *25:* 654–666, 1966.
23. Herren, R. Y., and Edwards, J. E. Diplomyelia (duplication of the spinal cord). Arch. Pathol., *30:* 1203–1214, 1940.
24. James, C. C. M., and Lassman, L. P. *Spina Bifida Occulta*, pp. 1–230. Grune & Stratton, New York, 1981.
25. Kapsenberg, J. G., and Van Lookeren Campagne, J. A. A case of spina bifida combined with diastematomyely, the anomaly of Chiari and hydrocephaly. Acta Anat., *7:* 366–388, 1949.
26. Kunitomo, K. The development and reduction of the tail and of the caudal end of the spinal cord. Contrib. Embryol., *8:* 161–198, 1918.
27. Lemire, R. J. Variations in development of the caudal neural tube in human embryos (Horizons XIV–XXI). Teratology, *2:* 361–370, 1969.
28. Lemire, R. J. Embryology of the central nervous system. In *Scientific Foundations of Paediatrics*, pp. 547–564. London, William Heinemann Medical Books, 1974.
29. Lemire, R. J., Loesser, J. D., Leech, R. W., and Alvord, Jr., E. C. *Normal and Abnormal Development of the Human Nervous System*, pp. 1–421. Harper & Row, New York, 1975.
30. Lemire, R. J., Shepard, T. H., and Alvord, Jr., E. C. Caudal myeloschisis (lumbosacral spina bifida cystica) in a five millimeter (Horizon XIV) human embryo. Anat. Rec., *152:* 9–16, 1965.
31. Lendon, R. G., and Emery, J. L. Forking of the central canal in the equinal cord of children. J. Anat., *106:* 499–505, 1970.
32. Lichtenstein, B. W. Spinal dysraphism, spina bifida and myelodysplasia. Arch. Neurol. Psychiatry, *44:* 792–810, 1940.
33. Marin-Padilla, M., and Marin-Padilla, T. M. Morphogenesis of experimentally induced Arnold-Chiari malformation. J. Neurol. Sci., *50:* 29–55, 1981.
34. McLetchie, N. G. B., Purves, J. K., and Saunders, R. L. de CH. The genesis of gastric and certain intestinal diverticula and enterogenous cysts. Surg. Gynecol. Obstet., *99:* 135–141, 1954.
35. Moore, K. L. *The Developing Human*, Ed. 3, pp. 1–479. Philadelphia, W. B. Saunders, 1982.
36. Osaka, K., Tanimura, T., Hirayama, A., and Matsumoto, S. Myelomeningocele before birth. J. Neurosurg. *49:* 711–724, 1978.
37. Padget, D. H. Spina bifida and embryonic neuroschisis—A causal relationship. Definition of the postnatal conformations involving a bifid spine. Johns Hopkins Med. J., *128:* 233–252, 1968.
38. Padget, D. H. Neuroschisis and human embryonic maldevelopment: New evidence on anencephaly, spina bifida and diverse mammalian defects. J. Neuropathol. Exp. Neurol., *29:* 192–216, 1970.
39. Padget, D. H. Development of so-called dysraphism, with embryologic evidence of clinical Arnold-Chiari and Dandy-Walker malformations. Johns Hopkins Med. J., *130:* 127–165, 1972.

40. Patten, B. M. Fusion of notochord to neural tube in a human embryo of the sixth week. Anat. Rec., *95:* 307–311, 1946.
41. Patten, B. M. Overgrowth of the neural tube in young human embryos. Anat. Rec., *113:* 381–393, 1952.
42. Patten, B. M. Embryological stages in the establishing of myeloschisis with spina bifida. Amer. J. Anat. *93:* 365–395, 1953.
43. Peach, B. Arnold-Chiari malformation with normal spine. Arch. Neurol., *10:* 497–501, 1964.
44. Peach, B. The Arnold-Chiari malformation: Morphogenesis. Arch. Neurol., *12:* 527–535, 1965.
45. Peach, B. Arnold-Chiari malformation: Anatomic features of 20 cases. Arch. Neurol., *12:* 613–621, 1965.
46. Penfield, W., and Coburn, D. F. Arnold-Chiari malformation and its operative treatment. Arch. Neurol. Psychiatry, *40:* 328–336, 1938.
47. Rokos, J. The pathogenesis of spina bifida and related malformations: In: *Recent Advances in Neuropathology*, pp. 225–245. Glasgow, Churchill Livingstone, 1979.
48. Saunders, R. L. de CH. Combined anterior and posterior spina bifida in a living neonatal human female. Anat. Rec., *87:* 255–278, 1943.
49. Smith, J. R. Accessory enteric formations: A classification and nomenclature. Arch. Dis. Child., *35:* 87–89, 1960.
50. Streeter, G. L. Factors involved in the formation of the filum terminale. Am. J. Anat. *25:* 1–12, 1919.
51. Thompson, M. W., and Rudd, N. L. The genetics of spinal dysraphism. In: *Current Controversies in Neurosurgery*, pp. 126–146. Philadelphia, W. B. Saunders, 1976.
52. Van Hoytema, G. J., and van den Berg, R. Embryological studies of the posterior fossa in connection with the Arnold-Chiari malformation. Dev. Med. Child. Neurol. (Suppl.), *11:* 61–76, 1966.
53. Variend, S., and Emery, J. L. The weight of the cerebellum in children with myelomeningocele. Dev. Med. Child. Neurol. (Suppl. 29), *15:* 77–83, 1973.
54. Veeneklaas, G. M. H. Pathogenesis of intrathoracic gastrogenic cysts. Am. J. Dis. Child., *83:* 500–507, 1952.
55. Walker, A. E., and Bucy, P. C. Congenital dermal sinuses; A source of spinal meningeal infection and subdural abscesses. Brain, *57:* 401–421, 1934.
56. Warkany, J. Morphogenesis of spina bifida. In: *Myelomeningocele*, edited by R. L. McLaurin, pp. 31–39. New York, Grune & Stratton, 1977.
57. Yamada, S., Zinke, D. E., Sanders, D. Pathophysiology of "tethered cord syndrome." J. Neurosurg., *54:* 494–503, 1981.

CHAPTER

18

Radiology of Spinal Dysraphism

THOMAS P. NAIDICH, M.D., DEREK C. HARWOOD-NASH, M.D., and DAVID G. McLONE, M.D., PH.D.

INTRODUCTION AND DEFINITIONS

Spinal dysraphism designates a heterogeneous group of spinal anomalies with the common feature of imperfect fusion of midline mesenchymal, bony, and neural structures. *Spina bifida* is a dysraphism of the osseous elements that normally form the closed spinal canal (60). Spina bifida aperta (synonym: spina bifida cystica) signifies posterior protrusion of all or part of the spinal contents through a posterior spina bifida to form (a) a meningeal sac (meningocele); (b) a midline plaque of exposed, unneurulated neural tissue which is flush with the skin surface (myelocele); or (c) a midline plaque of exposed, unneurulated neural tissue which is elevated above the normal skin surface by a variable expansion of the subjacent subarachnoid space (myelomeningocele; synonym: meningomyelocele). Occult spinal dysraphism designates the group of skin-covered spinal dysraphisms which have no exposed neural tissue and no obvious cystic mass (1, 60). In such patients, any associated mass is likely to be a subcutaneous lipoma. Occult spinal dysraphism encompasses diastematomyelia, the split notochord syndrome, dorsal dermal sinus, spinal lipoma, and "the tight filum terminale" syndrome (1, 60). This term replaces the term spina bifida occulta, which has come to mean simple failure of fusion of the lamina, usually at L5 and S1 (Fig. 18.1).

Spinal CT, particularly metrizamide CT myelography, now appears to provide the most precise and elegant depiction of the anatomic derangements which characterize these entities. Reference 31 provides a protocol for performing these studies.

SPINA BIFIDA APERTA

Simple Meningocele

The simple meningocele is a protrusion of dura, arachnoid, and subarachnoid fluid into the subcutaneous tissue of the back. The simple meningocele lies beneath an intact skin cover unless there is secondary

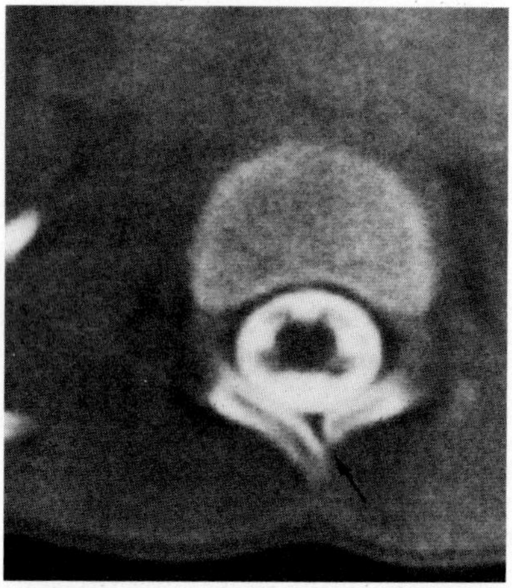

FIG. 18.1. Thoracic spina bifida occulta. Metrizamide CT myelography demonstrates the focal defect (*arrow*) in fusion of the posterior arch. The normal spinal cord, normal emerging paired nerve roots, and intact arachnoid sac rule out meningocele or neural dysraphism at this level.

ulceration and skin breakdown. By definition, the simple meningocele contains no intrinsic neural tissue (Fig. 18.2). A loop of nerve which arises within the spinal canal may occasionally herniate into the sac and return thereto prior to exiting through its normal root sleeve (54). Rarely, such roots may become adherent to the wall of the sac. The conus medullaris may lie in normal position or may lie abnormally low within the spinal canal (43). The filum terminale may insert into the neck of the sac.

The simple meningocele is lined by arachnoid mater. The arachnoid tends to fuse with dura at the dome of the sac and is most easily distinguished as a separate membrane at the neck of the sac (54). Filmy adhesions commonly traverse the sac. Denser adhesions may partially obliterate the neck of the sac (22, 54). The sac communicates with the intracanalicular subarachnoid space and may change size with patient position and Valsalva's maneuver.

Simple meningocele is usually associated with a relatively limited bony deformity: absence of a single spinous process, narrow spina bifida of a single lamina, or relatively focal multilevel spina bifida with widening of the spinal canal (Fig. 18.2). Neuroradiologic evaluation of the simple meningocele is undertaken to define the presence, size, and exact site of the meningocele; the precise relationship to the laminar defect(s); the absence of intrinsic neural structure; and the sites of the conus medullaris and filum terminale.

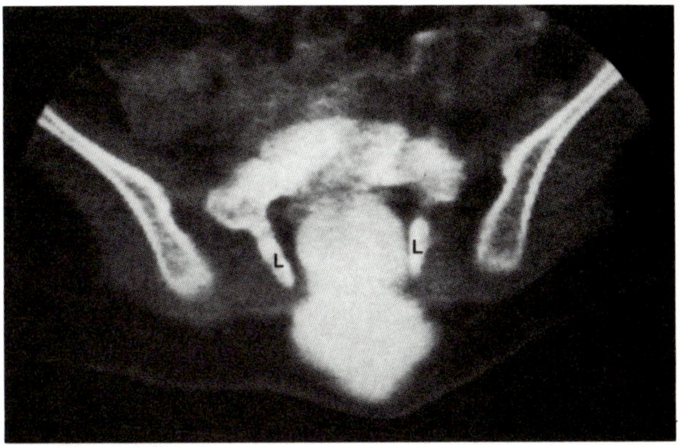

FIG. 18.2. Simple meningocele. Metrizamide CT myelography. The opacified subarachnoid space herniates posteriorly through the bifid laminae (*L, L*) and the separated paraspinal musculature to form a midline subcutaneous meningeal sac. Absence of the spinal cord, nerve roots, and mass within the sac (and termination of the spinal cord within the spinal canal on higher CT sections) identifies this sac as a simple meningocele.

Myelocele and Myelomeningocele

At present, there is no indication for detailed neuroradiologic evaluation of a newborn with straightforward clinical and neuroradiological signs of myelocele or myelomeningocele. Such patients typically exhibit slightly asymmetrical neurological deficits; show rapid, incomplete recovery after surgical closure of the back; and do not deteriorate thereafter, provided that hydrocephalus is controlled. Neuroradiological evaluation of these patients is best restricted to (a) the patient with *markedly* asymmetrical neurological deficits which may signify a hemimyelocele, and (b) the older patient with later deterioration of neurological function or progressive hydrocephalus which may indicate complicating neuropathology (33).

HEMIMYELOCELE

Cameron (11) and Emery and Lendon (20) have shown that 31–46% of patients with myelocele or myelomeningocele have an associated diastematomyelia (*vide infra*). The diastematomyelia involves the spinal cord cephalic to the myelomeningocele in 31% of cases, at the myelomeningocele in 22% of cases, and caudal to the myelomeningocele in 25% of cases (20). In 9% of patients with myelomeningocele (and 2.3% of all patients with spinal dysraphism), the myelocele or myelomeningocele affects the two hemicords at very different levels, producing very asymmetric clinical findings (17, 20). In most of these cases, only one of the two hemicords exhibits a myelocele, while the other is normal.

Infrequently, a myelocele is present on each hemicord at substantially different levels. Typically, these patients show normal neurological findings on the side of the normal cord. Metrizamide CT myelography in such cases demonstrates the diastematomyelia, the presence and (a)symmetry of the myelocele or myelomeningocele, any associated bone spur, and any other anomaly that may influence the surgical repair (Fig. 18.3).

Late postoperative deterioration of neurological functions is not part of the natural history of myelomeningocele. Such late deterioration suggests possible constriction of the reconstituted arachnoid and dural tubes, retethering of the spinal cord by scarring, cord compression by associated lipomas or implantation (epi)dermoid cysts, segmental cord infarction from vascular compromise, and/or hydrosyringomyelia. In patients whose myelomeningoceles were repaired by the older technique of simple dural closure, the neural plaque and adjacent spinal cord are densely scarred into the posterior dural-cutaneous closure and cannot be identified as separate structures (Fig. 18.4). Serial CT sections will show only the normal cord which exists below the closure and a thickening of

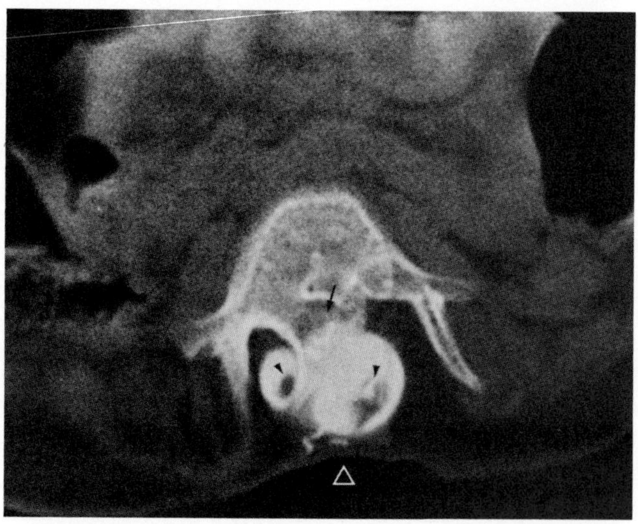

FIG. 18.3. Hemimyelocele. Metrizamide CT myelography. Thin skin and thin subcutaneous tissue mark the site where the myelocele of one hemicord was repaired (*open arrowhead*). Because the clinically evident midline hemimyelocele was taken to be a routine myelocele and the obliquely oriented bone spur (*arrows*) was taken to be the typical everted lamina, the diastematomyelia, occult hemicanal, and normal hemicord were not detected until later follow-up. In this patient, the hemicord and the hemimyelocele (*closed arrowheads*) lie in separate arachnoid and dural tubes. The bone spur passes medial to both dural tubes in the interdural cleft and divides the bifid canal into two very asymmetric hemicanals.

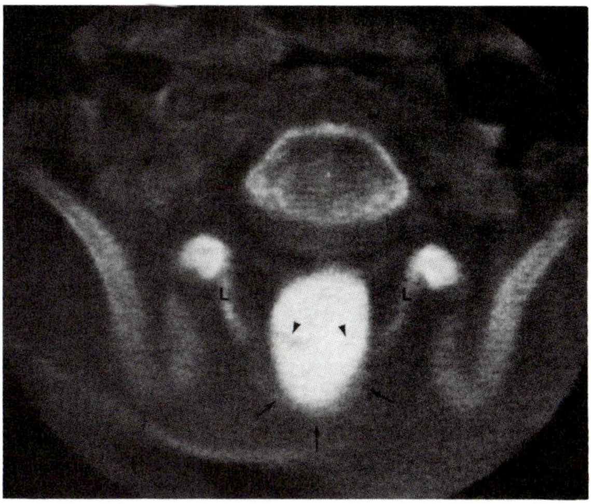

FIG. 18.4. Myelomeningocele with spinal cord tethering after old-style surgical repair. Metrizamide CT myelography. The opacified sac extends posterior to the bifid laminae (*L, L*). The gray "posterior wall" (*arrows*) of the sac represents the neural placode, completely scarred into the closure. Nerve roots (*arrowheads*) are seen faintly within the opacified CSF.

the posterior wall of the thecal sac at the level of the closure itself (Fig. 18.4). Emerging nerve roots may occasionally be defined and may help to distinguish this phenomenon from the simple meningocele radiologically (Fig. 18.4).

In patients closed by the McLone technique (47) and its variants, the surgically reconstructed closed neural tube and its emerging roots float within the cerebrospinal fluid (CSF) and are anchored only lightly by a surgically created dorsal midline pia-arachnoid pedicle which is analogous in some ways to the dentate ligament (Fig. 18.5). In such patients, "normal" or "base line" postoperative metrizamide CT scans demonstrate opacified CSF surrounding the low-lying spinal cord at all levels.

Patients with associated intracanalicular lipomas or inclusion (epi)dermoid cysts exhibit a lucent intraspinal mass which is often adherent to the spinal cord, roots of the cauda equina, and canal wall (Fig. 18.6). The lipoma or (epi)dermoid cyst tethers the cord and may compress the cord by mass effect. Abrupt focal reduction in the caliber of the cord suggests segmental cord infarction. Marked focal narrowing of the opacified subarachnoid space suggests that the dura was pulled together too tightly during closure, with consequent constriction of the arachnoidal-dural tube about the cord and cauda equina.

Hydromyelia is present in 29–77% of patients with myelomeningocele (11, 20). The exact incidence depends on the success of shunt therapy of

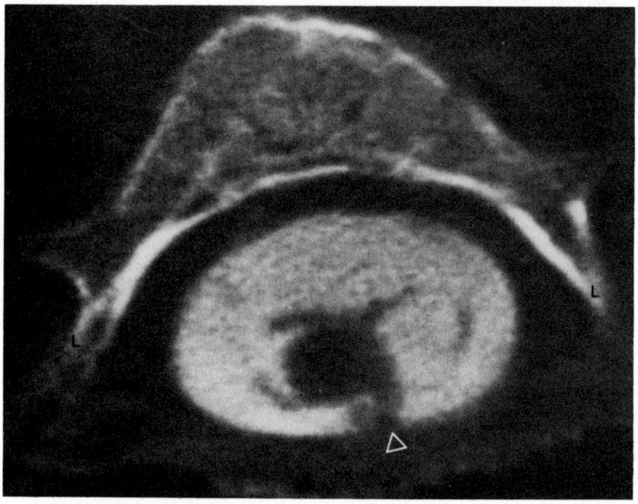

FIG. 18.5. "Normal" postoperative appearance of a myelomeningocele closed by the McLone technique (47). Metrizamide CT myelography. Wide eversion of the laminae (*L, L*) signifies spina bifida. The reconstructed spinal cord lies within the opacified subarachnoid space and gives off the paired nerve roots. A pia-arachnoidal pedicle (*open arrowhead*) suspends the cord from the posterior wall of the canal.

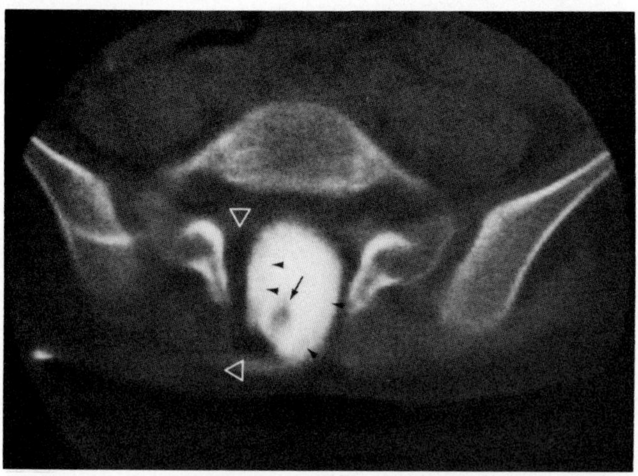

FIG. 18.6. Retethering of the spinal cord after myelomeningocele repair. Metrizamide CT myelography. A lucent lipoma (*open arrowheads*), situated behind and lateral to the opacified arachnoid sac, anchors the spinal cord (*arrow*) and nerve roots (*closed arrowheads*) at this and higher levels. Such lipomas may be difficult to distinguish from inclusion epidermoid cysts.

accompanying hydrocephalus (5, 28, 29). Because such hydromyelia results from passage of CSF through the obex and down the central canal of the spinal cord, the hydromyelia typically distends the entire length of the spinal cord above the neural placode and, by hydrostatic pressure, is most severe immediately above the placode (Fig. 18.7). Such hydromyelia is not present below the placode (20). Untreated hydromyelia may be responsible for extremely rapid development or progression of scoliosis (5, 28, 29). In patients with shunted hydrocephalus, rapidly developing scoliosis may be a sign of shunt malfunction (Fig. 18.7) or of isolation of the fourth ventricle and central canal of the cord from the lateral ventricles (5, 28, 29). Because such scoliosis may often be cured or reduced markedly and rapidly by shunt revision, by shunt decompression of untreated hydrocephalus, or by local decompression of the hydromyelia, all patients with rapidly progressive scoliosis deserve CT scans of the head and spine to rule out this easily remediable cause of scoliosis (5, 28, 29).

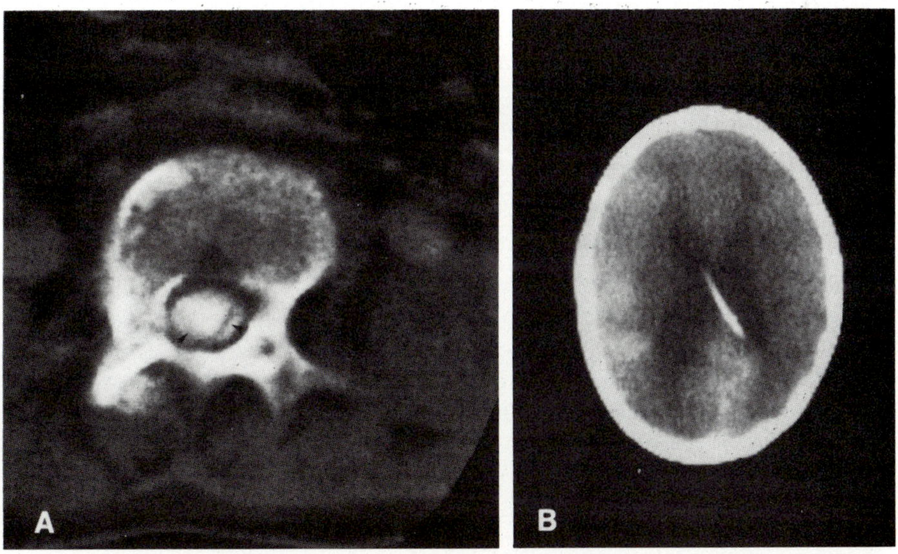

FIG. 18.7. Hydrocephalus with hydromyelia. Girl, 8½ years old, with repaired myelomeningocele and progressive scoliosis associated with shunt malfunction. (*A*) Metrizamide CT myelography, after direct puncture of the hydromyelic cavity, reveals the thin black ring of the extremely attenuated spinal cord (*arrowheads*), the dense metrizamide within the hydromyelia, and the less dense metrizamide in the subarachnoid space outside the cord. Obliquity of the vertebral body indicates scoliosis. (*B*) Simultaneous CT of the head reveals metrizamide in the subarachnoid space, nonfilling of the ventricles, and marked increase in ventricular size since slit-like ventricles were seen on prior CT. Revision of the shunt returned the ventricles to slit-like size and reduced the scoliosis by 30° within 1 week.

OCCULT SPINAL DYSRAPHISM

Diastematomyelia

Diastematomyelia is a sagittal clefting of the spinal cord into two not necessarily symmetrical "hemicords," each lined by its own pia mater (2, 15, 38, 40, 55, 56, 63, 64, 70). Such clefting may extend through the full thickness of the cord, may involve only the ventral half of the cord (partial ventral diastematomyelia), or may involve only the dorsal half of the cord (partial dorsal diastematomyelia) (27, 28, 58). Partial clefting is frequently observed as a transitional state at the cranial and caudal extremes of a full-thickness cleft (15, 51, 53).

The conus medullaris lies below L2 in 76% of patients with diastematomyelia (35). The filum terminale is thicker than 2 mm in 41% of cases of diastematomyelia and is believed to tether the cord in such cases. The cleft in the cord lies between T9 and S1 in 85% of cases (35). It is exclusively thoracic in 20%, is thoracolumbar in 18%, and is exclusively lumbar in 61% of cases (35). The two hemicords usually reunite into a single cord below the cleft (91%) (35). When the cleft extends unusually low, however, the hemicords may remain separate, forming two conuses and two fila.

The relationship of the hemicords to the arachnoid and dural tubes defines two different forms of diastematomyelia (15, 36, 37, 51, 53).

DIASTEMATOMYELIA WITH A SINGLE ARACHNOID TUBE AND A SINGLE COAXIAL DURAL TUBE (FIG. 18.8)

In 50% of all cases of diastematomyelia, the two, pia-lined hemicords lie side by side in a single undivided subarachnoid space and are encompassed within a single undivided tube of arachnoid mater. External to the arachnoid tube lies a single undivided coaxial tube of dura mater. The anterior spinal artery remains unfused and "duplicated" along the length of the two hemicords. This form of diastematomyelia is not associated with any bone spur or fibrous septum and is rarely symptomatic (37).

DIASTEMATOMYELIA WITH LOCAL DOUBLING OF THE ARACHNOID AND DURAL TUBES

In the other 50% of all cases of diastematomyelia, the arachnoid mater and dura mater also separate into paired arachnoid and dural tubes, one set surrounding each of the two hemicords (15, 36, 37, 51, 53). Thus, each hemicord has separate pial, arachnoid, and dural sheaths for a limited number of segments (Fig. 18.3). The medial walls of the two dural tubes form a double-layered dural partition between the two hemicords. The

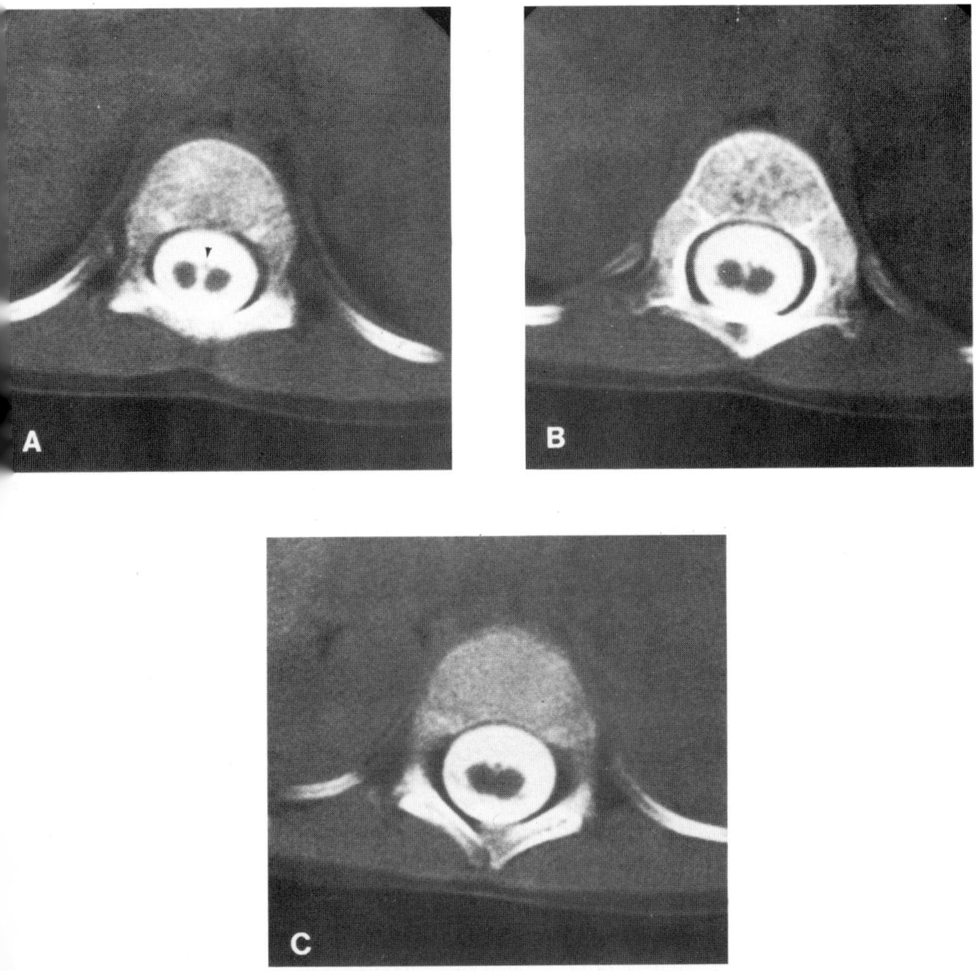

FIG. 18.8. Diastematomyelia with single arachnoid tube and single coaxial dural tube (*A–C*). Metrizamide CT myelography. (*A*) The two hemicords lie within a single subarachnoid space. The anterior spinal artery (*arrowhead*) is bifid. There is no bone spur or fibrous partition. (*B*) At the lower end of the diastematomyelia, the dorsal halves of the two hemicords have reunited partially, leaving a partial ventral diastematomyelia. (*C*) More inferiorly, the two hemicords have reunited nearly completely. The anterior spinal artery is single.

space between the two walls of the dural partition is the interdural cleft (51, 53). Most patients with this form of diastematomyelia have a fibrous band or osteocartilaginous spur which passes through the interdural cleft between and external to the medial walls of the two dural tubes (36, 37)

(Fig. 18.3). Fibrous adhesions frequently attach the bone spur to the adjacent dural walls. The bone spur typically lies at the lower end of the interdural cleft. If it does not, a second separate spur should be sought at the lower end of the interdural cleft (35). The cleft in the cord (*i.e.*, the diastematomyelia itself) is necessarily longer than the interposed dural partition by millimeters to centimeters, and so extends into the single arachnoid-single dural tube above the dural partition, sometimes for long distances (15, 51, 53). When the two hemicords reunite below the dural partition, the cleft in the cord may also extend into the single arachnoid and single dural tube below the partition.

The spinal column is nearly always grossly abnormal in diastematomyelia. The laminae are abnormal in 91% of patients with diastematomyelia (35). They are often thickened and are often fused with the adjacent laminae ipsilaterally or diagonally (intersegmental laminar fusion). Spina bifida of greater severity than nonfusion of the spinous processes of L5 and S1 is present in 86–100% of patients with diastematomyelia (35). Combined intersegmental laminar fusions and spina bifida are present in 60% of cases of diastematomyelia, and are highly suggestive of the diagnosis of diastematomyelia and the site of the clefting (35). The interpediculate distance is typically widened at the level of the diastematomyelia (35–37, 69).

Eighty-five percent of patients have abnormalities of multiple vertebral bodies, including hemivertebrae, butterfly vertebrae, block vertebrae, and narrowed intervertebral disk spaces (35). Scoliosis and kyphosis are present in 50–60% of patients with diastematomyelia and are directly related to the bony anomalies themselves (35). The incidence and severity of these curvatures increase with age. Diastematomyelia accounts for 4.9% of 392 cases of congenital scoliosis (35).

The bone spur is *not* a necessary feature of diastematomyelia. It is present in only one-half of cases, *i.e.*, most of those with double arachnoid and double dural tubes (37). The spur may traverse the entire, or nearly the entire, sagittal dimension of the canal and attach to the dorsal canal wall, the ventral canal wall, or both (35, 45, 68) (Fig. 18.9). The spur projects only partway into the canal in patients with partial diastematomyelia (27). The attachment of the spur to the canal wall may be a synchrondrosis (15), accounting for the small lucent gap demonstrated on CT. Similar lucent gaps between portions of the bone spur appear to represent cartilage between ossification centers in the spur (15). The spur may lie along the midsagittal plane and may divide the spinal canal into two equal hemicanals which lie side by side. Scoliosis may rotate such a spur off the midline, so the hemicanals lie more ventral and dorsal than side by side (51, 53) (Fig. 18.9). Occasionally, the spur crosses the

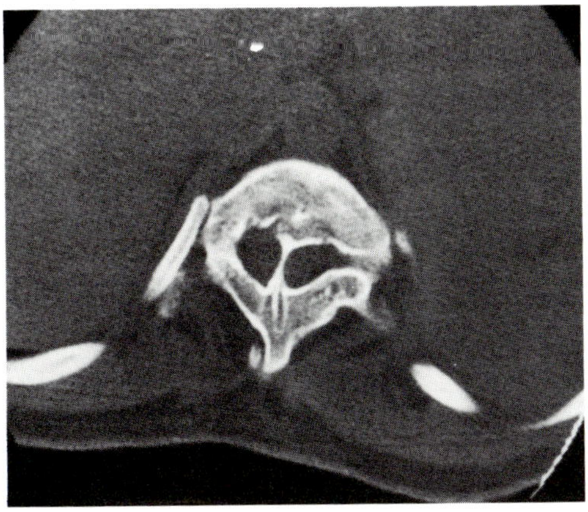

FIG. 18.9. Diastematomyelia with bone spur. Noncontrast CT discloses the typical bony changes of this form of diastematomyelia: a sagittally short, broad vertebral body; short, thick laminae; a stubby spinous process; a sagittally oriented bone spur which extends between the vertebral body and the lamina to form two nearly symmetrical hemicanals; and scoliosis which rotates the vertebral body and the spur away from the midsagittal plane.

canal very obliquely and inserts into an outwardly rotated lamina or pedicle to create two very unequal hemicords (Fig. 18.3). In such cases, the smaller hemicanal typically lies ventral to the larger hemicanal.

In combined series, the spur was observed at L1-L3 in 48% of cases, T7-T12 in 26% of cases, L4-L5 in 18% of cases, and T1-T6 in 5% of cases (41). Cervical spurs are rare. Two spurs at separate sites are observed in 5–6% of cases (35, 51).

The Split Notochord Syndrome

The split notochord syndrome is a term used to designate, collectively, the group of disorders believed to represent sequelae of splitting or deviation of the notochord with persistent communication between the gut and the dorsal skin (1). The archetype and most severe form of this abnormality is the dorsal enteric fistula: a persistent, patent track which extends from the mesenteric border of the intestine through the mesentery and the prevertebral tissue, vertebral bodies (or interspaces), spinal canal, meninges, spinal cord, dorsal elements of the spine, and dorsal raphe to the midline skin (7, 8, 10). As with the analogous vitelline duct remnants, any portion(s) of the dorsal enteric fistula may become obliterated, leaving isolated diverticula, duplications, cysts, fibrous cords, and/or sinuses at any point(s) along the segmental track of the anomaly (7, 8, 10). Because the track represents a segmental anomaly, and because the bowel segments migrate inferiorly and rotate, it is common to trace such enteric remnants far upward through the mesentery, diaphragm, and mediastinum to the cervical or high-thoracic vertebrae. Butterfly vertebrae, hemivertebrae, block vertebrae, diastematomyelia, anterior and posterior spina bifida, and enteric-lined cysts in the prevertebral, postvertebral, and intracanalicular compartments are natural consequences of this anomaly.

Patients with intraspinal enteric cysts usually exhibit CT evidence of an intraspinal mass with widened interpediculate distances and eroded laminae and bodies. Newborns and infants often exhibit the vertebral anomalies described above, whereas older patients often show no segmentation anomalies (Fig. 18.10). The cysts are thin- or thick-walled, are usually large at the time of presentation, and typically displace the cord dorsally. Less frequently, they lie between two hemicords, displacing them laterally, or they lie dorsally and displace the cord ventrally.

Dorsal Dermal Sinuses

Congenital dermal sinuses are epithelium-lined dermal tubes which extend from the skin surface for varying distances and which frequently connect with the central nervous system or its coverings (50). In Wright's

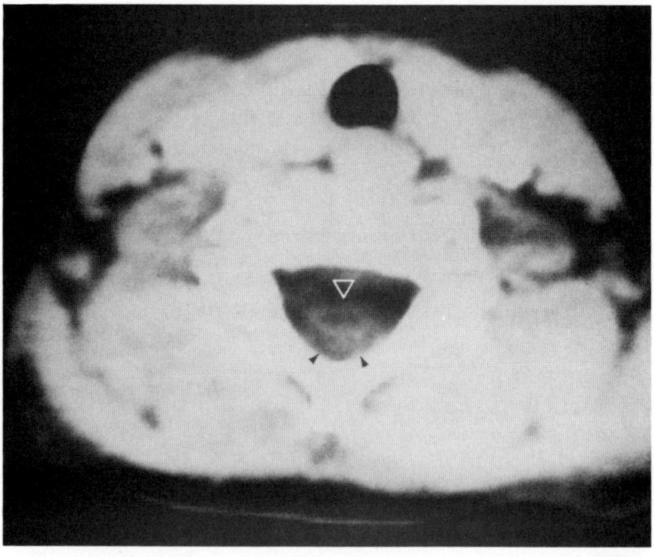

FIG. 18.10. Intraspinal enteric cyst, C7-T1. Split notochord syndrome. Highly processed (filtered) CT images disclose the upper pole of a thick-walled cyst (*open arrowhead*) which compresses the spinal cord (*black arrowheads*) and displaces it posteriorly. The cyst entered and attached to a defect in the body of T1, which was not detected in the CT sections obtained.

collected series of 127 dorsal dermal sinuses, 1 was sacrococcygeal, 72 were lumbosacral, 12 were thoracic, 2 were cervical, 30 were occipital, and 10 were at diverse loci (mostly ventral to the skull and spinal column) (71). Approximately 60% of dermal sinuses terminate in deep dermoid or epidermoid cysts (13). Conversely, 20–30% of dermoid tumors are associated with dermal sinuses (26, 30, 44). Nearly two-thirds of dermal sinuses become infected, potentially leading to epidural, subdural, subarachnoid, and/or extensive intramedullary abscesses (6, 13, 66). Dermal sinuses account for up to 3% of spinal cord abscesses (3).

The dermal sinuses are usually thin (0.5–7 mm), are lined by cutaneous elements and collagen, and extend deeply through the subcutaneous tissue, so that they appear on CT as thin, dense tracts which lead from the skin surface toward the spinal canal. One-half to two-thirds of dermal sinuses extend intraspinally (6, 13, 26, 30, 44). Because the dermal tracts follow a segmental distribution, and because the spinal cord normally "ascends" with respect to the vertebrae as the patient grows, the dermal sinus tract frequently ascends cephalad as it penetrates deeply from skin surface to the spinal cord (46) (Fig. 18.11). The full course of such sinuses must be defined on serial CT sections at and above the external ostium therefore (Fig. 18.12).

The sinuses may extend intracanalicularly (a) between two spinous processes, (b) along a groove in one spinous process, or (c) through a bifid spinous process. Expansion of the spinal canal usually signifies a coexistent (epi)dermoid cyst (46, 50). The dermal sinus tract penetrates to a variable depth. It may merge with the dura and stop. If it extends more deeply, a dorsally oriented sleeve of dura and arachnoid typically encompasses the entry of the tract (46). The sinus may terminate in the subarachnoid space and discharge (opacified) CSF (62). More commonly, the thin sinus tract traverses the subarachnoid space to terminate in the conus medullaris, the filum terminale, a nerve root, a fibrous nodule in the dorsal column of the cord, or an (epi)dermoid cyst (32, 46, 61, 62). Metrizamide CT then shows the filling defect of the dermal sinus in the subarachnoid space, any expansion of the cord and canal by concomitant (epi)dermoid cyst, and any discharge of opacified CSF into the tract (51, 62). Conversely, routine CT and metrizamide CT myelography can demonstrate that the tract is not connected with the spinal canal at all and does not require extensive surgery.

Spinal Lipomas

Spinal lipomas are collections of fat and connective tissue which appear at least partially encapsulated and which have definite connections with the meninges and spinal cord (19). These lipomas are composed of monotonous masses of mature fat cells which are divided into lobules by

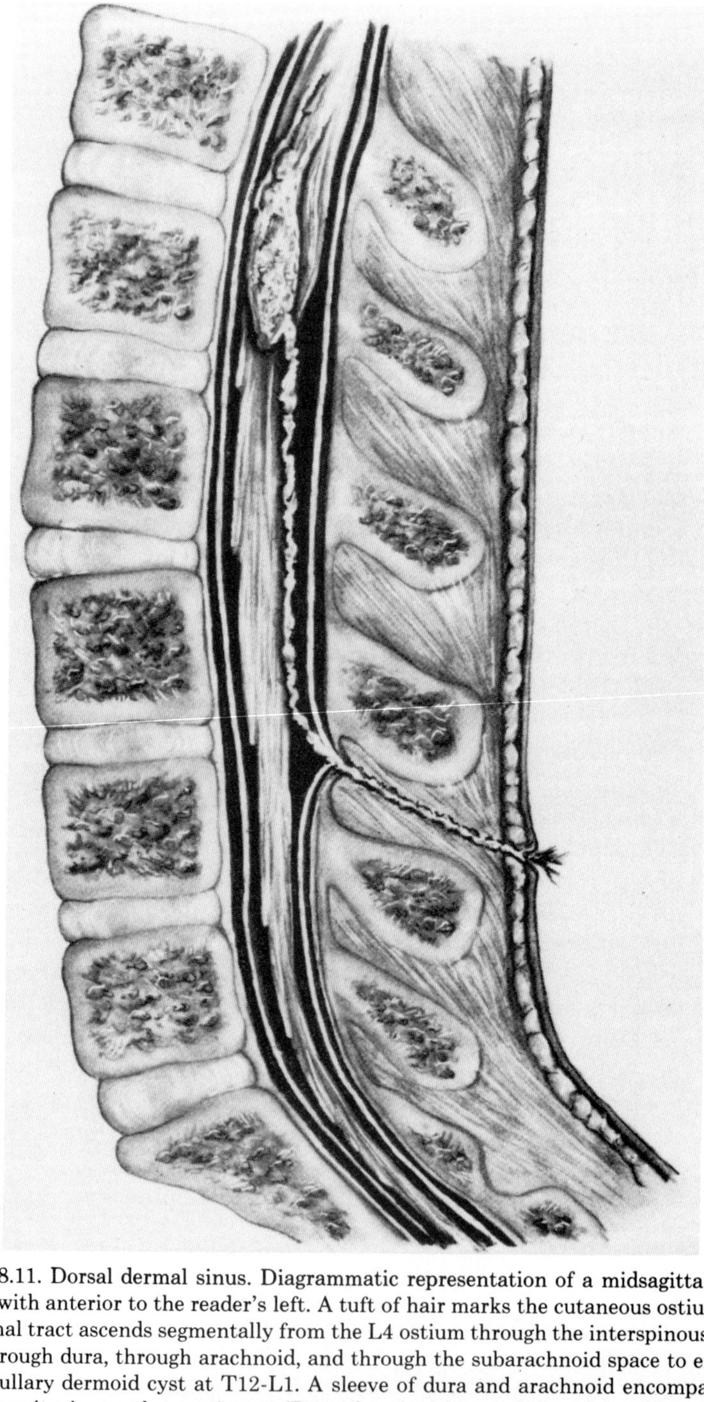

FIG. 18.11. Dorsal dermal sinus. Diagrammatic representation of a midsagittal section oriented with anterior to the reader's left. A tuft of hair marks the cutaneous ostium at L4. The dermal tract ascends segmentally from the L4 ostium through the interspinous median raphe, through dura, through arachnoid, and through the subarachnoid space to end in an intramedullary dermoid cyst at T12-L1. A sleeve of dura and arachnoid encompasses the tract where it pierces the meninges. (Reproduced with permission from D. D. Matson. *Neurosurgery of Infancy and Childhood*, Ed. 2. Springfield, Ill., Charles C Thomas, 1969.)

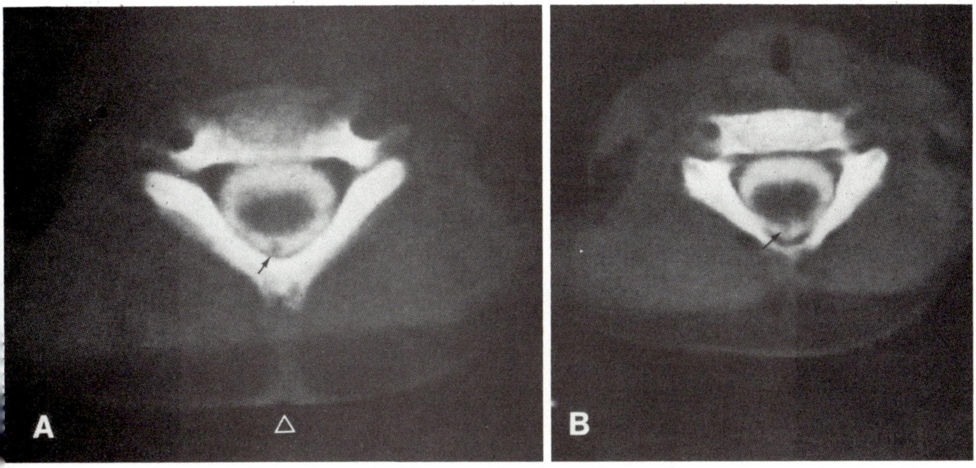

FIG. 18.12. Cervical dermal sinus. (*A* and *B*). Metrizamide CT myelography. The ostium (*open arrowhead*) of the dermal sinus and the subcutaneous portion of the sinus are shown by virtue of the greater density of cutaneous elements and collagen in the wall of the tract. The round, midline structure (*arrow*) in the posterior cervical subarachnoid space is the cross section of the subarachnoid portion of the tract. This passes superiorly to end just off the midline at a portion of the cervical spinal cord which appears to have deeper ventral and dorsal median sulci, suggestive of a very mild *forme fruste* of diastematomyelia.

variably heavy connective tissue strands. The proportion of connective tissue is greatest near the lipal-neural interface and least near the dorsal surface of lipoma (18, 43) (Fig. 18.13). Calcification and ossification are uncommon (23, 43, 67).

Spinal lipomas are commonly divided into three major groups: (a) "intradural" lipomas, (b) lipomyelomeningoceles, and (c) fibrolipomas of the filum terminale (16).

INTRADURAL LIPOMAS

The intradural lipomas are a group of juxtamedullary lipomas which remain nearly completely confined within a normal or narrowly bifid spinal canal. The subcutaneous tissue overlying these is often normal, or nearly so. As a group, the intradural lipomas constitute slightly less than 1% of primary intraspinal tumors (23).

Intradural lipomas typically involve the cervical and thoracic spinal cords (cervical 12%, cervicothoracic 24%, thoracic 30%) but may affect any part of the cord or cauda equina (14, 23) (Fig. 18.14). Most such lipomas affect the dorsal surface of cord (23, 59). Some 25% are described as affecting the lateral or anterolateral surfaces of the cord, but the degree of cord rotation induced by the lipoma is not described in these cases. The lipoma is usually predominantly juxtamedullary-subpial in

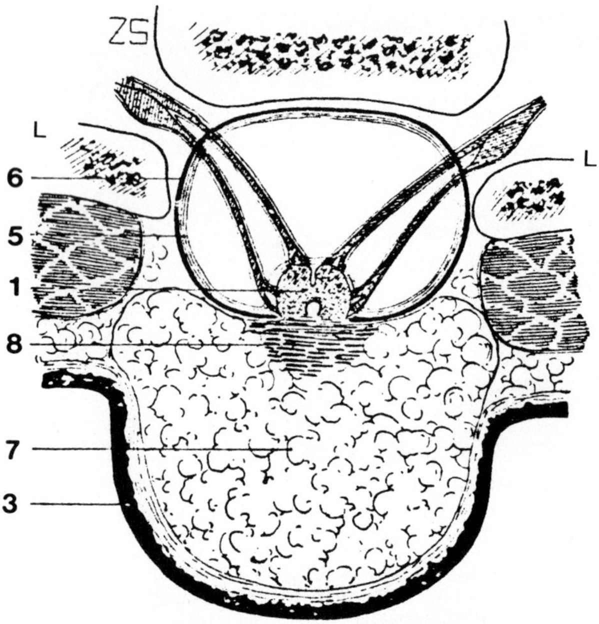

FIG. 18.13. Anatomic relationships in lipomyelomeningocele. The neural placode (*1*) shows partial dorsal myeloschisis and lies posterior to the bifid laminae (*L, L*). The dorsal nerve roots and ventral nerve roots arise from the placode (*1*), not the lipoma (*7*), and return to the spinal canal to exit normally. The dura (*dark line 6*) is deficient dorsally and attaches to the neural placode just posterior to the dorsal root entry zone. The pia-arachnoid (*fainter lines 5*) forms one continuous membrane which lines the ventral surface of the placode and extends ventrally, deep to dura, as the arachnoid sac. The lipoma attaches tightly onto the dorsal surface of the neural placode via a fibrous connective tissue (*8*) and is loosely approximated to the dura lateral to the placode. The skin (*3*) forms an intact layer over the lipoma. In the authors' opinion, the fibrous tissue is not as heavily concentrated at the placode as is depicted here. Rather, the fibrous tissue divides the lipoma into lobules and extends farther out into the fat, while the fat (contained within fibrous tissue) reaches far closer to the placode itself. The authors believe that the same anatomic relationships hold in many so-called "intradural" lipomas (Reproduced with permission from J. B. Leveuf (43).)

location (23). Approximately 45% of intradural lipomas also have an extramedullary component, often representing the upper or lower pole of the mass (23). Low-lying intradural lipomas may tether the conus medullaris.

Intradural lipomas have a fine, whitish capsule which divides the lipoma into lobules and which appears continuous at its margins with thickened pia-arachnoid. The dura is usually tense and displaced posteriorly by such lipomas (12). The dura is deficient posteriorly when the intradural lipoma is associated with an extradural-subcutaneous component of lipoma.

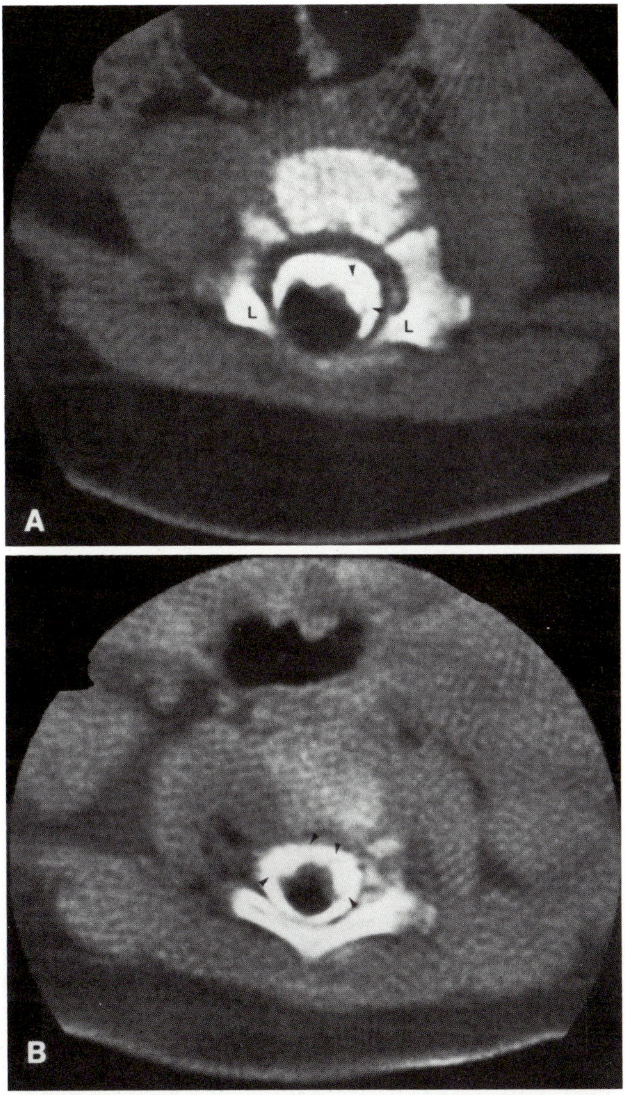

FIG. 18.14. "Intradural" lipoma (*A* and *B*) Metrizamide CT myelography. The anatomic relationships depicted correspond well to those diagrammed in Figure 18.13. The laminae (*L, L*) are bifid. The lucent lipoma appears to splay the unneurulated neural placode, to displace it anteriorly, and then to ascend along the dorsal myeloschisis to underlie an intact neural arch. The pia-arachnoid and opacified subarachnoid space, which appear to surround the lipoma in *B*, are actually seen to be reflected away from the lipoma and placode in *A*. The reflected pia-arachnoid extends ventrally to form the arachnoid sac. The dorsal and ventral nerve roots (*arrowheads*) emerge from the placode and pass forward through the opacified subarachnoid space.

Intradural lipomas may lie within a normal spinal canal. More commonly, they cause focal expansion of the spinal canal and, at times, the adjacent neural foramina (51, 52). Narrow or very focal spina bifida is frequently present. Segmentation anomalies are uncommon.

LIPOMYELOMENINGOCELES

Lipomyelomeningoceles are lipomas intimately attached to a neural placode which herniates through a widely bifid spinal canal to form a dorsal subcutaneous mass composed of fat, fibrous tissue, neural tissue, and meningocele (43, 48, 49, 51, 52) (Fig. 18.15). As a group, lipomyelomeningoceles account for 20% of skin-covered lumbosacral masses (42) and 20–56% of occult spinal dysraphism (65).

Lipomyelomeningoceles typically involve the lumbosacral spinal cord and typically tether it in low position (48, 51, 52). Anatomically, they are analogous to the myelomeningocele, with the additional features of a lipoma attached to the dorsal surface of the neural tissue and an intact skin cover. The neural tissue characteristically remains in the form of the unneurulated neural folds, with a midline groove representing the primitive neural groove of the placode (43, 48, 51, 52). The midline groove

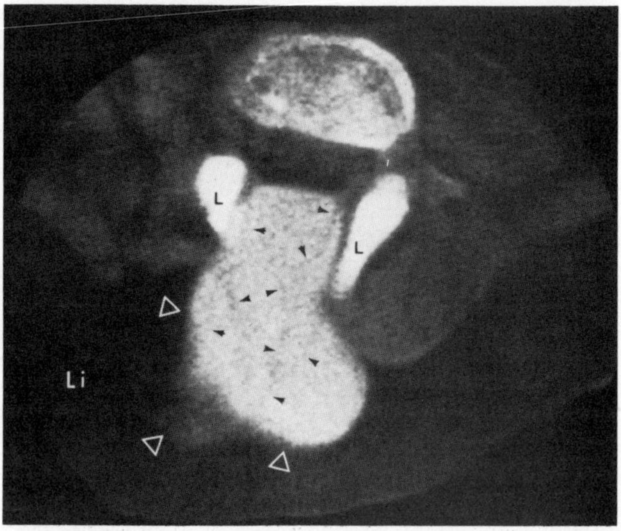

FIG. 18.15. Lipomyelomeningocele. Metrizamide CT myelography demonstrates the bifid laminae (*L, L*); the asymmetric, skin-covered lipoma (*Li*); the neural placode (*open arrowheads*); the opacified arachnoid sac, which herniates through the spina bifida and bulges to the side opposite the lipoma; and the nerve roots (*closed arrowheads*), which emerge from the placode and pass through the subarachnoid space to reenter the spinal canal.

is continuous superiorly and inferiorly with the central canal of the spinal cord. The lipoma is situated along the dorsal surface of the neural placode and may extend cephalad along the groove into the central canal of the intact cord above it (48, 51, 52). In the uncomplicated case, the lipal-neural junction appears deceptively smooth (48, 51, 52). Irregularity of this junction suggests the presence of other complicating dysraphic elements such as an associated epidermoid cyst (51, 52).

The dural tube is deficient dorsally in the region of the lipoma. The dura appears to attach to the lateral surface of the neural placode just dorsal to the root entry zones of the dorsal nerve roots (43, 51, 52). This leaves a dorsal dural deficiency through which the dorsal surface of placode is exposed to lipoma (43, 48, 51, 52). The pia-arachnoid forms a single continuous membrane which lines the ventral surface of the neural placode and continues ventrally, beneath the dura, as the arachnoid sac (43, 48, 51, 52). The dorsal and ventral nerve roots all arise from the ventral, pia-covered surface of placode and traverse the subarachnoid space prior to exiting via their root sleeves (43, 48, 51, 52). The lipoma itself lies outside the subarachnoid space, arachnoid sac, and dural sac (43, 48, 51, 52). The junction of lipoma, neural placode, and CSF lies along the lateral edge of the neural placode just dorsal to the dorsal root entry zone (48, 51, 52).

Expansion of the ventral subarachnoid space appears to displace the cord, placode, and lipoma dorsally through the spina bifida into the subcutaneous tissue as a lipomyelomeningocele. Because the lipoma is often asymmetric (40%) (9, 48) and anchors the dorsal surface of the placode, the dorsal surface of placode rotates toward the lipoma as the placode herniates (51, 52). The contralateral nerve roots then come to lie in the midline behind the protective laminae, where they are at increased risk for operative trauma (48, 51, 52). The meningocele typically bulges to the side opposite an asymmetric lipoma. The expanding subarachnoid space thins and invaginates the herniating placode and, in effect, converts the pancaked placode into a thin everted wall for the arachnoid sac. Such thinned areas of placode still give rise to functional nerve roots (48, 51, 52).

The spinal canal is typically wide at the site of the lipomeningocele. At the lipomeningocele, the posterior elements of the spine exhibit a sequence of progressive dysraphism consisting of (from above downward) (a) the lowest intact neural arch (possibly with a stubby spinous process), (b) zero to 2 *narrowly* bifid neural arch(es) with laminae that curve posterior to the spinal canal but just fail to fuse in the midline, and (c) one widely bifid neural arch with laminae that are joined by a fibrovascular band (51, 52). Below (c), the laminae are widely bifid for a variable length, often over the entire distal spine, and have no associated fibrovascular bands. If the laminae reform into a normal spinal canal below the lipomeningocele, then the abnormal vertebrae (a–c) usually reappear in reverse sequence (51, 52). The fibrovascular band, which joins the laminae of the most cephalic *widely* bifid laminae, forms the superior edge of the soft tissue defect through which the cord, placode, lipoma, and meningocele herniate (51, 52). This fibrous band tethers the herniated tissue; kinks the cord, placode, and/or sac sharply; and appears to compromise cord function, since section of the band is associated with increased amplitude and reduced latency of somatosensory-evoked potentials recorded during surgery (48, 51, 52). If the canal reforms below, a fibrovascular band joining the lowest widely bifid laminae often forms the inferior edge of the soft tissue defect through which the lipomyelomeningocele herniates.

Segmentation anomalies of the vertebral bodies are found in up to 43% of cases (24). Sacral asymmetry, confluent sacral neural foramina, partial sacral agenesis, and abnormally wide sacroiliac joints are present in up to 50% of patients (15, 51, 52, 57).

FIBROLIPOMAS OF THE FILUM TERMINALE

The normal filum terminale is a long, thin, fibrous stalk with both intradural and extradural components. It extends as a pia-lined, intradural stalk from the tip of the conus medullaris to the tip of the dural sac, pierces the dura, and then extends distally as an extradural fibrous cord to insert onto the dorsal aspect of the first coccygeal vertebra (19). A separate branch of the extradural filum occasionally extends dorsally to the skin, where it inserts into a dimple overlying the coccyx (19). A filar fibrolipoma may be detected as an incidental finding in 4–6% of postmortem evaluations of presumably normal spinal cords (19). James and Lassman (37) observed a filar lipoma only once (0.7%) in their series of surgically treated spinal dysraphism, but Emery and Lendon (19) identified filar fibrolipomas in 67% of 100 myelomeningocele patients examined at postmortem. In Emery and Lendon's series (19), 34% were limited to the intradural portion of the filum, and 27% were limited to the extradural portion of the filum; 39% involved both intradural and extradural portions of the filum in continuity. The intradural fibrolipomas are distinct, lucent, sausage-shaped masses which do not extend cephalad to the ventriculus terminalis and which taper where the filum pierces the dura (Fig. 18.16). The extradural fibrolipomas are usually larger and become less distinct where they expand into the adjacent extradural fat (19).

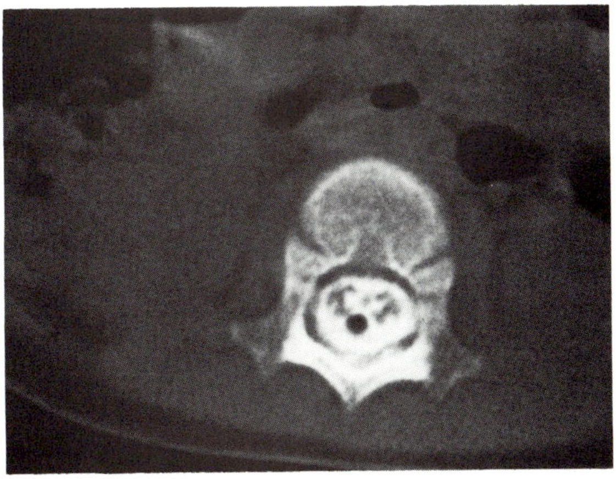

FIG. 18.16. Lipoma of the filum terminale. Metrizamide CT myelography demonstrates an intact spinal canal; the paired symmetrical roots of the cauda equina; and a very lucent, abnormally thick dorsal midline structure, representing the lipoma of the filum terminale.

TIGHT FILUM TERMINALE

The tight filum terminale syndrome designates a complex of neurologic and orthopedic deformities associated with a short, thick filum terminale and low position of the conus medullaris (21, 34, 39). Normally, the filum terminale measures less than 2 mm in thickness (25). Normally, the spinal cord reaches adult levels of L1-L2 by 48 weeks of gestational age (1–2 months postpartum) (4). With individual variation, however, the conus may reach adult levels by 31 weeks of gestation or may be found in unusually low position in apparently normal older individuals (L2-L3 in a 12-year-old child) (4, 30). As a rule, the conus should not lie below the mid-L2 level by age 12 years (30).

Patients with tight filum terminale syndrome may exhibit spina bifida occulta of limited numbers of lumbosacral vertebrae (34, 39). Congenital or developmental (kypho)scoliosis is present in 25% of patients. The filum is usually thickened to, perhaps, 5 mm in diameter. The spinal cord is characteristically tethered to the spinal canal by the tight filum and is stretched tightly across any kyphoscoliosis.

The arachnoid and dural sacs are frequently widened. They are tense and tented posteriorly by the taut filum terminale. The filum is so tightly applied to the posterior wall of the meningeal sac, however, that it may be detectable only by CT, not routine myelography.

Filar lipomas coexist in 23% of cases of tight filum terminale syndrome, and filar cysts coexist in 3% of cases (34). In 13% of cases, there is no distinct filum terminale and no distinct transition between conus medullaris and filum terminale. Rather, the spinal cord appears to extend all the way down to the caudal end of the thecal sac, where it ends in a small lipoma (34).

REFERENCES

1. Anderson, F. M. Occult spinal dysraphism: Diagnosis and management. J. Pediatr., *73:* 163–177, 1968.
2. Arredondo, F., Haughton, V. M., Hemmy, D. C., Zelaya, B., and Williams, A. L. The computed tomographic appearance of the spinal cord in diastematomyelia. Radiology, *136:* 685–688, 1980.
3. Arzt, P. K. Abscess within the spinal cord: Review of the literature and report of three cases. Arch. Neurol. Psychiatry, *51:* 533–543, 1944.
4. Barson, A. J. The vertebral level of termination of the spinal cord during normal and abnormal development. J. Anat., *106:* 489–497, 1970.
5. Batnitzky, S., Hall, P. V., Lindseth, R. E., and Wellman, H. N. Meningomyelocele and syringohydromyelia: Some radiological aspects. Radiology, *120:* 351–357, 1976.
6. Bean, J. R., Walsh, J. W., and Blacker, H. M. Cervical dermal sinus and intramedullary spinal cord abscess: Case report. Neurosurgery, *5:* 60–62, 1979.
7. Beardmore, H. E., and Wiglesworth, F. W. Vertebral anomalies and alimentary duplications: Clinical and embryological aspects. Pediatr. Clin. North Am., *5:* 457–473, 1958.
8. Bentley, J. F. R., and Smith, J. R. Developmental posterior enteric remnants and spinal malformations: The split notochord syndrome. Arch. Dis. Child., *35:* 76–86, 1960.
9. Bruce, D. A., and Schut, L. Spinal lipomas in infancy and childhood. Child's Brain, *5:* 192–203, 1979.
10. Burrows, F. G. O., and Sutcliffe, J. The split notochord syndrome. Br. J. Radiol., *41:* 844–847, 1968.
11. Cameron, A. H. The Arnold-Chiari and other neuro-anatomical malformations associated with spina bifida. J. Pathol. Bacteriol., *73:* 195–211, 1957.
12. Caram, P. C., Scarcella, G., and Carton, C. A. Intradural lipomas of the spinal cord with particular emphasis on the "intramedullary" lipomas. J. Neurosurg., *14:* 28–42, 1957.
13. Cardell, B. S., and Laurance, B. Congenital dermal sinus associated with meningitis: Report of a fatal case. Br. Med. J., *2:* 1558–1561, 1951.
14. Chapman, P. H. Congenital intraspinal lipomas: Anatomic considerations and surgical treatment. Child's Brain, *9:* 37–47, 1982.
15. Cohen, J., and Sledge, C. B. Diastematomyelia: An embryological interpretation with report of a case. Am. J. Dis. Child., *100:* 257–263, 1960.
16. Dubowitz, V., Lorber, J., and Zachary, R. B. Lipoma of the cauda equina. Arch. Dis. Child., *40:* 207–213, 1965.
17. Duckworth, T., Sharrard, W. J., Lister, J., and Seymour, N. Hemimyelocele. Dev. Med. Child Neurol., *10* (Suppl. 16): 69–75, 1968.
18. Ehni, G., and Love, J. G. Intraspinal lipomas: Report of cases, review of the literature, and clinical and pathological study. Arch. Neurol. Psychiatry, *53:* 1–28, 1945.
19. Emery, J. L., and Lendon, R. G. Lipomas of the cauda equina and other fatty tumours related to neurospinal dysraphism. Dev. Med. Child Neurol., *11* (Suppl. 20): 62–70, 1969.
20. Emery, J. L., and Lendon, R. G. The local cord lesion in neurospinal dysraphism (meningomyelocele). J. Pathol., *110:* 83–96, 1973.
21. Fitz, C. R., and Harwood-Nash, D. C. The tethered conus. Am. J. Roentgenol. Radium Ther. Nucl. Med., *125:* 515–523, 1975.

22. Friede, R. L. *Developmental Neuropathology*, pp. 266–271. Springer-Verlag, New York, 1975.
23. Guiffre, R. Intradural spinal lipomas: Review of the literature (99 cases) and report of an additional case. Acta Neurochir., *14:* 69–95, 1966.
24. Gold, L. H. A., Kieffer, S. A., and Peterson, H. O. Lipomatous invasion of the spinal cord associated with spinal dysraphism: Myelographic evaluation. AJR, *107:* 479–485, 1969.
25. Gryspeerdt, G. L. Myelographic assessment of occult forms of spinal dysraphism. Acta Radiol. [Diagn.] (Stockh.) *1:* 702–717, 1963.
26. Guidetti, B., and Gagliardi, F. M. Epidermoid and dermoid cysts: Clinical evaluation and late surgical results. J. Neurosurg., *47:* 12–18, 1977.
27. Guthkelch, A. N. Diastematomyelia with median septum. Brain, *97:* 729–742, 1974.
28. Hall, P. V., Campbell, R. L., and Kalsbeck, J. E. Meningomyelocele and progressive hydromyelia: Progressive paresis in myelodysplasia. J. Neurosurg., *43:* 457–463, 1975.
29. Hall, P., Lindseth, R., Campbell, R., Kalsbeck, J. E., and Desousa, A. Scoliosis and hydrocephalus in myelocele patients: The effects of ventricular shunting. J. Neurosurg., *50:* 174–178, 1979.
30. Harwood-Nash, D. C., and Fitz, C. R. *Neuroradiology in Infants and Children.* Vol. 3, pp. 1054–1227. C. V. Mosby, St. Louis, 1976.
31. Harwood-Nash, D. C. Computed tomography of the pediatric spine: A protocol for the 1980s. Radiol. Clin. North Am., *19:* 479–494, 1981.
32. Haworth, J. C., and Zachary, R. B. Congenital dermal sinuses in children: Their relation to pilonidal sinuses. Lancet, *2:* 10–14, 1955.
33. Heinz, E. R., Rosenbaum, A. E., Scarff, T. B., Reigel, D. H., and Drayer, B. P. Tethered spinal cord following meningomyelocele repair. Radiology, *131:* 153–160, 1979.
34. Hendrick, E. B., Hoffman, H. J., and Humphreys, R. P. Tethered cord syndrome. In: *Myelomeningocele*, edited by R. L. McLaurin, pp. 369–376. Grune & Stratton, New York, 1977.
35. Hilal, S. K., Marton, D., and Pollack, E. Diastematomyelia in children: Radiographic study of 34 cases. Radiology, *112:* 609–621, 1974.
36. James, C. C. M., and Lassman, L. P. Diastematomyelia: A critical survey of 24 cases submitted to laminectomy. Arch. Dis. Child., *39,* 125–130, 1964.
37. James, C. C. M., and Lassman, L. P. *Spinal Dysraphism: Spina Bifida Occulta.* Appleton-Century-Crofts, New York (Butterworth & Co., London), 1972.
38. James, H. E., and Oliff, M. Computed tomography in spinal dysraphism. J. Comput. Assist. Tomogr., *1:* 391–397, 1977.
39. Jones, P. H., and Love, J. G. Tight filum terminale. Arch. Surg. *73:* 556–566, 1956.
40. Kaiser, M. C., Pettersson, H., Harwood-Nash, D. C., Fitz, C. R., and Armstrong, E. Direct coronal CT of the spine in infants and children. Am. J. Neuroradiol., *2:* 465–466, 1981.
41. Keim, H. A., and Greene, A. F. Diastematomyelia and scoliosis. J. Bone Joint Surg. [Am.], *55A:* 1425–1435, 1973.
42. Lemire, R. J., Graham, C. B., and Beckwith, J. B. Skin-covered sacrococcygeal masses in infants and children. J. Pediatr., *79:* 948–954, 1971.
43. Leveuf, J. B. Spina bifida avec tumeur. In: *Etudes sur le Spina Bifida*, Chap. IV. Masson et Cie, Paris, 1937.
44. List, C. F. Intraspinal epidermoids, dermoids, and dermal sinuses. Surg. Gynecol. Obstet. *73:* 525–538, 1941.
45. Lohkamp, F., Claussen, C., and Schuhmacher, G. CT demonstration of pathologic changes of the spinal cord accompanying spina bifida and diastematomyelia. Prog. Pediatr. Radiol., *6:* 200–227, 1978.
46. Matson, D. D. *Neurosurgery of Infancy and Childhood*, Ed. 2. Charles C Thomas,

Springfield, Ill., 1969.
47. McLone, D. G. Technique for closure of myelomeningocele. Child's Brain, *6:* 65–73, 1980.
48. McLone, D. G., Mutluer, S., and Naidich, T. P. Lipomeningoceles of the conus medullaris. In: *Concepts in Pediatric Neurosurgery*, Vol. 3, edited by the American Society for Pediatric Neurosurgeons. S. Karger, Basel, 1983.
49. McLone, D. G., Mutluer, S., and Naidich, T. P. Lipomeningoceles of the conus medullaris. Presented at the 10th Annual Meeting of the International Society for Paediatric Neurosurgery, Philadelphia, Pennsylvania, September 1982.
50. Mount, L. A. Congenital dermal sinuses as a cause of meningitis, intraspinal abscess and intracranial abscess. JAMA, *139:* 1263–1268, 1949.
51. Naidich, T. P., McLone, D. G., and Harwood-Nash, D. C. Dysraphism. In: *Modern Neuroradiology*, Vol. 1, *Computed Tomography of the Spine and Spinal Cord*, Chap. 17, edited by T. H. Newton and D. G. Potts. Clavadel Press, San Francisco and New York, 1982.
52. Naidich, T. P., McLone, D. G., and Mutluer, S. Neuroradiology and surgical correction of lipomyeloschisis of the conus medullaris: An approach to understanding dorsal dysraphism with lipoma. Submitted for publication to Am. J. Neuroradiol., 1982.
53. Naidich, T. P., and Harwood-Nash, D. C. Diastematomyelia. Part I. Hemicords and meningeal sheaths. Single and double arachnoid and dural tubes. Presented at the XII Symposium Neuroradiologicum, Washington, D.C., October 1982.
54. Northfield, D. W. C. *The Surgery of the Central Nervous System: A Textbook for Postgraduate Students*, pp. 467–536. Blackwell Scientific Publications, Oxford, 1973.
55. Pang, D., and Wilberger, J. E., Jr. Tethered cord syndrome in adults. J. Neurosurg., *57:* 32–47, 1982.
56. Resjo, I. M., Harwood-Nash, D. C., Fitz, C. R., and Chuang, S. Computed tomographic metrizamide myelography in spinal dysraphism in infants and children. J. Comput. Assist. Tomogr., *2:* 549–558, 1978.
57. Roller, G. J., and Pribram, H. F. W. Lumbosacral intradural lipoma and sacral agenesis. Radiology, *84:* 507–511, 1965.
58. Scatliff, J. H., Till, K., and Hoare, R. D. Incomplete, false, and true diastematomyelia. Radiological evaluation by air myelography and tomography. Radiology, *116:* 349–354, 1975.
59. Schroeder, S., Lackner, K., and Weiand, G. Lumbosacral intradural lipoma. J. Comput. Assist. Tomogr., *5:* 274, 1981.
60. Schut, L., Pizzi, F. J., and Bruce, D. A. Occult spinal dysraphism. In: *Myelomeningocele*, edited by R. L. McLaurin, pp. 349–368. Grune & Stratton, New York, 1977.
61. Schwartz, H. G. Congenital tumors of the spinal cord in infants. Ann. Surg., *136:* 183–192, 1952.
62. Scotti, G., Musgrave, M. A., Harwood-Nash, D. C., Fitz, C. R., and Chuang, S. H. Diastematomyelia in children: Metrizamide and CT metrizamide myelography. Am. J. Neuroradiol., *1:* 403–410, 1980.
63. Scotti, G., Harwood-Nash, D. C., and Hoffman, H. J. Congenital thoracic dermal sinus: Diagnosis by computer assisted metrizamide myelography. J. Comput. Assist. Tomogr., *4:* 675–677, 1980.
64. Tadmor, R., Davis, K. R., Roberson, G. H., and Chapman, P. H. The diagnosis of diastematomyelia by computed tomography. Surg. Neurol., *8:* 434–436, 1977.
65. Villarejo, F. J., Blazquez, M. G., and Gutierrez-Diaz, J. A. Intraspinal lipomas in children. Child's Brain, *2:* 361–370, 1976.
66. Walker, A. E., and Bucy, P. C. Congenital dermal sinuses: Source of spinal meningeal infection and subdural abscesses. Brain, *57:*401–421, 1934.

67. Walsh, J. W., and Markesbery, W. R. Histological features of congenital lipomas of the lower spinal canal. J. Neurosurg., *52:* 564–569, 1980.
68. Weinstein, M. A., Rothner, A. D., Duchesneau, P., and Dohn, D. F. Computed tomography in diastematomyelia. Radiology *118:* 609–611, 1975.
69. Winter, R. B., Haven, J. J., Moe, J. H., and Lagaard, S. M. Diastematomyelia and congenital spine deformities. J. Bone Joint Surg. [Am.] *56A:* 27–39, 1974.
70. Wolpert, S. M., Scott, R. M., and Carter, B. L. Computed tomography in spinal dysraphism. Surg. Neurol., *8:* 199–206, 1977.
71. Wright, R. L. Congenital dermal sinuses. Prog. Neurol. Surg., *4:* 175–191, 1971.

CHAPTER

19

Meningomyelocele: "Pitfalls" in Early and Late Management

FRED EPSTEIN, M.D.

The emergence of spina bifida clinics, coupled with improved surgery, as well as medical and urological treatment, has been responsible for most dysraphic infants surviving the neonatal period. As a result of this, the complexion of the spina bifida clinic has evolved with the growing child. Originally intended for the neonate and very young child, the clinic is now also responsible for the long-term care of the older child and adolescent. On the basis of this experience, it has become clear that meningomyelocele is a dynamic disease process and that a spectrum of associated neurosurgical problems may become clinically manifest at any time between the neonatal period and adolescence, or even adulthood.

It is the purpose of this chapter to briefly discuss a few general problems referable to primary treatment and then describe the more recently recognized clinical entities of neonatal Arnold-Chiari malformation, tethered spinal cord, hydromyelia, and diastematomyelia which, occasionally, become symptomatic in the older myelodysplastic population. This report is based on the author's experience with a series of 300 patients with meningomyelocele treated in the Spina Bifida Clinic at the NYU Medical Center between 1977 and 1982.

TO TREAT OR NOT TO TREAT

A great deal of time and effort has been expended in discussing the moral and ethical responsibilities of the physician and society in making a decision as to whether or not to treat a severely disabled dysraphic child or to permit nature to take what is likely to be a long and drawn out course (6, 12, 13, 15–17). It is the perspective of the author that in a practical sense, this discussion is a waste of time inasmuch as there are few institutions that will accept a child with a growing head and leaking back, and there are few families that are willing to care for such a child in their home. It is also unrealistic for a physician to expect a father (mother is generally still hospitalized) to make such a difficult decision at a time of terrible emotional trauma. Invariably, in these circumstances, families make a decision based on information that is given to them by the pediatrician, pediatric neurologist, or neurosurgeon. The great likelihood is that any one of these physicians will have his/her own philosophy concerning what should be done and, therefore, whether intentional or unintentional, the information will be skewed. It is, therefore, the physician that is responsible for the immediate decision for or against surgery.

Even a highly intelligent family will have great difficulty in comprehending a detailed description of meningomyelocele and its potential sequelae. Although a general overview of the problem as it relates to a specific baby is indispensable, the most important part of the physician-family discussion is to emphasize that while it is not possible to predict the maximum severity of the future disability, the minimum future deficit may be described. For example, a paraplegic child with an L2 level will remain so and will be wheelchair bound but may have normal intelligence. A baby with an L3 level may walk with bracing, while an L4 level baby will probably be ambulatory with short leg braces. All of these children are likely to be incontinent of bowel and bladder. A baby born with macrocephaly and little cortical mantle will very likely be damaged, although this is notoriously difficult to predict, as many infants with even severe hydrocephalus are likely to have normal, or near normal, intelligence with appropriate treatment (1, 15, 18).

Finally, it is important to emphasize that the decision to treat does not commit the physician to treat any future life-threatening complication. Obviously, this is a subject to discuss with the family, following which any complication may be treated or not treated as the physician and the family shall agree upon.

TIMING OF SHUNT PLACEMENT

The various surgical techniques which may be employed in closing large meningomyeloceles have been well-described, and it is not the purpose of this chapter to address technical problems referable to primary closure.

It has been well-established that infection is the most important single event responsible for impaired intellectual development, and it is essential that every possible precaution be exhausted in an attempt to prevent its occurrence.

The size of the defect and the magnitude of hydrocephalus must be considered prior to primary repair of the meningomyelocele. Clearly, a poor repair in the presence of untreated advanced hydrocephalus is likely to become disrupted and serve as an avenue for local and disseminated spinal fluid infection. Therefore, the interrelationship of the hydrocephalus and the size of the meningomyelocele must be carefully considered prior to surgery. Although not always satisfactory, there are two therapeutic options: (a) placing a shunt simultaneously with the primary repair, or (2) repairing the meningomyelocele and carry out a shunting procedure sometime afterwards.

In the newborn infant with a leaking meningomyelocele and advanced hydrocephalus, it is advisable to carry out the shunt and repair the back at the same operation. However, if the baby is over 12 hours of age, it is essential to obtain ventricular CSF and only carry out simultaneous shunting in the absence of obvious infection.

When there is strong suspicion of infection, it has been my practice to insert a shunt with the distal end externalized in the lower abdomen. If cultures remain sterile, it may be internalized a few days later. It is important that the distal shunt be externalized far away from the ventricular catheter, as this makes secondary infection most unlikely and facilitates the later surgery.

It is unwise to attempt to place a shunt while the child is in the face-down position, as the necessary posterior tunneling of the distal catheter is a source of later pain along the shunt tract and even retrocollis. The procedures are performed sequentially, with the shunt performed first in the usual supine position.

In an infant in which the ventricles are only moderately enlarged, it is obviously preferable to perform the repair and only carry out a shunting procedure if significant hydrocephalus evolves.

Occasionally, a previously untreated child arrives from a foster home or chronic care facility. In these children, who usually have high motor levels and advanced hydrocephalus, the meningomyelocele, although often bulging, has spontaneously closed. In these cases, it is best to place a shunt prior to any neurosurgical and/or orthopedic surgical procedure directed towards the meningomyelocele or spine. This will facilitate the repair and make a postoperative CSF fistula unlikely. It is essential to study the spinal fluid prior to surgery to rule out a pre-existing chronic ventriculitis that may only become manifest following the surgical repair.

ARNOLD-CHIARI MALFORMATION

The Arnold-Chiari I malformation is characterized by downward displacement of the cerebellar tonsils into the cervical spinal canal while the vermis remains in its normal position. This anomaly *does not* occur in myelodysplasia. In contradistinction, the Arnold-Chiari II malformation *is* associated with myelodysplasia and is characterized by downward displacement of the anomalous vermis into the cervical spinal canal with or without associated displacement of the cerebellar tonsils. In addition, there are caudal displacement of the brain stem and a reduplication of the brain stem beneath the vermis. As a result of these structures being displaced into the cervical spinal canal, there is compression of the underlying brain stem by the posterior vertebral elements (2–4).

Although clinical diagnosis is the basis of treatment of neonates afflicted with the Arnold-Chiari malformation (11), Naidich (14) has described neuroradiological findings that are pathognomonic of the condition. The posterior fossa is invariably very small, and the CAT scan discloses a posteriorly concave configuration (scalloping) of the petrous pyramids which is secondary to pressure erosion by the anterior cerebellum as it extends around the brain stem. In addition, there is a "towering" anterior-superior cerebellar vermis which extends up through the incisural notch (Fig. 19.1).

The symptomatic neonatal Arnold-Chiari II malformation has required surgical decompression in 10 patients in the NYU series. The age range has been between 3 weeks and 3 months.

Respiratory stridor was the most common manifestation of the Arnold-Chiari malformation, having occurred in 43 patients. In the vast majority of cases, it has been intermittent and self-limited, resolving itself by 3

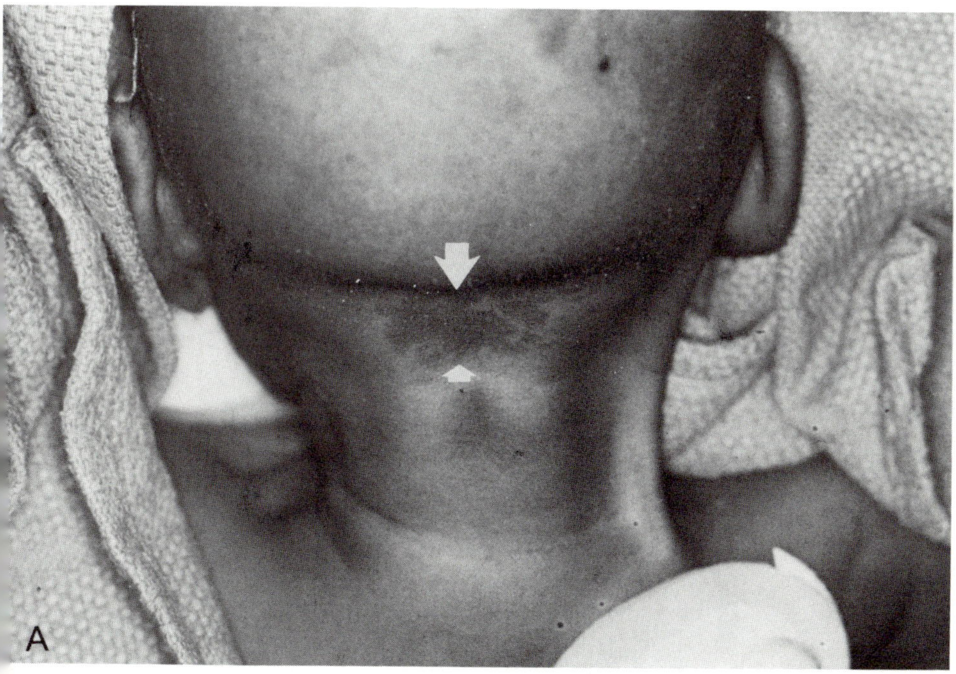

FIG. 19.1. Male, two months old, with symptomatic Arnold-Chiari malformation. (*A*) Small posterior fossa (*arrows*). (*B*) Scalloping of petrous pyramids. (*C*) Towering cerebella, extending superiorly through incisural notch. (*D*) "Beaking" of midbrain.

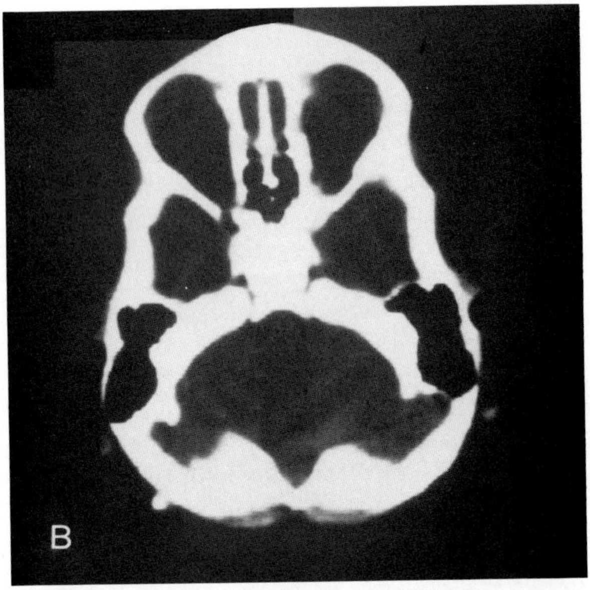

FIG. 19.1*B*

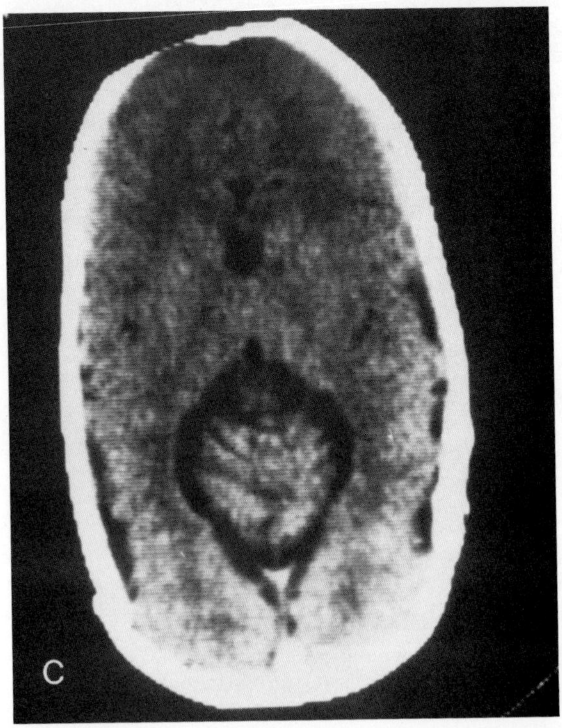

FIG. 19.1*C*

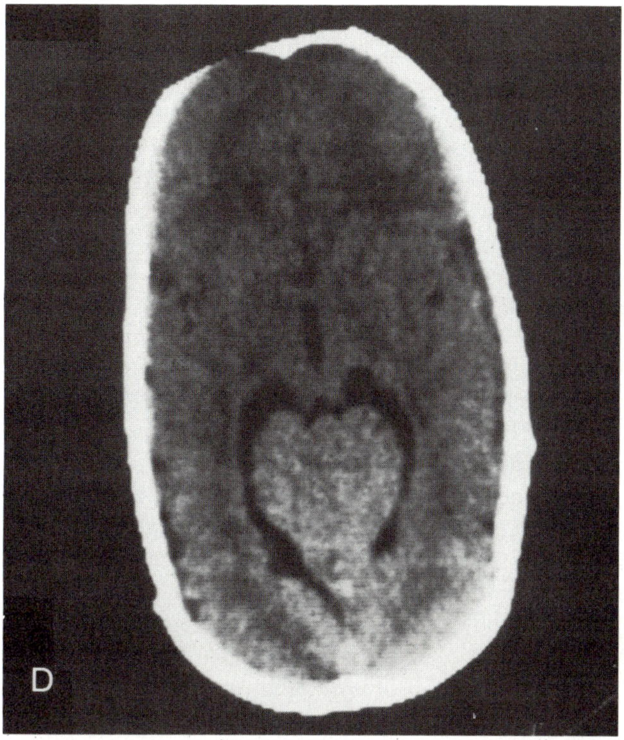

FIG. 19.1*D*

months of age. It was most problematic when associated with an upper respiratory infection, at which time life-threatening respiratory insufficiency may occur. It is my perspective that tracheostomy is to be avoided at all costs, and even in a life-threatening situation, a trial of several days of endotracheal intubation or surgical decompression of the malformation is preferable to a permanent tracheostomy.

Whereas respiratory stridor is most often a self-limited and relatively minor manifestation of the Arnold-Chiari malformation, there is a constellation of more threatening symptoms which are secondary to dysfunction of the lower cranial nerves. These include impaired ability to suck, difficulty in swallowing, drooling, and occasional regurgitation of fluids through the nose. The infant may have intermittent brief episodes of retrocollis, or even opisthotonus, associated with extreme irritability. Occasional brief apneic episodes with transient cyanosis are part of this syndrome and may be misinterpreted as a minor seizure. It is essential that a careful history be obtained, as transient retrocollis, drooling, and even apneic episodes may not be regarded as significant by a parent caring for a neurologically impaired infant. Neurological examination may or may not disclose dysfunction of the lower cranial nerves. Whereas respiratory stridor is generally self-limited, the more serious symptoms do not remit and, in fact, become more severe, often culminating in death. Infants manifesting any one of the major symptoms are in immediate danger of life and must be treated with relative dispatch.

In planning appropriate surgery, it is essential to understand the pathophysiology of the disorder. It is the result of downward displacement of the cerebellar vermis (with or without the tonsils), and the distorted brain stem into the cervicospinal canal. As a result of this pathological anatomical complex, there is brain stem compression beneath the anomalous cerebellum within the cervicospinal canal. It is, therefore, essential that the neurosurgeon recognize that the pathology is not intracranial but is within the cervical spinal canal. Treatment is directed towards decompression of the vermis and brain stem within the spinal canal by laminectomy and dural decompression. The foramen magnum is invariably greatly enlarged and need not be opened further. The laminectomy must extend caudal to the vermis and until normal posterior spinal cord has been visualized. Suboccipital craniectomy is not performed, and the dura is not opened over the cerebellar hemispheres. Indeed, this is hazardous as the transverse sinuses are much lower than normal and, in some cases, may be only 1–2 cm above the foramen magnum. Therefore, whereas the cervical dura is avascular, any additional rostral opening may be associated with serious bleeding and is unnecessary.

The following case histories are illustrative of the symptomatic neonatal Arnold-Chiari malformation.

Case 1

A male infant with an L4 motor level underwent repair of a meningomyelocele 18 hours after birth. A shunt was inserted a few days later, and the child was discharged. Three weeks later, the mother reported apneic episodes associated with transient cyanosis. In addition, she reported brief periods of retrocollis and irritability.

On physical examination, the baby appeared alert, cheerful, and comfortable. On the basis of the history, the child was admitted to the hospital, and all of the mother's observations were subsequently confirmed, although all of these episodes were transient. Neurodiagnostic studies confirmed the presence of an Arnold-Chiari malformation, and an upper cervical laminectomy and dural decompression were carried out. The vermis and tonsils were displaced to C5. The tonsils were white as a result of pressure necrosis (Fig. 19.2).

The postoperative course was uneventful, all symptoms were relieved, and the child is now asymptomatic 6 months after surgery.

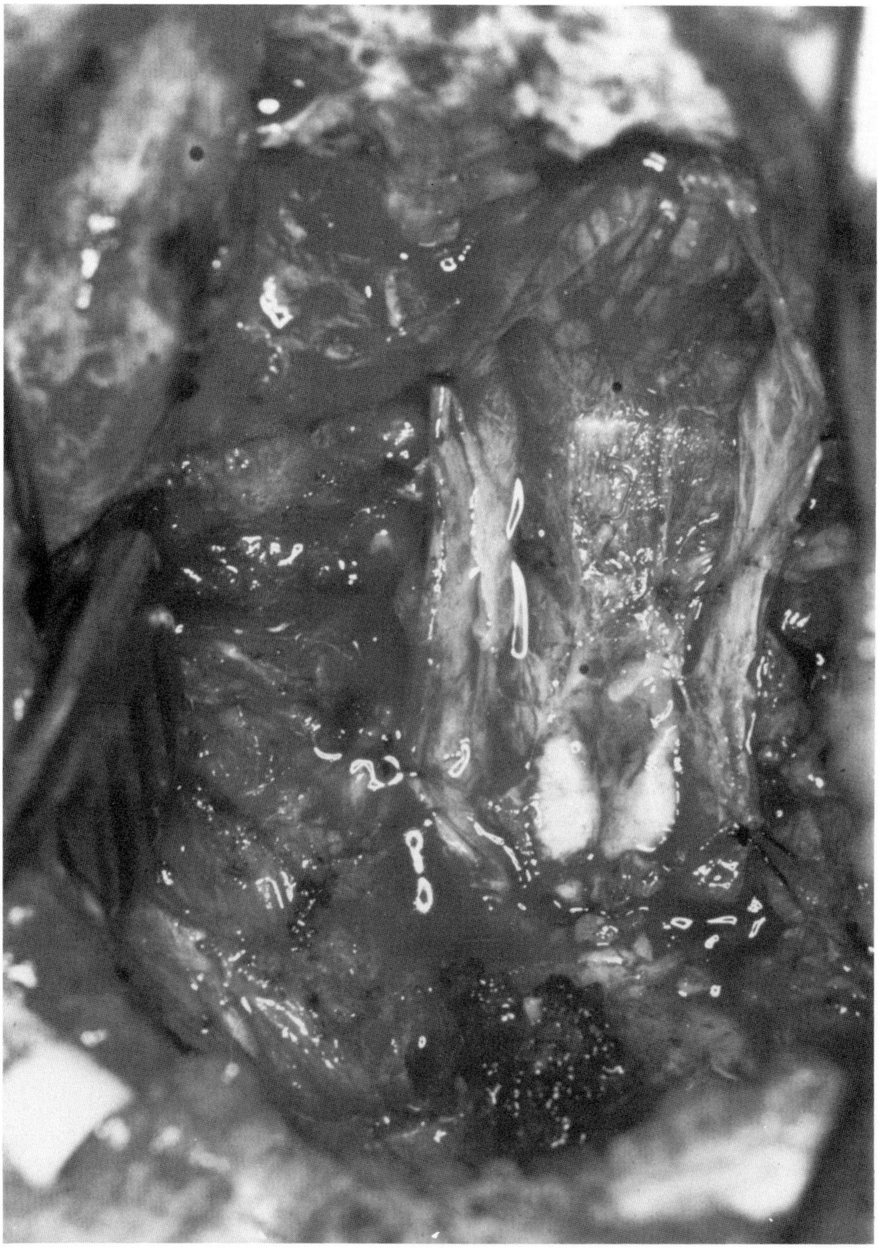

FIG. 19.2. Pressure necrosis of cerebellar tonsils. Note enlarged foramen magnum and anomalous vermis.

Case 2

A 12-day-old male with an L3 motor level underwent uneventful repair of a meningomyelocele 12 hours after birth. Hydrocephalus became manifest a few days later, and a right ventriculoperitoneal shunt was inserted. One week later, the mother described intermittent respiratory stridor and, 3 weeks after that, "peculiar seizures" manifested by transient apnea, cyanosis, and staring. She also stated that there were brief periods of time during which the infant arched the back and neck.

Neurological examination disclosed that the motor deficit was unchanged. There was a slightly impaired gag reflex, and fluid was occasionally regurgitated through the nose after feeding.

An upper cervical laminectomy and dural opening was performed. At surgery, the cerebellar tonsils were noted to extend to the C5 level (Fig. 19.3).

The apneic episodes did not recur postoperatively. Swallowing difficulties remained problematic, and the child died of an associated aspiration pneumonia 6 months later.

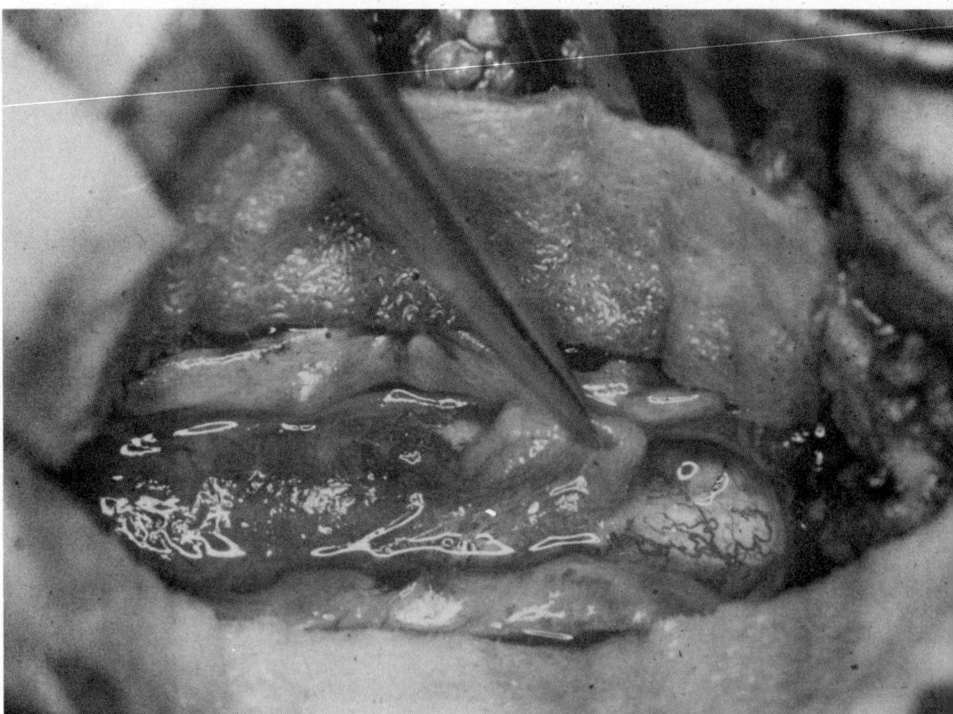

FIG. 19.3. Vermis displaced to C5. The laminectomy has been extended caudal to vermis, to the level of normal-appearing posterior surface of spinal cord.

In most cases, the operative procedure has led to significant improvement, and three of the patients are asymptomatic other than the motor deficits resulting from the primary problem. However, in an overall sense, it has been our experience that it is the most afflicted children who become symptomatic from this malformation, and the prognosis in most situations is not favorable. Nevertheless, occasionally a child will fare well and, assuming that there are not other multiple problems, there is no alternative to surgical decompression.

The second most common age when the Arnold-Chiari II malformation becomes symptomatic is during adolescence. Twelve patients between the ages of 12 and 18 have undergone surgical decompression in the NYU series. In this group of children, the most common symptom has been very severe suboccipital pain. The pain is described as most intense over the occiput and cervical spine, and it radiates forward towards the eyes (Fig. 19.4). In occasional cases, the family has described the onset of a "seizure" disorder manifested by transient apnea, dusky color, and loss of consciousness. Because these patients commonly suffer from occasional seizures, these new symptoms may not be regarded with alarm, although it is in this group of adolescents that sudden death may occur as the result of this malformation.

Surgery may be considered for severe suboccipital pain, and it is mandatory for respiratory irregularities. As in the neonate, the surgery is a cervical laminectomy which is carried caudad to the displaced cerebellar tissue. The foramen magnum is congenitally very large and need not be enlarged further. Markedly hypertrophic ligaments overlying the foramen magnum contribute to the symptomatic compression of the underlying neural structures. As in the neonate, following laminectomy the dura is incised from the foramen magnum to below the displaced vermis. It must be emphasized that the dura need *not* be opened rostral to the foramen magnum. It is not necessary to excise the vermis or cerebellar tonsils.

Surgery invariably results in complete relief of pain and, in most situations, respiratory problems are corrected as well. It is in the adolescent group of children that the long-term surgical results have been most satisfactory.

TETHERED SPINAL CORD

Irrespective of the surgical technique utilized at the time of the primary repair, the raw surface of the neural plate becomes enveloped in scar and fixed to surrounding tissue. Therefore, a tethered spinal cord is a certainty in all children who have undergone surgery for meningomyelocele. Children that are paraplegic, or nearly so, do not manifest signs and symptoms as a result of the already high motor level and sensory

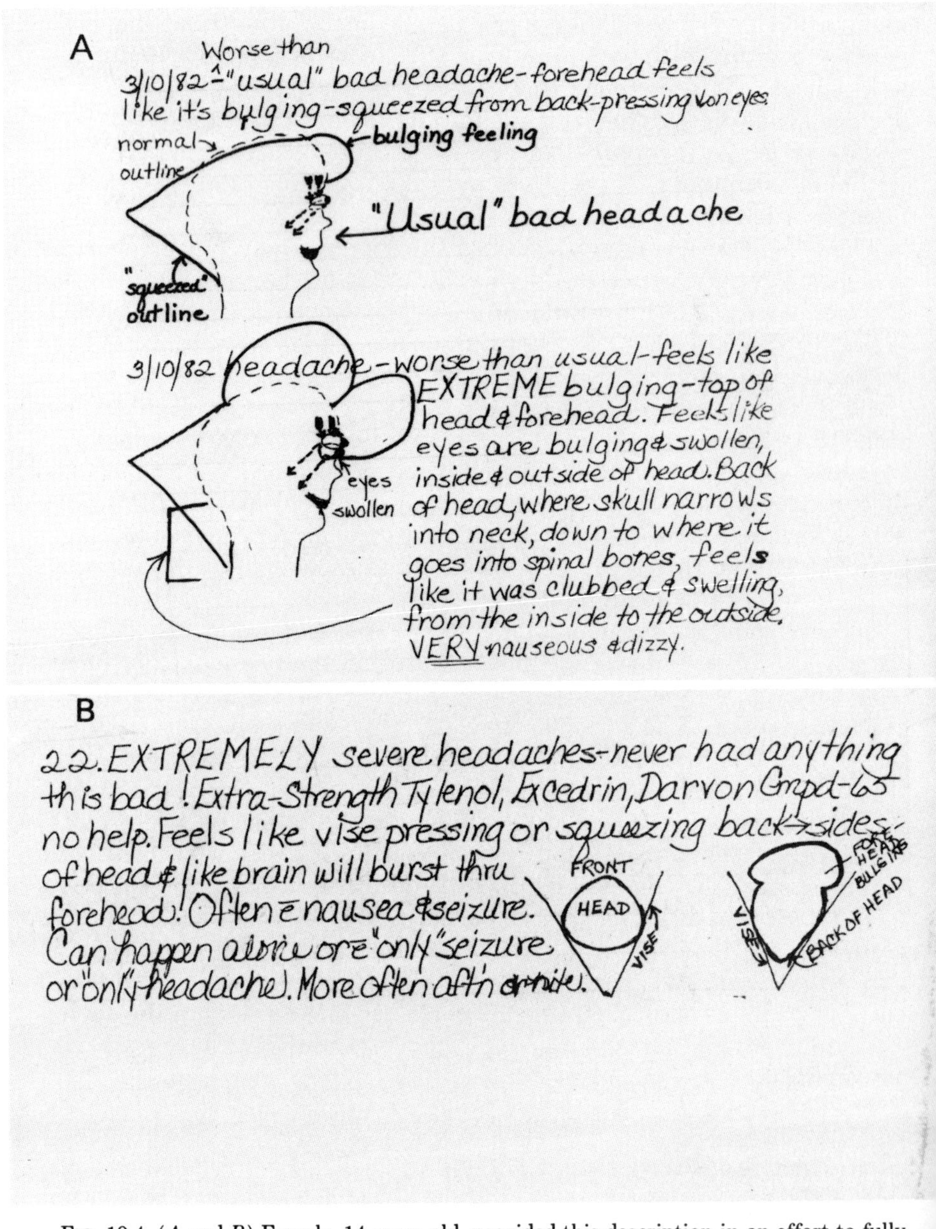

FIG. 19.4. (*A* and *B*) Female, 14 years old, provided this description in an effort to fully describe her subjective symptomatology.

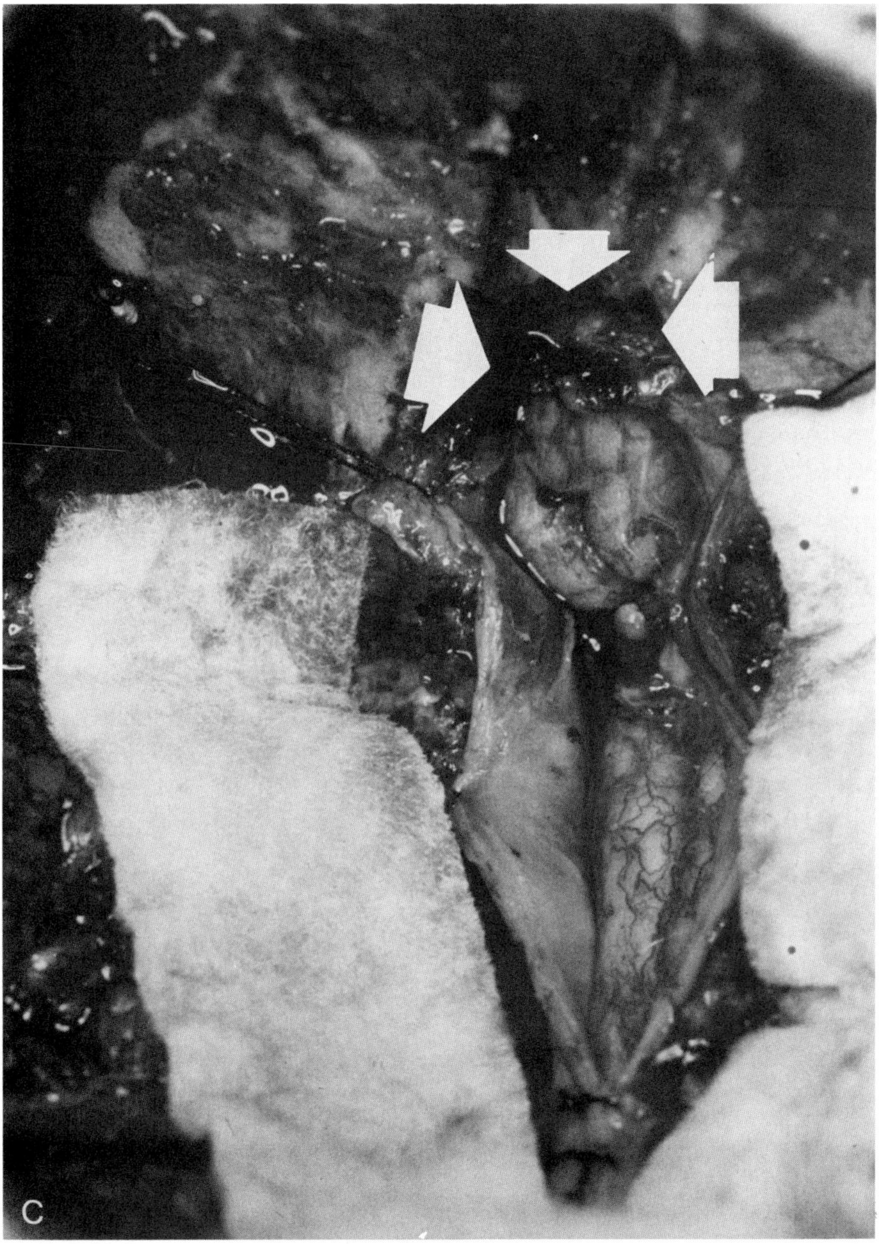

FIG. 19.4. (*C*) Note impaction of anomalous cerebellum into rostral cervical canal. Foramen magnum enlarged (*arrows*). Patient had complete symptomatic relief.

impairment. However, less afflicted children with L4 and L5 levels may occasionally have significant neurological deterioration as a result of this condition.

There are two major manifestations of the tethered cord syndrome in myelodysplastic children—pain and motor-sensory deterioration. Although most often occurring together, either may occur individually. The most common symptom in the NYU series of 8 patients (ages 3–8) has been severe local pain over the site of the previous repair. The pain, which is constant and boring in quality, interferes with normal sleep and results in personality aberrations as a result of continued distress. Neurological deterioration is most commonly manifest by an ascending motor deficit. This is asymmetric at first but may become symmetric over a period of a few months. The evolution of progressive motor dysfunction is often very slow and extremely difficult to detect at its onset. Most commonly, the parents or physiatrist first become aware of it. The episodic examination by the neurologist or neurosurgeon almost invariably overlooks the subtle deterioration. In some centers, myelodysplastic children are followed with sequential somatosensory evoked potentials in an attempt to objectively document progressive tethering. Although at present this is a research technique, it is likely to become of established clinical value in early diagnosis of this syndrome.

Surgery is directed towards neurolysis of the neural plate and terminal spinal cord. At operation, it will be noted that dense adhesions envelop the most normal caudal spinal cord and neural plate (Fig. 19.5). It is not completely clear as to whether the evolving neurological deficit is secondary to tethering of the spinal cord, or entrapment in dense scar tissue of functional nerve roots egressing at the lowermost part of the normal spinal cord. In any event, the surgery will relieve the pain, and many patients will have improved neurological function if there has not been a prolonged delay between the time deterioration was first observed and the time surgery is carried out.

HYDROMYELIA

Infants and young children with myelodysplasia often have an associated hydromyelia (7). The dilatation of the central canal may extend from the obex to the neural placode. Progressive enlargement of the hydromyelic central canal is the cause of three different clinical syndromes. The most common is progressive scoliosis, which may be secondary to denervation of paraspinal muscles as a result of destruction of anterior horn cells (9, 10). Symptomatic hydromyelia must be considered in any child in which there is evolving spinal deformity in segments that are rostral to the motor level and, therefore, are not a result of the primary motor deficit.

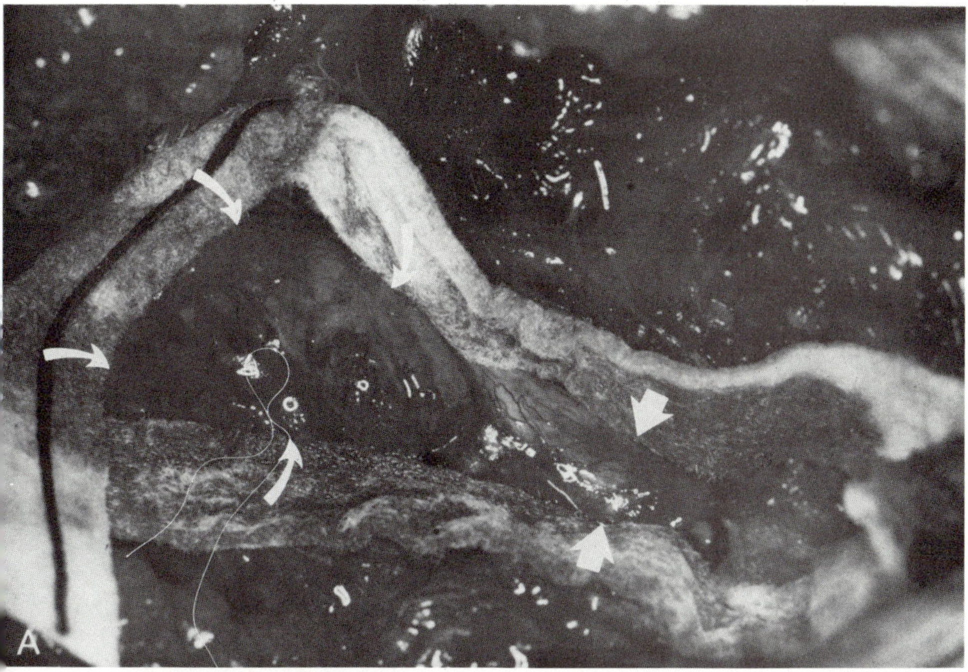

FIG. 19.5. (*A*) Tethered neural plate and cord in a 3-year-old child with local pain and progressive motor impairment.

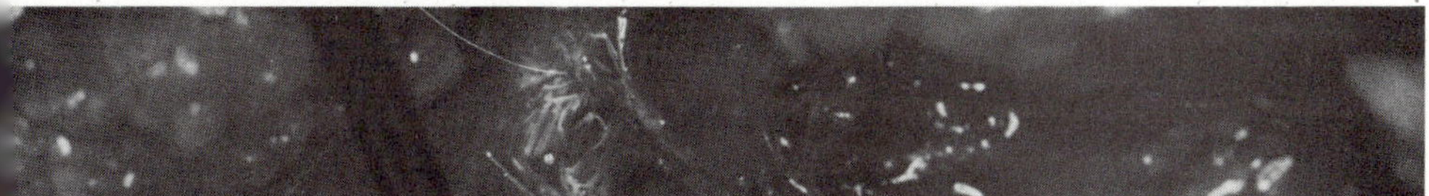

FIG. 19.5. (*B*) Neurolysis of neural plate complete. Note relative relaxation of terminal cord. Child was completely relieved of pain and recovered much neurological function.

The clearest constellation of signs and symptoms caused by hydromyelia are secondary to its occurrence in the cervical spinal cord. In these cases, there is weakness of the upper extremities and dissociated sensory loss with or without dysfunction of the lower cranial nerves.

The third possible manifestation is a sudden increase in motor deficit at the time of shunt malfunction. It is likely that when shunt obstruction occurs, there is the acute transmission of increased pressure down the hydromyelic central canal which in some way damages nerves in the lowermost spinal cord, or functional neural elements of the neural placode, resulting in further disability. There are three surgical approaches to this condition.

1. Placement of a Shunt If Hydrocephalus Is Present and the Child Has Not Been Previously Treated for It. If a shunt is already in place, it should be revised if there is any question concerning its function. In other words, a functioning shunt in many situations will ameliorate the signs and symptoms caused by hydromyelia. The exception is the situation in which there is aqueductal stenosis and there is no free communication between the lateral ventricular system and the fourth

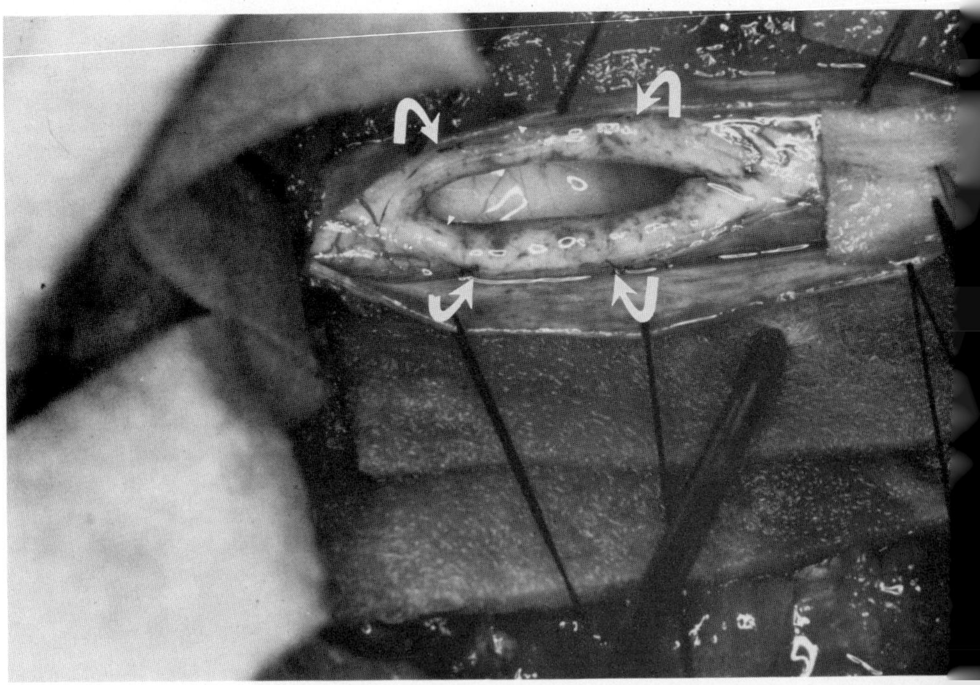

FIG. 19.6. Typical hydromyelic central canal. The pia has been sutured to the anterior lateral dura (*arrows*).

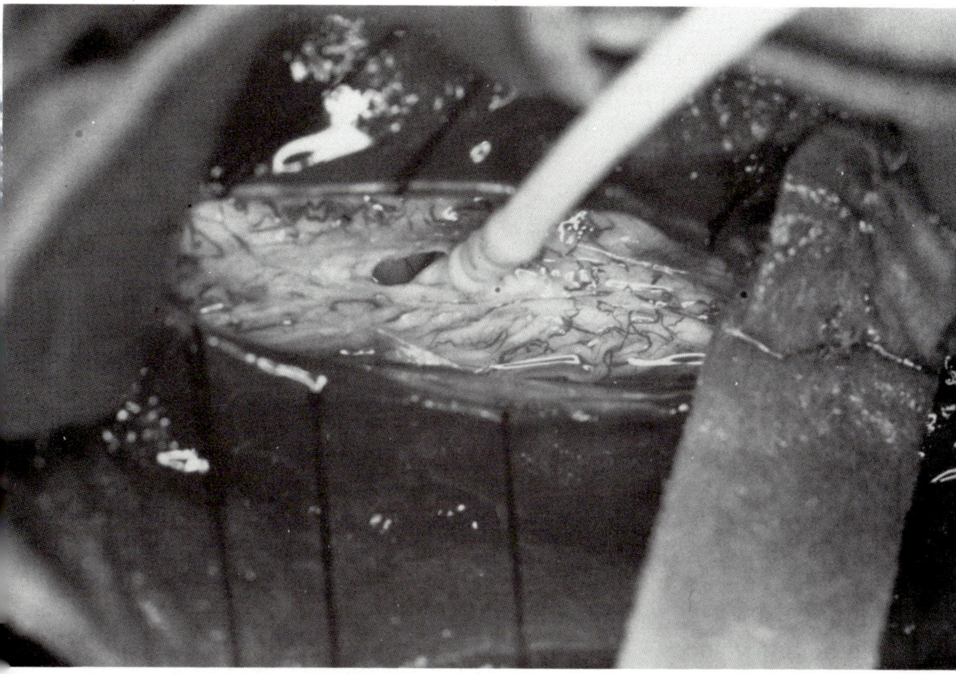

FIG. 19.7. "T" tube shunt has been inserted into hydromyelic cavity. Distal end may be extended to pleural or peritoneal cavity.

ventricle. In these rare cases, the fourth ventricle may be massively enlarged ("double compartment hydrocephalus"), and a posterior fossa shunt may resolve the problem (8).

2. Midline Myelotomy with Wide Opening of the Dilated Central Canal. The pia may be sutured to the anterior lateral dura, and the latter may be closed. In this way, the hydromyelic cavity is marsupialized to the subarachnoid space (Fig. 19.6). Another approach is the insertion of a shunt tube into the hydromyelic cavity, with the distal end of the catheter extending to either the pleural or peritoneal cavity (Fig. 19.7).

3. Upper Cervical Laminectomy with Direct Exposure of the Floor of the Fourth Ventricle. The communication between the fourth ventricle and the hydromyelic central canal (obex) is plugged with muscle (7). Because an Arnold-Chiari II malformation is always associated with hydromyelia, the obex is below the foramen magnum, and it is not necessary to explore the more rostral regions of the fourth ventricle.

It is my perspective that symptomatic hydromyelia should be primarily treated by the least hazardous surgical procedure. Therefore, a shunt or shunt revision is the first choice, followed by the other described procedures. It must be emphasized that no surgical procedure has been consistently satisfactory. The goal of surgery is to stabilize the condition and, although improvement may occur, it cannot be taken for granted.

DIASTEMATOMYELIA

Symptomatic diastematomyelia is very rarely a concurrent condition with myelodysplasia, and it occurred only three times in the NYU series. The age range was between 2 and 5. In all cases, the bony or cartilaginous spicule transected the spinal cord within two segments of the rostral bifid vertebrae. The clinical presentation was similar to that of tethered cord, with severe local spine pain associated with asymmetric deterioration of neurological function in the lower extremities. Plain spine films disclosed multiple anomalous vertebrae one or two segments above the first bifid spine. In addition, there was a large protuberant spinous process overlaying the actual diastematomyelic spur. Surgical removal of the spur relieved the pain and resulted in improved neurological function in all three children (Fig. 19.8).

The New York University series has underscored the long-term vul-

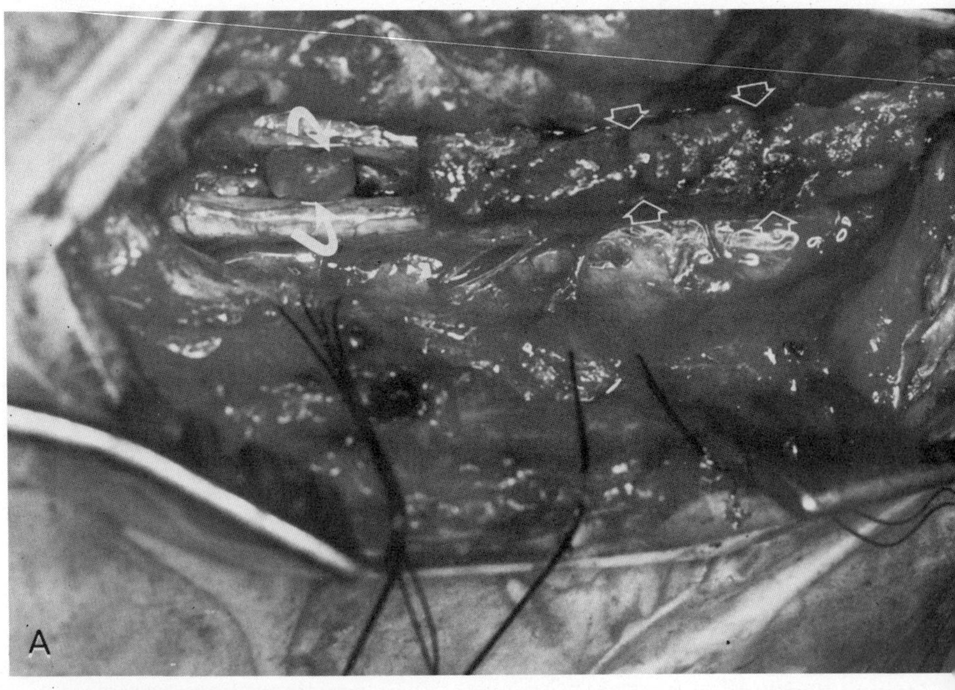

FIG. 19.8. (*A*) Symptomatic diastematomyelia in an 18-month-old child. Note that cartilaginous spicule is one segment above neural plate (*closed* and *open arrows*).

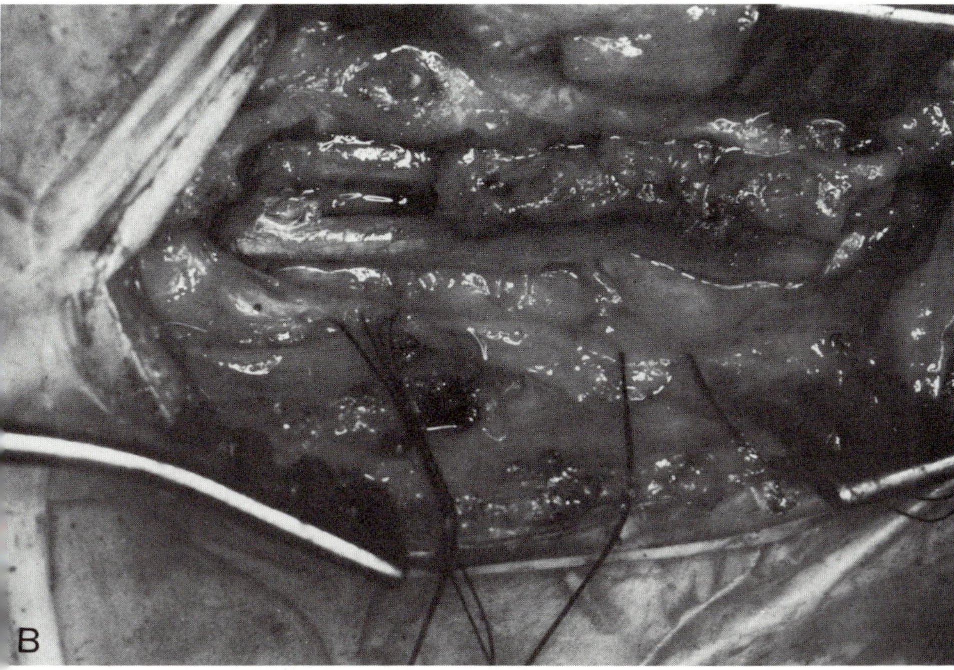

FIG. 19.8. (*B*) Cord following removal of the spicule.

nerability of myelodysplastic children to a variety of related pathological processes, the common denominator of which is progressive motor deficit. The differential diagnosis must include tethered spinal cord, hydromyelia, diastematomyelia, as well as a variety of congenital tumors which are associated with dysraphism. More recently, Findler and Hoffman (5) described the association of huge midline cysts of the velum interpositum with spasticity and progressive weakness of the lower extremities. All of these conditions may become clinically manifest at any age. A complete neurodiagnostic evaluation is the basis of a correct diagnosis and must include plain x-rays and metrizamide followed by myelography and immediate and delayed CT scans of the spine. It seems certain that with increased recognition of the vulnerability of these children to a diversity of pathological processes, the etiological list will continue to grow.

SUMMARY

Meningomyelocele is a dynamic ever evolving disease. Children surviving the neonatal period remain at risk for a variety of related neurosurgical problems which are only being recognized as that affected population grows larger and older. The least afflicted children are the most vulnerable, as they have more function which may be further impaired. It is essential that the spina bifida clinic be aware of these potential problems and remain responsive to the changing medical and surgical needs of this "aging" patient population.

REFERENCES

1. Badell-Ribera, A., Schulman, D., and Paddock, N. The relationship of nonprogressive hydrocephalus to intellectual functioning in children with spina bifida cystica. Pediatrics, *39:* 787–793, 1966.
2. Daniel, P. M., and Strich, S. J. Some observations on the congenital deformity of the central nervous system known as the Arnold-Chiari malformation. J. Neuropathol. Exp. Neurol., *17:* 255–266, 1958.
3. Emery, J. L., and Levick, R. K. The movement of the brain stem and vessels around the brain stem in children with hydrocephalus and the Arnold-Chiari deformity. Dev. Med. Child Neurol. (Suppl. 11): 49–60, 1965.
4. Emery, J. L., and MacKenzie, N. Medullo-cervical dislocation deformity (Chiari II deformity) related to neurospinal dysraphism (meningomyelocele). Brain, *96:* 155–162, 1973.
5. Findler, G., and Hoffman, H. J. Intracranial midline cyst in association with myelodysplasia. Neurosurgery, *7:* 520–525, 1980.
6. Freeman, J. M. To treat or not to treat: Ethical dilemmas of treating the infant with a myelomeningocele. Clin. Neurosurg., *20:* 134–146, 1973.
7. Gardner, W. S. Hydrodynamic mechanism of syringomyelia. Its relationship to myelocele. J. Neurol. Neurosurg. Psychiatr., *28:* 247–259, 1965.
8. Hawkins, J. C., Hoffman, H. J., and Humphreys, R. P. Isolated fourth ventricle as a complication of ventricular shunting. J. Neurol. Surg., *49:* 910–913, 1978.
9. Hall, P. V., Kalsbeck, J. E., Wellman, H. N., Blanitsky, S., Campbell, R. L., and Lewis, S. Clinical radioisotope investigation in hydrosyringomyelia and myelodysplasia. J. Neurosurg., *45:* 188–194, 1976.
10. Hall, P. V., Kalsbeck, J. E., Wellman, H. N., Campbell, R. L., and Lewis, S. Radioisotope evaluation of experimental hydrosyringomyelia. J. Neurosurg., *45:* 181–187, 1976.
11. Holinger, P. D., Holinger, L. D., Reichert, T. J., and Holinger, P. H. Respiratory obstruction and apnea in infants with bilateral abductor vocal cord paralysis, meningomyelocele, hydrocephalus, and Arnold-Chiari malformation. J. Pediatr., *92:* 368–373, 1978.
12. Lorber, J., and Zachery, R. B. Primary congenital hydrocephalus: Long-term result of controlled therapeutic trial. Arch. Dis. Child., *43:* 516–527, 1968.
13. Lorber, J. Spina bifida cystica: Results of treatment of 270 consecutive cases for selection criteria for the future. Arch. Dis. Child., *47:* 845–873, 1972.
14. Naidich, T. Computed tomography of the spine and spinal cord, In: *Modern Neuroradiology*, Vol. 1, Chap. 17. Clavadale Press, San Francisco, in press, 1982.
15. Raimondi, A. J., and Soare, P. Intellectual development in shunted hydrocephalic children. Am. J. Dis. Child., *127:* 664–680, 1974.
16. Shurtleff, D. B., Foltz, E. L., and Loeser, J. D. Hydrocephalus: A definition of its progression and relationship to intellectual function, diagnosis and complications. Am. J. Dis. Child., *125:* 688–693, 1973.
17. Shurtleff, D. B., Hayden, P. W., Loeser, J. D., and Kronmal, R. A. Myelodysplasia: Decision for death or disability. N. Engl. J. Med., *291:* 1005–1010, 1974.
18. Young, H. F., Nulsen, F. E., Weiss, M. H., and Thomas, P. The relationship of intelligence and cerebral mantle in treated infantile hydrocephalus (IQ potential in hydrocephalic children). Pediatrics, *52:* 37, 44–54, 60, 1973.

CHAPTER

20

Management of the Chiari Malformations in Childhood

PETER W. CARMEL, M.D.

A wide range of anomalies affect the cerebellum and brain stem of infants and children. Unfortunately, these hindbrain malformations are generally grouped together under the term "Arnold-Chiari malformation," creating a pathological grab bag which has often confused the understanding and therapy of these disorders. This spectrum of anomalies can be appropriately subdivided, and two major types of hindbrain malformations may be descerned in the pediatric age group. These two groups are most conveniently termed the Chiari Type I and Chiari Type II anomalies, following original descriptions from Chiari's papers (10, 11).

Chiari defined the Type I anomaly as a "peg-like elongation of the tonsils and the medial part of the inferior lobes of the cerebellum, which go along the medulla into the cervical canal." This abnormality is usually limited to the inferior portion of the cerebellum, while the medulla is normal in its location and configuration. Because of the lack of displacement of the cervical-medullary junction, there are rarely abnormalities of the cranial and upper cervical nerves. These nerves are not elongated and take a normal course to their root foramina. The upper cervical cord is frequently compressed by the overlying portions of the inferior cerebellum. Tonsillar tissue is often abnormal, and there is frequently scarring at the tips of the tonsillar herniations. In perhaps one third of the Chiari Type I anomalies, an associated syringomyelia may be present.

The Type II anomaly was described by Chiari in 1896 as "displacement of part of the lower vermus, displacement of the pons and displacement of the medulla oblongata into the cervical canal and elongation of the IV ventricle into the cervical canal" (11). This description emphasizes brain stem displacement and cerebellar dysplasia as the major components of the malformation. The downward prolongation of the medulla may override the unyielding upper cervical cord and form a "kink-like" deformity. Because of caudal migration of the brain stem, the lower cranial nerves are often stretched and take abnormal courses to their

TABLE 20.1

Comparison of Chiari Type I and Type II Malformations

	Type I	Type II
Anatomic anomaly		
Caudal dislocation of medulla	Unusual	Yes
Caudal dislocation of inferior vermis	No	Yes
Spina bifida	May be present	Rarely absent
Hydrocephalus	May be present	Rarely absent
Medullary "kink"	Absent	Present in 55%
Course of upper cervical nerve roots	Usually normal	Usually cephalad
Clinical syndromes		
Onset of symptoms	Adolescent/adult	Infant
Progressive hydrocephalus	Occasional	Over 90%
Brainstem compression signs	May be present	Rare
Surgery		
Relief by shunting	Occasional	Usual
Posterior fossa decompression	May be needed	Occasional
Decompression (if needed)	Elective	Urgent

root foramina. The upper cervical nerve roots frequently stretch upward to exit from the spinal canal. Additional characteristic deformities are seen in the telencephalon, the diencephalon, and the mesencephalon. A comparison of the Type I and Type II anomalies is seen in Table 20.1.

Arnold's contribution to the understanding of this disorder was quite limited and was restricted to a single case report without any real consideration of the nature of the cerebellar abnormality (2). The case that Arnold described most closely fits into the Chiari Type I description. An earlier description of the Chiari Type II anomaly by Cleland (12) in 1883 has been largely overlooked. A fuller evaluation of Cleland's contribution has been undertaken elsewhere (8).

Although both the Type I and Type II anomalies are found in childhood years, they are very different in their clinical presentation, their surgical management, their prognosis, and their underlying embryogenesis. The Type II anomaly is largely found in infants and neonates, is almost invariably associated with hydrocephalus, and is initially treated by a shunting procedure. The Type I anomaly most often becomes apparent later, usually in the adolescent or early adult period, and is frequently found without concomitant hydrocephalus. In addition to these obvious disimilarities, the two types have quite different implications as to the presence of other central nervous malformations and bone anomalies.

EMBRYOGENESIS

The Type II anomaly usually has the greater morphological abnormality. Its genesis almost certainly occurs earlier in gestation than the Type I abnormality. It seems likely that the Type II anomaly has its embryogenesis at the time of the major changes in the rhombencephalic cavity. These changes are associated with the formation of the pontine flexure and take place in stage XIV, at about the 35th day of gestation (30). These hindbrain changes immediately follow closure of the posterior neuropore, stage XII, which takes place several days earlier. Thus, common association of myelomeningocele and Chiari Type II anomaly probably reflects a common period for their embryogenesis.

The Type I anomaly occurs much later in gestational life. Available data indicate that the Type I malformation occurs after the major portion of the cerebellar hemispheres has formed. A period of rapid vermian and hemispheric growth follows formation of the primary cerebellar fissure, in the period from the 10th to 14th weeks of gestation. The embryo at this stage has a crown-rump length between 65 and 120 mm.

Several different theories have been proposed for the cause of the Type II anomaly. Cleland felt that the malformation was due to a primary dysgenesis of the brainstem (12). Chiari (11) attributed the presence of all of the anomalies to hydrocephalus. The hydrocephalus theory has been given a new and provocative form by Gardner (14, 15). Other authors have felt that the Type II malformation is caused by tethering of the lower end of the spinal cord by the associated myelomeningocele (26). It is postulated that tethering would result in caudal displacement of the brain stem and cerebellum.

Daniel and Strich (13) and Peach (24, 25) have each reviewed the pathological features of a large group of Chiari Type II deformities. Both series reach similar conclusions. These authors attributed the hindbrain abnormality to failure of the pontine flexure to form in early embryonic life. Failure of this flexure would account for the marked elongation of the brain stem seen in this abnormality. Certain features of the anomaly, including beaking of the tectum and thickening of the intrathalamic connexus, were related to upward movement of the brain stem towards the mesencephalon. Herniation of the medulla and vermis into the upper cervical canal and abnormal courses for the cranial and cervical nerves were related to elongation of the rhombencephalon in a caudal direction. Figures 20.1*A* and *B*, based on drawings of Bartelmez and Dekaban, illustrate this mechanism. In Figure 20.1*A* the flexure has formed in normal fashion, bringing the following cerebellum to a position which overlies the more caudal rhombencephalon. Figure 1*B* is a reconstruction showing the results of failure of the flexion to form. Here, the roof of the rhombencephalic fossa is brought downward below the level of the cervical flexure. As the cerebellum continues to develop, its attachment to the posterior membrane causes it to grow caudally along the membrane into the upper portion of the cervical canal.

Each of these theories are confounded by individual cases which do

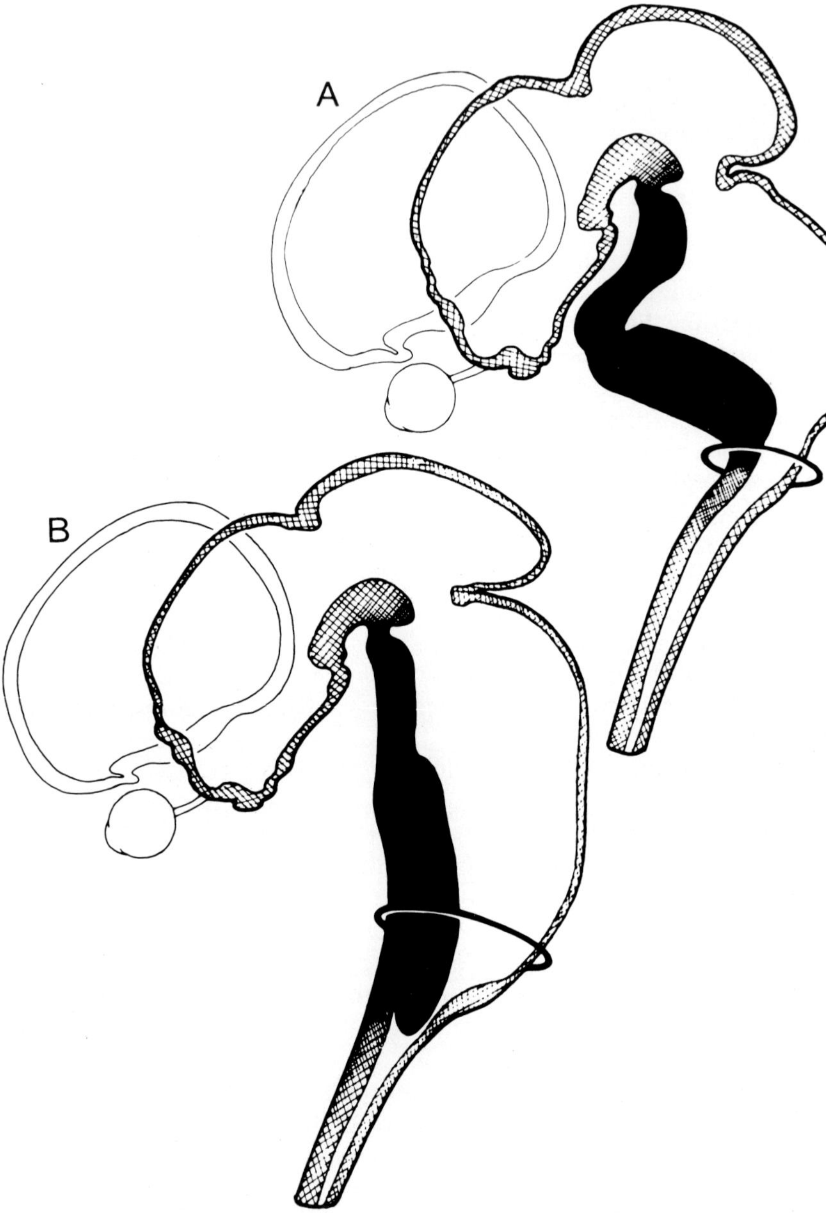

FIG. 20.1. (*A*) Midsagittal representation of brain of embryo approximately 25-mm crown-rump length (horizon XXII). The pontine flexure has formed (*black areas*) and the cerebellum is starting to form in the roof of the IVth ventricle. Foramen magnum at circle. (Modified from G. W. Bartelmez and A. S. Dekaban (4).)

FIG. 20.1. Reconstruction showing changes that might occur if pontine flexure failed to form. The hindbrain is elongated forcing the tegmentum to a more rostral position and causing a beak-like deformity of the tectum. Caudal portions of the hindbrain are displaced downward below the cervical flexure, and the medulla overrides the cervical cord. The roof of the ventricle is carried caudally as well, and at a later period cerebellar tissue will form in this position.

not seem to fit the authors schemes. It is likely that there is a broad spectrum of anomalies, and that cases may be found giving support to each of these theories. A full discussion of the reasons for supporting or discounting each of these theories has been presented elsewhere (9, 25).

It is evident that an entirely different mechanism must be responsible for the Type I anomaly. In this type there is no distortion of the brain stem, and these patients frequently present without hydrocephalus. Whether the abnormally formed cerebellar tonsils are caused by a local overgrowth of cerebellar tissue, or are related to a failure of the normal invagination of midline cerebellar structures as growth proceeds is not clear. What is apparent is that the anomaly is initially quite limited in its abnormal morphology. Later destructive changes of cord and medulla are seen associated with medullary or cord compression and the development of syringomyelia. It is likely that these changes occur with growth and need not be present at the time of birth (21).

CLINICAL PRESENTATION

The Type II anomaly, with widespread anatomic abnormality, is usually noted early in life. Although a small number of cases of Type II abnormality with normal spinal canals have been reported (7, 32), almost all of these children have a myelomeningocele. The myelomeningocele is noted at birth, and the child's initial surgical treatment is repair and closure of the defect. Type II anomalies are also associated with other bony malformations of the upper cervical spine.

More than 90% of these children go on to develop hydrocephalus (22). Hydrocephalus may become apparent immediately after the closure of the spinal deficit, or within the ensuing months. More than 80% of these children who eventually develop hydrocephalus do so within 6 months. The Type II anomalies generally cause hydrocephalus syndromes undistinguishable from hydrocephalus due to other factors. However, a specific syndrome, marked by laryngeal stridor and weakness or paralysis of the vocal cords, is seen occasionally in Type II children who become hydrocephalic (18, 28). It is these children who are perhaps at greatest risk, as laryngeal paralysis may threaten the child with rapid onset of asphyxia and death. Other brain stem anomalies associated with the Type II malformation include degeneration of the nuclei of the lower cranial nerves (28, 29).

Treatment of hydrocephalus by shunting usually relieves most of the signs of brain stem dysfunction. However, Hoffman *et al.* (17) have reported a group of infants who required direct posterior fossa decompression for their malformations. In these children, apneic spells, loss of gag reflex, and upper extremity weakness were noted. In 4 children, hydrocephalus had been treated by shunting but had failed, and decompression was required.

Rare instances of Chiari II malformations without spinal dysraphism have been reported (7, 32). These patients do not become symptomatic in early childhood, and their clinical syndromes may be identical to those described below for the Type I anomaly.

The Type I malformation, in striking contradistinction to Type II, is rarely symptomatic in infancy, and the clinical syndromes associated with this anomaly usually appear in adolescent or young adult years (1, 27). The most common presenting sign is pain, often in the distribution of the occipital nerves. These patients may undergo treatment of many kinds before the anomaly is recognized (1, 21). Occipital headache syndromes associated with cerebellar anomalies are often increased by coughing or sneezing and may be relieved by lying down (1).

Motor syndromes may be the initial symptom and usually involve the upper extremities. Most frequently, arm weakness is entirely unilateral or more pronounced on one side and involves the lower motor neuron primarily. Lower extremity signs are usually bilateral, spastic, and fairly symmetrical. Malis *et al.* (20) found that motor syndromes were the most common clinical picture associated with the Chiari syndrome in adults.

Finally, there are a group of patients who present with signs and symptoms of raised intracranial pressure. In this group, obstruction of outlets of the IVth ventricle leads to progressive hydrocephalus.

Three pathophysiological mechanisms are seen in patients with the Type I anomaly; direct compression of the spinal cord by overlying tonsils, obstruction of the IVth ventricle, and syringomyelia. In many cases a puzzling combination of these clinical groups is found. Attribution of the major clinical problem to one or another mechanism may be difficult, and these patients are not uncommonly subjected to a number of surgical procedures.

RADIOLOGICAL EXAMINATION

Skull films of the child with Chiari Type II malformation and associated hydrocephalus reveal characteristic enlargement of the cranium and cephalofacial dysproportion. Cranila lacuna, or lückenschädel, are found in approximately 85% of children with the Type II malformation. The posterior fossa characteristically is small, and the insertion of the transverse sinuses is low. There is enlargement of the foramen magnum and elongation of the laminar arches of the upper cervical vertebrae (Fig. 20.2). Plain films may also reveal platybasia, basalar impression, assimilation of the atlas, or the Klippel-Fiel deformity. Hemivertebra are found in almost 20% of cases.

In marked distinction to these abnormalities, children with the Type I malformation show few plain radiographic abnormalities. Less than 10% of this group of children have a skull or cervical spine abnormality.

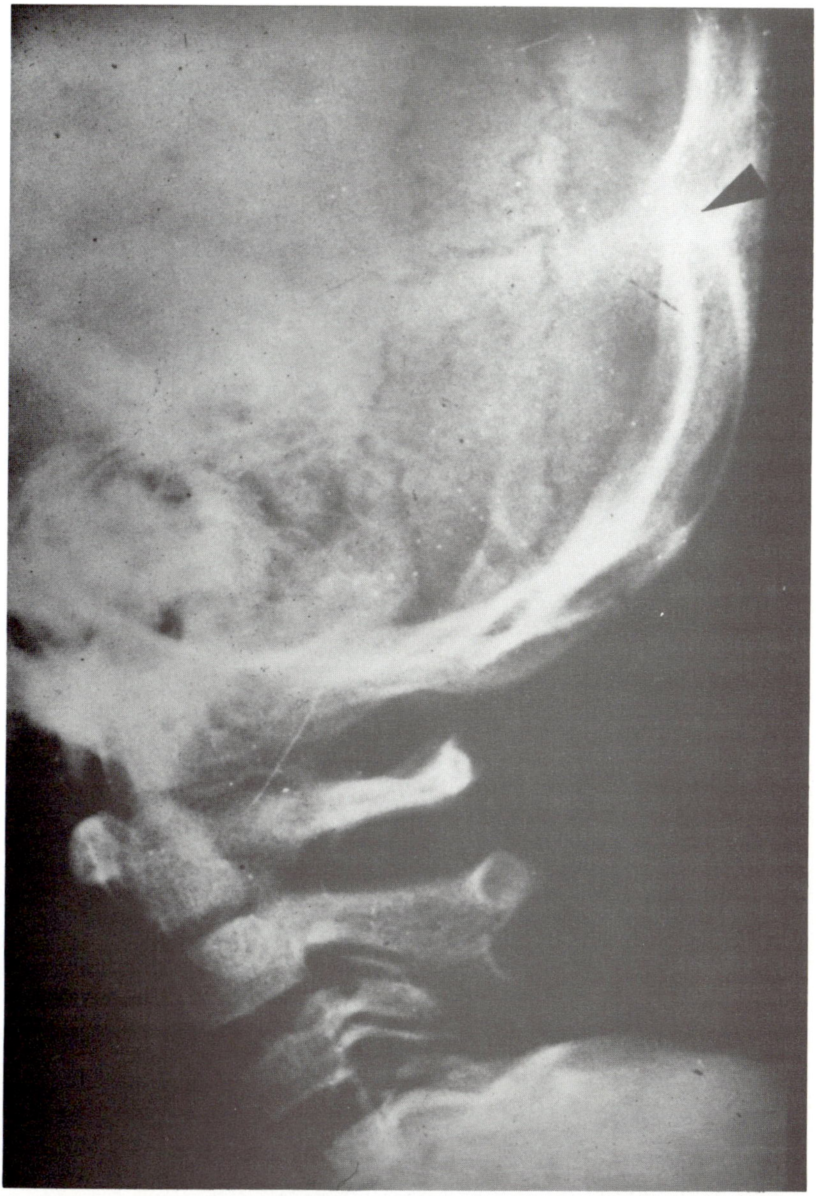

FIG. 20.2. Lateral cervical spine film of child with myelomeningocele repaired shortly after birth. The posterior fossa is small, as outlined by bone density at transverse sinus, and insertion of tentorium is low (*arrow*). The foramen magnum is enlarged, and the laminae of C1 and C2 are elongated. (Reproduced with permission from P. W. Carmel (9).)

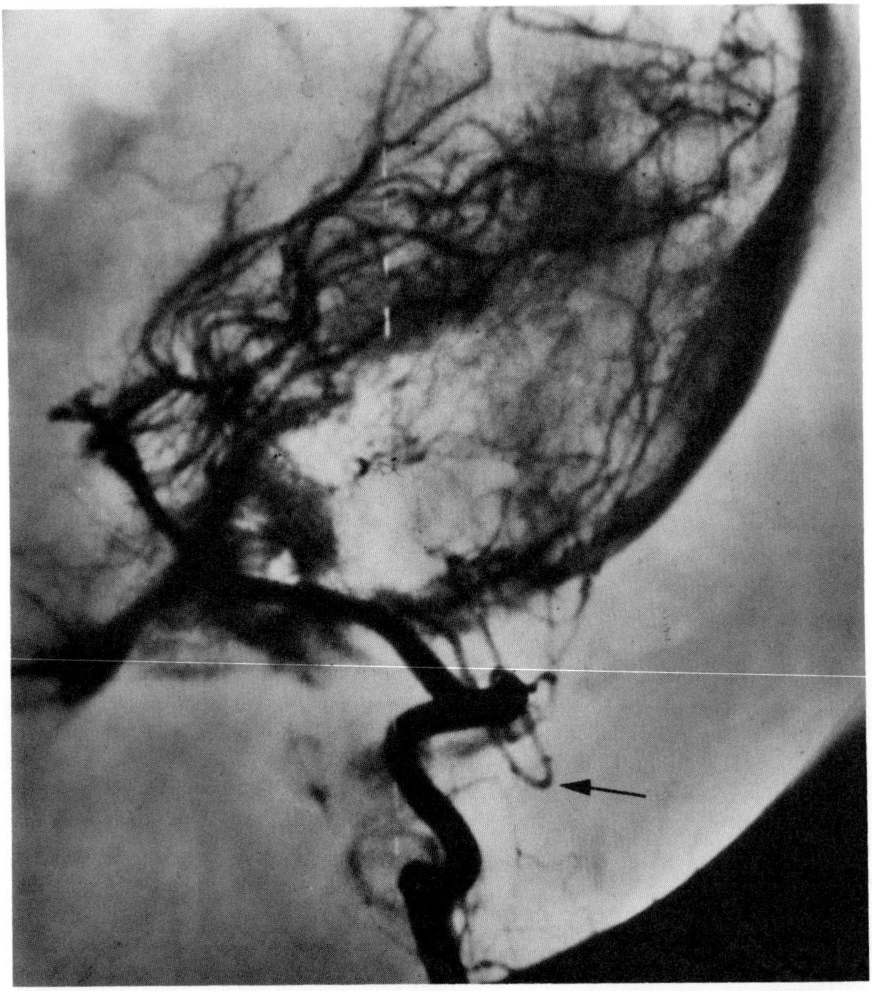

FIG. 20.3. Lateral view of vertebral angiogram in a 15-year-old girl with progressive dorsal column sensation loss and increasing spasticity. Tonsillar branch of posterior inferior cerebellar artery has descended to the C2 level (*arrow*). At operation, the tonsil was a full level below C2.

The typical features of both the Type I and Type II anomalies are most readily found on contrast x-ray studies. In the past these have included ventriculography, pneumoencephalography, and Pantopaque or air myelography. Angiography is occasionally useful to delineate the descent of tonsils into the cervical canal (Fig. 20.3). As the tonsils descend, the tonsillar loop of the posterior inferior artery is usually pushed both laterally and caudally, and this loop may not accurately represent the lowermost pole of the descended tonsil.

In the last few years, use of contrast-enhanced cisternography, utilizing water-soluble material and CT scanning, has largely replaced other forms of contrast radiological studies for this anomaly (23). The changes on routine unenhanced posterior fossa scanning are often quite subtle. They may reveal elongation of the brain stem and upward movement of the mesencephalon (Fig. 20.4). Careful investigation of the nonenhanced

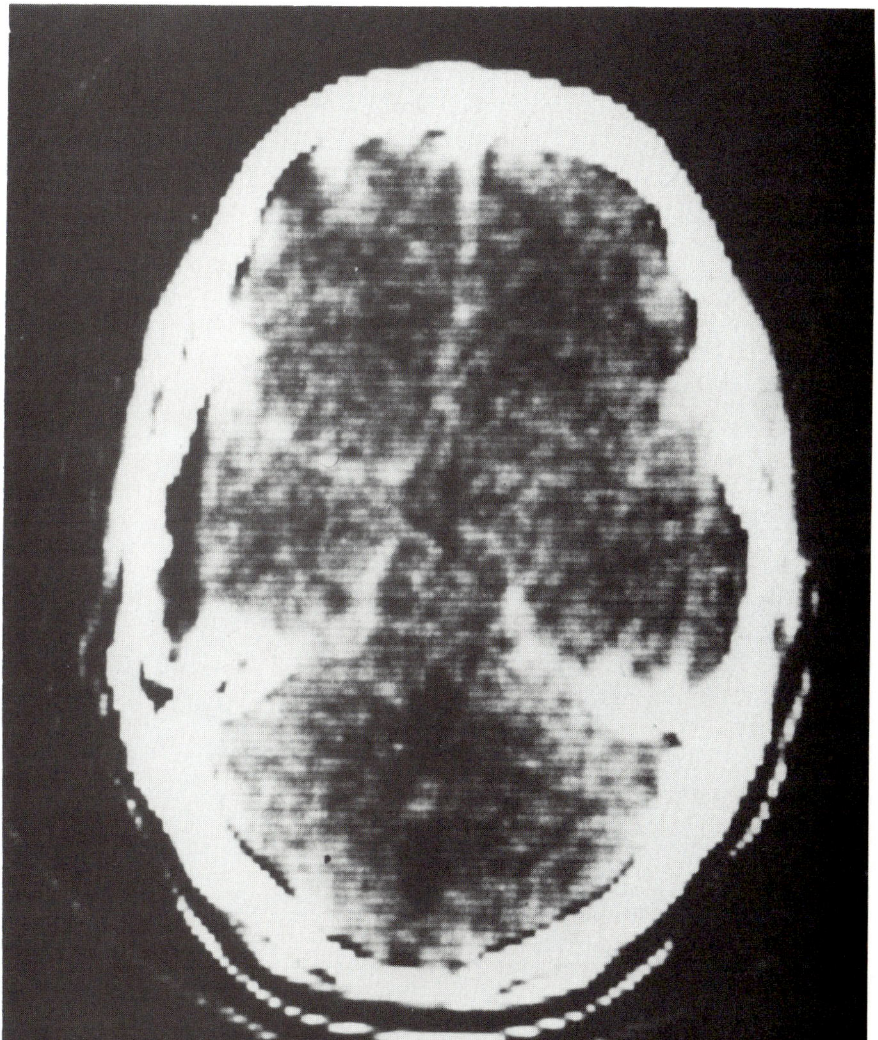

FIG. 20.4. Enhanced axial scan of adolescent with Type II anomaly and abnormal sacral spine. The IVth ventricle is elongated, and the roof (indicated by tuft of enhancing choroid plexus) is flattened. There is upward displacement of the mesencephalon, compressing the interpeduncular and suprasellar cisterns.

scan shows the characteristic changes in CSF cisterns that indicate mesencephalic beaking, transincisural extension of the cerebellum, and a growth of the cerebellum around the brain stem (23).

Injection of intrathecal metrizamide in small doses has proven to be a powerful tool in computerized investigation of these anomalies. Axial sections demonstrate the low position of the tonsils, downward migration of cerebellar tissue, and distortion of the IV ventricle (Fig. 20.5*A*). Compression of the cervical cord is easily appreciated (Fig. 20.5*B*). In cases where an associated syrinx has formed, a widened cervical cord may be identified (Fig. 20.5*C*). Delayed scan, 6–12 hours after intrathecal injection, will occasionally show penetration of syrinx by contrast.

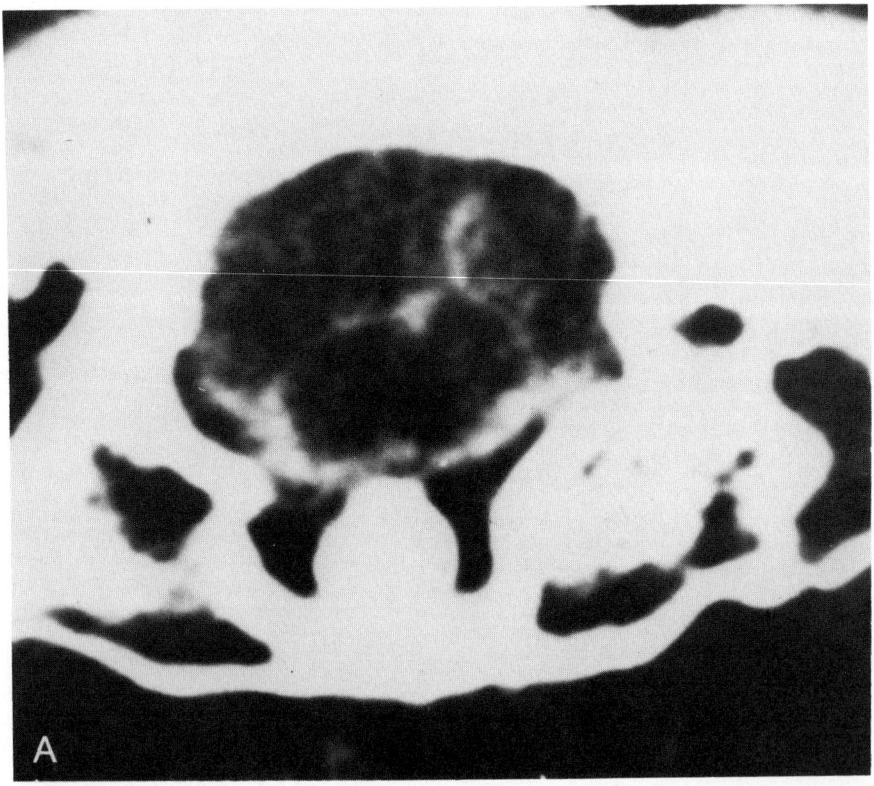

FIG. 20.5. (*A*) Intrathecal metrizamide enhanced scan at foramen magnum level in a 12-year-old boy with assymetrical weakness in upper extremities and spasticity in legs. Distortion of the caudal IVth ventricle and compression of lower medulla by overlying cerebellar tissue is seen.

FIG. 20.5. (*B, opposite*) Same case as in 20.5*A*. Intrathecal metrizamide axial scan below cervical-medullary junction level. There is compression of cord due to tonsillar descent. Tonsils are assymetrical, with greater herniation at left of image.

FIG. 20.5. (*C, opposite*) Same case as in Figure 20.5*A* and *B*. Metrizamide scan at upper cervical level, below level of tonsils, showing marked cord dilatation by syrinx.

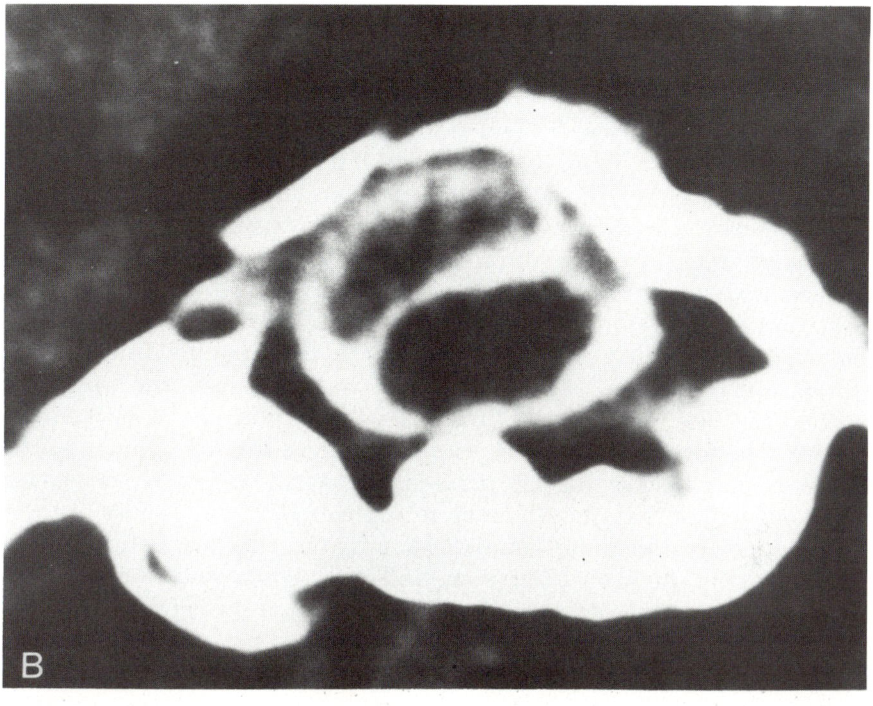
B
C

SURGICAL PROCEDURES

Most of the children who require neurosurgical decompression of the posterior fossa have the Type I anomaly. Children with the Type II anomaly may have symptoms referable to hindbrain compression appear as they progressively develop hydrocephalus. These symptoms usually recede when the hydrocephalus is controlled by shunting. In a small number of cases, direct posterior fossa surgery is required. Lapras and Lotfi reviewed several large series of children with Chiari Type II malformation and myelomeningocele, and found only 5 instances where these children had decompressive procedures (19). Operated infants were generally extremely ill due to apnea or quadriparesis, and operative mortality in these series ranged from 20 to 40%. Hoffman *et al.* reported a series of children with both the Type I and Type II lesions who required decompression. These authors pointed out that it was rarely necessary to remove any of the occipital bone in younger children because of their enlarged foramen magnum and felt that the neurological deficit due to compression of the lower brain stem and upper cord could be relieved by decompressive laminectomy alone. Decompression was always effective if carried out early, and they emphasized the need for speed of intervention once symptoms of pressure on medulla and cord become apparent. They also noted that the venous drainage at the foramen magnum in infants is particularly profuse and that great care is required when opening the dura at this level in childhood years.

In our institution, decompressive operation for adolescents is generally performed in the sitting position with the head fixed in a 3-point headrest, whereas younger children require 4-point fixation in a modified halo. The patient is always intubated and kept on controlled respiration. Care is taken not to flex the head any further than possible while the patient is awake. A suboccipital craniectomy is performed which is much more limited than that used in exploring midline posterior fossa lesions. The thickened bone at the edge of the foramen magnum is carefully removed. There is frequently a thickening of the atlantooccipital membrane and an increased tenacity of its attachment to the edge of the foramen magnum, and care must be taken in the removal of this membrane. Laminectomy of the upper cervical vertebra is performed to below the level of the herniated tonsils. It must be remembered that the tonsils may be caudal to the position indicated on contrast myelography. Barnett *et al.* (3) pointed out that it is not necessary to carry the laminectomy low enough to expose an associated syrinx. Extensive laminectomy in patients with neurological deficits associated with syrinx may be followed by severe flexion deformity of the cervical spine.

The dura is opened in Y-shaped fashion, and it is often tightly bound to the underlying arachnoid at the levels of the greatest constriction by

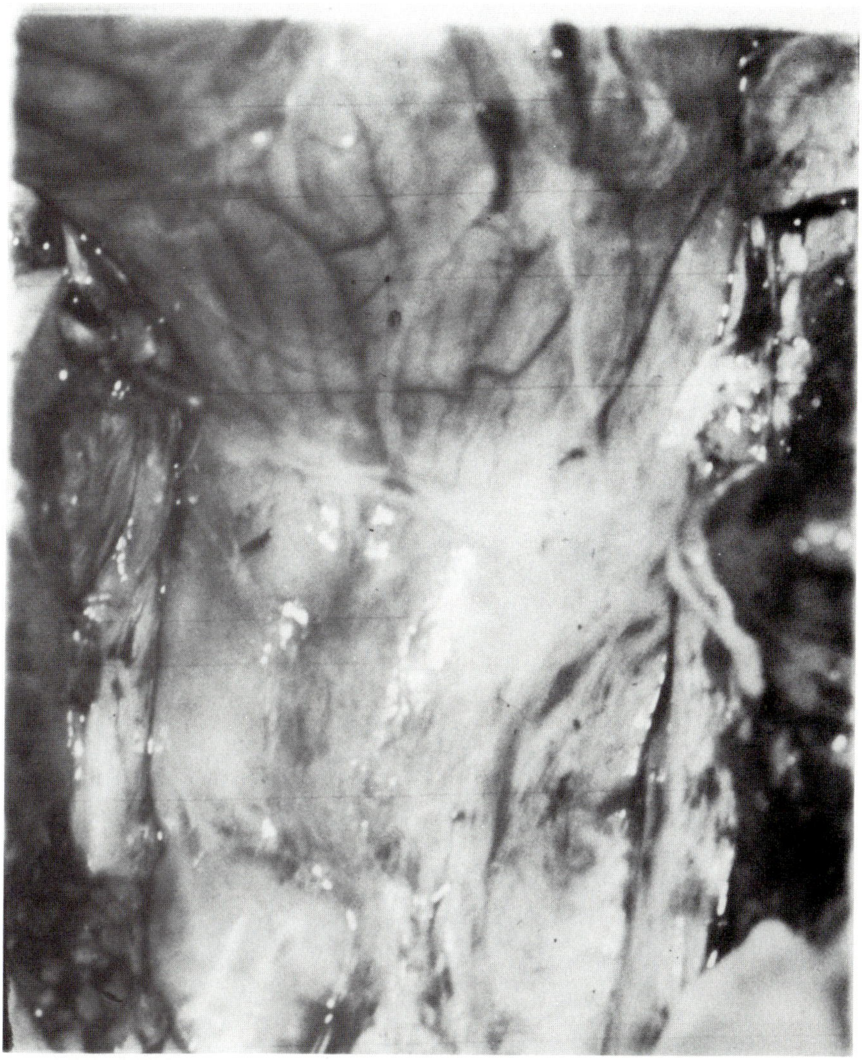

FIG. 20.6. Tough band of fibrous tissue extending from the level of the foramen magnum and below in a Chiari Type I anomaly. This tissue constricts the tonsils and cord and must be adequately opened for decompression.

cervical laminae or the foramen magnum. The underlying arachnoid may be unusually thickened, and there is frequently a band of tough fibrous tissue overlaying the inferior outlet portion of the vallecula cerebelli. This tight band may not only obstruct the outflow of CSF through the foramen of Magendie but also may be thick and tough enough to contribute to the compressive forces encircling the tonsils and brainstem (Fig. 20.6).

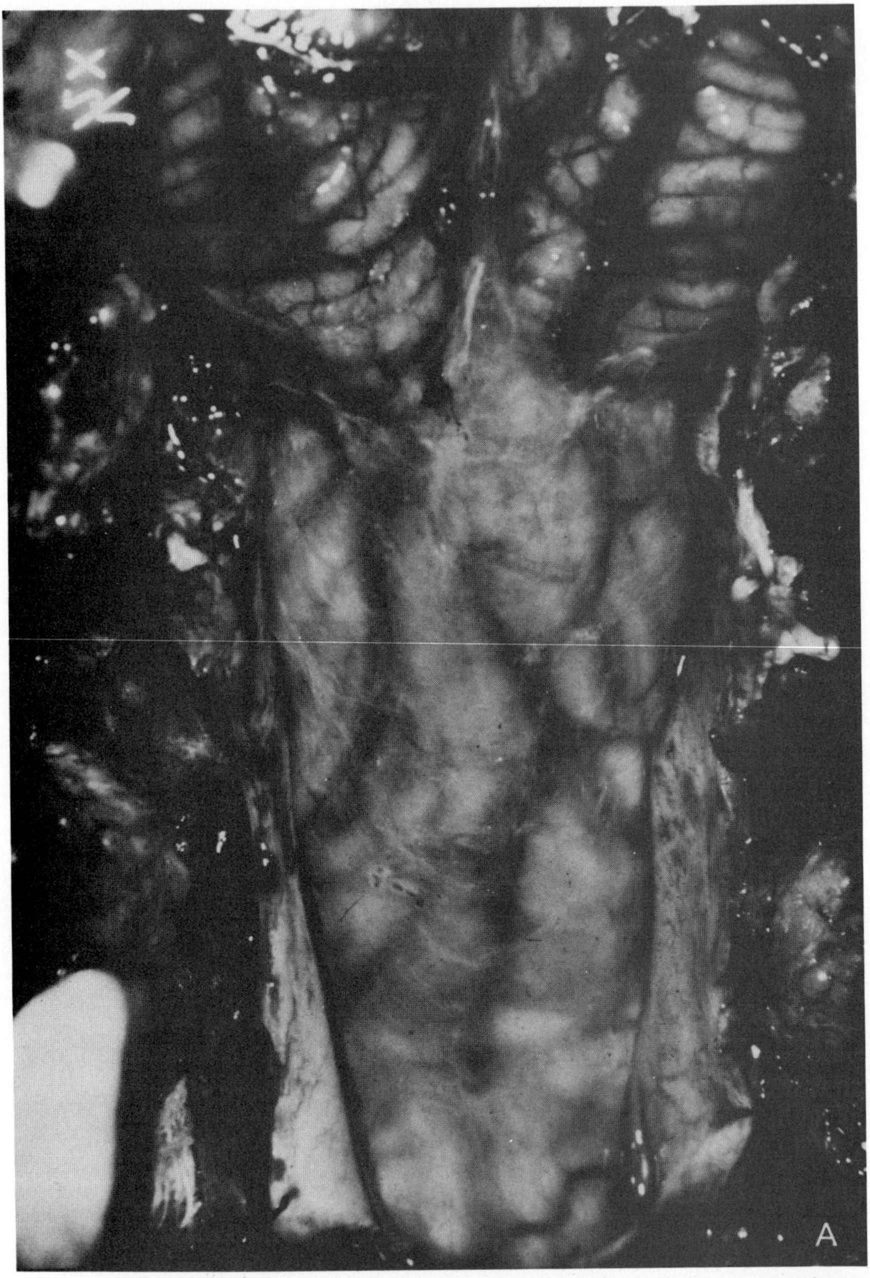

FIG. 20.7. (*A*) Dense fibrous tissue extending from the level of the foramen magnum to below the level of the C2 dorsal spine. Total laminectomy of C1 and C2 had been carried out. (Reproduced with permission from P. W. Carmel (9).)

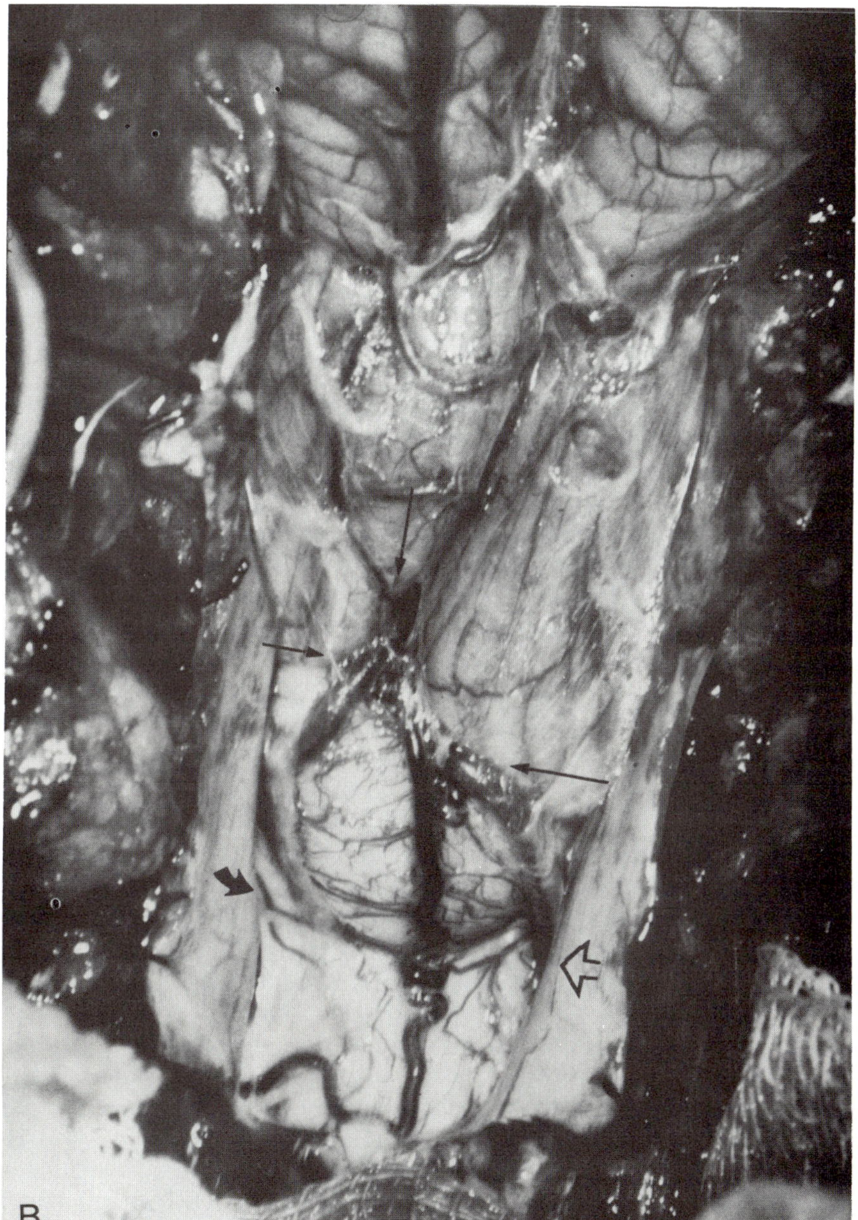

FIG. 20.7. (*B*) Same case as in Figure 20.7*A*, after removal of some of the dense connective tissue. The *small horizontal arrows* indicate the lower poles of the left and right tonsils. These tonsils are densely adherent to the underlying medulla and should not be dissected further. The caudal pole of the inferior vermis is indicated by the ventrical arrow. Beneath this point is the opening of the IVth ventricle, which drained CSF adequately. (*Open arrow, left*) the C1 nerve root can be detected running upward toward its foramen. (Reproduced with permission from P. W. Carmel (9).)

The aim of the operation is to decompress the cerebellar tonsils and upper cervical region and to permit egress of CSF from the IVth ventricle. These principles should be kept in mind when undertaking removal of the arachnoid at the caudal end of the cerebellar tonsils. Current enthusiasm for microdissection has occasionally led to overzealous attempts at microscopic removal of this tissue. It is not necessary to remove all of this tissue but merely to provide adequate decompression. Figures 20.7*A* and *B* indicate a pitfall that may await the unwary microscope surgeon. In this patient, dissection of the arachnoid over the "tonsils" revealed a very prominent and bulging medullary kink which would have resulted in surgical disaster if included in the dissection.

Tonsillar displacement need not be symmetrical around the cervical cord (Fig. 20.8). In some instances the tonsils not only compress the cord from its dorsal surface but also slide around the lateral portions of the cord in both directions to compress its sides. Adequate decompression may still be achieved simply by bony laminectomy, and it has never been necessary in our series to decompress by removal of tonsillar tissue. The most terminal portion of the herniated tonsils, which Chiari termed "peg-like," is often atrophic and scarred at the terminal portions of this appendage (Fig. 20.9). In some instances, these white, fibrotic tips may be freely elevated from the underlying cord, while in others they are so densely adherent to the cord itself that further dissection would be quite hazardous.

In many instances the foramen of Magendie is located quite rostrally to the tonsillar terminus (Fig. 20.10). It is not necessary in these instances to perform extensive microdissection of the tonsils but rather to open up the ventricular outlet. A band-like membrane is often found over the foramen of Magendie (6 of 47 cases of Barnett *et al.*) (3). This fibrous tissue must be opened to enter the IVth ventricle itself. Adequate flow of CSF through an opening held apart by retractors may not signify that the IVth ventricle will continue to drain after closure.

Gardner (15) has advocated exposure of the dilated opening of the central canal in patients with syringomyelia and plugging of this opening with a piece of muscle. Review of several series would indicate that there is not sufficient proof of the benefit of canal closure to make extensive dissection and ticklish manipulation of the floor of the IVth ventricle worth the risk. Most authors plug the central canal only when it is readily available (3), but it has not been our practice to utilize this step.

When the cervical cord is clearly dilated in the sitting position, it is likely that a syringomyelic cavity of some size exists. A number of procedures for draining this cavity have been proposed, and it is the purpose of another chapter in this book to review these techniques. Rhoton (27) has described incision of the cavity through the region of the dorsal root entry zone on the more dilated side.

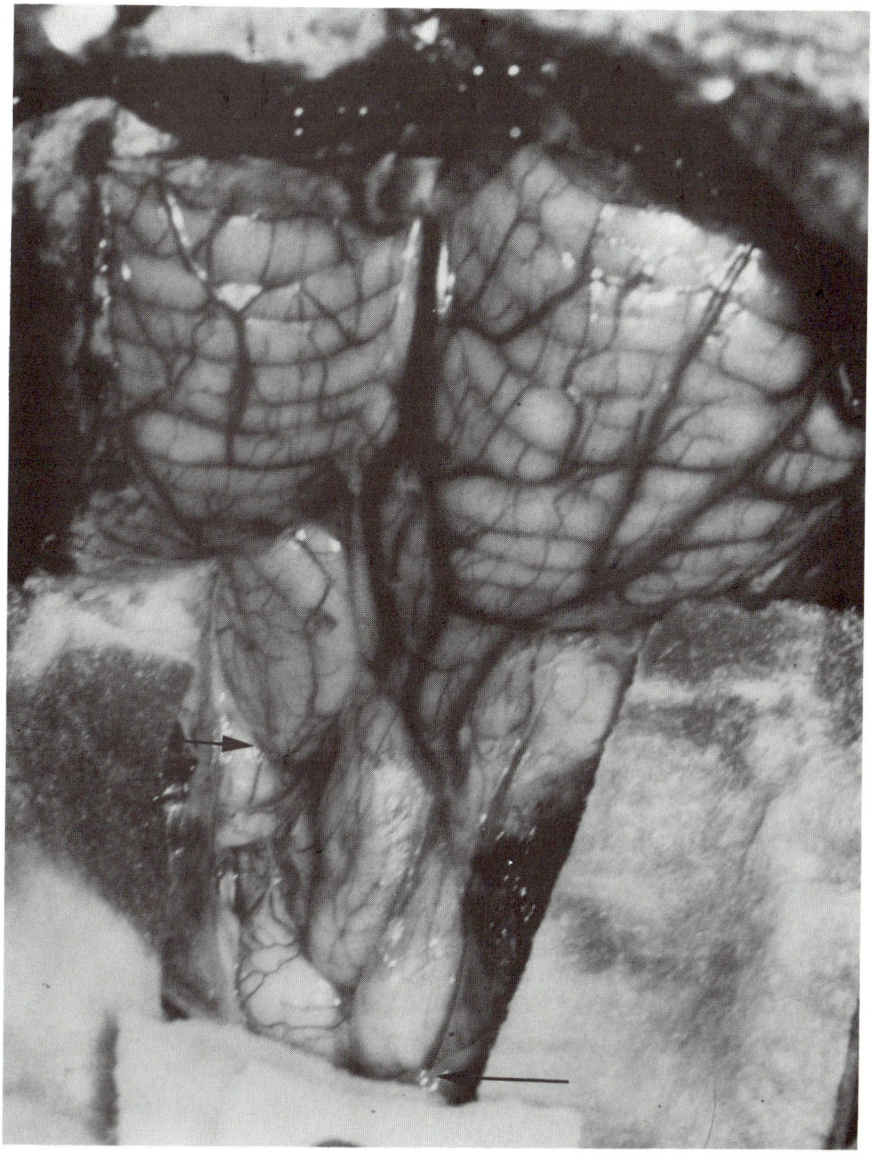

FIG. 20.8. Asymmetry of tonsillar descent, as indicated by the *two small arrows* which are at the lower pole of each tonsil. On the left, the tonsil descended to C1. The right tonsil was bilobed and extended caudal to the C2 lamina.

Decompression of the dura can be ensured by use of a dural graft sutured into the dural opening in watertight fashion. Barnett *et al.* (3) point out that when the dura was left opened the postoperative course was rather stormy, probably as a result of contamination of the CSF with blood and transudate. These patients experienced severe headache, neck

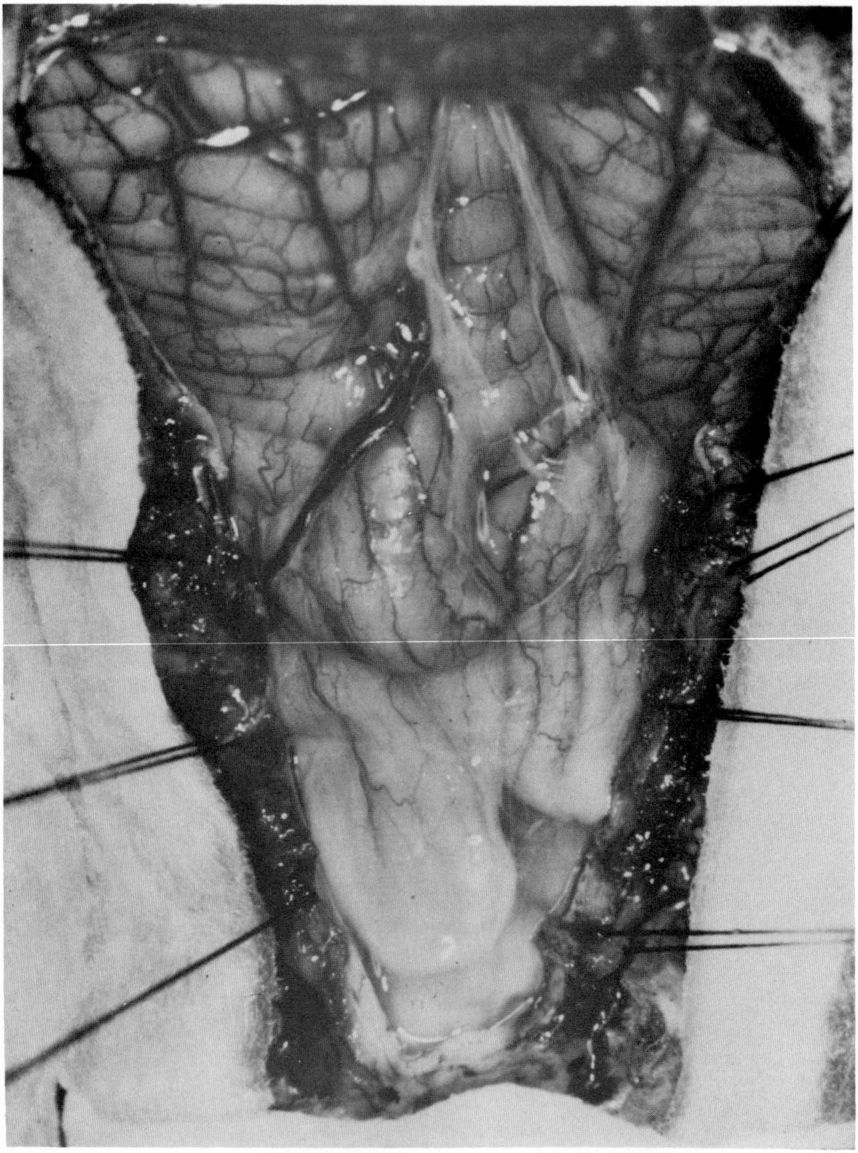

FIG. 20.9. Atrophic whitish tonsillar tips, described by Chiari as "peg-like." Note that in this case the overlying arachnoid is not unusually thickened, nor are the tonsils adherent to the cord. There was no obstruction to CSF flow from the IVth ventricle.

stiffness, and fever with elevated spinal fluid protein content. This "posterior fossa syndrome" has been reviewed elsewhere (6).

Calliauw and Dehaene (5) evaluated surgical risk in the treatment of these malformations. Their extensive review of the literature indicated

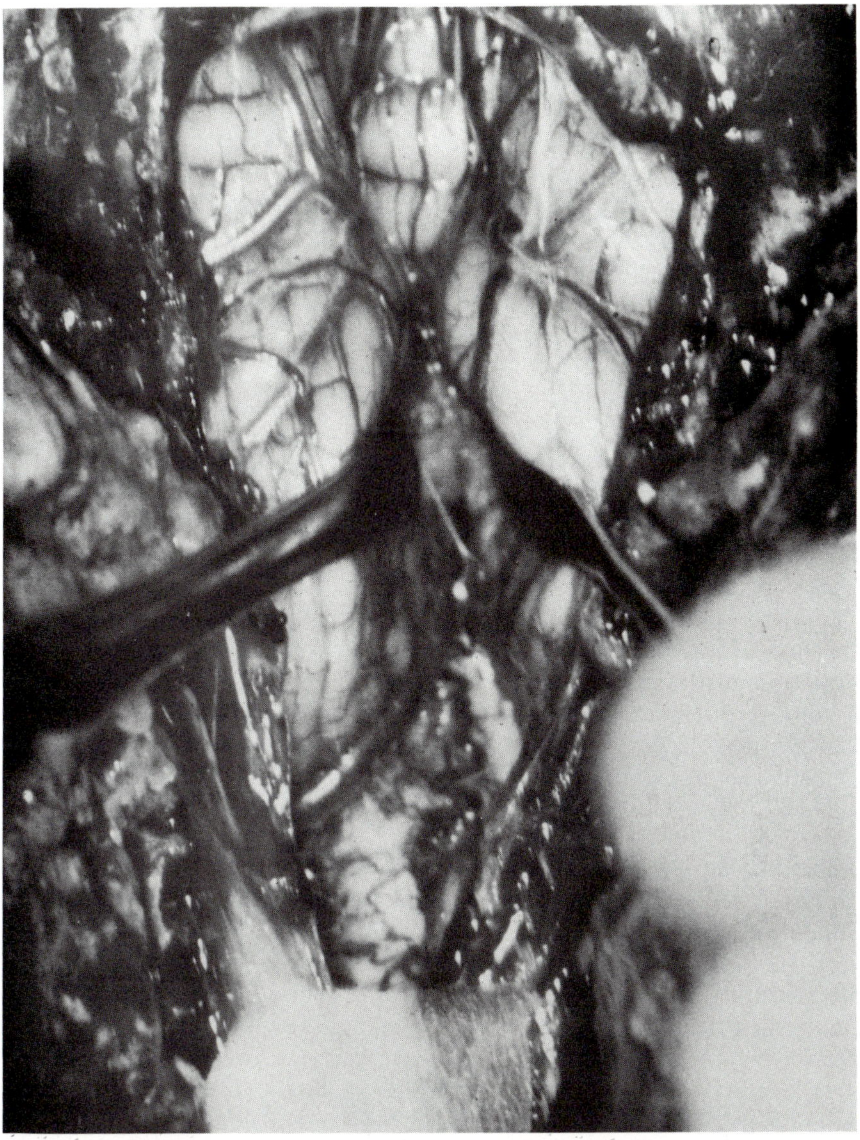

FIG. 20.10. Chiari Type I anomaly, with lower pole of tonsils at C1-C2 level. However, the outlet of the IVth ventricle was above the level of the foramen magnum beneath the inferior vermis. The obex of the ventricle is seen between the retracting instruments.

that mortality rates for these procedures ranged from 5 to 10%, with 27 of 243 patients reported up until 1974 as dying in the postoperative period. The major cause for these deaths and for other operative complications was respiratory compromise. Gardner (15) attributed respiratory arrest in 3 of 5 patients that died to closure of dura over the descended tonsils and advised that the dura should be left opened (15).

Another major complication is tetraplegia. This was felt to be a possible consequence of an excessively flexed posture of the head as the patient was positioned on the table (5). Hyperflexion leading to compression occurs especially in patients with pronounced basilar impression as they are positioned to facilitate removal of the inferior part of the squamous occipital bone.

In patients who have an obstructive syndrome, with moderate or progressive hydrocephalus, a shunting procedure is the operation of choice and often relieves all symptoms. However, further postoperative decompression of the posterior fossa may be required (3). Patients with uncontrolled hydrocephalus are at increased risk during the time of posterior fossa surgery.

In several cases, decompression of the posterior fossa, allowing the cerebellum to push further caudally after decompression, stretched an already compromised aqueduct. Thus, patients who had no preoperative indication of hydrocephalus may develop it following adequate posterior fossa decompression (7).

Gol and Hellbusch (16) have recently pointed out that compromise of the cervical root function in this anomaly may be in part caused by bony structures of the cervical canal. They have rerouted cervical nerve roots by removing part of the floor of the neural canal or by facetectomy (16). This unusual approach has been carried out in few patients, and its possible role in treatment of this disorder has not yet been determined.

CONCLUSION

Two major types of cerebellar and hindbrain anomaly are found in childhood and adolescent years. Both follow definitions first outlined by Chiari nearly a century ago.

The Chiari Type II malformation features caudal displacement of both the medulla and inferior cerebellum and is usually associated with myelomeningocele. These children have defects noted at birth, and over 80% develop symptomatic hydrocephalus within the first 6 months. Brain stem compressive symptoms are usually a late consequence of hydrocephalus and often respond to shunt procedures. However, in rare cases, direct posterior fossa decompression may be required and should be done immediately.

Chiari Type I malformation demonstrates caudal displacement of cerebellar tonsils and inferior lobes, without a major anomaly of the brain stem. These patients become symptomatic late in childhood, either in adolescence or in their young adult years. Hydrocephalus may be present, but most of these patients present with signs of compression at brain stem or upper cervical levels. Early signs due to an associated syringomyelia may be present. Shunting procedures occasionally relieve all symptoms in those children with associated hydrocephalus, but direct posterior fossa decompression is most often required. Although the type of operation remains controversial, its aims should be decompression of brain stem and cervical cord, and opening of CSF egress from the IVth ventricle. Extensive microdissection of tonsils or resection of cerebellar tissue is rarely indicated and may be dangerous. Additional procedures for treatment of syringomyelia may be needed.

REFERENCES

1. Appleby, A., Foster, J. B., Hankinson, J., and Hudgson, P. The Chiari anomalies in adult life. Brain, *91:* 131–139, 1968.
2. Arnold, J. Myelocyste, transposition von gewebskeimen und sympodie. Beitr. Pathol. Anat., *16:* 1–28, 1894.
3. Barnett, H. J. M., Foster, J. B., and Hudgson, P. Syringomyelia. W. B. Saunders, London, 1973.
4. Bartelmez, G. W., and DeKaban, A. S. The early development of the human brain. Contrib. Embryol., *37:* 13–32, 1962.
5. Calliauw, L., and Dehaene, I. The surgical risk in the treatment of Arnold-Chiari malformations. Acta Neurochir., *39:* 173–179, 1977.
6. Carmel, P. W., Fraser, R. A. R., and Stein, B. M. Aseptic meningitis following posterior fossa surgery in children. J. Neurosurg., *41:* 44–48, 1974.
7. Carmel, P. W., and Markesbery, W. R. Arnold-Chiari malformation in an elderly woman. Arch. Neurol., *21:* 258–262, 1969.
8. Carmel, P. W., and Markesbery, W. R. Early descriptions of the Arnold-Chiari malformation. The contribution of John Cleland. J. Neurosurg., *37:* 543–547, 1972.
9. Carmel, P. W. Arnold-Chiari malformation. In: *Pediatric Neurosurgery: Surgery of the Developing Nervous System,* edited by Robert McLaurin, Grune & Stratton, New York, 1982.
10. Chiari, H. Ueber Veranderungen des Kleinhirns infolge von Hydrocephalie des Grosshirns. Deutsch Med. Wochenschr. *17:* 1172–1175, 1891.
11. Chiari, H. Ueber Veranderungen des Kleinhirns, des Pons und der Medulla Oblongata in folge von Congenitaler Hydrocephalie des Grosshirns. Denschr. Akad. Wiss. Wien *63:* 71–116, 1896.
12. Cleland, J. Contribution to the study of spina bifida, encephalocele, and anencephalus. J. Anat. Physiol., *17:* 257–291, 1883.
13. Daniel, P. W., and Strich, S. J. Some observations on the congenital deformity of the central nervous system known as the Arnold-Chiari malformation. J. Neuropathol. Exp. Neurol., *17:* 255–266, 1958.
14. Gardner, W. J. Anatomic features common to the Arnold-Chiari and the Dandy-Walker malformations suggest a common origin. Cleveland Clin. Q., *26:* 206–222, 1959.
15. Gardner, W. J. The dysraphic states. Excerpta Medica, Amsterdam, 1973.
16. Gol, A., and Hellbusch, L. C. Surgical relief of progressive upper limb paralysis in Arnold-Chiari malformation. J. Neurol. Neurosurg. Psychiatry, *41:* 433–437, 1978.
17. Hoffman, H. J., Henrick, E. B., and Humphreys, R. P. Manifestations and management of Arnold-Chiari malformation in patients with myelomeningocele. Child's Brain, *1:* 255–259, 1975.
18. Kirsch, W. M., Duncan, B. R., Black, F. O., *et al.* Laryngeal palsy in association with

myelomeningocele, hydrocephalus and Arnold-Chiari malformation. J. Neurosurg., *28:* 207–214, 1968.

19. Lapras, C., and Lotfi, M. Surgical management of Chiari II malformation in children. Mod. Probl. Paediatr., *18:* 142–145, 1977.
20. Malis, L. I., Cohen, I., and Gross, S. W. Arnold-Chiari malformation. Arch. Surg., *63:* 783–798, 1951.
21. Mohr, P. D., Strang, F. A., Sambrook, M. A., and Boddie, H. G. The clinical and surgical features in 40 patients with primary cerebellar ectopia (Adult Chiari malformation). Q. J. Med., *181:* 85–96, 1977.
22. Mori, K., Handa, H., Okuno, T., and Hazama, F. Arnold-Chiari type II malformation. A clinicopathological study with special reference to its surgical treatment. Neurochirurgia, *21:* 9–14, 1978.
23. Naidich, T. P., Pudlowski, R. M., Naidich, J. B., Gornish, M., and Rodriquez, F. Computed tomographic signs of the Chiari II malformation. Part I. Skull and dural partitions. Radiology *134:* 65–71, 1980.
24. Peach, B. Arnold-Chiari malformation: Morphogenesis. Arch. Neurol., *12:* 527–535, 1965.
25. Peach, B. Arnold-Chiari malformation: Anatomic features of 20 cases. Arch. Neurol., *12:* 613–621, 1965.
26. Penfield, W., and Coburn, D. F. Arnold-Chiari malformation and its operative treatment. Arch. Neurol. Psychiatry, *40:* 328–336, 1938.
27. Rhoton, A. L., Jr. Microsurgery of Arnold-Chiari malformation in adults with and without hydromyelia. J. Neurosurg. *45:* 473–483, 1976.
28. Schut, L., and Bruce, D. A. The Arnold-Chiari malformation. Orthoped. Clin. North Am., *9:* 913–921, 1978.
29. Sieben, R. L., Hamida, M. B., and Shulman, K. Multiple cranial nerve deficits associated with the Arnold-Chiari malformation. Neurology, *21:* 673–681, 1971.
30. Streeter, G. W. Developmental horizons in human embryos. Description of age groups XV, XVI, XVII, XVIII, being third issue of a survey of the Carnegie collection. Contrib. Embryol., *32:* 133–203, 1948.
31. Venes, J. L. Multiple cranial nerve palsies in an infant with Arnold-Chiari malformation. Dev. Med. Child Neurol., *16:* 817–820, 1974.
32. Verbiest, H. The Arnold-Chiari malformation. J. Neurol. Neurosurg. Psychiatry, *16:* 227–233, 1953.

CHAPTER

21

Results of Treatment of Children Born with a Myelomeningocele

DAVID G. McLONE, M.D., PH.D., F.A.C.S.

INTRODUCTION

As new operative procedures, medications, and ancillary care develop, the natural history of a disease can be progressively altered. The impact of cerebrospinal fluid shunting on hydrocephalus and the even more recent utilization of computed tomography (CT) to diagnose and assess treatment of hydrocephalus are good examples of this type of progress. Periodically, the effect of progress on the outcome of treatment of children born with a myelomeningocele needs to be determined.

We would argue that it is moral and ethically correct to treat all children born with a myelomeningocele and that no valid criteria exists for the selection of infants for nontreatment. Certainly, as the "quality of survival" improves through meidcal progress, the poor outcome which the selection criteria (3) purport to accurately predict becomes less distasteful. An added scientific benefit of treating all children is that it affords the opportunity to measure the effectiveness of treatment without the bias of selection.

The initial decision to operate on a newborn child with a myelomeningocele rests on the premises that: (a) the physician informing the parents is familiar with the disease; (b) the information available concerning outcome is current; and (c) the outcome is predictable, based on the clincial condition of the newborn. The first is often lacking, the third is not true, and the second is the subject of this paper.

CLINICAL MATERIAL

Beginning in 1975 and extending through 1978, 100 consecutive unselected newborn children with a myelomeningocele were transferred to Children's Memorial Hospital of Chicago. Extensive data were collected in a prospective study for evaluation of outcome of treatment by a multiple-discipline team. All children had their myelomeningocele repaired following evaluation by the team. Orthopedic and urological treatment was begun during the initial hospitalization. Specialists in nursing, occupational and physical therapy, diet, psychology, and social work were involved as part of the team from the outset. After discharge, the children were followed closely by the same team in the outpatient clinic. Education of the child and of the parents and assistance to the family in habilitation of the child in order to attain the most independent competitive adult life possible were the ultimate goals of the team.

RESULTS

The period of follow-up is from 3.5 years to 7 years. Two of the children have been lost to follow-up and 14 have moved, but a recent evaluation is known to us, and the remaining living children are being followed in our clinic.

Eighty-nine percent of the children had their backs closed in the first 24 hours of life. The other 11 children were transferred later than 48 hours of life and were assumed to be infected. Following antibiotics and cleansing of the back, the repair was undertaken when cultures of the back were negative.

Preoperative motor function is summarized in Figure 21.1. Following surgery, at 10 days of life a repeat motor examination showed a significant improvement in motor function. Motor improvement was considered significant if the functional improvement added function across the next joint and functional improvement persisted beyond the 1-year follow-up examination. Deterioration in function is considered an indication for diagnostic study. Hydromyelia, tethered cord, and inclusion dermoids

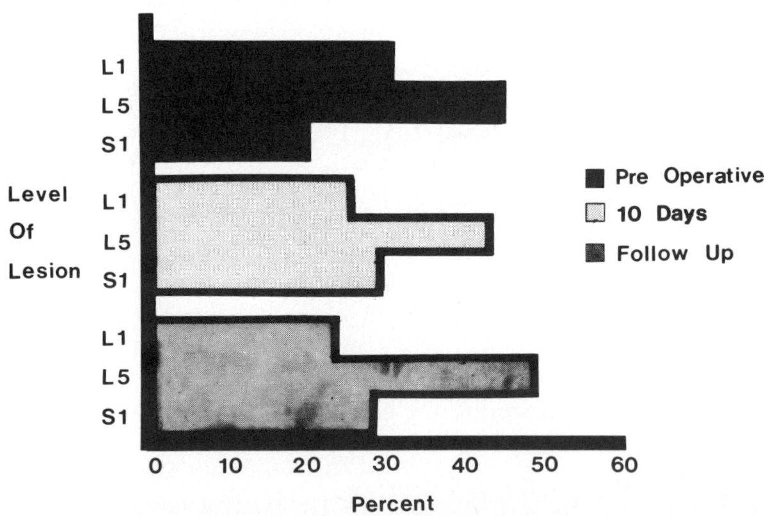

FIG. 21.1. Graph illustrates the preoperative, 10-day postoperative, and follow-up motor evaluation.

have explained deterioration in children followed in our clinic, but not as part of this series, and deterioration has been reversed by appropriate treatment.

Hydrocephalus requiring a shunt developed in 80% of the children. The ventricular volume was abnormally large in an additional 15%, but no shunt was inserted if the ventricles were stable on sequential CT scans and if the child's development was on time.

Almost half (48%) of the children with a shunt have not required a shunt revision. One revision was required in 16%, 2 in 16%, 3 in 8%, 4 in 8%, and 5, 7, and 9 each in 1%. A shunt infection occurred in 10.3% of the procedures. The majority of Gram-negative infections occurred in the first month of life and were significantly higher in children with delayed back repair.

Yearly developmental assessments, including intelligence, were obtained on most of the children. Development was normal in 73% of the surviving children.

One half (54%) of the children are community ambulators, and only 8% are confined to a wheelchair at the present time. Some 24% are exercise ambulators, and 14% use a wheelchair in the community but not in their home.

Urinary continence has been achieved in 87% of the children who are over 4½ years of age. We do not feel that incontinence prior to 4½ years predicts continence at school age. Urinary diversions to the abdominal wall were performed in 5 of the earlier cases, and 3 of these were subsequently undiverted. Clean intermittent catheterization in combination with pharmacotherapy has led to the high continency rate and has made urinary diversion rarely necessary.

The surgical mortality is 2%. One child died immediately after surgery of respiratory distress and another died of sepsis following breakdown of the back repair.

The overall mortality is 14% at 3.5–7 years of follow-up. Twelve children died subsequent to discharge; 7 of these deaths were associated with hindbrain problems of the Chiari II malformation. Three children died because of respiratory problems caused by compromise of the thoracic cavity by hemivertebra and fused ribs limiting the development of the hemithorax. Attempts at surgical correction on children not part of this series have not been successful, and it was therefore decided not to operate on these children.

Apnea, stridor, and reflux with aspiration—one of these or in some combination—were significant in 32% of the children. Chiari II symptoms are more severe in our series in those children with low lumbosacral lesions and function in their legs. Posterior fossa decompression was performed in 4 of these children. Subsequent to decompression, 2 died, 1 still requires a tracheostomy, and 1 has become asymptomatic. Of the remaining 28, 9 have died, 1 continues to require a tracheostomy, and the problem has resolved in the other 18 children. Thus, 11 of 32 have died, for an overall mortality of 34%. It should be pointed out that 2 of these are the children considered operative deaths, and 3 are the children with compromise of their hemithorax.

Of the 86 survivors who are older than 4½, 47% are intellectually normal, are continent of urine, and are community ambulators. An additional 28% older than 4½ are intellectually normal and continent but do not ambulate in the community. The total percentage of children who could be independent and competitive is approaching 70–80%.

DISCUSSION

This study represents an unselected consecutive series of patients. The extent of prior selection by the physicians who refer to Children's Memorial Hospital is unknown. All children were aggressively treated initially. In about 10% of the cases it ultimately became clear that continuation of aggressive therapy was inappropriate. The operative mortality should be near 0 in this group of children. Renal failure as a primary cause of death has almost been eliminated. Symptomatic Chiari II problems continue to be the major cause of death in these children.

Close scrutiny of these children reveals that almost all of the children have some symptoms of hindbrain problems. Mothers relate that they "spit up" more, choke easily, tolerate changes in food texture poorly, and have occasional respiratory pauses. In about one-third of the children the symptoms will present a significant problem. About 5% (5 of 100) will progress toward persistent apnea, and we have performed posterior fossa decompression in that group. In one-third of this symptomatic group, about 10% of the total 100, death will be directly or indirectly attributed to these problems. In almost two-thirds of the children the condition resolves with time. Resolution would appear to be the natural history of the hindbrain problem. The value of posterior fossa decompression is still debatable. In all 4 of our children who were decompressed (decompression carried into the posterior fossa), an immediate improvement was noted. Two subsequently died, and 1 continues to have significant problems. To advocate posterior fossa decompression on all symptomatic children, a success rate greater than two-thirds must be demonstrated.

The majority of children with severe Chiari II symptoms would have escaped selection criteria commonly used because of their lack of hydrocephalus at birth, low level of the lesion, and functional lower extremities.

We may be placing too great an emphasis on intellectual development. It would seem that if our primary goal is the most competitive independent adult possible in a technologically advanced society, normal intelligence is a requisite. Obviously, those individuals with less than normal intelligence have great human value, and everything must be done to make their lives comfortable and meaningful. Many of the children with less than normal IQs, although requiring some care, should make significant contributions to our society.

In a previous publication we demonstrated that retardation is acquired in most of these children as a result of shunt complications (4). Unfortunately, our shunt infection rate in this series was still too high. Children closed late were at greatest risk for Gram-negative ventriculitis. Every effort should be made to keep the shunt infection rate at a minimum.

Management of the hydrocephalus in reviewing the data was much less of a problem than the author thought. We tend to remember the child with 9 revisions and forget that 20% were not shunted, 50% of the shunted children have not required a revision, and only 10% have required between 4 and 9 revisions.

Motor deterioration in a child with a myelomeningocele dictates further diagnostic studies. Tethered cord, hydromyelia, and dermoid tumors have explained motor deterioration in children followed by our team but not included in this series. Recovery followed appropriate surgical intervention. Postoperative improvement after myelomeningocele repair noted at 10 days of life has persisted through the period of this study. Improvement followed by deterioration to the previous level, as a natural history of the disease described in the literature, was not borne out by this study (1).

The final ambulatory status of many of these children will be determined during their teenage years. The projected rate of community ambulation may be too high, but with improved orthosis and habilitation techniques this level may be reached.

The mortality rate, now at 14%, should stabilize within a few percentage points of 14%. Most of the children with severe problems have died. The children most at risk are those with hydrocephalus. All of the children who have died in this study had hydrocephalus. A shunt malfunction or a complication of a revision may cause the death of children in the future.

The survival and functional status of this group of children is superior to most studies in the literature, including those evaluating only patients selected for treatment (2, 5, 6). Aggressive management by a knowledgeable team and close follow-up ensure both survival and improved function.

CONCLUSION

Although we are far from a cure, the future becomes progressively optimistic for these children. Only time will confirm what is in store for these 86 surviving children. The mortality rate is low in this series, and the quality of survival for the majority of the children appears good. Habilitation, accessible housing, and job opportunities remain as societal problems to be solved.

REFERENCES

1. Brocklehurst, G., Gleave, J. R. W., and Lewin, W. Early closure of myelomeningocele, with special reference to leg movement. Br. Med. J., *1:* 666–669, 1967.
2. Lorber, J. Early results of selective treatment of spina bifida cystica. Br. Med. J., *4:* 201–204, 1973.
3. Lorber, J. Results of treatment of myelomeningocele, an analysis of 524 unselected cases, with special reference to possible selection for treatment. Dev. Med. Child. Neurol., *13:* 279–303, 1971.
4. McLone, D. G., Czyzewski, D., Raimondi, A. J., and Sommers, R. C. Central nervous system infections as a limiting factor in the intelligence of children with myelomeningocele. Pediatrics, *70*(3)*:* 338–342, 1982.
5. Shurtleff, D. B., Hayden, P. W., Loeser, J. D., and Kronmal, R. A. Myelodysplasia: Decision for death or disability. N. Engl. J. Med., *291:* 1005–1011, 1974.
6. Stark, G. D., and Drummond, M. Results of selective early operation in myelomeningocele. Arch. Dis. Childhood, *48:* 676–683, 1973.

CHAPTER

22

The Orthopedic and Orthotic Management of the Spina Bifida Child

NORRIS CARROLL, M.D.

INTRODUCTION

Total Care

The overall goal in management of a child with spina bifida is to achieve a pattern of development as near normal as possible. This cannot be attained by an orthopedist working in isolation. The total care for a child with spina bifida requires the coordinated efforts of a team of specialists in a multidisciplinary clinic (9).

The Combined Spina Bifida Clinic at the Ontario Crippled Children's Centre is really a group of clinics running simultaneously and organized by a nurse coordinator. For each combined clinic there is a patient roster. Beside the name of each patient, there is a list of the special services to be provided at that clinic.

The patients arrive at a reception area early in the morning. Some may have to go to X-ray for an IVP. All of the 30–40 patients that attend each clinic go to therapy, where they are assessed. Each therapist sees 5 or 6 children. The therapist, who assesses a child in the morning, then goes with the child and parents and acts as an ombudsman when the child is being reviewed by each specialist in the afternoon. If there are any conflicts in the plans for future care, the therapist notifies the coordinator so that the overall care can be more appropriately organized.

Below (Table 22.1) is a scheme of the organization of the Combined Spina Bifida Clinic.

INITIAL ASSESSMENT

A newborn with spina bifida cannot be assessed properly unless the child is warm and hungry. A check-off sheet in the nursery is useful for recording observations. What is the child's general condition? Has he a strong cry? What is his muscular tone? Head and chest sizes are recorded. Is the fontannel tight? Are the sutures wide? The child with hydroceph-alus will have an enlarged head, the fontanel will be tight, and the sutures will be split. The spine is inspected; the size and the level of the defect

TABLE 22.1

Scheme of the Organization of the Combined Spina Bifida Clinic

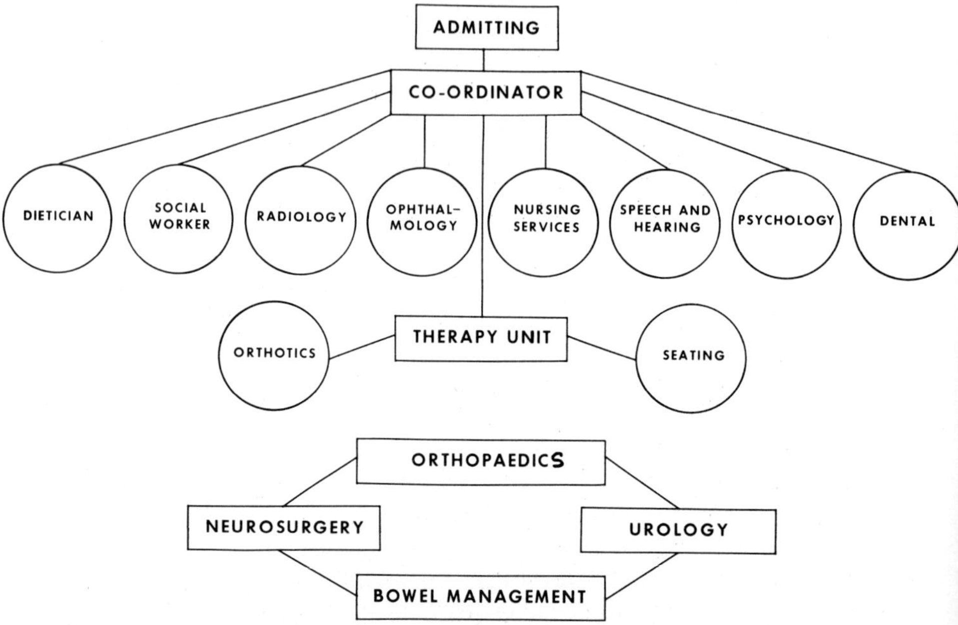

are recorded. Is the lesion skin covered or are the dura and neuroplacode exposed? Is the lesion dry, draining CSF, or bulging? Is there an associated spinal deformity? Thoracolumbar lesions in a child with hydrocephalus are commonly accompanied by kyphosis at birth.

The upper limbs are examined for range of motion and spontaneous movement. If the child has an Arnold-Chiari malformation (11), there will be upper motor neuron signs in the arms.

The lower limbs are watched for spontaneous movement. Then stimulate the limb and look for movement. Remember that movement which is initiated by stimulating the limb may be a reflex movement produced by an isolated segment of cord distal to the neural tube defect. Now scratch the trunk and look for limb movement again. Movement initiated by stimulation proximal to the site of the defect is more likely to be voluntary. The hips are assessed for range of motion and stability. Deformity at the hip, knee, and foot is recorded. The knees and ankles are assessed for range of motion.

In a newborn, grading motor power is difficult, but one should be able to tell whether a muscle is working and whether it is weak, strong, or spastic. The perineum is inspected for tone. Is the anal sphincter closed or patulous? Is there an anal wink? As the child cries, does he dribble urine?

The lower limbs are assessed for sensation. One can tell whether or not there is withdrawal when the feet and lower limbs are stimulated.

The needs of the newborn are largely met by the neurosurgeon who closes the lesion. These needs include explanations, counseling, and perhaps putting the parents in touch with the spina bifida association. Treatment of foot and knee deformities may start with serial casts. A therapist shows mother how to put weak lower limbs through a daily range of movement and prevent postural deformities (9).

PRACTICAL CLASSIFICATION

There is more to spina bifida than paraplegia. The treatment and outcome depend mostly on general development, which in turn depends on home circumstances, shunts, lengthy illnesses, hydrocephalus, hydromyelia, and Arnold-Chiari malformation. However, infants with the highest neurosegmental lesions tend to be the ones with the most developmental delay.

Neurosegmental Levels

Spina bifida children have patterns of ability that vary with the severity of the motor and sensory deficit. In planning the total care for these children, it is useful to group them into 5 neurosegmental levels: upper thoracic, lower thoracic, upper lumbar, lower lumbar, and sacral. The neurosegmental level is defined as the lowest active motor root (15).

UPPER THORACIC

A child with an upper thoracic level does not have enough trunk power to sit without support. Despite a spinal support for hands-free sitting, they frequently develop spinal deformities, which may require surgical stabilization. The strength of the upper limbs, which are often mildly spastic, determines the functional peak. All children will require help with the activities of daily living and will become wheelchair users.

The goals for children with upper thoracic level disability are (a) good sitting balance, (b) ambulation during the first decade if there is good upper limb function, (c) ability to transfer from a chair, (d) wheelchair propulsion, (e) self-care, and (f) an education and social acceptability.

LOWER THORACIC

These children have sufficient innervation of their trunk musculature to be better sitters. They usually have enough upper limb strength to transfer independently and use a wheelchair well. As children they often ambulate during the first decade with a standing brace or parapodium but at puberty become wheelchair users. They have a high risk of trophic ulceration under their ischial tuberosities. Good skin care, parent and child education, and prophylactic skin assessment are necessary to prevent the social, educational, vocational, and psychological setbacks that can occur as a result of skin breakdown.

UPPER LUMBAR

These children have active hip flexors and adductors and weak quadriceps. Muscle imbalance frequently causes hip and knee flexion deformities and hip instability (3).

Their goal is household ambulation in long leg braces. (See upright mobility for a defintion of types of ambulation.) They require crutches to maintain an upright stance and may choose to ambulate using a 4-point or a swing-through gait. When they become teenagers and adults, wheelchairs provide quick mobility.

LOWER LUMBAR

The hip flexors, adductors, and quadriceps are normal. The medial hamstrings will usually flex the knee against gravity. Despite some motor function below the knee, this is not sufficient to balance the feet or avoid below knee bracing. Hip abductor power varies. Very weak abductors necessitate forearm crutches or a cane. Hip instability is common, and surgical correction is worthwhile. The majority require surgery to keep their feet plantigrade (17). Their strong quadriceps give them a better quality of life than children with higher lesions. They should become community ambulators.

SACRAL LEVEL

These children should be community ambulators without braces. They may require surgery to correct foot deformities.

Developmental Evaluation

Motor development tends to be delayed in children with spina bifida. The major developmental landmarks are head control, sitting balance, prone mobility, upright stance, and upright mobility.

BIRTH TO HEAD CONTROL

Management objectives, *e.g.*, myotomy for a hip adduction contracture are listed below:

1. Correct deformities. Manipulations and serial casts for club feet.
2. Avoid contractures. Tight hip adductors can be stretched with the hips in flexion; a calcaneus deformity can be manipulated. A splint will prevent the hips from lying in flexion, abduction, and external rotation.
3. Promote developmental stimulation. The parents are encouraged to

handle and play with their baby, as they would in the case of a normal infant.

4. Complete a base line urological assessment.

HEAD CONTROL TO SITTING

Management objectives are listed below:

1. Avoid contractures, for example, stretching the knees with the hips in abduction to overcome tight hamstrings.
2. Encourage sitting balance.
3. Encourage elementary hand skills and eye-hand coordination.
4. Protect anesthetic skin.

SITTING TO PRONE MOBILITY

The management objectives are listed below:

1. Avoid contractures, *e.g.*, the hip flexors can be stretched with the child prone and with the hips abducted and internally rotated.
2. Encourage upper limb use to improve strength.
3. Encourage bilateral hand function.
4. Expand the child's environmental horizons through mobility.

UPRIGHT STANCE

The management objectives are listed below:

1. Continue to avoid contractures.
2. Assess weight-bearing potential.
3. Ensure adequate footwear to protect anesthetic skin.
4. Promote social stimulation through preschool groups.

UPRIGHT MOBILITY

The management objectives are listed below:

1. Achieve upright mobility in childhood so as to avoid contractures and osteoporosis and to promote eye level contact with peers.
2. Predict quality of ambulation in the short and long term.
3. Select appropriate orthosis.
4. Use surgery to facilitate the use of an orthosis or progress to a simpler orthosis.

CLASSIFICATION OF AMBULATION

1. Nonambulators are wheelchair-bound but can usually transfer from a chair to a bed.

2. Nonfunctional ambulator. A wheelchair is used for mobility, but walking is possible in supervised therapeutic sessions at home, in school, and in hospital.

3. Household ambulators walk short distances with apparatus. They are able to get in and out of a chair and bed with little, if any, assistance. They may use the wheelchair for some indoor activities at home and school and for all community activities.

4. Community ambulators walk much of the day but may need crutches or braces. A wheelchair is used for long trips (8).

Orthotic Devices and Mobility Aids

Mobility implies more than walking. It must provide the means for a child to explore his environment, to develop his perceptual skills and his body image in space, and to make possible quick transportation from place to place. Aids such as parallel pushers, H-frame crutches, strollers, or hand-driven bicycles reduce the energy required to be mobile. Mobility is essential in order to attain social maturation and educational, vocational, and avocational goals.

There is a tendency to regard the mobility problems of children with spina bifida as unchanging. However, their neurological deficit may increase due to hydrocephalus, hydromyelia and tethering or scarring of the cord, or it may improve. Investigation, in addition to a new orthotic prescription, is required.

A long-term study of patients with spina bifida, 12–29 years old, indicated that the eventual ambulatory status was primarily dependent upon the neurosegmental level of the lesion, the motor power within a given neurosegmental level, and the extent and degree of the orthopaedic deformity (5). Other important factors are age and the stature of the patient, upper limb strength, the design and effectiveness of the orthosis, the intelligence and motivation, spasticity, obesity, and possibly the sex of the child.

Struggling about with long leg braces and two crutches requires more energy than wheeling a chair (as Hoffer *et al.* (8) have shown). Hence, many children who can walk come to prefer a wheelchair.

We will now look at the choice of aids available.

INFANT SEAT

An infant seat, whether custom made or commercially made, provides the child with an upright position from which to view his world, and it makes a parent's job easier. It can be designed to give the spine some support (Fig. 22.1).

HIP ABDUCTION SPLINT

A hip abduction splint is indicated for children with an upper lumbar neurosegmental level who tend to develop hip flexion-abduction-external

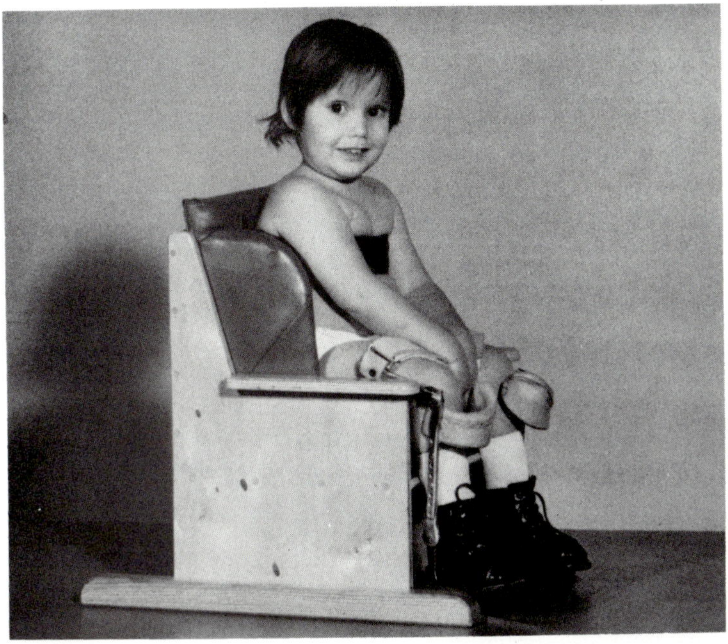

FIG. 22.1. Custom made infant seat.

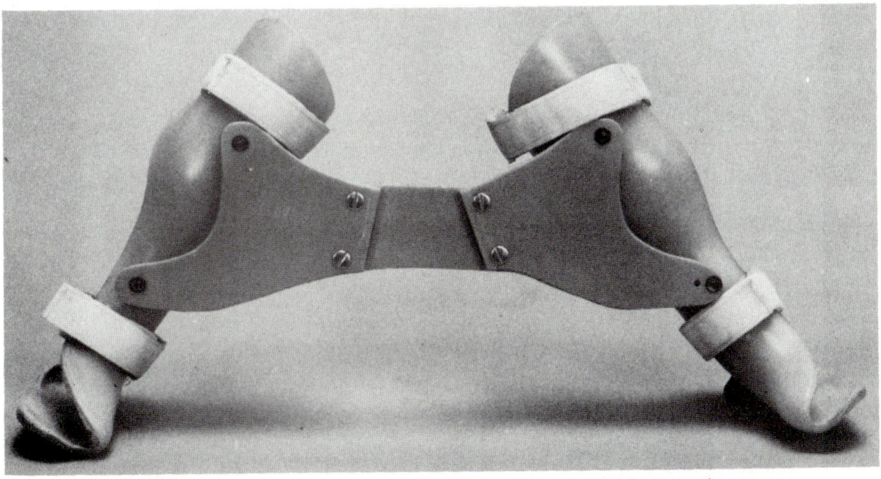

FIG. 22.2. Hip abduction splint used during child's unattended hours.

rotation contractures (10). It maintains hip stability while avoiding contractures. A child in an abduction splint should receive extra developmental stimulation. The splint is worn during the child's unattended hours, for example, during naps and at night (Fig. 22.2).

RESTING SPLINTS

The posterior half of a hip spica made of thermoplastic is often used following hip surgery to prevent the child from flipping over in bed, only to sustain a fracture. Posterior thermoplastic back slabs are used to maintain knee extension postoperatively. Denis Browne splints are used to correct internal tibial torsion deformities (Figure 22.3). Good skin care is necessary for all resting splints.

CASTER CART

This mobility device has a seat with a low center of gravity close to the floor (2). Pushing replaces crawling. A child with thoracic or upper lumbar lesion who has difficulty moving from place to place can learn to use his hands to manipulate the wheels and explore his environment. His skin is protected. Spinal support systems can be built into the orthosis, and a handle can be attached to enable the parent to push the child about (Fig. 22.4).

STANDING BRACE

The standing brace is an inexpensive prefabricated orthosis that allows the child to maintain an upright stance. Fitting can be completed in less than 2 hours. The standing brace allows hands-free standing; swivel walking is achieved by shifting the center of gravity from side to side. With a pusher or H-frame crutches, the child can learn to do a swing-to or swing-through gait. As a preliminary device, it enables the clinic team to assess the child in standing. This device is usually prescribed for children with thoracic or upper lumbar level lesions (Figure 22.5).

When a child is ready for upright mobility, what should be prescribed? Children who cruise furniture need little or an ankle-foot orthosis. All

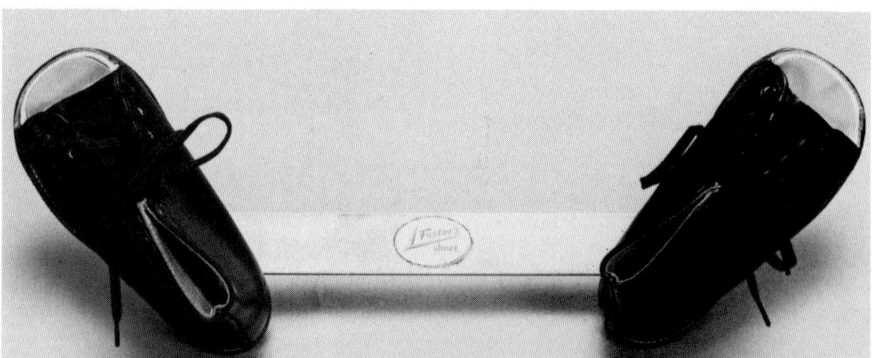

FIG. 22.3. Denis Browne splint used for internal tibial torsion.

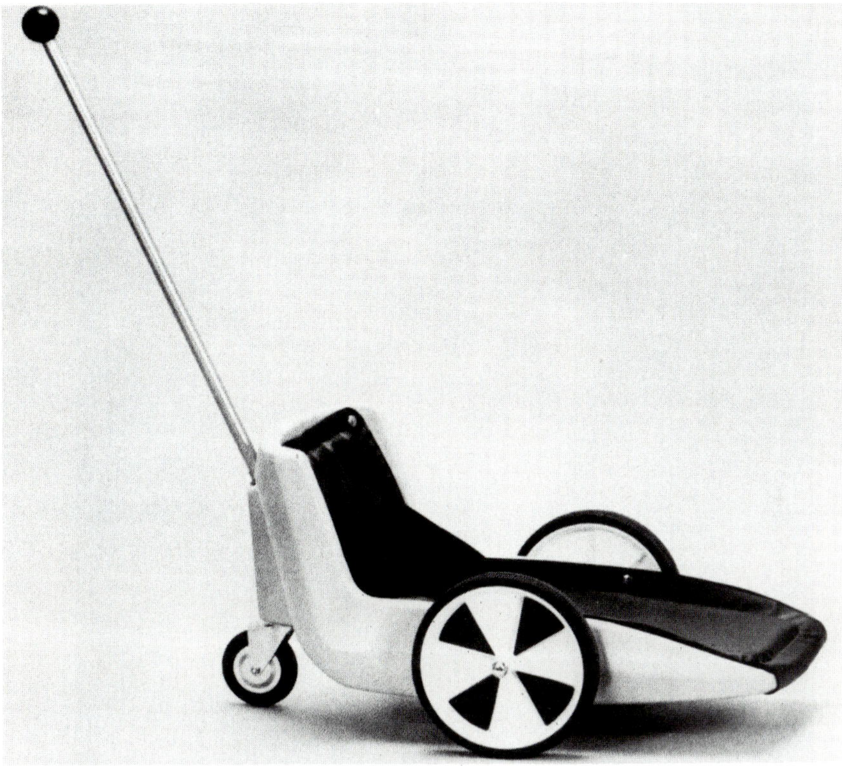

FIG. 22.4. Caster cart. Replaces crawling for a paraplegic child.

the rest are best in a standing brace. We prefer to start with hands-free standing and reduce the extent of bracing as a child demonstrates improved function.

PARAPODIUM

The parapodium is a modular orthosis designed to support the spine in standing and sitting positions. The alignment enables a child to stand without crutches; hinges at the hip and knee permit standing. The brace is easy to assemble and align from a prefabricated kit. Growth adjustments are easy (Fig. 22.6). Its weight is usually one-eighth to one-tenth of the body weight. With the parapodium the shoe, in a sense, becomes part of the child, not part of the brace. Crutchless walking can be achieved by attaching a pivot walker or swivel walker platform to the footplate. Special attachments can be designed and mounted easily. For example, an attachment may be necessary to control a spinal deformity, or a raise can be added to the footplate to compensate for a leg length discrepancy.

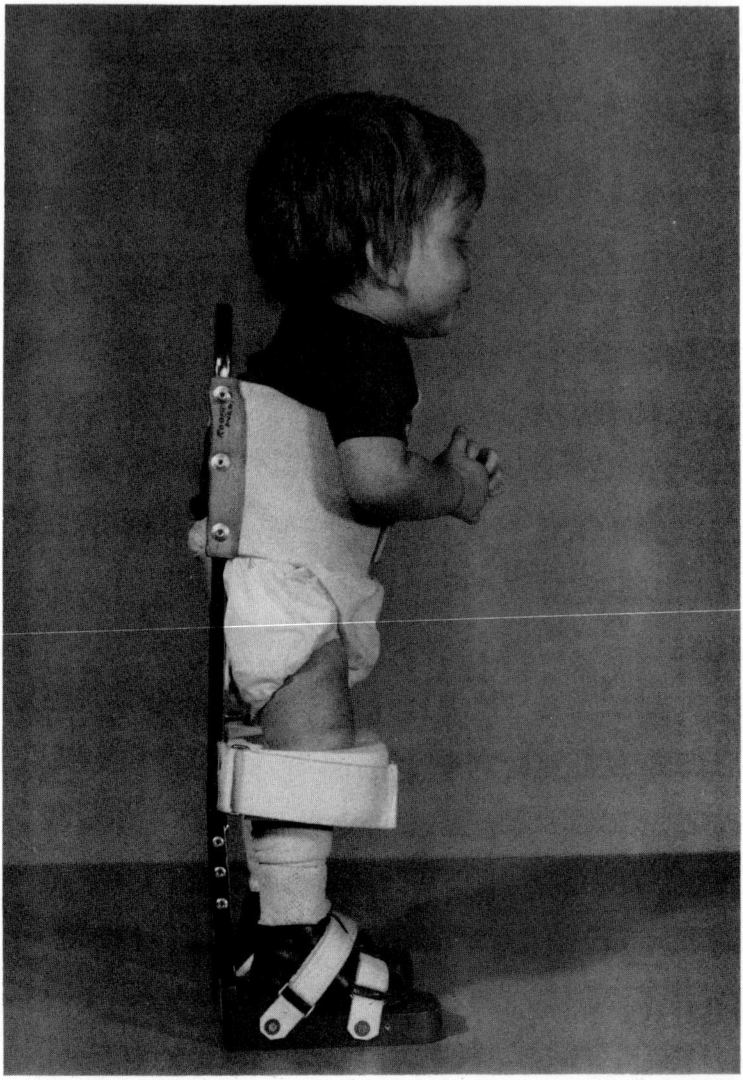

FIG. 22.5. Standing brace. This orthosis allows a paraplegic child to maintain an upright stance.

With crutches the child is capable of a swing-to or a swing-through gait. This orthosis is prescribed for the older child with a thoracic or upper lumbar lesion, particularly the preschool child who needs the option of sitting or standing in a classroom. An orthosis such as the parapodium that braces the spine, hips, knees, and feet is frequently rejected between

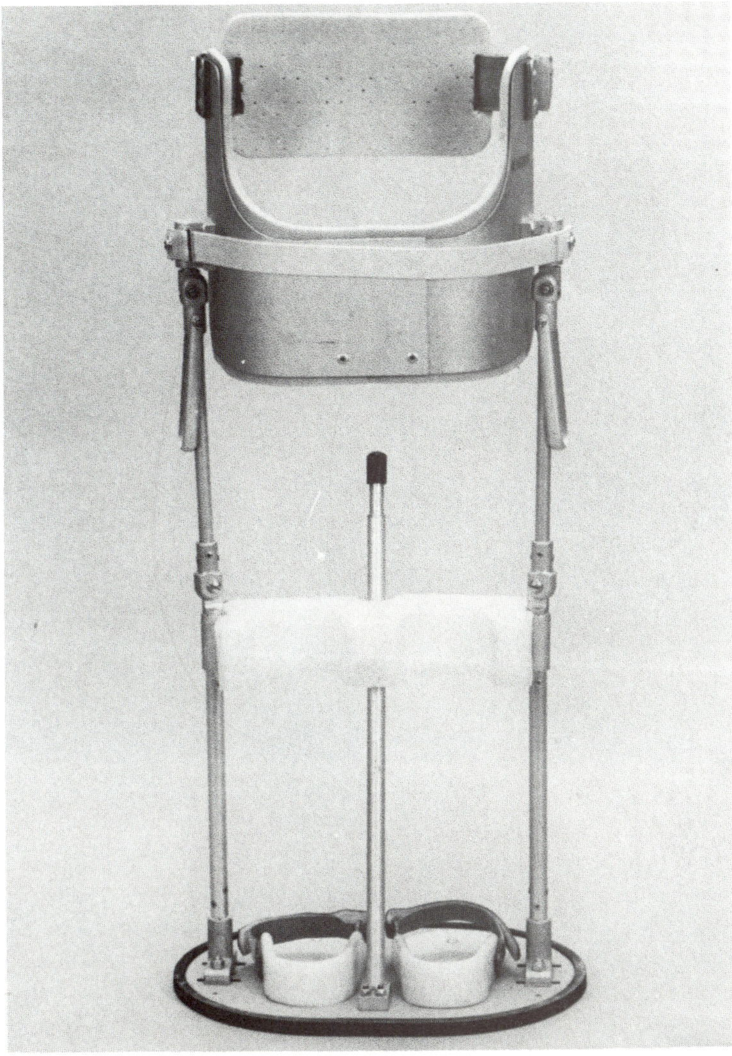

FIG. 22.6. Parapodium. This "exoskeleton" enables a paraplegic child to maintain an upright. It has (locking) hip and knee hinges which allow the child to sit in the brace.

the ages of 8 and 12 because of the energy required to be mobile in the upright position. Some children object to the appearance of such an orthosis.

We prefer this system of bracing to long leg braces with a pelvic band because better hip and spine control is achieved. Adjustments and repair are easier.

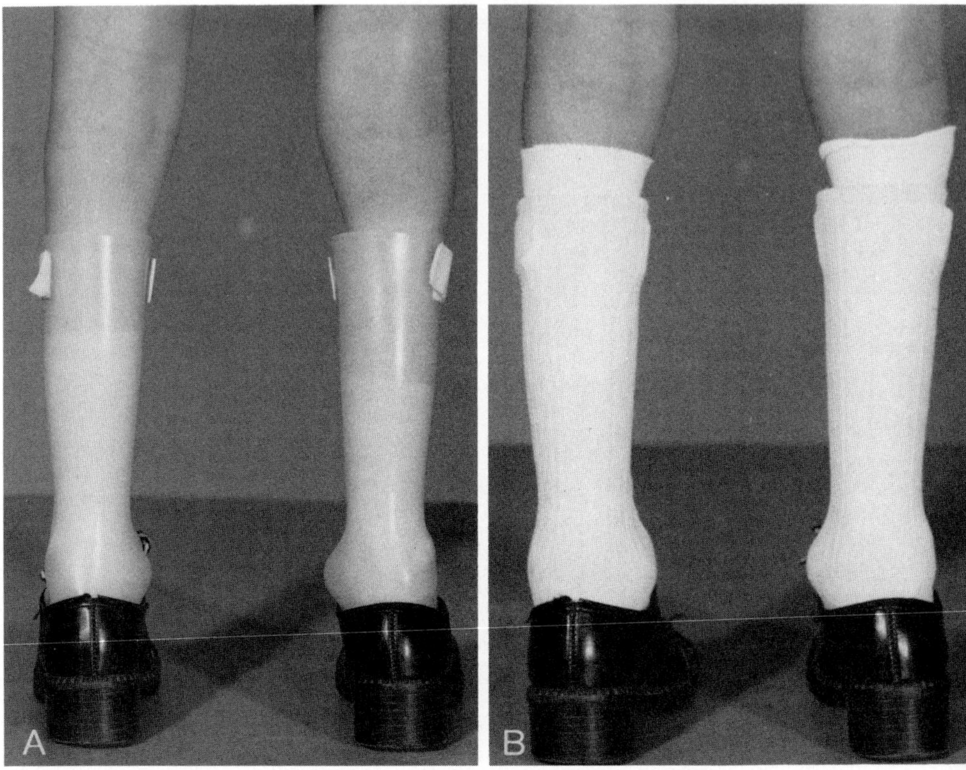

FIG. 22.7. Ankle-foot orthosis (AFO).

POLYPROPYLENE SPLINTS

For the past 11 years we have been using vacuum-formed polypropylene ankle-foot orthoses for control of ankle-foot instability. These splints are prescribed for children with good quadriceps and medial hamstring power but without enough power below the knee to control the ankle-foot complex. The child's foot must be checked regularly in the splint for red marks which are early warning signs of excessive pressure. We have found these splints extremely effective, light weight, and cosmetically acceptable because they can be worn with regular shoes.

A vacuum-formed splint constructed with the foot at a 90° angle to the long axis of the leg causes a problem with weight transfer from the heel to the toe when walking. Gait is improved by casting the foot in slight dorsiflexion or by contouring the sole of the shoe that is being worn over the splint (Fig. 22.7).

The child with weak quadriceps or a knee which tends to go into varus or valgus requires a knee-ankle-foot orthosis. The original ankle-foot orthosis can be extended by a single- or double-upright bar with a hinge.

A knee pad is attached to one or both bars and is designed to apply pressure to the proximal tibial flare and over the patellar tendon (Fig. 22.8).

SHOE MODIFICATIONS

Children with low lumbar or sacral lesions sometimes present with a foot deformity that is not severe enough to require an ankle-foot orthosis. A slight calcaneus deformity in a young child can be managed by

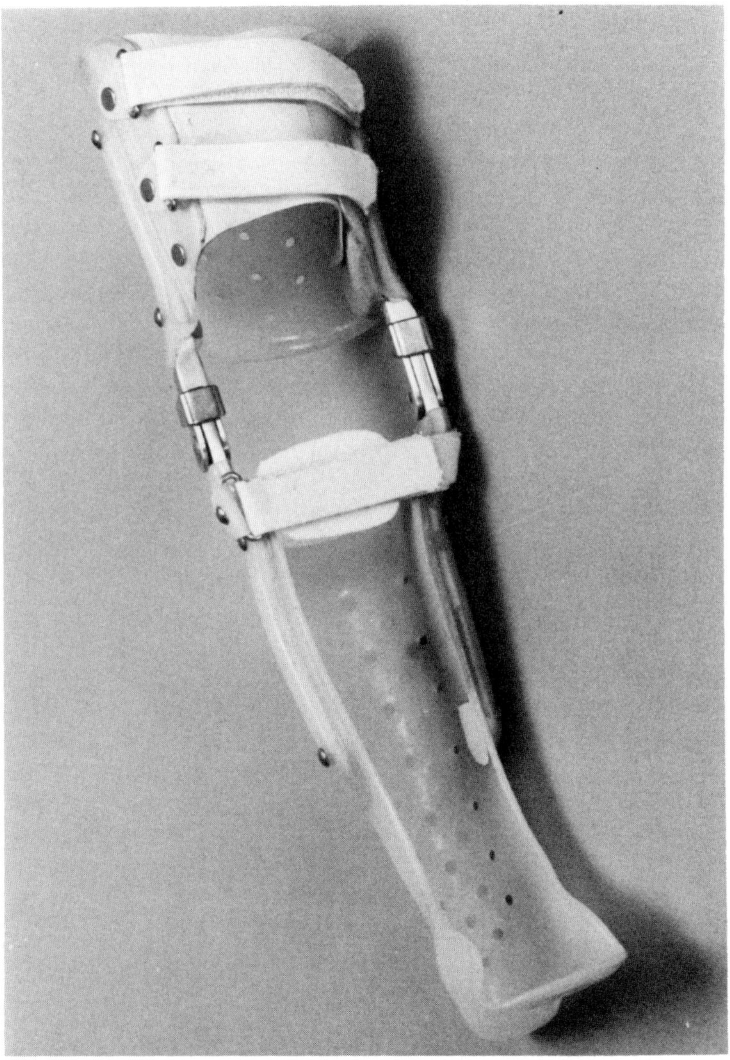

FIG. 22.8. Knee-ankle-foot orthosis (KAFO).

reinforcing the tongue of the boot with Plastozote. A vacuum-formed polypropylene slipper is useful for the control of forefoot adduction and supination. A mild valgus heel can be controlled either by wrapping polypropylene around the heel counter or by a vacuum-formed insert with projections under the longitudinal arch. Wedges applied to the sole of the shoe are only useful for minor deformities. They become more effective if the sole of the shoe is made rigid by inserting an aluminum plate between the layers of leather. Children much prefer inserts, which may be hidden inside any shoe, to visible shoe modification.

SPINAL ORTHOTICS

The main goal in managing spinal deformities in spina bifida is the maintenance of a stable posture for sitting and standing. Bracing the spine of a child with myelomeningocele is an unresolved problem in orthotics because of the many causes of the deformity. There are structural problems with the spine's "foundation," "superstructure," and "walls and insulation." Among the problems that can occur with the foundation are (a) sacral agenesis; (b) pelvic obliquity due to muscle imbalance, hip instability, or leg length discrepancy; and (c) the petite pelvis providing little grip for a brace. Superstructure problems include deficient pedicles, laminae and dorsal spinous processes, hemivertebrae, congenital unsegmented bars, fused ribs, muscle weakness, muscle spasticity, hydromyelia, diastematomyelia, and tethered cords. Wall and insulation problems include scarred skin, insensitive skin, and either too much or too little subcutaneous tissue.

The type of spinal bracing required to improve function depends on the neurosegmental level.

Upper Thoracic. The neonate with an upper thoracic level lesion can have a spinal deformity that defies bracing. Some of these children can be helped with a trough bed.

The spine of a child with lower thoracic lordosis and thoracolumbar kyphosis usually collapses when he/she sits so that the rib cage rests on the thighs. A bucket insert supports the spine, improves chest expansion by getting the ribs off the thighs, and enables the child to sit with his hands free. A bucket insert can be used on a car seat, on a chair at home, or in a caster cart (Fig. 22.9). Poor head stability may be assisted by an attachment to support the head.

Older children with a collapsing paralytic scoliosis are best prescribed a thermoplastic body jacket designed so that it can fit inside a parapodium (Fig. 22.10). The jacket controls the spinal deformity and prevents the child from collapsing like an accordion inside his parapodium.

A wheelchair is usual for the child with an upper thoracic level lesion when he is of school age. These wheelchairs require more than a standard

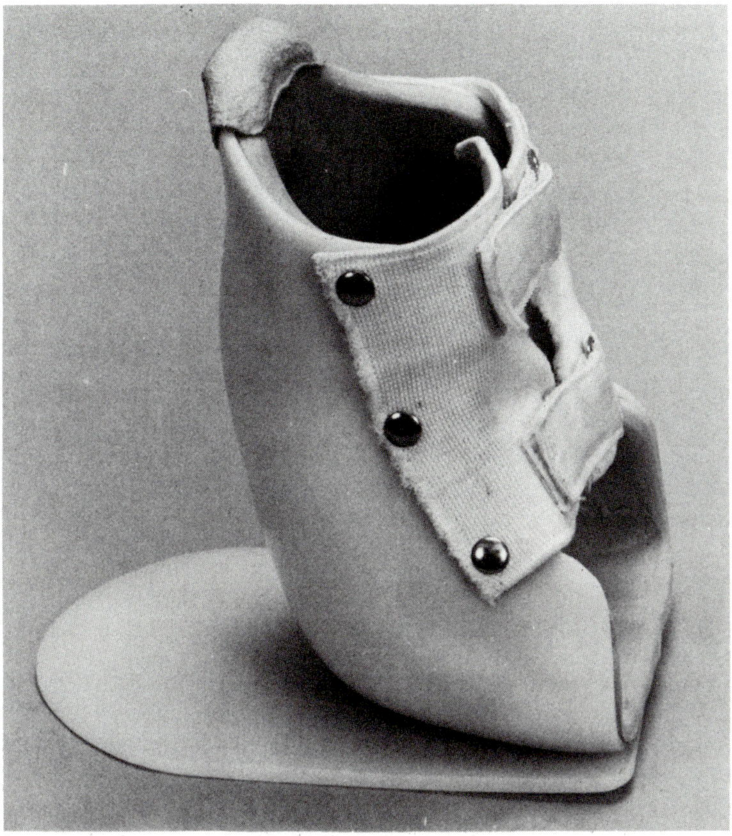

FIG. 22.9. Bucket insert for use on a car seat, in a chair, or in a caster cart.

sling seat and sling back. A plywood seat is put in the chair and is covered with T-foam; an upholstered upright is placed in the back of the chair, and foam wedges are used to keep the child from habitually leaning to one side as he propels the chair.

We have used suspension systems in wheelchairs to unload the buttocks. Some of the child's weight is taken by the flare of the rib cage. Buttock pressure and spinal collapse should be reduced. Although the idea seems good, it is not very effective for the active child.

Lower Thoracic. Trunk musculature is better. Severe deformities do not develop at such an early age, as in upper thoracic level lesions. There are no problems until children want to be mobile in the sitting position. Care must be taken that weight is borne equally through both buttocks while sitting, so as to avert the development of a lumbar scoliosis and pelvic obliquity. These children are less mobile than those with lumbar lesions and, therefore, do more sitting. They usually require a back

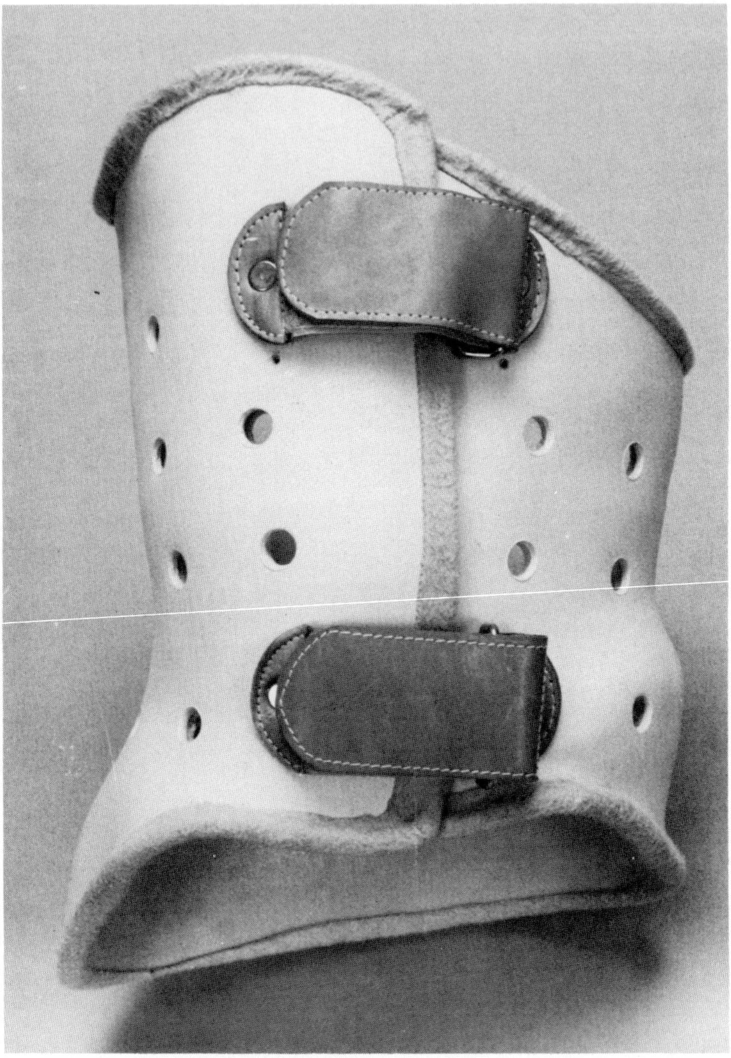

FIG. 22.10. Thermoplastic body jacket.

support in the caster cart with an anterior chest strap and foam wedges to provide lateral stability.

Upper Lumbar. Children who walk with long leg braces and forearm crutches often start to develop a spinal deformity by age 4. A total contact body jacket can be prescribed for such a child, although these are quite restrictive and tend to impede function. A total contact body jacket is made from a plaster mold of the child while he lies prone with 3-point pressure and longitudinal traction applied to correct deformity. If there is a significant lumbar or rib hump, a section can be cut out of the jacket, and a pad can be applied which is held in position by adjustable laces or Velcro straps. Children who do not walk need a wheelchair with foam wedges to support the spine.

A lumbar lordosis often develops with hip flexion deformities. The lumbar lordosis cannot be controlled by an orthosis until the hip flexion deformity is corrected.

Lower Lumbar and Sacral. Severe spinal deformities at an early age are unusual. Developing curves can be treated in a total contact body jacket. More powerful lower limbs compensate for the restriction in trunk motion produced by the jacket. . Spinal braces may be used as a temporary device to improve function, but surgery often proves necessary to completely control the deformity. An orthosis cannot compete with a curve produced by a congenital unsegmented bar, severe spasticity, or severe muscle weakness.

When a child who has rejected his or her leg braces and spends all his time sitting in a wheelchair develops a collapsing scoliosis, an increasing neurological deficit should be suspected and investigated.

Surgical Problems

In the past, children with spina bifida could look forward to one operation after another. Infection, pathological fracture, pseudarthrosis, and failure were common. Today's better orthotics are often preferable to an operation. Today, the unstable hip is either ignored or treated better than it was 10 years ago. Most foot deformities are treated early by soft tissue procedures. The use of standing postoperative casts has dramatically reduced the frequency of pathological fractures. There is much less surgery for spina bifida than formerly. Today's indications are (a) to correct deformity that precludes braces and (b) to control deformity that cannot be controlled by braces.

THE FOOT IN SPINA BIFIDA

The common foot deformities are equinovarus, calcaneus, valgus, cavus, and rocker bottom deformity due to vertical talus. The overall aim in managing such foot deformities is to achieve a plantigrade foot with stable skin (12). Spina bifida Olympians appreciate that:

1. Many feet are insensitive.
2. Concentrated pressure leads to skin breakdown.
3. The load of weight bearing must be evenly distributed.
4. Plantar skin was designed for weight bearing.
5. Surgical procedures must correct muscle imbalance and must completely correct deformity.
6. Valgus feet cause splint pressure over the navicular and medial malleolus.

NEUROGENIC CLUB FOOT

During the first 3 months of age this deformity is managed by serial manipulations and casting. A cast will not produce pressure sores if the manipulations are done carefully, with the foot and leg painted with tincture of benzoin and held in the corrected position while wrapped in cotton flannelette, followed by a below knee plaster.

After the age of 3 months, plan operation when and if the child's general condition is good and casting has failed or plateaued.

CALCANEUS DEFORMITY

Children with a lower lumbar lesion often have a calcaneus deformity produced by active function in the tibialis anterior and toe extensors that is not balanced by adequate calf function (17). During the first 3 years of life, this deformity can be controlled by stretching exercises and a sansplint or polypropylene reinforced tongue in the boot. By age 3 there is usually enough of a contracture of the anterior capsule to permit posterior transfer of the tibialis anterior through the interosseous membrane to the os calcis without an equinus deformity developing. If the heel is going into calcaneovalgus, then the tendon is sutured to the medial side of the os calcis and to the medial side of the insertion of the tendo achillis. If the heel is going into calcaneovarus, then the tibialis anterior is sutured to the lateral side of the os calcis and tendo achillis. The foot is immobilized in plaster for a period of 6 weeks followed by a polypropylene ankle-foot orthosis.

CAVUS FOOT

Children with a sacral neurosegmental level can develop a significant cavus deformity by the age of 5. The first choice is an adequate plantar release. When weakness of the tibialis anterior produces clawing of the great and small toes, then the plantar release can be supplemented by a transfer of the extensor hallucis longus into the first metatarsal and extensor digitorum communis into the fourth metatarsal, bringing the tendons anterior to the extensor retinaculum at the ankle so that they have a more effective dorsiflexor pull.

When there is a severe cavus deformity, the heel may be elevated or realigned by an osteotomy of the os calcis (6).

VALGUS DEFORMITY

A standing anteroposterior x-ray should be obtained to determine whether the valgus deformity is at the distal tibia, the subtalar joint, or both. Correction of deformity in the distal tibia requires a supramalleolar osteotomy.

A valgus subtalar joint is frequently seen in children with a low neurosegmental level who have some spasticity in their calves. With weight bearing, the os calcis swings into valgus. Subtalar valgus in the older child can be managed satsfactorily by selective lengthening of the tendo achillis, together with a varus displacement osteotomy of the os calcis or a triple arthrodesis.

NEUROGENIC VERTICAL TALUS

A neurogenic vertical talus which is more common than an idiopathic vertical talus is initially managed with serial stretching exercises and casts. Occasionally, this is enough, but surgical correction is commonly required at 3–6 months of age, depending on the child's general condition.

THE KNEE

Several problems are common (14):

1. Knee flexion deformity—usually the result of quadriceps weakness and hamstring spasticity.
2. Recurvatum—which is usual in newborns with an L4 lesion who are commonly born as an extended breech. The hamstrings are weak, and the quadriceps are strong.
3. Limited knee flexion—seen at a later age due to imbalance between quadriceps and hamstring muscles.
4. Valgus deformity—may develop in children with low lumbar lesions who walk in ankle-foot orthoses. At midstance, the hips adduct and internally rotate. The knees are overflexed due to weak quadriceps. The feet externally rotate. The line of weight bearing lies lateral to the knee producing a progressive valgus.

By and large, knee surgery in spina bifida children is limited to three types of procedures: (a) quadriceps plasty to gain flexion; (b) posterior soft tissue release to overcome flexion contractures; and (c) realignment supracondylar osteotomies.

A child may present at age 2 with an upper lumbar level lesion and may be frustrated by the fact that he does not have enough function to permit an upright stance. His therapist may feel that he is ready to stand, but he may have a knee flexion deformity that would make it difficult for him to get into a standing brace. We have found that it is possible to overcome a 40° flexion deformity by a posterior release at the knee.

Residual flexion deformities following posterior soft tissue releases and residual valgus deformities following iliotibial tract releases can be corrected by supracondylar osteotomies.

THE HIP

The problems include:

1. Hip instability—This condition is due to imbalance between the paralyzed hip abductors and extensors and the powerful adductors and flexors (3). Instability can present in the following ways. Sublux-

ation with a lax hip capsule; subluxation with a lax hip capsule and a saucer-shaped acetabulum, fetal dislocation (occurring *in utero*), dislocation with a saucer-shaped acetabulum, dislocation with a deficient acetabulum, pelvic obliquity, and abnormalities of the neck-shaft angle.

2. Deformity—Flexion is frequent when psoas is the only muscle working. In children with flail hips, the legs lie in abduction and external rotation, which is followed by contractures. Spastic extensors and external rotators are unusual but may provide fixed extension. An adduction contracture follows dislocation.

The orthopedic goal is a hip that will allow walkers to walk and sitters to sit.

Children who can achieve upright stance and upright mobility require a stable posture. Menelaus has shown that the prognosis for upright mobility is best in those children whose center of gravity is balanced over their feet and who have minimal flexion deformity at their hips and knees (12). A major goal therefore is to correct deformity completely and to ensure that deformity does not recur.

Containment surgery in spina bifida is contentious. At best, it rarely results in a "normal" hip as assessed by the standards we use in congenital dislocation. Failure and complication have been frequent; hence, stabilization procedures, by and large, are reserved for children who will be household or community ambulators or those with unilateral hip dislocation. This means that most children undergoing major reconstructive hip surgery have lower lumbar neurosegmental levels with strong quadriceps muscles.

Children without good quadriceps power should have soft tissue releases to rid them of deformity. The cost of putting the hip in joint is not repaid by better function.

SPECIFIC PROBLEMS—THE NEWBORN

In the newborn without hip abductors and extensors, the adductors are stretched by physiotherapy. Tight adductors that are causing subluxation are released subcutaneously. In a neonate with a lower lumbar lesion and unstable hips, there may be a place for adductor release, closed reduction, and immobilization in a splint that keeps the hips abducted and internally rotated. This splint is used during the child's unattended hours. There is evidence to suggest that splinting of a reduced hip can produce an improvement in stability (10). Abduction-internal rotation splints are difficult to fit in young children and need to be changed frequently as the child grows. If a spina bifida child with absent abductors and extensors is put in a Frejka pillow or plaster with the hip in Salter's "Human Position" (15), one of fairly full flexion and 45° of abduction, the child will tend to develop a hip flexion abduction and external rotation contracture as the iliopsoas is allowed to shorten and as the degenerating hip abductors and extensors become fibrotic.

A neonate may present with one good lower limb with a stable hip and one poor limb with a dislocated hip. If the unstable hip is not reduced with an adductor release, reduction may be accomplished by opening the capsule medially as described by Fergusson (7), such a child should not be subjected in the neonatal period to open reduction and capsulorraphy via the anterior approach.

PROBLEMS AT 18 TO 24 MONTHS

A child with a thoracic or upper lumbar neurosegmental level may be a candidate for a standing brace but for hip deformities. Habilitation for this child will be much easier if his hips are rendered flail by tendon division or excision (12). Containment procedures will not improve the child's function and are therefore contraindicated. However, a unilateral dislocation in a child with an upper lumbar lesion should be stabilized to avoid a leg length discrepancy and the possibility of pelvic obliquity and a spinal deformity.

In the child with lower lumbar neurosegmental level function, major hip surgery, including muscle balancing procedures, is delayed until the clinic team has agreed that the child is, in fact, going to be a household or community ambulator. If muscle imbalance is producing a mild hip subluxation, it is possible to achieve hip stability with either a Mustard (13) or Sharrard iliopsoas tendon transfer (16) together with an appropriate adductor release. A child without hip subluxation but with a positive Trendelenburg sign who walks without aids should not undergo iliopsoas tendon transfers because there will be more functional impairment from the weakening of the hip flexors (for instance, inability to step up into a school bus) than functional improvement in the lurching gait.

Subluxation with a lax hip capsule requires a capsulorraphy at the time of iliopsoas tendon transfer.

A potential community ambulator with muscle imbalance, a lax capsule, and a saucer-shaped acetabulum demands an operation combining capsulorraphy, acetabuloplasty (1), and iliopsoas tendon transfer.

It is important to treat all components of the hip problem at one sitting; inadequate surgery will fail, and multiple operations will result in excessive scarring and stiffness.

THREE YEARS AND LATER

A child with a low lumbar lesion causing the hip to dislocate in the newborn period has a small deficient acetabulum. This type of hip requires an open reduction, capsulorraphy, Chiari osteotomy (4), and iliopsoas tendon transfer. In these cases it is easier to use the Sharrard technique in which the tendon is taken back through a hole in the posterior ilium. By and large, an innominate osteotomy is not a useful procedure because if the deficient acetabulum is rotated forward and laterally the hip will tend to dislocate posteriorly.

Occasionally, even after dealing with the problems of muscle imbalance, capsular laxity, and poor acetabular development, the normal neck shaft angle may require a femoral osteotomy.

Following any reconstructive procedure, the spica cast must permit weight bearing on a tilt table. This reduces osteoporosis and decreases the incidence of pathological fractures. Five to 10 days postoperatively the children are transferred from the Hospital to the Rehabilitation Centre, where they stand daily as part of their therapy. The spica is removed at 4 to 6 weeks. Mobilization exercises are then commenced, often in a pool, and the appropriate orthosis is fitted.

REFERENCES

1. Carroll, N. Hip instability in children with myelomeningocele. Orthop. Clin. North Am., *9*(2): 403, 1978.
2. Carroll, N. The orthotic management of the spina bifida child. Clin. Orthop., *102:* 108, 1974.
3. Carroll, N. C., and Sharrard, W. J. W. Long-term follow-up of posterior iliopsoas transplantation for paralytic dislocation of the hip. J. Bone Joint Surg., *54A:* 551, 1972.
4. Chiari K. Ergebnisse mit der Beckenosteotomie als Pfannendachplastik. Z. Orthop., *87:* 14–26, 1955.
5. De Souza, L. J., and Carroll, N. C. Ambulation of the braced myelomeningocele patient. J. Bone Joint Surg., *58A:* 1976.
6. Dwyer, F. C. Osteotomy of the calcaneum for pes cavus. J. Bone Joint Surg., *41B:* 80, 1959.
7. Ferguson, A. B. The medial adductor approach for congenital dislocation of the hip. J. Bone Joint Surg. *54A:* 1799, 1972.
8. Hoffer, M. M., Ferwell, E., Perry, J., and Bennett, C. Functional ambulation in patients with myelomeningocele. J. Bone Joint Surg., *55A:* 137–148, 1976.
9. Kupka, J., Geddes, N., and Carroll, N. Comprehensive management in the child with spina bifida. Orthop. Clin. North Am., *9*(1): 97, 1978.
10. McKibbin, B. The use of splintage in the management of paralytic dislocation of the hip in spina bifida cystica. J. Bone Joint Surg., *55B:* 163–172, 1973.
11. McLaurin, R. L. *Myelomeningocele*, pp. 241–260. New York, Grune & Stratton, 1977.
12. Menelaus, M. B. *The Orthopedic Management of Spina Bifida Cystica*, Ed. 2. Edinburgh, Churchill-Livingstone, 1980.
13. Mustard, W. T. Iliopsoas transfer for weakness of the hip abductors. J Bone and Joint Surg., *34A:* 647, 1952.
14. von Parsch, K., and Schulitz, K-P. *Das Spina Bifida Kind.* Stuttgart, Georg Thiem Verlag, 1972.

15. Salter, R. B. *Textbook of Disorders and Injuries of the Musculoskeletal System.* Baltimore, Williams & Wilkins, 1970.
16. Sharrard, W. J. W. Posterior iliopsoas transplantation in the treatment of paralytic dislocation of the hip. J. Bone Joint Surg., *46B:* 426–444, 1964.
17. Sharrard, W. J. W., and Grosfield, I. The management of deformity and paralysis of the foot in myelomeningocele. J. Bone Joint Surg. *50B*(3): 456–465, 1968.

CHAPTER

23

Diastematomyelia

ROBIN P. HUMPHREYS, M.D., F.R.C.S.(C), E. BRUCE HENDRICK, M.D., F.R.C.S.(C), and HAROLD J. HOFFMAN, M.D., F.R.C.S.(C)

The unknown noxious stimuli which act on the developing and closing neural tube between the 24th and 28th days of gestation can bring about a wide variety of pathological consequences to the forming spinal cord. Diastematomyelia (DSM) is one of the less common but more intriguing forms of closed spinal dysraphism. The term "diastematomyelia" was first used in 1837 by Ollivier to describe an abnormality of the spinal canal in which the dura is perforated by a bony spike or fibrous band to create two sleeves, each containing a portion of the spinal cord which is divided in two parts sagittally, joining together above and below the spike (24, 25).

Very few cases of DSM were clinically described before 1950, and reports thereafter contained limited numbers of patients (7, 20, 23, 25). In 1969, Matson (21) updated his series to 31 children and enunciated many principles of care, some of which are still applicable. By the mid-70s, there was sufficient information obtained through clinical, radiologic, operative, and necropsy studies to detail the increasingly diverse features of DSM. For example, while the Greek derivative of "diastematomyelia" means "cleft" of the "medulla," the term does not apply to the median septum nor even imply its presence (9, 14). Nor should the term be used interchangeably with "diplomyelia," a true rarity indeed.

At one time, the diagnostic confirmation of DSM and its treatment decisions appeared straightforward (14, 21–23). However, detailed study of the problem, especially in the last decade, has highlighted its neuroradiologic variants, such as the frequent appearance of "second lesions" within the spinal canal, and has examined priorities for operative treatment as well as the need for "prophylactic" surgery.

There has been substantial change in the state of art during these past few years, so the discussion which follows is based on the analysis of 50 children with DSM from the Hospital for Sick Children at Toronto (HSC) who were treated between 1970 and 1982.

EMBRYOGENESIS AND PATHOLOGY

One of the enchantments of DSM is the analysis of its abnormal embryology. The profusion of causation theories is obvious testimony that no one satisfies all pathologic components. Hypotheses advanced in the past tried to explain the division of the cord as well as the development of the midline septum (14).

The *split notochord syndrome* was proposed by Bentley and Smith (2) to explain not only DSM but also the formation of a spinal neurenteric cyst. It supposed that a primary split of the notochord allows invaginating entoderm (ventrally) and neural plate (dorsally) to become juxtaposed. The endodermal tract is eventually obliterated whereas the neuroectodermal component becomes filled in with mesodermal tissue of the vertebral body, thereby creating the septum.

Bremer's *accessory neurenteric canal* thesis was offered for the same reason and presumes that an accessory neurenteric canal splits the neural plate and notochord and doubles the mesodermal blocks which then attempt to form two vertebral bodies (14). These mesodermal precursors merge, heaping up a median septum which projects into the anterior spinal canal. Persistence of the accessory neurenteric canal dorsally leaves the neural plate cleaved and sets the stage for development of a congenital dermal sinus.

Gardner's *hydromyelic theory* makes it unnecessary to hypothesize a primary dysgenesis of other germ cell layers (10). Overdistention of the neural tube results in the rupture of its roof and floor plates and distortion of the surrounding mesoderm. The neural tube splits and two smaller tubes are formed. Coalescence of mesodermal cell layers then accounts for the bony spur which develops between the separated tubes.

The *overgrowth hypothesis* suggests that the apposing folds of the neural plate, unable to reach each other and fuse in the dorsal midline, curve inwards instead and develop two separate neural tubes (18). The mesoderm, in subsequently directing the formation of the vertebral laminae, causes them to also curve in medially and to fuse in the midline and form the septum. The *twinning theory* adopts much the same premise (15).

By contrast, Lichtenstein (19) suggested that a *primary mesodermal abnormality* acts as the provocateur which then splits the flat neural plate and causes development of two neural tubes (19).

The last opinion notwithstanding, most pediatric practitioners would agree with Willis "that the primary fault lies in the formation of the neural tube and not in its investing mesoderm" (28). However, when one considers the pathological variants of DSM (most recently summarized by French (9)), there are many questions which are not served by the existing hypothesis. For example, why, with all the proposed splitting and reformation of the neural tube, is the entity of diplomyelia not more common? That is, the pathological anatomy of DSM is separated equal (or unequal) portions of one spinal cord. Why are the proposed duplicated neural tubes incapable of producing two identical cords with matching pairs of dorsal and ventral roots, especially if, among other things, the neural crest cells must also be split?

Most of the theses presume a midaxial crisis which triggers a split in the developing neural tube. Why then do some cord segments end up of unequal size, why do they rotate inwards through 90°, and why in some instances is the median septum so eccentrically placed (26)? It seems certain that at some time in the dysraphic evolution, a mesodermal event occurs which results in the formation of a median septum—a bony, cartilaginous, or fibrous spur (N.B. the terms "median septum" and "spur" will be used interchangeably hereafter). However, what is the explanation for an apparent abortion of septum formation in those children who have cord splitting but no penetration by a spur? And how can a split in the neural tube be responsible for those examples of DSM occurring caudad to the conus tip and involving only the cauda equina?

While many children with DSM have a median septum and cord cleft which extends over 1 to 3 segments, the bony vertebral abnormality is usually far more extensive, suggesting considerable early mesodermal commotion. Why did the neural maldevelopment not follow pari passu, and why is it this degree of mesenchymal disruption that the dural tube, doubled though it may be, is usually very well constructed?

Of all the theories proposed, those of Bentley and Bremer perhaps best explain the occurrence at the level of the DSM, although neither one seems to account for the longitudinal events which occur above and/or below the DSM and which consist of secondary neural lesions and multiple bony anomalies.

PATHOGENESIS OF CLINICAL DETERIORATION

The presence of a bony spur in a child with a DSM syndrome has in the past piqued the attractive cause-and-effect relationship of the spur to local spinal cord insult with resultant clinical deterioration. This mechanical explanation is probably too simple, and one must now take into consideration the complexity of the entire dysraphic condition. Thus, there are a number of possible explanations for the child's clinical findings related to DSM.

Multilevel Spinal Vertebral Abnormality

Scoliosis by itself may be the reason for evaluation of children with DSM, as it was in 11 patients in the present series. When there is no neurological deficiency, then clearly the congenital scoliosis is an expression of maldevelopment of the mesodermal segments of the spine, which varies from localized hemivertebrae and block vertebrae to widespread areas of dysraphism and failure of segmentation (11, 16). Thus, one need not invoke any form of neural compromise for these children who present with congenital scoliosis.

Traction by the Spur

One would expect that when the spur is impacted in the lower end of the spinal cord cleft, that the neurologic signs are directly related to the traction effect of the spur, impeding the normal upward migration of the cord (21, 23). Furthermore, it was argued that the continued differential growth of spinal column and cord exaggerates the traction, especially during periods of rapid acceleration of linear growth such as occurs during early adolescence. One would expect neurologic and/or orthopedic worsening at those times.

While the surgeon will be impressed by the tight adherence of the median septum against the lower cleft in many children's DSM, the traction theory may nevertheless be too simplistic. For example, Barson's study of normal fetuses suggests that the conus ends at the adult level (L1-2) between birth and 2 months of age (1). If such is the case in children with DSM, then should they not present at, or shortly after, birth with their maximum neurologic or orthopedic condition? Alternatively, if children escape the early months, then one might anticipate that many would come to diagnosis in adolescence. The average age of the child's presentation with DSM is 3.5 years in Matson's report, 6.5 years in the HSC review, and 17 months in Guthkelch's series (12, 21). There were no children over 12 years of age reported by Matson, only 1 by Guthkelch, and 5 in the present series. The majority of patients with DSM will present before the patient reaches age 5, but well after the early neonatal months (9). Thus, how can a traction thesis be held solely responsible?

Finally, the traction theory does not adequately explain the appearance of neurologic signs in patients with the spur located at the midportion of the cleft (two in the present series) nor in those in whom the septum is surrounded by cauda equina (one in the present series) (11). Whatever the role of traction, and it is not negligible, there must be other contributing explanations for the altered neurologic function in children with DSM.

Traction by Bands

There is no doubt that the bands described by James and Lassman (17) exist in many patients with spinal dysraphism, particularly DSM.

Those authors have at operation traced the bands both outside and inside spinal dura, sometimes running in continuity and proceeding dorsally to neural arch joints or other tissues which substitute for bone in the defective neural arches. Their "importance lies in their tethering or traction effect upon the intrathecal structures" (17).

This author has also witnessed those bands, which are likely aberrant dorsal nerve roots, but was never impressed that they were sufficiently numerous, taut enough, nor creating adequate distortion of intradural structures to account *by themselves* for the traction syndrome. Their effect is likely additive to the other insults, and so these bands must be severed at operation.

Traction by Associated Tight Filum

Till (27) has stressed that some children with DSM will deteriorate after its correction, because of a second lesion, the most common of which in his experience was an elongated tethered conus (27). Computed tomographic metrizamide myelography has confirmed his observation in that a substantial number of dysraphic children, even those without a median septum or spur, will have coexistent tethering of the spinal cord (26).

There were 8 children in the present series who had, in addition to the DSM, a thick filum and tethered conus. This tight filum adds another insult to the DSM syndrome and raises the provocative question as to which entity should be corrected first.

Compression Ischemia by the Spur

Instead of subscribing to the theory of the local anchoring effect of the spur on the cord, perhaps one should consider the metabolic and ischemic changes which occur regionally in cord tissue about the spur. Yamada *et al.* (29) have examined the mitochondrial oxidative metabolic changes in spinal cord, which is subject to stretching. Lumboscral neuronal dysfunction may result in local structural damage, unless the tethering is released, in which case the oxidative metabolism is improved. This may be the explanation for the signs in those children whose spur is jammed into the lower end of the cleft.

Axial Distortion of Fiber Tracts

DSM is likely the only form of spinal dysraphism (excluding associated cervicomedullary or cervical anomalies) in which the examiner will encounter some signs of an upper motor neurone lesion. If regional forces acting on the conus medullaris were entirely responsible, then one would *always* expect lower motor signs. Breig (3) has thus suggested that the provocative influence of the median septum, regardless of its position, is the axial distortion of the descending and ascending fiber bundles as they are deviated away from the midline around the contained mass (3). Such long tract involvement would produce the hyperresponsive or pathologic reflexes which are encountered from time to time in DSM.

Associated (Covert) Abnormality

Guthkelch (12), Matson (21), and Till (27) have documented in their series the "second lesion" which can be present in children with DSM. Some are obvious, such as meningocele or dermal sinus, while others (lipoma, tethered conus) are detected by myelography or at operation. Moreover, some children followed through spina bifida clinics after treatment of their myelomeningocele may show secondary neurologic deterioration related to a DSM. There were 9 such children in the HSC series.

The important contribution in the paper by Scotti *et al.* (26) is the discovery in 15 of 21 children with a DSM clinical syndrome that the spinal cord was split but lay within an unsplit dural sac. Four children in the present review had such myelographic features and were operated on. In each, there was no median septum, but the split cord segments were anchored in two instances by bands, one each by lipoma and hibernoma.

Furthermore, detailed study of computed tomographic metrizamide myelography (CTMM) has outlined asymmetric splitting of the cord structures with no correlation between the smaller cord segment and the involved leg (26). In view of the absence of a central spur in many of these patients, one wonders about inherent myelodysplasia at the ultrastructural level and, dating from early gestation, about its being responsible for the clinical features.

In summary, there is probably a multifactorial explanation for the clinical features in children with DSM. It is a dynamic process in these children and, in the author's opinion, relates to a combination of tethering (by spur and/or associated lesion) and developmental and metabolic ultrastructural events. The excision of the spur and/or release of the thick filum in disabled children seems to halt the progress of their neurologic deterioration, but it is seldom that the child completely regains normal function.

CLINICAL PRESENTATION

If there has been any constancy with DSM, it exists for the clinical features, which for the children in the HSC series (Tables 23.1 and 23.2) are very similar to those reported previously (12, 17, 21). DSM is three

TABLE 23.1

Diastematomyelia: Cases from The Hospital for Sick Children

50 Patients (1970–1982)	
1. Sex—girls, 37; boys, 13	
2. Age—newborn to 17 years ($\bar{X}$:6½ yr)	
3. Cutaneous hallmark	
Hair,	13
Meningocele,	8
Nevus,	1
Lipoma,	1
4. Spur	
All but 1 below T7	
L3, L4, L1, and T9 (commonest levels)	
Sacral, 3	
None in 4	

TABLE 23.2

Presentation of Diastematomyelia: HSC

Orthopedic syndrome	11
Neurologic syndrome	20
Other dysraphism	13
Normal	6

times more common in girls than in boys, and its presence (and location) is often tipped-off by the cutaneous hallmark. The most frequent skin abnormality is the hairy patch, reportedly seen in as many as 81% of cases of DSM (12, 17). It was present in only 26% of the HSC review. DSM may be associated with nevoid pigmentation of the underlying skin or, less frequently, with a subcutaneous lipoma or dermal sinus. There are a small number of infants who will have a DSM within or adjacent to a myelomeningocele. The spur may or may not be visible at the time of early closure of the open tube defect. In those instances in which it is not obvious, it can account for secondary neurologic deterioration occurring a few years later. On occasion, the DSM may be discovered incidentally when the skin abnormality is evaluated or when x-rays are taken for other reasons and include the involved segment of the spine (6 of 50).

Invariably, the child with symptomatic DSM comes to the attention of an orthopedist or neurosurgeon. James and Lassman (17) and Guthkelch (12) have devised the "orthopedic" and "neurologic syndromes" which classify the clinical abnormalities. There is inevitably overlap between the two categories, and for the purposes of this review, those syndrome types were modified slightly (Table 23.3).

Children with the orthopedic syndrome may have scoliosis alone, or in association with a stiff back and the foot abnormalities described. The

TABLE 23.3

Orthopedic and Neurologic Syndromes

Orthopedic Syndrome	Neurologic Syndrome
Scoliosis	Wasted calf/foot
Stiff back	Weak ankle motors
Cavovarus foot	Absent ankle reflex
Cock-up toe(s)	Sphincter impairment
Failed skin nutrition	Back/radicular pain

latter, as well as the problem of chronic skin ulceration and poor wound healing in the feet, have presumably occurred on a neurogenic basis, but the neurologic examination of these children is normal, apart from a mild discrepancy in ankle reflex testing. Some authors indicate that the incidence of DSM in patients with congenital scoliosis is 5% (9). It is a moot point as to whether all children with congenital scoliosis should have myelography prior to orthopedic spinal surgery. One would certainly advocate it in the presence of deficient posterior elements and/or widened interpediculate distance.

Patients who have neurologic abnormalities, show it more frequently in one leg only, and they manifest it as calf wasting, weakness of one or more of the prime movements of the ankle, and an absent ankle reflex. These features would suggest a lower motor neurone lesion, implying that the conus medullaris is directly compromised. However, it is not exceptional to find that the knee reflexes and opposite ankle jerk are quite brisk and that there is a contralateral Babinski response. There can be therefore a blend of upper and lower motor signs.

While some children will have overt urinary sphincter difficulties (enuresis, urgency) at the time of first assessment, others will not but will show abnormality on preoperative urodynamic testing. A considerable number of children (11 of 20) with the neurologic syndrome will also have scoliosis.

There is substantial reason to be suspicious of more than one spinal lesion in these children. Fifteen of Guthkelch's 37 children had obvious meningocele or dermal sinus (12). In the HSC review, 13 (26%) first came to attention because of an open tube defect, lipoma, or dermal sinus. Such occurrence seems to support multiple factors acting at multiple levels of the spinal axis during early development.

When all the testing is concluded, it is usually (although not always) possible to isolate the level of the median septum. Again, there is agreement as to the frequency of the level of spinal involvement, the lumbar canal in 70% of all patients (9). The septum is infrequently found above T7, and the three commonest sites in major series are L2, L3, L1 (9), L3, L1, L2 (16), L4, L2, L3 (21), and L3, L4, and L1 (HSC).

Thus, the clinical appraisal of children with DSM remains fairly standard and can be summarized by the *"Rule of S"*—if not *Silent*, it presents with *Scoliosis*, *Skin* (hallmark), *Stiffness* (of back), *Sluggish* (of ankle motors and reflex), *Sphincters* (maybe), and *Spinal* dysraphic changes (extensive).

RADIOLOGIC FEATURES

The radiologic assessment of a child with DSM is now so precise, that neurosurgeons and neuroradiologists must be cautious as to whether they are analyzing exactly the same patient populations. Scotti *et al.* (26) in a recent radiologic review of 21 children examined because of neurologic and/or orthopedic syndromes, stated that a bony or cartilaginous spur was an uncommon finding and that, more frequently, the split spinal cord occurred within an *unsplit* dural sac. With such information, the gauntlet is tossed to the neurosurgeon, who must try to explain the clinical features and, more importantly, determine the course of therapy, if any. Meanwhile, the critic must be aware that patients in radiologic reports of DSM are culled from multiple sources—orthopedic, neurologic, neurosurgical, general pediatric—whereas the neurosurgical accounts, this one included, comprise patients in whom a traditional lesion was identified and operated on.

Plain radiographs of the spine can no longer be relied on to outline the bony spur, the established hallmark of DSM. Such x-rays, as well as plain tomography, are best at revealing the full complexity of dysraphic changes in the spinal column, and scoliosis, if present (Fig. 23.1). In this and other surgical reports of proven DSM, all patients had abnormalities such as anterior or posterior fusion defects, hemivertebrae, butterfly vertebrae, widened interpediculate distance, partial or complete vertebral fusion, or narrowed bodies (13, 16). The actual site of the spur is often signalled by the adjacent narrowed intervertebral disc space (Fig. 23.2).

The standard spinal radiographs may show the bony spur, but if a complex posterior block fusion is present, the spur can be difficult to discern from the other associated bony abnormalities, themselves creating the appearance of the spur. The spur usually projects upward and forward and can unite dorsally with nearby normal bony structures, such as the remaining intact laminar arch on one side, or even a rib. Many bony spurs have the shape of a mushroom, with the puffy head capping the dural tube at the involved level. That mushroom component is often not appreciated on plain films, tomography, or even routine myelography.

Patients with suspect DSM are best assessed with computed tomographic metrizamide myelography (CTMM). It demonstrates the abnormalities of the spinal cord, particularly the site, extent, and asymmetry

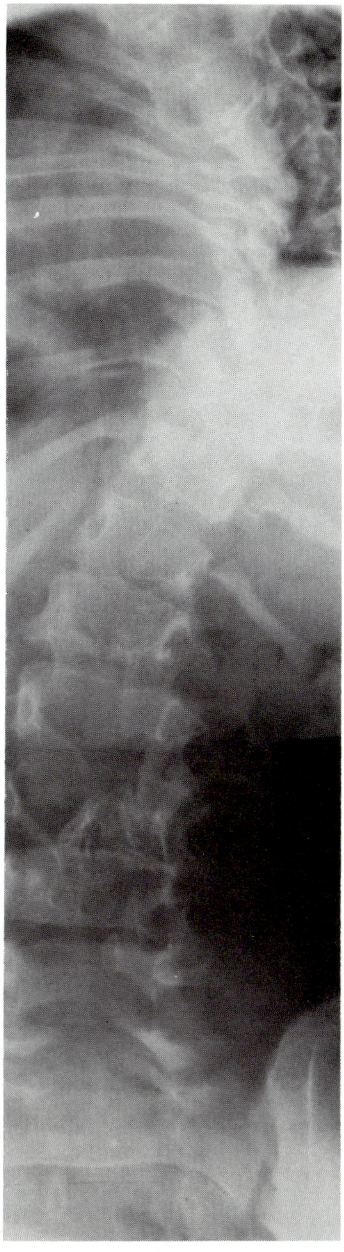

FIG. 23.1. The plain spinal AP radiograph is shown, in addition to the scoliosis, multilevel dysraphism, hemivertebrae, and posterior arch defects. This examination suggests but does not confirm that the spur is at L3–4.

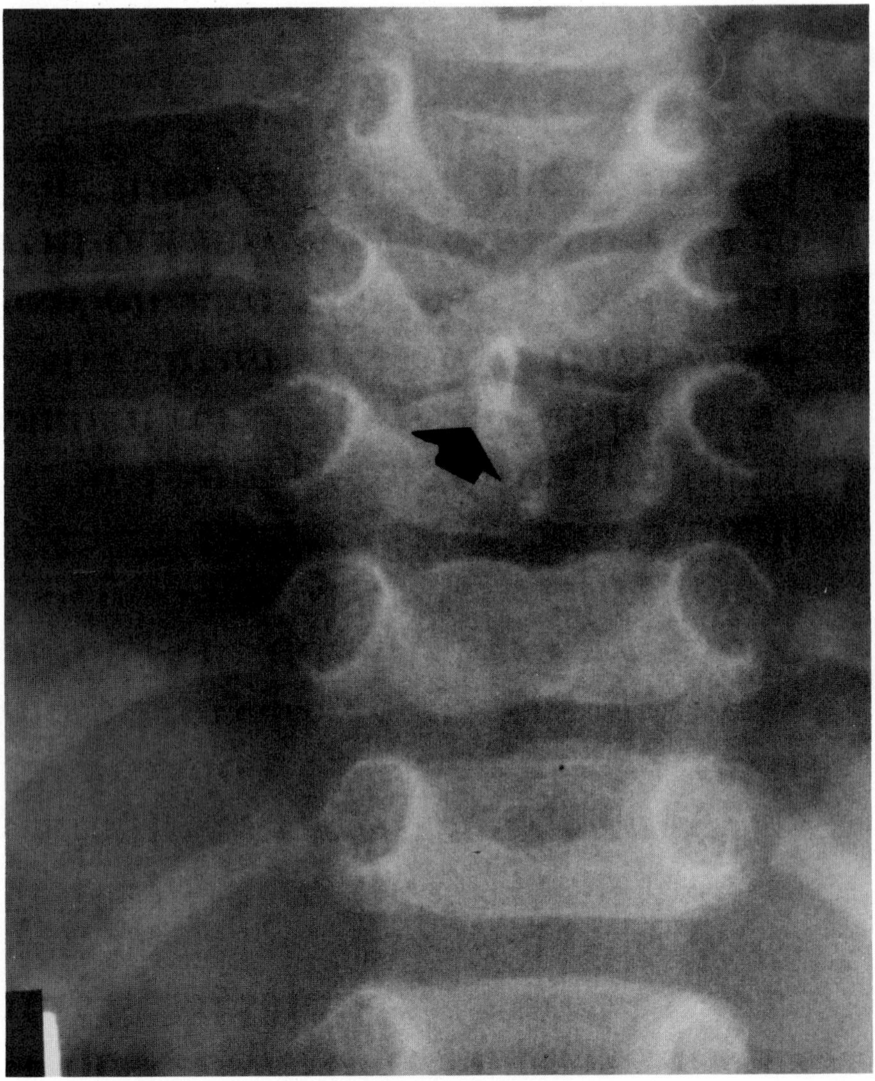

FIG. 23.2. The spur (*arrow*) is signaled by the adjacent narrowed disc space and dysraphism of the two cephalad vertebrae.

of the spinal cord. The CT examination shows the dysraphic anomalies of the vertebral bodies and, when present, the axial development of the fibrous, cartilaginous, or bony spur as it penetrates the divided cord or cauda equina, as well as its dorsal connections (Fig. 23.3). The spur does not necessarily arise or terminate in the midaxis of the spinal canal (26).

The metrizamide myelogram by itself is complimentary to the CTMM not only by providing accurate localization of the lesion to be studied

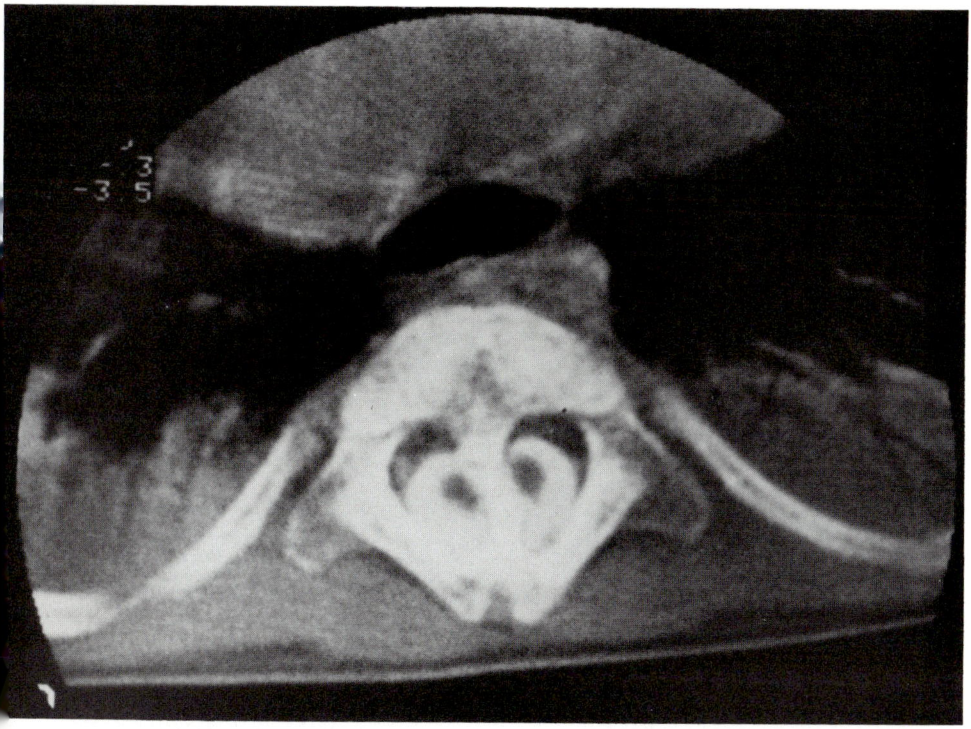

FIG. 23.3. CTMM outlines two dural sacs, evenly split cord, and centrally placed bony spur passing dorsally to unite with minimally bifid lamina.

with CTMM (Fig. 23.4) but also by outlining the associated abnormality, if present, such as tethering of the conus, thickened filum, or intradural lipoma. These combined studies may thus provide the neurosurgeon with unexpected information, *viz.*, absence of spur with splitting of cord in a single dural tube, tethering of spinal cord, or the presence of other coexistent dysraphic lesions. The treatment dilemma is thus extended beyond the consideration of the asymptomatic patient with the demonstrated bony spur, to include now the symptomatic child with cord splitting but no spur.

AIMS OF SURGERY

The aims of surgical correction of DSM are:

1. Stabilize scoliosis
2. Improve gait
3. Reverse neurologic deterioration
4. Improve sphincter function
5. Relieve a pain syndrome
6. Correct the associated dysraphic lesion(s)

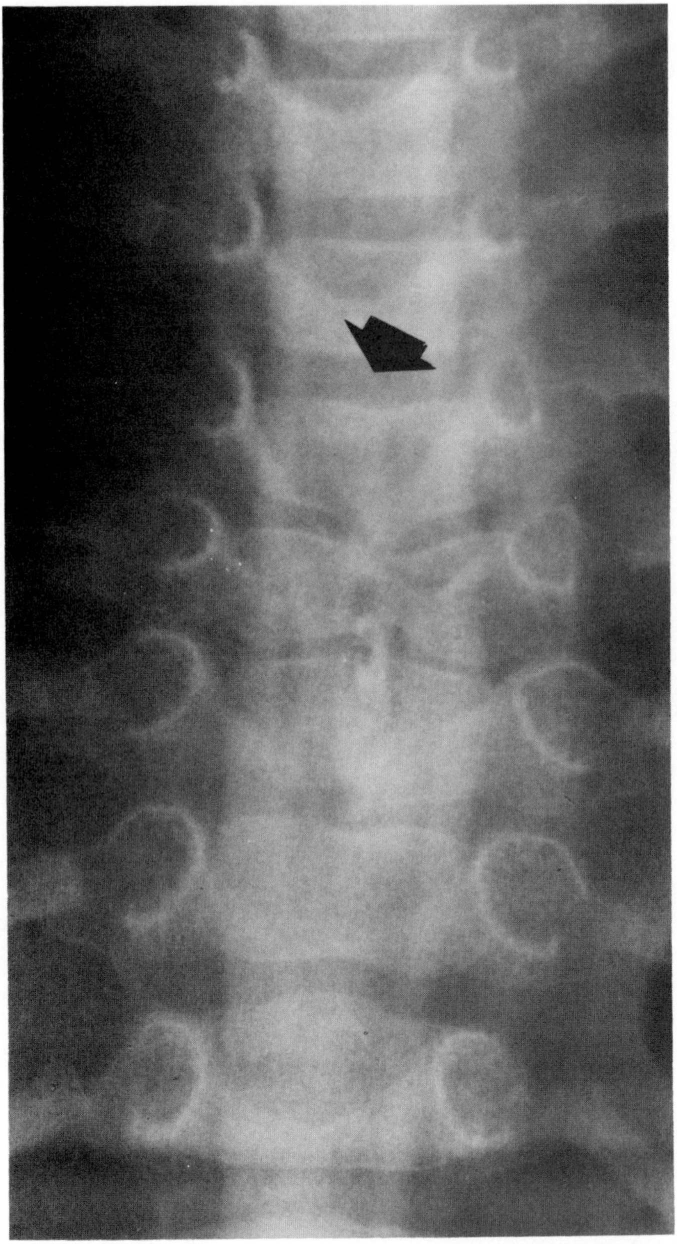

Fig. 23.4. Metrizamide myelogram completed just prior to CT study. The longitudinal aspect of the DSM is outlined with the cord cleft (*arrow*) extending two segments above the spur.

Such an itemization may seem presumptuous and connotes that there is no option other than operative correction of DSM. "Prophylaxis" is the key word used by experienced pediatric neurosurgeons to justify surgery, and implies, of course, not prevention of DSM but prevention of the inevitable clinical deterioration from that condition present at first assessment (12, 16, 21, 22, 27). Guthkelch (12) has confirmed that the majority of patients who present either with the normal or with the orthopedic syndrome and are managed expectantly, will develop "evidence of progressive spinal cord dysfunction" (12). He believes that a child is at an 83% risk of developing cord symptoms by adolescence and thus "removal of the spur should be considered at whatever age it is discovered." Matson (21) and Till (27) share that opinion. It may also happen that children who do not become symptomatic, are liable to deterioration in adulthood, as suggested by English and Maltby (8).

The contrary view determines the need for surgery by the relationship of the septum to the caudal exteme by the cleft, especially in the asymptomatic patient (9). The patient is managed nonoperatively if the septum lies in the midportion of the cleft. This recommendation can be challenged on the basis that the spur position is not the only noxious factor capable of producing symptoms, as previously discussed, and that patients may not be safe if left untreated.

When considering the treatment decisions on DSM, the surgeon will come to rely, as always, on the patient's clinical presentation, and will determine what can be accomplished with surgery to influence that. For the patient who is asymptomatic, it is tempting to ascribe to the belief of "firstly do no harm" and then to observe the child. Guthkelch's argument in this regard has been stated. In the HSC review, two patients were managed expectantly and deteriorated, and then they required neurosurgical care. Four other children were clinically normal but had spurs and were operated on "prophylactically." They remained normal.

The detail of CTMM may be capable of easing the treatment decision. It will accurately define the presence and position of the septum, as well as of the associated lesions, such as cord(s) tethering. To the contrary, it may demonstrate a split cord at normal levels, in a single dural sac with no septum, which even in a symptomatic patient, favors an expectant treatment program.

More often, the question arises as to what can be expected for the child symptomatic with orthopedic or neurologic syndromes from DSM and for whom operative correction is recommended. If scoliosis is the prevailing symptom, then the DSM requires first attention and a delayed decision made about the need for spinal fusion (11, 16). However, unlike other spinal dysraphic or neoplastic conditions which first declare themselves with scoliosis which improves after correction of the primary lesion, such may not be the case with DSM. The surgical treatment of the DSM *per se* does not alter the more extensive abnormal architecture of the spinal column and, so, not unexpectedly the scoliosis is often not improved, and may worsen. Seven of the 11 children in the HSC review who presented with the orthopedic syndrome required interval spinal fusion.

Matson (21) urged that "patient's parents should understand that operation is undertaken not so much in an attempt to reverse changes already present as to permit subsequent normal growth and maturation of the nervous system and thus prevent, if possible, increase in loss of function" (21). That dictum is still true with regard to gait performance, neurologic deterioration, sphincter function, and pain syndromes. The latter, incidentally are uncommon, and are almost always improved after surgery.

One can usually be assured that children who present with fixed orthopedic or neurologic syndromes will not be worse after proper surgical care, although they may be no better. In fact, unless there is an associated and more severe dysraphic lesion, the child's gait motion, power, foot dexterity, and skin nutrition are usually improved. Muscle bulk, tendon responses, skin anesthesia, and chronic sphincter disturbance are not influenced but fortunately seldom worsen.

A final aim of surgery is to correct the associated dysraphic lesion, an increasingly prevalent component of the DSM syndrome (12, 27). If an open tube defect existed at birth, it may already have been operated upon, but require re-exploration when the DSM is removed. In these situations, it is the myelomeningocele which determines the permanent neurologic handicap, and the DSM is treated to preserve whatever limited function may exist.

Similarly, there is little dispute concerning the need for early correction if the associated lesion is a dermal sinus or intraspinal lipoma (5, 6, 21). The more difficult decision is what to do for the occult and secondary spinal lesion, if it is at a distance from the DSM (*e.g.* DSM at L1 and tethered conus with thick filum at S1). Once again, the surgeon is guided by basic principles and is advised to operate on the lesion which best accounts for the patient's symptoms and signs.

In summary, the recommendations for treatment of children with DSM are the same as those for lipomyelomeningocele, dermal sinus, and tethered cord. Neurologic and/or orthopedic deterioration is inevitable and, as it is only a matter of time, prophylactic operative correction is advocated when the diagnosis is confirmed.

SURGICAL TECHNIQUE

Having analyzed the aims of the operative correction of a child's DSM, the surgeon must then plan the anatomical approach, especially if there are two lesions present. If they cannot be reached via the same skin incision and limited laminectomy, then it is advisable to operate *first on the clinically important or threatening* (*e.g.*, dermal sinus, meningocele) *lesion* and to plan a delayed procedure for the second.

Whatever the decision, the procedure will almost certainly begin as a laminectomy sited somewhere across the lumbosacral junction and centered at the level of the cord cleft. The patient is placed prone. While controlled ventilation is required, the neuromuscular junctions must not be pharmacologically paralyzed in case the surgeon wishes to stimulate anomalous roots during the procedure. If the skin incision extends down over the sacrum, then the perianal region should be draped and isolated from the surgical wound.

The techniques beautifully outlined 15 years ago by Meacham (22) are still quite appropriate and are modified now only by the use of microinstrumentation and magnified vision (22). In some respects, the most difficult part of the procedure will be the laminectomy which should aim to take one, but not more than two, laminae cephalad and caudal to the spur. By virtue of the multiple-level and form of the bony anomalies, the surgeon should *expect the laminectomy to be confusing.* The median septum frequently unites with some portion of the posterior neural arch, bringing about the appearance of the mushroom cap lying over the dorsal dura. The bifid spinous processes are found adjacent to this broad flat cap from which the muscles and soft tissues can be released. As in the dissection of other spinal dysraphic conditions, the surgeon must not be seduced into going down the inner face of the bifid arches when reflecting the paraspinal musculature. Recall that the interpediculate distance is wider at the level of the cleft and that the dysraphic arches lie more horizontal; therefore, the dissection must proceed more laterally than otherwise would be the case.

The normal dural tube rostral and caudal to the septum are identified (Fig. 24.5), and the limits of the septum are determined. The intimidating bony cap is removed *centripetally*, first by blunt dissection beneath its overhang (Fig. 24.6) and then with excision using a series of small, sharp-biting rongeurs. Avoid twisting or tugging motions during this bony removal; the force should not be transmitted to the cord segments.

The object at this stage is to remove the dorsal bulk of the septum, so that its vertical descent through the dural cleft is apparent. The adherence of dura and/or bands to the spur is released with sharp dissection, and one should expect a degree of venous bleeding in this extradural plane. At this time, *microscopic visualization* is of great value, and the spur may be further reduced with a high speed drill (Fig. 24.7). The latter is especially useful if the septum is jammed against the lower end of the cleft, where dissection about the caudal pole is difficult.

In most situations, it is best to leave the dural tubes intact for as long

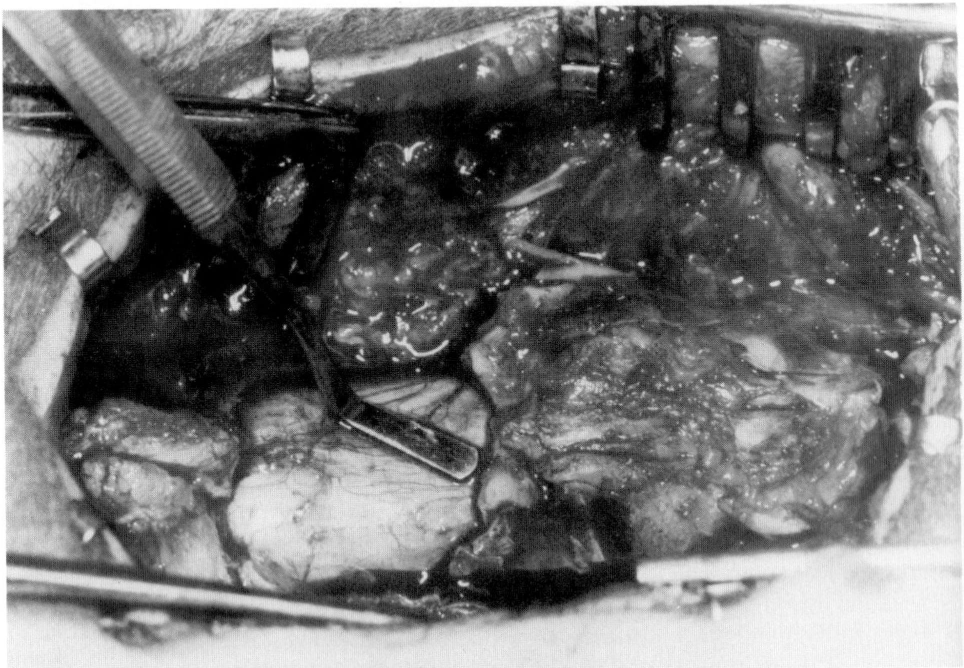

FIG. 23.5. The normal dural sleeve caudal (*left*) to the suspect spur is identified, and the extent of the latter is probed with an angled, blunt dental dissector.

as possible while the spur is debulked ventrally to the posterior surface of the vertebral body. If the dura has been released from the spur, then one need not worry about the effect of adhesions joining with cord segments. Eventually, the dura will have to be opened around the septum, and the relationship between the residual portion of spur with the spinal cord needs to be determined (Fig. 24.8). The rest of the septum can be burred away, and the central cuff of dura can be trimmed to lessen its bulk. Sometimes, it is possible to close it anteriorly. The medial and lateral aspects of the cord segments are inspected, any bands or adhesions are severed, and stray roots are repositioned. If there is no need to pass caudad to section a thickened filum, then the dura is closed in traditional fashion. Such a maneuver reapproximates the previously separated spinal cord segments.

If the DSM is associated with another major dysraphic condition, then the operation becomes tedious, and the surgeon must improvise. The septum may be uncovered by chance in the center of a myelomeningocele or intraspinal lipoma, and it is then removed judiciously. If the DSM declares itself in a child with a previously repaired myelomeningocele, it is usually found rostral to the latter, sometimes 1 or 2 segments away.

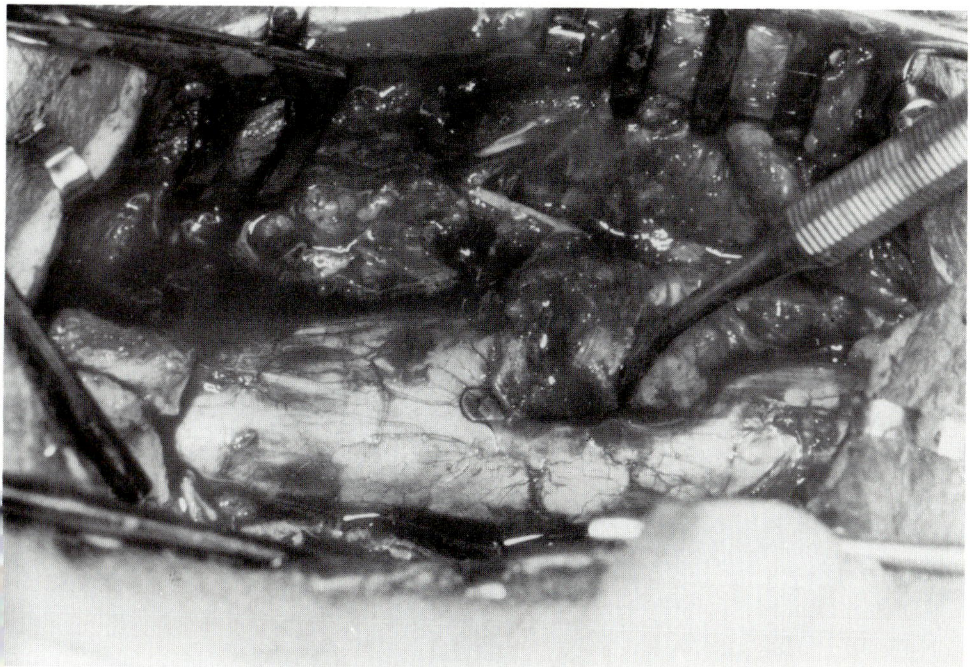

FIG. 23.6. Dissection and removal of the bony mushroom cap proceeds in a centripetal fashion, first on one side, then on the other. The foot of the dissector is halted by the vertical spike of the spur beneath the remaining cap.

The exploration thus begins cephalad and proceeds caudal toward the DSM and myelocele.

Finally, if the decision is taken to explore the dural sac of a child with a divided but tethered cord and no median septum, then the exposure by contrast wil be low, over the sacrum. A 2-level laminectomy is sufficient, duplication of the dural sac is determined at this site, and the dura is opened appropriately. The filum is identified, and it is stimulated and divided and the dura is closed.

Whatever the situation, the child must be followed during the postoperative months by the orthopedist and urologist conjointly with the neurosurgeon. As a rule, the decision about the need for a spinal fusion in patients with scoliosis is held in abeyance for at least 12 months after the DSM surgery.

CONCLUSIONS

1. DSM is a complex form of spinal dysraphism of uncertain embryogenesis and consists of multiple lesions of neuroectodermal and mesodermal development.

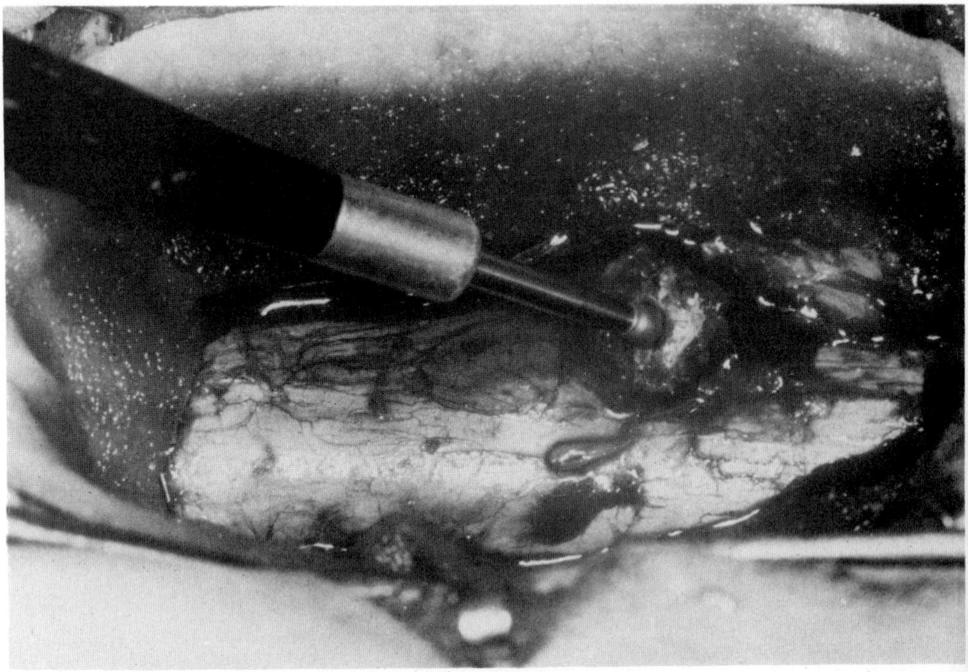

FIG. 23.7. Once the cap has been removed, the bulk of the spur is further reduced with a high speed drill.

2. DSM is a dynamic process in which a combination of factors—tethering and ultrastructural abnormalities—provokes eventual clinical features.

3. The median septum or spur is not the sine qua non of DSM, although it will likely be the demonstrated anatomic fault which brings the child to the neurosurgeon.

4. Computed tomographic metrizamide myelography and increasing operative experience have each demonstrated that DSM may exist without a median septum, as cord segmentation in a single dural tube, or in association with one or more dysraphic lesions of other types; it is usually located caudad.

5. The child with DSM who seeks a neurosurgeon's advice is usually a girl between 3 and 6 years of age who has lumbar hypertrichosis, scoliosis, and a mixed neurologic syndrome prominent in one leg.

6. Operative release of the median septum and associated tethered cord, if present, is indicated for all children, regardless of the mode of clinical presentation. Surgery is performed on the appropriate lesion(s) with the expectation that no patient will be neurologically worsened, and

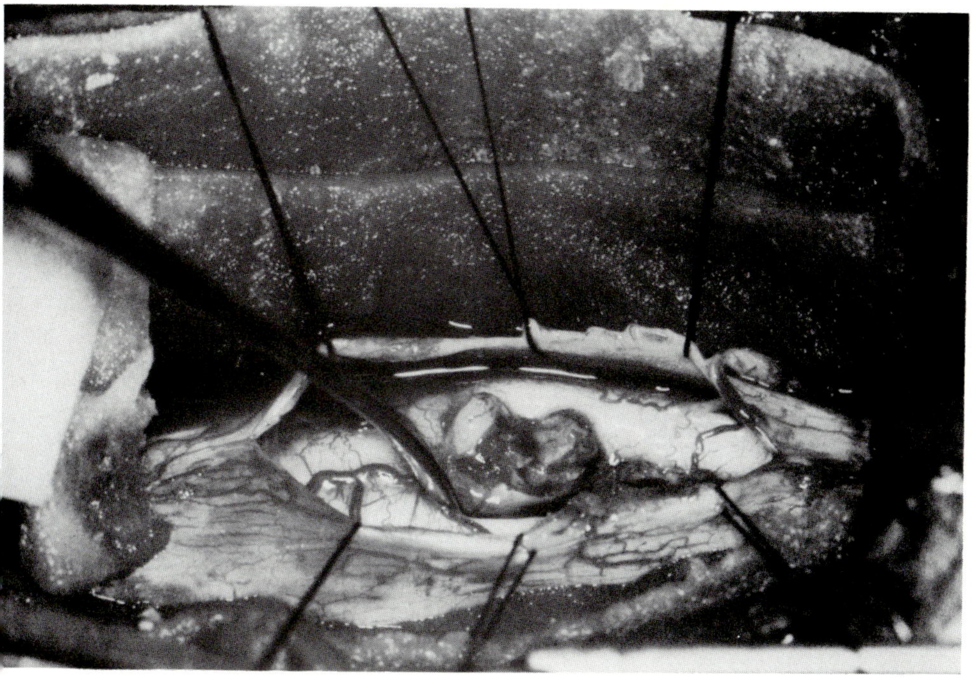

FIG. 23.8. With the cord exposed, the dural cuff about the spur is detached, and the mobility of the cord segments around the spike are noted. The cleft extends rostrally (*right*). The spike is burred ventrally, to vertebral body surface.

some will show areas of improvement, although the scoliosis may continue to deteriorate.

REFERENCES

1. Barson, A. J. The vertebral level of termination of the spinal cord during normal and abnormal development. J. Anat., *106:* 489–497, 1970.
2. Bentley, J. F. R., and Smith, J. R. Developmental posterior enteric remnants and spinal malformations: The split notochord syndrome. Arch. Dis. Child., *35:* 76–86, 1960.
3. Breig, A. Personal communication, 1972.
4. Bremer, J. L. Dorsal intestinal fistula: Accessory neurenteric canal; diastematomyelia. Arch. Pathol., *54:* 132–138, 1952.
5. Bruce, D. A., and Schut, L. Spinal lipomas in infancy and childhood. Child's Brain, *5:* 192–203, 1979.
6. Chapman, P. H. Congenital intraspinal lipomas. Anatomic considerations and surgical treatment. Child's Brain, *9:* 37–47, 1982.
7. Dale, A. J. D. Diastematomyelia. Arch. Neurol., *20:* 309–317, 1969.
8. English, W. J., and Maltby, G. L. Diastematomyelia in adults. J. Neurosurg., *27:* 260–264, 1967.
9. French, B. N. Midline fusion defects and defects of formation. In: Neurological Surgery, editd by J. R. Youmans, Ed. 2, pp. 1236–1380. W. B. Saunders, Philadelphia, 1982.

10. Gardner, W. J. Myelocele: Rupture of the neural tube? Clin. Neurosurg., *15:* 57–79, 1968.
11. Gillespie, R., Faithfull, D. K., Roth, A., and Hall, J. E. Intraspinal anomalies in congenital scoliosis. Clin. Orthop. Related Res., *93:* 103–109, 1973.
12. Guthkelch, A. N. Diastematomyelia with median septum. Brain, *97:* 729–742, 1974.
13. Harwood-Nash, D. C., and Fitz, C. R. Neuroradiology in infants and children, pp. 1098–1099. C.V. Mosby, St. Louis, 1976.
14. Hendrick, E. B. On diastematomyelia. Prog. Neurol. Surg., *4:* 277–288, 1971.
15. Herren, R. Y., and Edwards, J. E. Diplomyelia (duplication of the spinal cord). Arch. Pathol., *30:* 1203–1214, 1940.
16. Hood, R. W., Riseborough, E. J., Nehme, A. M., Micheli, L. J., Strand, R. D., and Neuhauser, E. B. D. Diastematomyelia and structural spinal deformities. J. Bone Joint Surg. (Am), *62:* 520–528, 1980.
17. James, C. C. M., and Lassman, L. P. Spinal dysraphism: Spina bifida occulta, pp. 61–76. Butterworths, London, 1972.
18. Kapsenberg, J. G., and Van Lookeren Campagne, J. A. A case of spina bifida combined with diastematomyely, the anomaly of Chiari and hydrocephaly. Acta Anat., *7:* 366–388, 1949.
19. Lichtenstein, B. W. Spinal dysraphism, spina bifida and myelodysplasia. Arch. Neurol. Psychiatry, *44:* 792–810, 1940.
20. Matson, D. D., Woods, R. P. Campbell, J. B., and Ingraham, F. D. Diastematomyelia (congenital clefts of the spinal cord); Diagnosis and surgical treatment. Pediatrics, *6:* 98–112, 1950.
21. Matson, D. D. *Neurosurgery of Infancy and Childhood*, Ed. 2, pp. 84–95. Charles C Thomas, Springfield, Ill., 1969.
22. Meacham, W. F. Surgical treatment of diastematomyelia. J. Neurosurg., *27:* 78–85, 1967.
23. Moes, C. A. F., and Hendrick, E. B. Diastematomyelia. J. Paediatr., *63:* 238–248, 1963.
24. Ollivier, C. P. Triate des maladies de la moelle epiniere, Ed. 3 Vol. 1, p. 189. Paris, 1837.
25. Perret, G. Diagnosis and treatment of diastematomyelia. Surg. Gynecol. Obstet., *105:* 69–83, 1957.
26. Scotti, G., Musgrave, M. A., Harwood-Nash, D. C. F., Fitz, C. R., and Chuang, S. H. Diastematomyelia in children: Metrizamide and CT metrizamide myelography. AJNR, *1:* 403–410, 1980.
27. Till, K. Occult spinal dysraphism. The value of prophylactic surgical treatment. In: *Recent Progress in Neurological Surgery*, edited by K. Sato, S. Ishii, and D. Levay, pp. 61–66. Excerpta Medica, Amsterdam, 1974.
28. Willis, R. A. *The Borderland of Embryology and Pathology*, Ed. 2, p. 154. Butterworths, London, 1962.
29. Yamada, S., Zinke, D. E., and Sanders, D. Pathophysiology of "tethered cord syndrome." J. Neurosurg., *54:* 494–503, 1981.

CHAPTER

24

The Tethered Spinal Cord

E. BRUCE HENDRICK, M.D., F.R.C.S. (C),
HAROLD J. HOFFMAN, M.D., F.R.C.S. (C), and
ROBIN P. HUMPHREYS, M.D., F.R.C.S. (C)

The tethered spinal cord or the tight filum terminale syndrome has been recognized for a long time. The neurological deterioration which occurs as a result of traction on the conus medullaris by a thickened tight filum terminale was brought to the general attention by Anderson's article (1) in 1975 and a subsequent review of our experience at the Hospital for Sick Children (6) in 1976. There have been many articles since, describing tethering as a result of intradural fibrous adhesions, diastematomyelia, dermal sinus tracts, intradural lipomas, lipomyelomeningoceles and adhesive arachnoiditis at the site of the previous neonatal myelomeningocele repair. Indeed, the term has been used as a very loose diagnosis to include all the previously mentioned surgical pathological entities.

CASE MATERIAL

The development of neurological deficits, as well as scoliosis, due to a short thickened filum terminale associated with a low conus is a definite entity, and this chapter summarizes our experience with 86 cases in the past 12 years in which the physical disabilities were due exclusively to a tethered cord produced by a tight filum terminale alone. All other pathology has been excluded from the group.

The sex distribution was 37 males and 49 females, precisely what one might expect in dealing with a congenital abnormality of the lower back. There is no significant sex distribution. There is no significant sexual predilection as in other anomalies associated with spina bifida (Table 24.1).

The age spread was from one newborn to a patient 21 years old. The major groupings, however, were in the age ranges of 5–10 and 10–15 yr. Both groups involved periods of rapid growth spurts which produced increased traction on the cord, resulting in the development of the presenting symptoms and signs.

PRESENTING SIGNS AND SYMPTOMS

As one would expect, the majority of the patients presented first to a urologist or an orthopedic surgeon because of the predominance of lower extremity, back, or urological problems. As a result of the growing awareness by urologists and orthopedic surgeons of the possibilities of a neurological basis for changes in bladder control as well as the development of scoliosis and lower foot problems, there have been very few patients in whom long-term treatment of their particular presenting problems has been carried out prior to recognizing the basic spinal entity. This, of course, is at variance with our previous experience with diastematomyelia, in which many years of urological treatment or orthopedic operative procedures might go by before the original problem is properly diagnosed. Early recognition of the tethered cord syndrome is reflected in the good results of surgical treatment in this series.

The presenting symptoms and signs in this group of patients were similar to those in our original survey. The large number associated with signs of motor or sensory loss in the lower extremities or with bladder dysfunction presenting with pain alone was surprising. Thirty-six patients in the group had pain in some form as a major component of their presenting disability. Scoliosis associated with either lower limb involvement or bladder dysfunction occurred in 12 patients. Sixty-five patients demonstrated some motor deficit in the lower extremity, and 30 patients had some form of bladder dysfunction (Table 24.2).

TABLE 24.1

Sex and Age Distribution of 86 Patients with Tethered Spinal Cord

Sex	*Males*	*Females*					
	37	49					
Age	*Newborn*	*Under 1 yr*	*1–3 yr*	*3–5 yr*	*5–10 yr*	*10–15 yr*	*15–21 yr*
	1	2	8	10	27	34	4

TABLE 24.2

Tethered Cord: Symptoms and Signs

Scoliosis	12
Painful scoliosis	3
Back pain	8
Back and leg pain	6
Leg pain	8
Motor weakness of lower limb(s)	65
Sensory deficit of lower limb(s)	18
Bladder dysfunction	3
Bladder dysfunction—lower limb deficit	16
Bladder dysfunction—lower limb deficit—back pain	11

Fifty percent of patients on examination revealed some form of cutaneous stigmata associated with the diagnosis of spina bifida occulta. The most common sign was the presence of a small skin dimple in the midline, followed in frequency by a capillary hemangioma or abnormal hair growth in the lumbar area.

Duration of the symptoms varied in the group from 5 days (the case of the newborn) to 8 years. The average length of time from the development of symptoms to diagnosis and treatment was 14 months. The interval was longer in the younger child, particularly those under the age of three in whom gait disturbance or loss of bladder control were not readily recognized, either by the family physician or the pediatrician. In all cases, the onset of symptoms and signs was subtle and progressive and was not related to an abrupt onset or to trauma as described in adults by Pang and Wilberger (7). The motor deficit was invariably a result of spinal cord rather than cauda equina involvement. The presence of structural deformities such as a pes cavus foot or a tight tendo achillis with exaggerated deep tendon reflexes was diagnostic in many cases before any further investigation had been carried out. The urinary tract dysfunction was usually that of incontinence rather than retention and overflow. The hypertonic neurogenic bladder often produced urinary reflux with upper tract involvement as described by Fukui and Kakizaki (4).

RADIOGRAPHIC DIAGNOSIS

Every patient in this series showed a spinal defect in the form of a malformation of the neural arch at one or more levels in the lower lumbar, lumbosacral, or sacral area. The commonest levels involved were L4, L5, and S1. The authors feel that the presence of a normal spinal x-ray almost excludes the possibility of a tethered cord syndrome, and one must look for other intraspinal lesions (Table 24.3).

Myelography was carried out on all patients. Surprisingly, myelograms were read as normal in 12 of the 86. These patients, however, had such classical symptoms and signs, including the presence of spina bifida, that surgery was carried out in all cases. In all 12 patients, a demonstrably thick tight filum was identified which sprang apart when transected.

In 74 patients, myelography demonstrated a low conus which was

TABLE 24.3

Tethered Cord: Radiological Findings

Spina bifida (one or more levels)	86
Myelogram	
Abnormal	74
Normal	12

considered abnormal if the tip lay below the lower border of the L2 vertebral body. In some cases, the conus lay as low as the L4 and L5 interspace. In almost all cases of abnormal myelography, one could visualize the thickened filum terminale.

Early myelography had been carried out by the use of Pantopaque (iophendylate). With this technique, the contrast material was injected with the patient in the prone position; the needle was then removed, and the patient was turned into the supine position. This allowed for easier visualization of the dorsally located conus and filum terminale and also required the use of less contrast material in the young child. Since 1973, metrizamide myelography has been used exclusively. This has eliminated the supine position and has allowed the use of computerized tomography. The advantages of combining computerized tomography with metrizamide myelography were described by Harwood-Nash and associates (5) in 1978. Fitz and Harwood-Nash (3) had previously described the myelographic appearance of the tethered conus, using varied techniques. Myelography showed the presence of a lipoma in the filum terminale in 18 of the 25 cases, and it was confirmed at surgery. We have no explanation as to why the lesion was not demonstrated on myelography in 12 cases.

TREATMENT

Some 86 patients were treated by laminectomy, usually of L4, L5, and S1 (Table 24.4). On opening the dura the conus, unless abnormally low, was not usually visualized, but the thick tight filum with its associated lipoma (in 25 cases) could be identified in the majority of cases. In patients in whom the filum was not grossly thickened, it was obviously tight. An associated large vein was on occasion helpful in identification of the structure.

Intraoperative monitoring in the form of a pressure transducer in the anal sphincter attached to a video display terminal allowed us to record in detail the results of nerve stimulation. On several occasions, this was of great value in identifying a filum terminale which was enmeshed in the roots of the cauda equina.

The intraoperative appearance of the horizontally dispersing cauda equina, which then assumed a normal downward path following section

TABLE 24.4

Tethered Cord: Operative Findings

Low conus with tight filum	12
Tight filum	49
Filum containing lipoma	25

of and release of the tight filum, was *not* a constant feature in this group of patients.

RESULTS

The results of operative treatment were dramatic in most cases (Table 24.5). In all patients who had pain, there was either a total disappearance of their symptoms (23 patients), or a significant improvement (in 10). In no case was the pain made worse. The three cases of painful scoliosis were dramatically improved, and none required a subsequent Harrington rod procedure. In 12 cases of scoliosis without pain and associated bladder or bowel function, two patients were improved, but all required some form of spinal instrumentation and fusion.

Two-thirds of the patients with weakness in the lower extremities were improved to such a degree that no orthopedic surgery was required. They either developed a normal gait or required a minor surgical procedure, such as a plantar fasciotomy in the case of pes cavus. Eighteen patients had no improvement in their motor deficit. In no case was there any progression of their symptomatology following surgery. The degree of motor improvement was almost directly related to the length of time the symptoms had been present prior to operative treatment.

There was a significant improvement in the sensory deficit in all 18 patients with this finding. Eight had return of normal sensation, and 10 were significantly improved, so that in five patients with trophic ulcers, there was no longer any problem with skin healing. No patients suffered sensory loss as a result of surgery.

Improvement of bladder dysfunction was dramatic. In the three patients who presented with bladder dysfunction alone, there was reversion to normal control. Fifteen patients who presented with bladder and associated lower limb or back pain had a return of normal bladder

TABLE 24.5

Tethered Cord: Results

	No. of Cases	Normal	Improved	No Change
Scoliosis	12		2	10
Painful scoliosis	3	3		
Back pain	8	8		
Back and leg pain	6	6		
Leg pain	8	2	6	
Motor weakness	65	26	21	18
Sensory loss	18	8	10	
Bladder dysfunction	3	3		
Bladder—lower limb	16	8	4	4
Bladder—lower limb—back pain	11	7	4	

function, and eight other patients were improved. There was no change in four patients with severe lower urinary tract disability, which is in accord with the experience of Bruce and Schut (2). Patients who have long-standing neurogenic bladders with recurrent infection and reflux diverticuli generally do not revert to more normal function. However, there was a dramatic improvement in one 17-year-old girl who had lost one kidney as a result of reflux and infection. Following section of her filum terminale, there was a return to normal of her upper collecting system and bladder function within 8 months.

DISCUSSION

The literature is in agreement that it is the degree of traction on the conus that determines the age at which symptoms appear. In the developing fetus, before the 15-mm stage, the cord extends to the lower end of the sacrum, as described by Streeter in 1919 (8). Subsequently, the developing vertebral column lengthens more rapidly in a caudad direction, and the spinal cord and the conus ascend the canal to reach approximately the L3 level at about 30 weeks of gestation. When the embryo has reached the 30-mm stage, the conus formed by the caudally placed cell mass regresses to become the filum terminale, which normally should remain thin and slightly redundant to allow for further ascent of the cord and the conus.

If the filum develops abnormally into a short thick anchor, the conus may be trapped at an abnormal level. Certainly, the neurological disturbance which usually appears during a rapid growth period in early childhood and adolescence would suggest an increase in the degree of tethering and stretching of the conus.

Yamada and his associates (9), in an excellent paper in 1981, demonstrated on an experimental model that the progressive neurological deficit results from a metabolic dysfunction of the lumbosacral neurones. They felt that untethering of the conus proved to be an effective means of improving oxidative metabolism, which corresponded to the neurological improvement following surgery.

The tethered cord syndrome, which probably occurs more commonly than is recognized and whose diagnosis is dependent on an alert group of clinicians of various specialties, results in a reversible neurological deficit in most patients. It is apparent that even delayed recognition and treatment will prevent further progression of lower extremity disability and, in the case of bladder involvement, will prevent a probable life-threatening situation in the patient's later years. As with most developmental anomalies which present during the growth period, it is imperative that all involved in the treatment of children persist in investigation of progressive neurological disability and spinal deformity until a diagnosis is made.

REFERENCES

1. Anderson, F. M. Occult spinal dysraphism: A series of 73 cases. Pediatrics, *55:* 826–835, 1975.
2. Bruce, D. A., and Schut, L. Spinal lipomas in infancy and childhood. Child's Brain, *5:* 192–203, 1979.
3. Fitz, C. R., and Harwood-Nash, D. C. The tethered conus. Am. J. Radiol., *125:* 515–523, 1975.
4. Fukui, J., and Kakizaki, T. Urodynamic evaluation of the tethered cord syndrome including tight filum terminale. Urology, *15:* 539–552, 1980.
5. Harwood-Nash, D. C. F., Fitz, C. R., Resjo, I. M. *et al.* Congenital spinal and cord lesions in children and computed tomographic metrizamide myelography. Neuroradiology, *16:* 69–70, 1978.
6. Hoffman, H. J., Hendrick, E. B., and Humphreys, R. P. The tethered spinal cord: Its protean manifestations, diagnosis and surgical correction. Child's Brain, *2:* 145–155, 1976.
7. Pang, D., and Wilberger, J. E. Tethered cord syndrome in adults. J. Neurosurg., *57:* 32–47, 1982.
8. Streeter, G. L. Factors involved in the formation of filum terminale. Am. J. Anat., *25:* 1–11, 1919.
9. Yamada, S., Zinke, D. E., and Sanders, D. Pathophysiology of "tethered cord syndrome." J. Neurosurg., *54:* 494–503, 1981.

CHAPTER

25

The Management of the Child with a Lipomyelomeningocele

LUIS SCHUT, M.D., DEREK A. BRUCE, M.B., Ch.B., and LESLIE N. SUTTON, M.D.

INTRODUCTION

The term *spina bifida* is applied to a dysraphic state of the osseous elements that enclose the vertebral canal. *Dysraphism* defines the failure of closure of two structures that are normally fused. Willis (8), in 1958, divided spina bifida into two groups, *spina bifida cystica* and *spina bifida occulta.* The former term describes the familiar meningocele in which meninges or neural elements protrude through a bony spinal defect and are usually not covered by skin. The term *spina bifida occulta* has been reserved for a state in which similar vertebral defects are present, but in which there is no visible exposure of meninges or neural tissue. Included among the many forms of occult spinal dysraphism are diastematomyelia, congenital dermal sinus and tracts, neurenteric cyst, hydromyelia, tethered cord syndromes, redundant nerve roots, and myelolipomas or lipomyelomeningoceles.

In order to ascertain the relative frequency of these disorders, wc have reviewed our series of congenital malformations of the spine for the period from 1975 to 1981 (Table 25.1). During this time, 132 myelomeningoceles were operated on at the Children's Hospital of Philadelphia. Over the same period, 68 cases of occult spinal dysraphism were studied and operated on. Included among these were 34 lipomyelomeningoceles, 10 teratomas, 7 diastomatomyelias, 14 dermal sinuses and tracts, and 3 tethered cords with thickened filum terminale.

Lipomyelomeningocele is thus the most common form of occult spinal dysraphism seen in our clinic. Between 1958 and 1981, 76 cases of this pathological entity were studied and operated on (Table 25.2). Of these, 42 were seen in the period from 1958 to 1975 and 34 in the period from 1975 to 1981, reflecting increased awareness of this entity and the willingness of pediatricians and pediatric neurologists to refer these problems to the attention of the pediatric neurosurgeon.

Recently, interest in the studies of these lipomatous masses of the

TABLE 25.1

Myelomeningoceles (132 Cases from 1975 to 1981)

Occult Spinal Dysraphism (68)	
Lipomeylomeningocele	34
Teratoma	10
Diastematomyelia	7
Congenital dermal sinus and tract	14
Tethered spinal cord	3

TABLE 25.2

Lipomyelomeningocele (76 Cases)

1958–1975
42
1975–1981
34

spinal canal has increased. At the last meeting of The International Society for Paediatric Neurosurgery, 10 papers were presented dealing with the problem of occult spinal dysraphism, and 4 specifically addressed the issue of lipomyelomeningoceles. As recently as 10 years ago, the senior author presented his experience with lipomas of the spinal cord at a national meeting of neurological surgeons, and the majority of those present stated that they would not study and would not operate on a child with a skin-covered mass in the low back. When the author polled those present at a recent meeting of the American Society for Paediatric Neurosurgery, however, 21 of 22 stated that they would obtain myelogram and/or CT scan of a child so affected and would recommend prophylactic surgery.

While these spinal lipomas have been recognized for more than a century, it was Bassett (1) in 1950 who brought them to the general attention of the neurosurgical community. Subsequent reports included those of Ingraham *et al.* (5), in 1943, Groff and Yaskin (4) in 1947, and Till (7) in 1968.

In a classical paper published in 1969, Emery and Lenden (3) studied the histopathology of the lipomas of the cauda equina and other fatty tumors related to neurospinal dysraphism. They divided them into (a) fibrolipomas of the filum terminale, which could be intrathecal, extrathecal, or combined; (b) dural fibrolipomas, which could be a layer of fat (en plaque), lateral or attached to other sites; and (c) leptomyelolipomas, which are large fatty masses attached to the conus medullaris and are frequently intermingled with the spinal cord and nerve roots in such a way as to make a distinction between the spinal cord and the lipomatous mass impossible.

CLINICAL DATA

As mentioned above, the present series of children reviewed at the Children's Hospital of Philadelphia consisted of 76 cases and did not include those adult cases (over 18 years old) that were seen in other institutions. The children were separated into two definite groups: those who presented in the newborn period or within the first few months of life because of a fluctuating or semifluctuating mass in the back (Fig. 25.1), usually in the lumbosacral area, and older children over the age of 1 referred because of orthopedic deformity (4.8%) (Fig. 25.2), neurological deficit (4.8%), urological complaints (33%), or leg pain (2.4%). Several patients carried the diagnosis of sacrococcygeal teratoma, and one case was referred to our Oncology Clinic for treatment of a possible malignancy of the sacrum. There was a preponderence of females over males, and no family history of spinal dysraphism or other congenital malformations of the central nervous system was obtained.

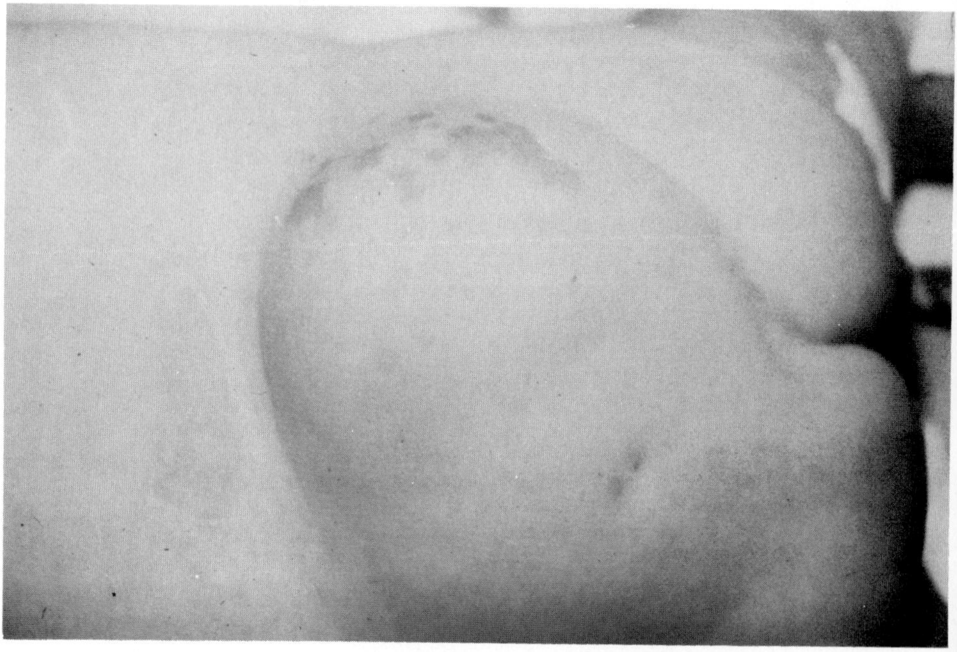

FIG. 25.1. Three common cutaneous abnormalities associated with the entity of lipomyelomeningocele: subcutaneous mass, hemangioma, and sacral dimple.

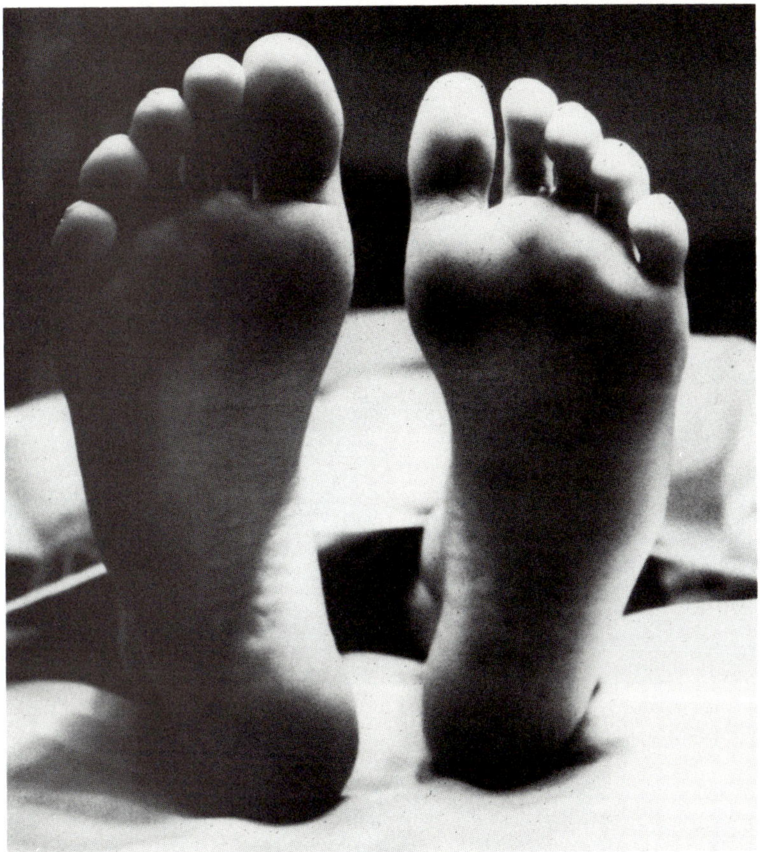

FIG. 25.2. **Orthopedic deformity associated with occult spinal dysraphism. There is an** obvious inequality in the size of the feet.

PHYSICAL AND RADIOLOGIC EXAMINATION

Practically all of the children had semifluctuant masses in the midline or paramedian, usually in the lumbosacral area. There were only 3 thoracic lipomas in the series. Other cutaneous abnormalities such as skin marks, hemangiomas, dimples, or skin tags were noted in one-half of the cases examined. There were no cases of hydrocephalus associated with leptomyelolipomas, and no patients showed clinical evidence of the Arnold-Chiari malformation. X-rays commonly revealed spina bifida and, not infrequently, striking deformities of the sacral region with hemisacrum, hemivertebrae, partial fusion of the vertebrae, or "scimitar" deformity of the sacrum (Fig. 25.3). Urological examination, including

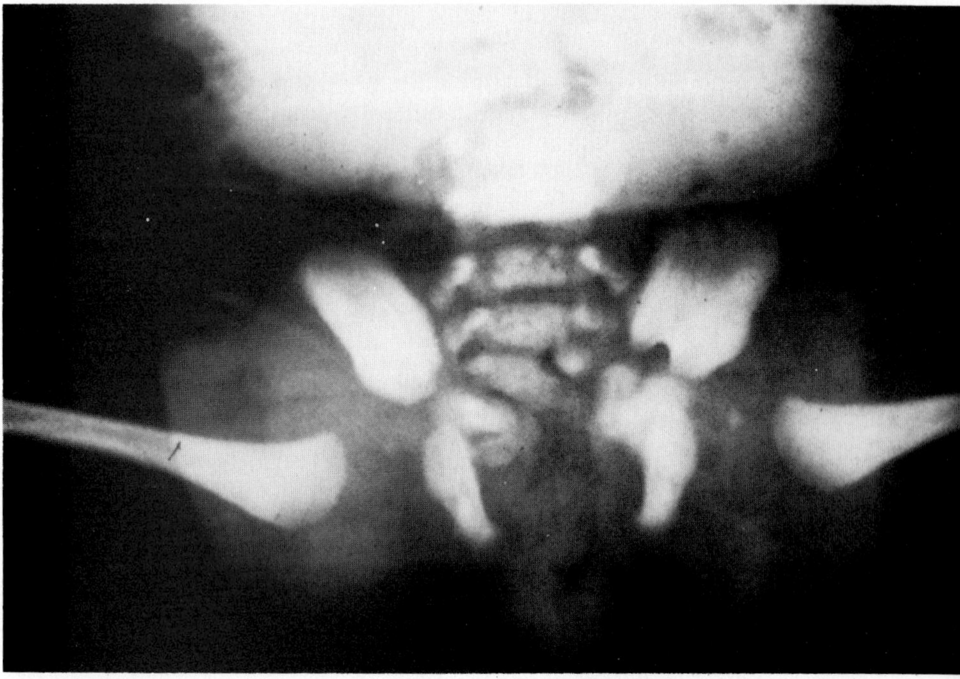

FIG. 25.3. Spine x-ray in spinal dysraphism. This patient shows a hemisacrum and multiple vertebral anomalies.

intravenous pyelogram (IVP) was obtained in most patients, revealing that in 60% of the cases, there was evidence of urinary tract infection or abnormal radiological studies, including bladder dysfunction with retention, thick-walled bladder or trabeculated bladder, large bladder with retention, poor emptying, destruction of the kidney tissue, hydronephrosis, and severe pyelonephritis. The incidence of abnormal urologic findings in children with lipomyelomeningocele was exactly the same as the incidence of urinary infections in patients with myelomeningoceles (2, 6). All patients were studied with myelography. Significant findings included dural ectasia, low-lying conus medullaris, extradural or intradural soft tissue masses, horizontally running nerve roots, and, in 60% of the cases, a large communication between the lumbosacral subarachnoid space and a subcutaneous space within the lipoma (Fig. 25.4). Frequently during myelography, a large portion of the lipomatous mass could be identified entering the spinal canal and attaching itself intimately to the neural tissue. Infiltration of the spinal cord could be seen as widening of the shadow of the spinal cord (Fig. 25.5). In recent years,

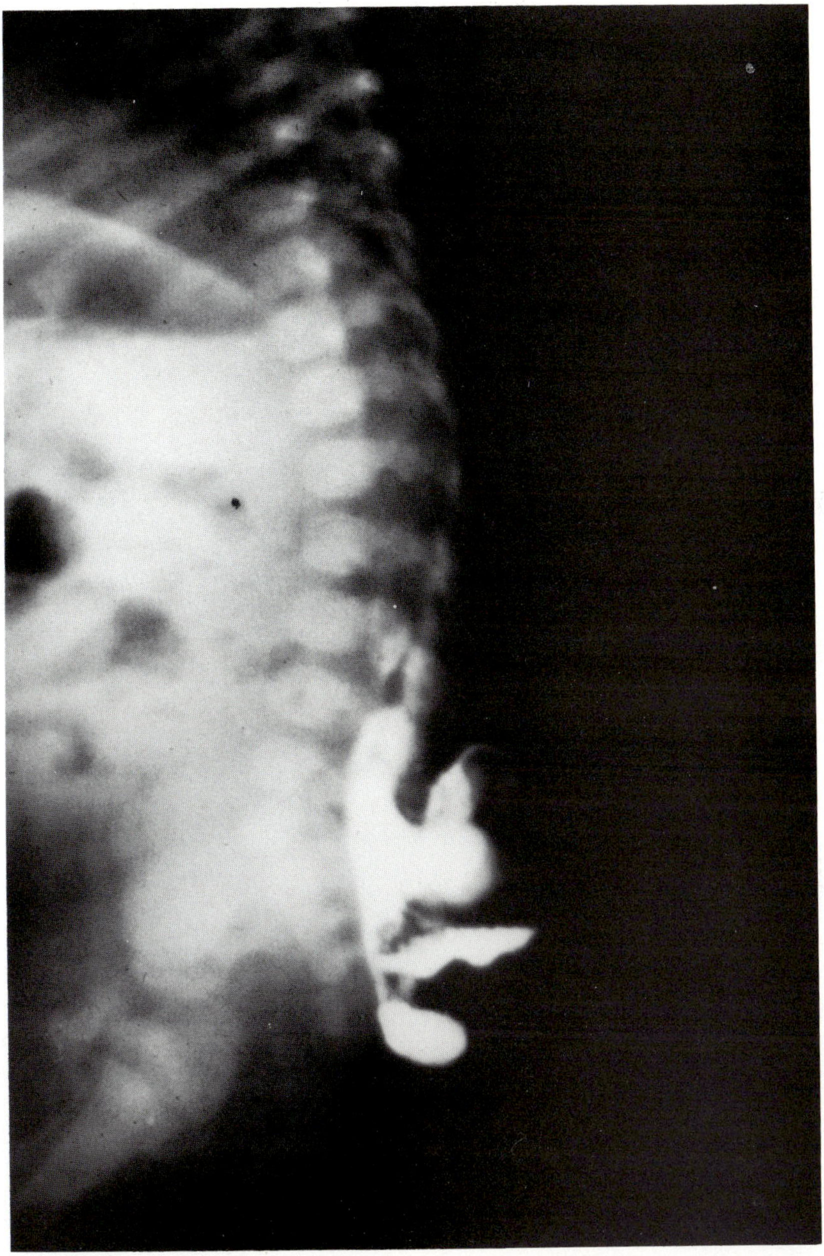

FIG. 25.4. Myelogram of patient with lipomyelomeningocele. Contrast material can be seen extravasating through the dural defect and into the lipoma.

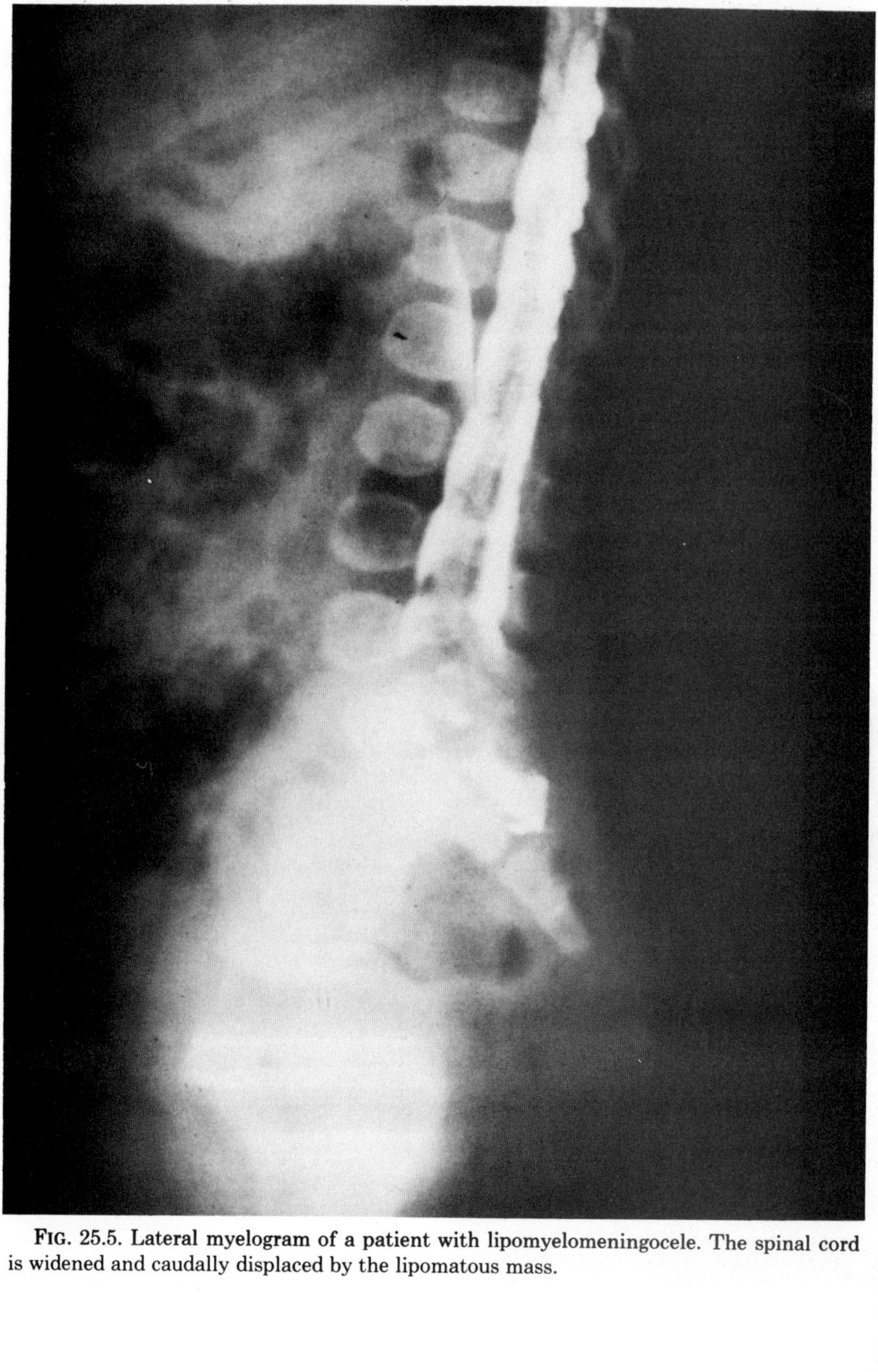

FIG. 25.5. Lateral myelogram of a patient with lipomyelomeningocele. The spinal cord is widened and caudally displaced by the lipomatous mass.

CT examination of the spinal canal has corroborated the presence of lipomas with the spinal canal.

MANAGEMENT

To illustrate the problems encountered in the management of these cases, 2 clinical cases will be presented.

The first is that of an infant (Fig. 25.6) born with severe congenital malformations, the most striking of which was a visible mass at the lower end of the spine and also an independent mass visible in the region of the left buttock. Many studies were performed, including an IVP, a barium enema, and ultrasonography. It was finally determined that the mass of the buttock did not connect to the abdominal cavity in any way, and a myelogram demonstrated the classical picture of a leptomyelomeningocele. At the age of 3 weeks, both masses were explored. A lipomatous mass was found at the lower end of the spine, funneling through a fascial defect measuring 2.5 cm across. The pedicle continued through a defect in the lamina and into the intradural space. A laminectomy was performed one segment above the bony defect and, through the translucent dura, a lipoma could be seen infiltrating the spinal cord. The dura mater was then opened circumferentially above the mass, and the lipoma was sectioned as low as possible, just short of the conus medullaris (Fig. 25.7). The region of the filum was also explored, and another lipoma of the

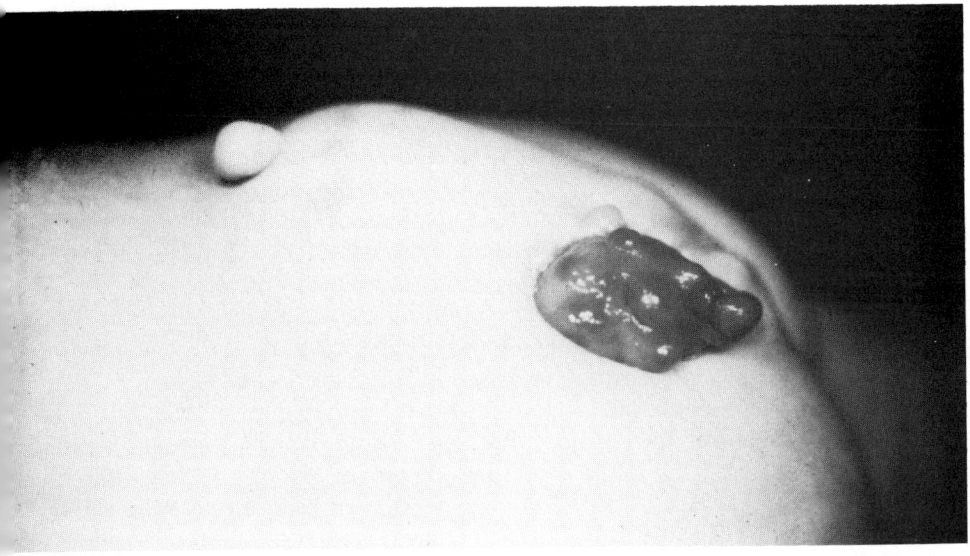

FIG. 25.6. (Case 1) There is a subcutaneous mass with overlying hemangioma as well as a bowel-like tissue protruding through a skin defect of the left buttock.

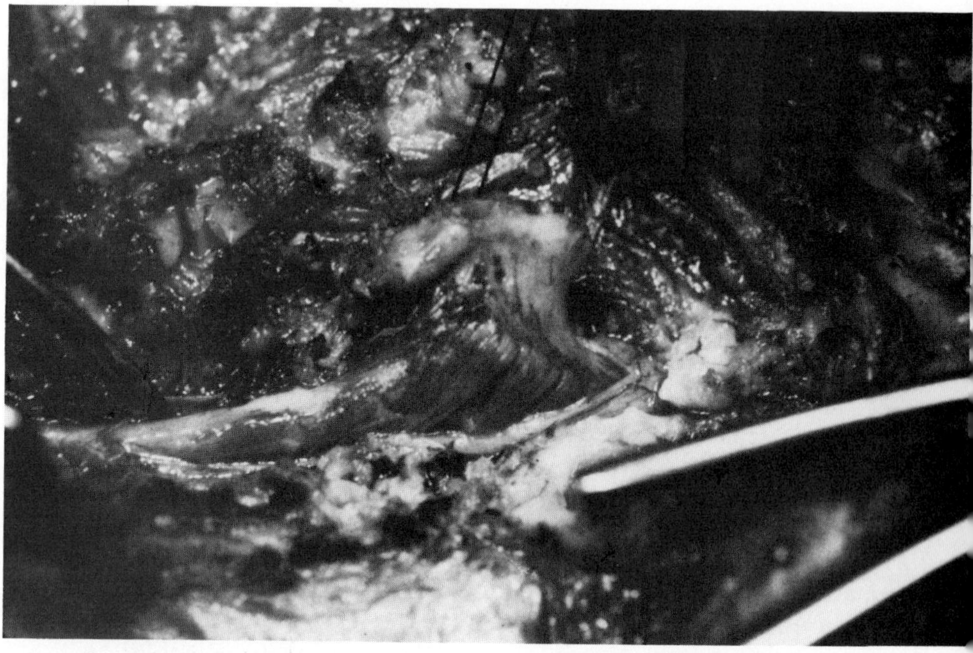

FIG. 25.7. (Case 1) At surgery, the lipoma was intimately attached to the spinal cord and numerous nerve roots.

filum terminale was encountered. This was sectioned, completely untethering the lower end of the spinal cord, which is the primary purpose of the operation in these cases. The dura mater was closed in a watertight fashion with a graft of lyophilized dura, which is reconstituted in the operating room by soaking it for 30 minutes in a sterile saline solution. Later, the incision was extended to include the mass of the buttock, which had the gross appearance of a piece of bowel with a mucoid material, and was attached to the fascia and partially to the muscle itself. Figure 25.7 shows the mass removed in one piece. Pathological examination of this specimen revealed abundant fatty fibrous tissue covered by thin relatively normal collagen bands. The center of one of the masses contained a cyst with connective tissue lining (lipomatous mass attached to the spinal cord). The second mass in the region of the buttock contained an abundance of intestinal epithelium of both large and small bowel type, lymph node-like structures, layers of smooth muscle characteristic of GI tract, fat, Vater-Pacini type structures, lymphangioma-like structures, mature and immature cartilage, and squamous epithelium, which was continuous in places with other intestinal epithelium. No neural tissue of central origin was seen in this portion of the specimen. The first specimen was consistent with lipomyelomeningocele; the second

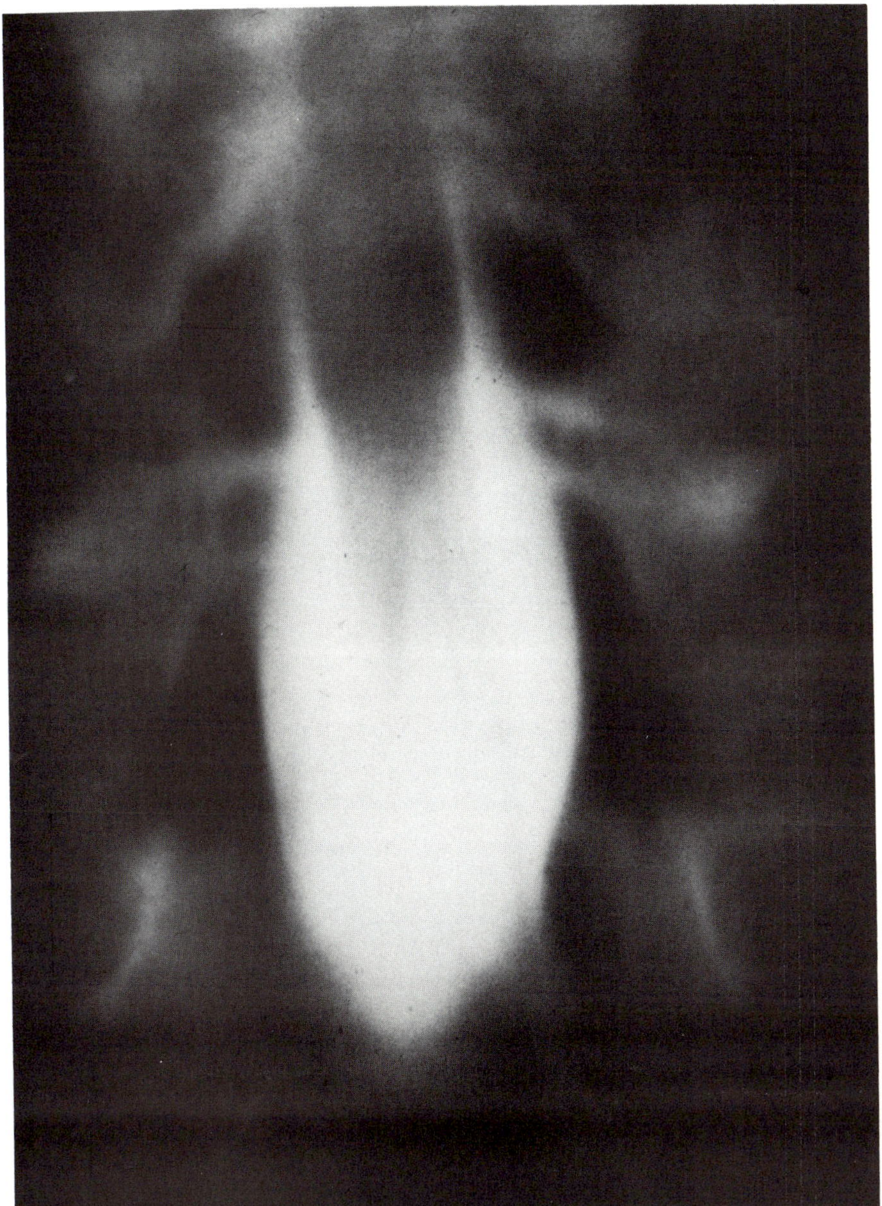

FIG. 25.8. (Case 2) A lumbar myelogram demonstrates that the conus medullaris is at the L5-S1 interspace.

was described as a mixed hamartoma or choristoma. The wounds healed by primary closure, and no neurological deterioration has been noted.

The second case illustrates the opposite end of the age spectrum. This 27-year-old female was neurologically intact for many years when she suddenly developed findings consistent with tethering of the spinal cord. She had noted since early childhood the presence of a lump in the lumbosacral area but had experienced no neurologic, orthopedic, or urologic problems. She had been seen several times by general and plastic surgeons who advised against surgical removal of the presumed lipoma. Just prior to our seeing the patient, she was examined by a gynecologist for the possibility of genital herpes. She was placed in stirrups for examination and, almost immediately, noticed numbness of the left leg in a stocking-like distribution and also weakness of the left leg when she tried to ambulate. This was much more noticeable on trying to walk up stairs, and the numbness eventually extended to include the vaginal area and rectal and sacral dermatomes. On examination, she had weakness which included the psoas muscle and all of the leg musculature below that level on the left side, and numbness of the left lower extremity. An IVP demonstrated residual urine in the bladder after emptying. A myelogram was performed (Fig. 25.8) which demonstrated tethering of the spinal cord by a mass entering the canal and attaching itself to the low-lying conus medullaris. At surgery, a lipomatous mass (Fig. 25.9) was demonstrated and excised. The dura mater was closed in a watertight fashion without use of a dural patch, and the patient has experienced no further deterioration of her neurological condition.

DISCUSSION

In recent presentations, both Dr. Chapman of the Massachusetts General Hospital and Dr. McLone of the Chicago Children's Memorial Hospital have emphasized the same points we would like to make in this publication.

1. A thorough understanding of the physiopathology of the lipomyelomeningoceles is necessary before undertaking surgery for this disorder, and a predetermined plan should be followed at surgery.
2. The primary goal of operation is to untether the spinal cord, either from the filum terminale or the lowermost point attachment of the lipoma.
3. It is necessary to reconstruct the dura mater, either with normal tissues taken from the patient, such as fascia, or with lyophilized dura, which we have been recently using, to prevent the retethering of the spinal cord by the formation of adhesions between the remnants of the lipoma and the lowermost portion of the spinal cord.

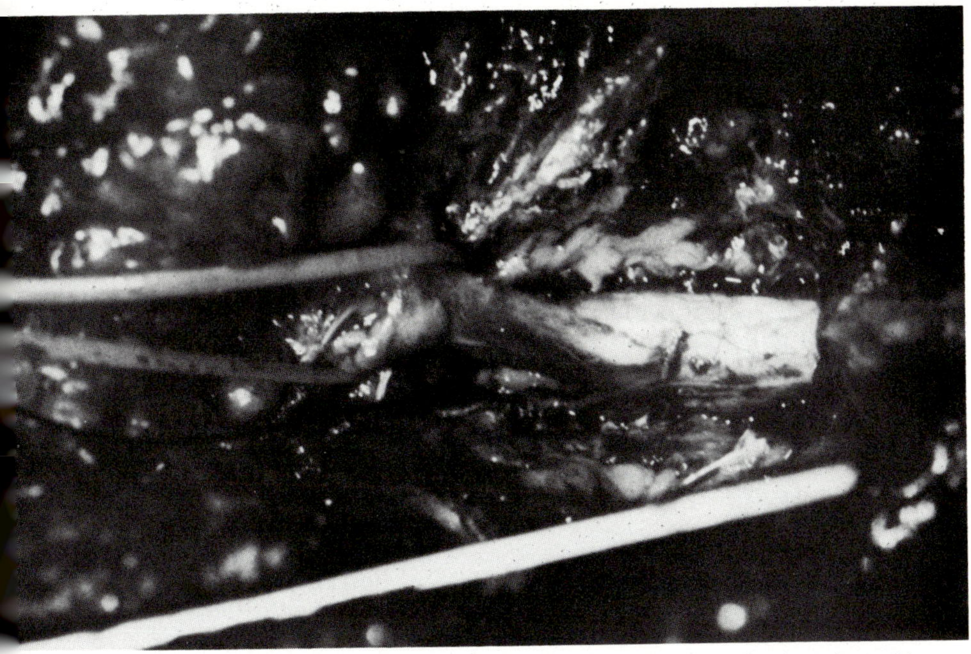

FIG. 25.9. (Case 2) At surgery, the lipoma is seen to attach to the dural sac by a thin pedicle.

Surgery is relatively safe, and we have had no mortality in these 76 cases. The major postoperative complications have been cerebrospinal fluid leaks, as it is at times extremely difficult to obtain good tissue for surgical repair. Because of this, we would like to stress, once again, the need for a watertight closure of the dura mater. We maintain our patients in the prone postion, with the head lower than the buttocks, for at least 72 hours.

It is our contention that, in children born with large lipomatous mass of the lumbar or sacral region, investigation should be instigated as early as possible. If studies reveal the presence of transdural adhesion of the lipoma to the spinal cord, prophylactic surgery should be recommended. It has been our experience that if these children are not operated on in infancy all will have some degree of neurological, urological, and orthopedic problems. It is also our experience that when neurological deficit has already occurred, surgery will usually prevent the progression of the deformity or deficit, but in very few cases will there be improvement of the neurological condition after surgery. It has been postulated that continuous traction and pressure over the neural elements could produce changes, either mechanical or metabolic, which will produce permanent destruction of the neuronal elements and irreversible damage. Because of this, we recommend that patients with leptomyelolipomas be investigated and operated on at the time they come to the attention of the pediatric neurosurgeon and that they not be allowed to wait until problems develop later on.

REFERENCES

1. Bassett, R. C. The neurological deficit associated with lipomas of the cauda equina. *Ann Surg., 13:* 109–116, 1950.
2. Cooper, D. W. G. Urinary tract infections in children with myelomeningocele. *Arch. Dis. Child., 42:* 521, 1967.
3. Emery, J. C., and Lenden, R. G. Lipomas of the cauda equina and other fatty tumours related to neurospinal dysraphism. *Dev. Med. Child Neurol., 20:* 62–70, 1969.
4. Groff, R. A., and Yaskin, J. C. Late occurrence of sphincter and other neurological disturbances associated with congenital malformations of the vertebral column. *Trans. Am. Neurol. Assoc.*, 218, 1947.
5. Ingraham, F. D., Swan, H., Hamlin, H., Lowrey, J. J., Matson, D. D., and Scott, H. W., Jr. *Spina Bifida and Cranium Bifidum.* Harvard University Press, Cambridge, Mass., 1943.
6. Sokol, G. M., and Schwartz, M. W. Urinary complications of lipomyelomeningocele. Arch. Dis Child, *48*(7)*:* 560–562, 1973.
7. Till, K. Spinal dysraphisms, a study of congenital malformations of the back. *Dev. Med. Child Neurol., 10:* 470, 1968.
8. Willis, R. A. *The Borderland of Embryology and Pathology.* Butterworth, London, 1958.

V

Spinal Surgery

CHAPTER

26

Spine-Spinal Cord Relationships in Spinal Cord Trauma*

CHARLES H. TATOR, M.D., Ph.D., F.R.C.S.(C)

An important source of difficulty in the diagnosis and treatment of patients with acute spinal cord injury is the multitude of combinations of spinal cord and spinal column injuries which the clinician encounters. Not only are there variations with respect to cause of injury, age of patient, and delay between injury and admission, but also with spinal injuries there are an almost infinite number of additional variations among three factors peculiar to spinal injuries. These factors are: (a) the severity of the neurological injury; (b) the level of injury; and (c) the type of dislocation or fracture, including the direction and severity of dislocation.

There have been very few attempts to document the frequency of each of the combinations of cord and vertebral injuries (1, 2, 4), or to analyze the possible effects which these cord-column injury combinations may have on recovery of neurological function. It was felt that the management of acute cord-injured patients would be improved by the identification of any relationships which might exist between the neurological and bony injuries and their effect on recovery. For example, diagnosis of the injuries in the acute stage, selection of the most favorable treatment, and establishment of prognosis might be improved by a knowledge of the frequencies with which various neurological injuries and vertebral injuries may be associated and the effect of these relationships on recovery.

Thus, the present study was designed to provide answers to two questions:

1. What is the relationship, if any, between the type of spinal column injury and the type of spinal cord injury?
2. What is the relationship, if any, between the spinal column injury, the spinal cord injury, and the recovery of neurological function?

---

* Supported by a Demonstration Model Grant to the Acute Spinal Cord Injury Unit, Sunnybrook Medical Centre, from the Ontario Ministry of Health.

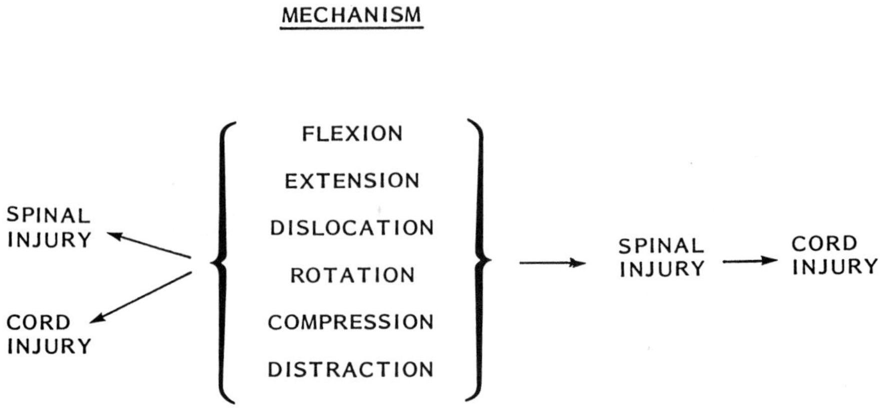

FIG. 26.1. Possible relationships between mechanism of injury, spinal injury, and spinal cord injury.

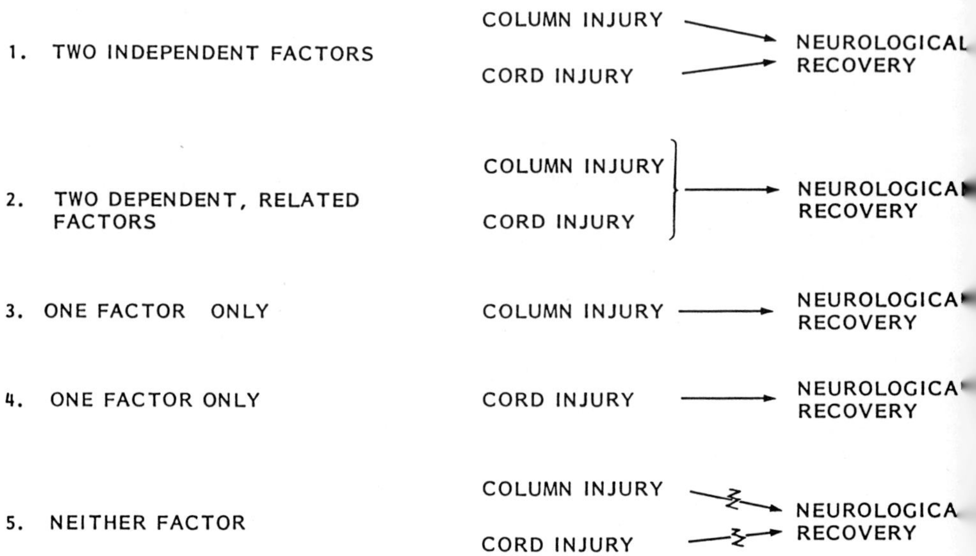

FIG. 26.2. Possible relationships between spinal injury, cord injury, and recovery.

The possible relationships are shown in Figures 26.1 and 26.2. It is quite likely that in some instances the same mechanism that injures the spine injures the cord. For example, a compression or axial loading force which causes a burst fracture may also cause compression of the cord due to the posteriorly protruding fragment of the vertebral body. In other instances, the mechanism that injures the spine will differ from that which injures the cord. For example, a force which strikes the head from behind and produces an anterior dislocation of the cervical spine at C5-C6 may injure the cord by compression when the cord is pinched between the posterior superior edge of the body of C6 and the anterior edge of the lamina of C5. Thus, the mechanism of injury to the cord and column may be the same or may differ.

With respect to recovery, the cord and column injuries may be important independent or dependent factors affecting recovery; only one factor may affect recovery, or neither factor may affect recovery as shown in Figure 26.2. The unravelling of these possible relationships was one of the purposes of the present study.

METHODS

The Study Population

The records of patients with acute spinal cord injuries admitted to either the Toronto General or Sunnybrook Hospitals during the 25 year period from 1948 to 1973 were analyzed. For inclusion in the study, a patient must have been admitted to either hospital within 30 days of injury, and the record must have contained complete documentation of the cord injury, treatment, and result. Patients who had major treatment in other institutions prior to referral or who had spinal injuries without cord involvement were excluded. Similarly, those with only root involvement or those with injuries at L2 or below were excluded. A total of 358 patients were included in the study. The information was computer processed by the University of Toronto Department of Statistics under the direction of Dr. David Andrews. An epidemiological analysis of these 358 patients has been published previously (6).

Level of Spinal Column Injury

In most cases, the level of spinal column injury was established from the initial radiological examination. However, when there was no spinal column injury detectable on the initial x-rays, the level was assigned on the basis of one or more of the following: the neurological examination, operative findings, subsequent x-ray results, or postmortem examination. For some analyses, the cases were grouped into three areas of injury: cervical (C1 to C7-T1); thoracic (T1 to T11); and thoracolumbar (T11–T12 to L1–L2). There were eight cervical injuries in which the level was designated as "cervical-undefined" because a precise cervical vertebral level could not be determined. In these cases, there was no detectable vertebral column injury, and in most the neurological deficit was mild and rapidly improving.

Classification of Type of Spinal Column Injury

Information about the spinal column injury was obtained from the radiological reports and clinical records and in a few cases by review of the films by the author. In patients with no detectable injury to the spinal column, the x-rays were designated "normal." Dislocations were graded as to degree: mild, 1–3 mm; moderate, 4–6 mm; and severe, equal to or greater than half the anteroposterior width of the involved vertebral body. The direction of dislocation was recorded as anterior, posterior, lateral, or combinations of these directions. The anterior or posterior dislocations were named with reference to the more superior vertebra. For example, if C4 was dislocated anterior to C5, this was designated as a C4-C5 anterior dislocation. Up to four features of the spinal column injury were recorded for each patient, with the most prominent or important recorded as first feature, and so on. For example, in most instances the dislocations or burst fractures were recorded first, and less important features such as spinous process fractures were recorded last. When the degree or direction of dislocation was not recorded, the case was excluded from the analysis of these factors. When there was more than one level of spinal column injury, the level which was deemed to have caused the cord injury was recorded as the neurologically significant vertebral level, and the other level (or levels) was designated as a remote or contiguous level of spinal column injury. For the present study, only the injuries at the neurologically significant vertebral level were analyzed.

Description and Classification of the Spinal Cord Injury

Table 26.1 shows the classification of the neurological deficit used in the present study. The injuries are classified according to severity of the motor and sensory deficit. Motor deficits were judged complete or incom-

TABLE 26.1

Neurological Grade: The Sunnybrook Cord Injury Scale for the Severity of the Neurological Injury

Grade	Description
1	Complete motor loss. Complete sensory loss.
2	Complete motor loss. Incomplete sensory loss.
3	Incomplete motor useless. Complete sensory loss.
4	Incomplete motor useless. Incomplete sensory loss.
5	Incomplete motor useless. Normal sensory.
6	Incomplete motor useful. Complete sensory loss.
7	Incomplete motor useful. Incomplete sensory loss.
8	Incomplete motor useful. Normal sensory.
9	Normal motor. Incomplete sensory loss.
10	Normal motor. Normal sensory.

plete, with the latter group divided into "motor useless" and "motor useful." Complete motor loss was defined as total loss of voluntary motor function below the level of the lesion. Motor useless was defined as the retention of some motor power below the level of the lesion but not sufficient to be of practical use to the patient. For example, if the retained motor power in the lower extremities was limited to the ability to wiggle the toes, it was considered to be of no practical use to the patient. In general, motor useless includes grades 1 and 2 of the MRC scale. Useful motor power was defined as sufficient voluntary power to be of practical use to the patient, such as sufficient strength in the legs to bear weight or to walk with or without aids. In general, useful motor power encompasses grades 3–5 on the MRC scale. Frankel *et al.* (3) have used similar definitions of motor useless and useful. Sensory deficits were defined as complete or incomplete loss below the level of the lesion without regard to the modalities involved. Retention of normal position and vibration sense, but partial loss of pain sensation was classified as incomplete sensory loss.

The 10 neurological grades listed in Table 26.1 are placed in sequence of severity, with grade 1 the most severe neurological deficit and grade 10 normal. The neurological grade in each patient was established on admission, at discharge from the acute treatment center, either Toronto General or Sunnybrook, and at final follow-up which in the case of complete lesions (grade 1 patients) was at least 1 year from the time of the injury, and in the case of incomplete lesions (grades 2–9 patients) was at least 1½ years from the time of the injury. These follow-up times were felt to be sufficiently long to have encompassed most of the neurological recoveries (or deteriorations) which might have occurred.

Measurement of Neurological Improvement or Deterioration

Three methods were used to assess any changes in the neurological function of patients in this study. The basis of the first method was the neurological grade (Table 26.1) and involved a comparison of the neurological grade at three time points—admission, discharge, and final follow-up. Changes were converted to a percentage of the possible changes which that patient could make. For example, a patient who deteriorated from grade 7 to grade 2 deteriorated 5 of 6 possible grades and would be considered to have deteriorated 5 of 6 × 100, or 86%. A patient improving from grade 1 to grade 2 would have improved 1 of 9 possible grades and would be considered to have improved 1 of 9 × 100 (11%). In this way a numerical percentage change was calculated for each patient, and by adding them, the changes in selected groups of patients or in the entire population were determined.

The second method involved a stepwise tabulated display of the number of patients who showed each of the possible types of improvements and deteriorations at any two selected time points, such as between admission and final follow-up.

The third method was based on the assessment of 17 possible neurological changes between any two time points, such as between admission and follow-up. The 17 changes shown in Table 26.2 were selected to represent the most important ways in which patients' neurological status can change after spinal cord injury. A numerical value for change was determined by calculating changes as a percentage of the total possible change which a patient with that particular neurological grade (Table 26.1) could make. For example, a grade 1 patient with complete motor loss and complete sensory loss who improved to an incomplete motor loss and normal sensory function would be considered to have improved from neurological change number 9 to number 15. This represents an improvement of 6 of 8 possible levels, or a 75% improvement. A detailed description of the use of the Sunnybrook Cord Injury and Recovery Scales has been published recently (7). In general, the neurological change method is more effective for showing changes in patients with complete cord injuries who rarely change their grade but who frequently recover function at the level of the injury due to nerve root recovery.

TABLE 26.2

Neurological Change Method for Assessment of Neurological Improvement or Deterioration after Acute Spinal Cord Injury: The Sunnybrook Cord Injury Recovery Scale

Neurological Change No.	Description of Neurological Change
1	Deteriorate to complete motor, complete sensory loss.
2	Deteriorate to complete motor, incomplete sensory loss.
3	Deteriorate to incomplete motor, complete sensory loss.
4	Deteriorate to incomplete motor, incomplete sensory loss.
5	Deteriorate to incomplete motor, normal sensory.
6	Deteriorate to normal motor, incomplete sensory loss.
7	Deteriorate to higher level, but grade the same.
8	Deteriorate at same level, but grade the same.
9	No change.
10	Improve at same level, but grade the same.
11	Improve to lower level, but grade the same.
12	Improve to complete motor, incomplete sensory loss.
13	Improve to incomplete motor, complete sensory loss.
14	Improve to incomplete motor, incomplete sensory loss.
15	Improve to incomplete motor, normal sensory.
16	Improve to normal motor, incomplete sensory loss.
17	Improve to normal.

TABLE 26.3

Level of Spinal Cord Injury (Neurologically Significant Level)

	No. of Patients	%
Cervical		
C1 to C7–T1	202	56.5
Thoracic		
T1 to T11	71	19.7
Thoracolumbar		
T11–12 to L1–L2	85	23.8
	358	100.0

RESULTS AND DISCUSSION

Level of Injury

Table 26.3 shows the level of injury in the 358 cases. Cervical injuries were present in 202, or 56.5%, and were approximately three times more frequent than either thoracic (19.7%) or thoracolumbar injuries (23.8%). The most frequent level of injury was C5-C6, which occurred in 53 patients, or 14.8% of the total. Patients with injuries at C4-C5, C5, or C5-C6 totaled 110, or 30.7%, of the entire series. In the thoracic region, the injuries tended to be evently distributed, while in the thoracolumbar injuries, T12-L1 was injured most frequently, accounting for 35 injuries, or 9.8% of the total.

Classification of Type of Spinal Column Injury

Table 26.4 shows the frequency of the main types of spinal column injuries. Fifty-eight patients had no demonstrable radiological evidence of injury to the spinal column. Dislocations, without accompanying fracture, were encountered in 24 patients, and all of these were anterior dislocations. The anterior fracture-dislocation was the most frequently encountered of the designated types of spinal column injury being present in 115 patients (32.1%). Also common were posterior fracture-dislocations (39 patients, or 10.9%) lateral fracture-dislocations (30 patients, or 8.4%), and burst fractures (24 patients, or 6.7%). Of the 30 lateral fracture-dislocations, 12 were lateral only, 12 were anterolateral, and 6 were posterolateral. The burst fractures were frequently accompanied by posterior displacement of fragments of the vertebral body into the spinal canal. Simple linear vertebral body fractures occurred as a first feature in 8 cases and were present in a total of 40 cases. Of the body fractures there was posterior dislocation of bone fragments into the spinal canal in 8 cases, 7 posteriorly and 1 anteriorly and posteriorly.

Compression fracture was the main injury in 49 patients and was

TABLE 26.4

Main Types[a] of Spinal Column Injury as Seen on X-rays

Type	No. of Patients	%
False normal	7	2.0
True normal	51	14.2
Anterior dislocation	24	6.7
Anterior fracture-dislocation	115	32.1
Posterior fracture-dislocation	39	10.9
Lateral fracture-dislocation	30	8.4
Compression fracture	49	13.7
Burst fracture	24	6.7
Body fracture	8	2.2
Lamina, spinous process, facet, etc.	6	1.7
Foreign body	5	1.4
	358	100.0

[a] These groupings were selected to emphasize the most important features. The lateral dislocations include all the anterolateral and posterolateral cases. The compression fractures are those in which this feature existed without other major injuries, such as a fracture-dislocation.

present as a 2nd, 3rd, or 4th feature in an additional 120 patients, mainly those with fracture-dislocations, where the compression fracture was present in the lower of the two vertebrae. Thus, a compression fracture was present in 169 patients, or 47.5%, of all cases, making compression fracture one of the most frequent spinal column injuries.

Bilateral facet reversal, or "locked facets," occurred in 40 patients (11.2%), and unilateral facet reversal occurred in 15 (4.2%). Facet fractures occurred in 30 patients, 16 unilaterally and 14 bilaterally.

Increased interpedicle width was present in 42 patients (4.8%) and fractured spinous processes in 26. Laminar fractures were present in 30 patients, or 10.7% of the total. Probably more laminar fractures would have been detected if tomography had been used more often. Foreign bodies were present in the spinal canal in only 5 patients, and all were bullets.

Of the 58 patients designated as normal with no traumatic features on the radiological examination, four were later found to have fractures or dislocations on a subsequent radiological examination; two were discovered at operation, one at autopsy. Thus, these seven cases were designated as "false normals," leaving 51 cases, or 14.2%, with no detectable injury to the spinal column who were classified as "true normals."

Relationship between Region and Type of Spinal Column Injury

Table 26.5 is a cross-tabulation showing the relationship between the three regions of injury and the five main types of spinal column injury. There was a highly significant difference ($p < 0.0001$) demonstrated

TABLE 26.5
Relationship between Level and Type of Spinal Column Injury

Type of Column Injury	Level			Total No. of Patients
	Cervical (C1 to C7–T1)	Thoracic (T1–T11)	Thoracolumbar (T11–12 to L1–L2)	
	No. of Patients	No. of Patients	No. of Patients	
Normal	48 (83)[a] [25][b]	8 (14) [12]	2 (3) [2]	56
Anterior Dislocation	22 (92) [12]	1 (4) [1]	1 (4) [1]	24
Fracture-dislocation	98 (53) [52]	38 (21) [56]	48 (26) [59]	184
Compression fracture	15 (30) [8]	19 (39) [28]	15 (31) [18]	49
Burst fracture	6 (25) [3]	2 (8) [3]	16 (67) [20]	24
Total no. of patients	189	68	82	339

[a] (Row %).
[b] [Column %].

between the distribution of types of injury among the three regions, although in all three regions the most frequent injury was the fracture-dislocation (52%, 56%, and 59% in the cervical, thoracic, and thoracolumbar regions, respectively). One striking difference between the regions was the fact that of all the patients whose x-rays were diagnosed as normal, 83% were cervical. Many of these patients were elderly and had cervical spondylosis, but they had no detectable bony injuries. We have recently reviewed the issue of spinal cord injury in patients with cervical spondylosis and found that 25% of a recent series had no detectable bony injury (5).

Conversely, in patients with thoracic or lumbar cord injuries, it was rare not to find a bony lesion. The anterior dislocations without fracture also showed a marked preponderance for the cervical region (92%). These were mainly patients with bilaterally dislocated facets. Another regional difference was that 67% of the burst fractures occurred in the thoracolumbar region.

Relationship between the Direction and Degree of Dislocation

Table 26.6 shows the relationship between the direction and degree of dislocation in the 124 cases in which both features were recorded and

TABLE 26.6

The Relationship between the Direction and Degree of Dislocation

Degree	Direction			Total
	Anterior (No. of Patients)	Posterior (No. of Patients)	Lateral[a] (No. of Patients)	
Mild (1–3 mm)	12 (33.3)[b] [13.8][c]	18 (50.0) [75.0]	6 (16.7) [46.2]	36
Moderate (4–6 mm)	10 (76.9) [11.5]	2 (15.4) [8.3]	1 (7.7) [7.7]	13
Severe (>6 mm)	65 (86.7) [74.7]	4 (5.3) [16.7]	6 (8.0) [46.2]	75
Totals	87	24	13	124

[a] Includes anterolateral and posterolateral dislocations.
[b] (Row %).
[c] [Column %].

TABLE 26.7

Relationship between Severity of Spinal Cord Injury and Level of Spinal Column Injury

Neurological Grade at Admission	Level of Spinal Column Injury						Totals
	Cervical		Thoracic		Thoracolumbar		
	No. of Patients	%	No. of Patients	%	No. of Patients	%	
1	122	60.4	55	77.5	55	64.7	232
2–10	80	39.5	16	22.5	30	35.3	126
Totals	202	100.0	71	100.0	85	100.0	358

indicates that there were significant differences ($p < 0.0001$). In 74.7% of cases, the anterior dislocations were severe, whereas only 16.7% of the posterior dislocations and 46.2% of the lateral dislocations were severe. Thus, anterior dislocations would appear to place the cord at greatest risk. Of the mild dislocations, 50.0% were posterior while only 33.3% were anterior and 16.7% were lateral.

Relationship between Severity of Spinal Cord Injury and Level of Injury

Table 26.7 shows the proportion of cases in each region of the spinal cord that were complete (grade 1) or incomplete (grades 2–10) injuries at admission. The thoracic injuries contained a significantly higher proportion (77.5%) of complete injuries than the cervical (60.4%) or thoracolumbar regions (64.7%) ($p < 0.05$), indicating that thoracic injuries as a group were more severe cord injuries.

Relationship between Severity of Spinal Cord Injury and Type of Spinal Column Injury

Table 26.8 shows the relationship between the five main types of spinal column injury in 330 patients and the neurological grade at admission. Major differences were found ($p < 0.0001$), especially with respect to the normal group, wherein only 29.3% were grade 1. In contrast, with the anterior dislocations and fracture-dislocations, 70.8% and 78.3%, respectively, were grade 1. Patients with fracture-dislocations had the lowest mean neurological grade (1.5). The compression fractures had the lowest incidence of complete cord injuries (57.1%). Of the grade 1 cases, 70.2% were fracture-dislocations. Thus, the neurological deficit at admission was significantly related to the type of spinal column injury.

Relationship between Severity of Spinal Cord Injury and Direction and Degree of Dislocation

Table 26.9 shows an analysis of 124 patients who had anterior, posterior, or lateral dislocations and in whom the degree of dislocation was known. The results show that as the degree of dislocation (in millimeters) increased, the likelihood of sustaining a complete cord injury increased ($p < 0.05$). For example, in the 75 patients with severe dislocations, 84.0% were grade 1 whereas in the 36 patients with minor dislocations only 55.6% were grade 1. Beatson (1) and Burke and Berryman (2) reported similar findings in patients with anterior dislocation. In the current series of anterior dislocations, 81.6% were grade 1, whereas only 58.3% of the posterior dislocations were grade 1. Although this difference was not statistically significant ($p > 0.05$), there is a strong suggestion that anterior dislocations produced more severe neurological deficits.

Relationship between Neurological Recovery and Level of Spinal Column Injury

Numerous factors have been analyzed to determine which spine-spinal cord relationships might be related to neurological recovery. This paper will only discuss the effect of the level of the injury on neurological recovery, but subsequent reports will deal with the effect on neurological recovery of the following factors: type of spinal column injury; direction and degree of dislocation; presence of an accompanying compression fracture; and effect of treatment. Table 26.10 shows the relationship between the level of spinal column injury and neurological recovery between admission and follow-up, as measured by the Sunnybrook Cord Injury Recovery Scale shown in Table 26.2. Data for 264 patients are shown. Among these patients are those who have survived sufficiently

TABLE 26.8

Relationship between Severity of Spinal Cord Injury and Type of Spinal Column Injury

Neurological Grade at Admission	Type of Injury					Total
	Normal	Anterior Dislocation	Fracture-Dislocation	Compression Fracture	Burst Fracture	
	No. of Patients ((Mean Grade))	No. of Patients ((Mean Grade))	No. of Patients ((Mean Grade))	No. of Patients ((Mean Grade))	No. of Patients ((Mean Grade))	
1	17	17	144	28	16	222
	(7.7)[a]	(7.7)	(64.9)	(12.6)	(7.2)	
	[29.3][b]	[70.8]	[78.3]	[57.1]	[66.7]	
	((1.0))	((1.0))	((1.0))	((1.0))	((1.0))	
2–10	41	7	40	21	8	117
	(35.0)	(6.0)	(34.2)	(17.0)	(6.8)	
	[70.7	[29.2]	[21.7]	[42.9]	[33.3]	
	((5.3))	((4.3))	((3.5))	((3.9))	((4.5))	
Total	58	24	184	49	24	339
Overall mean grade	4.1	2.0	1.5	2.2	2.2	

[a] (Row %).
[b] [Column %].

TABLE 26.9

Relationship between Severity of Spinal Cord Injury and Direction and Degree of Dislocation

Degree of Dislocation	Direction of Dislocation			Total (No. of Patients)
	Anterior (No. of Patients)	Posterior (No. of Patients)	Lateral[a] (No. of Patients)	
Mild	12	18	6	36
(1–3 mm)	(75.0)[b]	(44.4)	(50.0)	(55.6)
	[1.7][c]	[2.6]	[1.5]	
Moderate	10	2	1	13
(4–6 mm)	(90.0)	(100.0)	(0.0)	(84.6)
	[1.1]	[1.0]	[7.0]	
Severe	65	4	6	75
(>6 mm)	(81.5)	(100.0)	(100.0)	(84.0)
	[1.5]	[1.0]	[1.0]	
Totals	87	24	13	124
	(81.6)	(58.3)	(69.2)	(75.8)
	[1.5]	[2.2]	[1.7]	

[a] Includes anterolateral and posterolateral dislocations.
[b] (% Grade 1).
[c] [Mean neurological grade].

long to have an adequate follow-up time as defined above. It may be seen that for Grade 1 patients, there was a 13.2% recovery in those with cervical injuries, whereas in the thoracic and thoracolumbar region, patients with complete cord injury showed virtually no ability to recover. With respect to grades 2–9, patients with cervical, thoracic, or thoracolumbar injuries all showed an increasing ability to recovery as the grade increased. In other words, the less the deficit at admission, the greater the ability to recover. When grades 1 to 10 were considered as a group, the cervical injuries showed the best ability to recover, followed by the thoracic injuries, while the thoracolumbar injuries showed the lowest group percent neurological change between admission and follow-up.

SUMMARY OF SPINE-SPINAL CORD RELATIONSHIPS IN SPINAL CORD TRAUMA

Thus, a number of significant relationships between the spinal column injury and the spinal cord injury have been identified. In many instances, the spinal column injury was significantly related to the initial neurological deficit. However, the sequence could not be determined with certainty. In some instances, it would seem that the same force which injured the spinal column, caused injury to the spinal cord, whereas in others the force injuring the cord may not have been the same. It would appear that both mechanisms shown in Figure 26.1 may occur, although the former seems to occur more frequently. In addition, there are rela-

TABLE 26.10

Effect of Level of Spinal Column Injury on Neurological Recovery (Sunnybrook Recovery Scale) between Admission and Follow-up

Neurological Grade at Admission	Cervical (% Neurological Change) (No. of Patients)	Thoracic (% Neurological Change) (No. of Patients)	Thoracolumbar (% Neurological Change) (No. of Patients)	Total No. of Patients
1	13.2	1.9	0.7	
	(73)	(39)	(53)	
2	32.5	38.9	−12.5	
	(21)	(6)	(8)	
3	0	0	33.4	
	(0)	(0)	(2)	
4	26.3	51.4	31.1	
	(16)	(7)	(9)	
5	0.0	0.0	0.0	
	(0)	(0)	(0)	
6	0.0	0.0	50.0	
	(0)	(0)	(1)	
7	62.5	0.0	63.3	
	(16)	(0)	(6)	
8	100.0	0.0	0.0	
	(2)	(0)	(0)	
9	100.0	0.0	100.0	
	(2)	(0)	(1)	
10	0.0	0.0	100.0	
	(1)	(0)	(1)	
Totals				
Grade 1	13.2	1.9	0.7	
	(73)	(39)	(53)	(165)
Grades 2–10	43.2	45.6	26.6	
	(58)	(13)	(28)	(99)
Grades 1–10	26.5	12.9	9.6	
	(131)	(52)	(81)	(264)

tionships between cord-column factors and neurological recovery. The following relationships between the spine and spinal cord injuries have been identified.

1. Cervical injuries are approximately 3 times as common as thoracic or thoracolumbar injuries.
2. Beware the false "normal" x-ray. All of the present examples occurred in patients with cervical cord injuries.
3. The true "normal" x-ray without evidence of spinal trauma is usually seen in older people with cervical spondylosis. Conversely, it is rare in patients with thoracic or thoracolumbar injuries to have normal x-rays.
4. The fracture-dislocation is the commonest spinal injury which injures the cord.

5. Anterior dislocations without fracture occur almost exclusively in the cervical region.
6. Burst fractures are most common in the thoracolumbar region, but the most common spinal column injury in the thoracolumbar region was the fracture-dislocation.
7. Anterior dislocations are generally severe in degree.
8. Anterior fracture-dislocations are much commoner than lateral or posterior.
9. Posterior dislocations are generally mild in degree.
10. Lateral dislocations are severe in half and mild in half in degree.
11. Thoracic injuries contain the highest percent of complete cord injuries (77.5%).
12. Cervical injuries contain the lowest percent of complete cord injuries (60.4%).
13. In cord injuries, complete cord injury followed ¾ of the cases of anterior dislocation, ¾ of the cases of fracture-dislocation, ½ of the cases of compression fracture, and ¼ of the patients with "normal" spinal x-rays.
14. The greater the degree of dislocation, the greater the neurological deficit.
15. The neurological deficit varies with the direction of dislocation or fracture-dislocation. The percentage of patients with complete cord injury was highest with anterior dislocations, next highest with lateral dislocations, and least common with posterior dislocations.
16. Complete cervical cord injuries show more ability to recover than either complete thoracic or complete thoraco-lumbar injuries. This is mainly due to the ability of the cervical nerve roots to recover, allowing many patients with complete cervical injuries to show some improvement at the level of the injury although they remained the same grade (neurological change No. 10 on Table 26.2).
17. Incomplete cervical and incomplete thoracic injuries showed more recovery than incomplete thoracolumbar injuries.
18. In all three regions, patients with incomplete injuries showed an increasing ability to recover, depending on the grade at admission: the higher the grade, the greater the neurological recovery.

It should be noted that the 358 patients included in the present study sustained their injuries and received their initial treatment between 1948 and 1973. A subsequent study of patients injured since then reveals several differences. For example, the relative incidence of complete cord injuries has diminished, and the incidence of certain types of injuries has increased, for example, burst fractures. The latter is most likely due to the use of conventional tomography and computerized tomography, which have shown that many fractures previously considered to be compression fractures are, in fact, burst fractures. The recent study also showed a lower incidence of "normal" spinal columns, which is probably also due to improved radiological methods. The more recent cases also appear to be showing better recovery than did the 1948–1973 series. These differences will be the subject of a subsequent report.

REFERENCES

1. Beatson, T. R. Fractures and dislocations of the cervical spine. J. Bone Joint Surg., *45B:* 21–35, 1963.
2. Burke, D. C., and Berryman, D. The place of closed manipulation in the management of flexion-rotation dislocations of the cervical spine. J. Bone Joint Surg., *53B:* 165–182, 1971.
3. Frankel, H. L., Hancock, D. O., Hyslop, G., Melzak, J., Michaelis, L. S., Ungar, G. H., Vernon, J. D. S., and Walsh, J. J. The value of postural reduction in the initial management of closed injuries of the spine with paraplegia and tetraplegia. I Paraplegia, *7:* 179–192, 1969.
4. Marar, B. C. The pattern of neurological damage as an aid to the diagnosis of the mechanism in cervical spine injuries. J. Bone Joint Surg., *56A:* 1648–1654, 1974.
5. Rowed, D. W., and Tator, C. H. Cervical spondylosis in acute cervical cord injuries. In: *Early Management of Acute Spinal Cord Injury*, edited by C. H. Tator, Chap. 28, pp. 335–347. Raven Press, New York, 1982.
6. Tator, C. H., and Edmonds, V. E. Acute spinal cord injury: Analysis of epidemiologic factors. Can. J. Surg., *22:* 575–578, 1979.
7. Tator, C. H., Rowed, D. W., and Schwartz, M. L. Sunnybrook Cord Injury Scales for assessing neurological injury and neurological recovery. In: *Early Management of Acute Spinal Cord Injury*, edited by C. H. Tator, Chap. 2, pp. 7–24. Raven Press, New York, 1982.

CHAPTER

27

Recovery from Spinal Cord Injury

THOMAS B. DUCKER, M.D., JOHN T. LUCAS, M.D., and CONSTANCE A. WALLACE, R.N.

It is believed that around 1700 B.C., Imhotep, a physician to Pharoah Zoser III of Egypt, was the first to classify spinal cord injuries. The classification system contained three subdivisions based on the severity of the lesion: (a) readily treatable disease, (b) disease to fight, and (3) disease which cannot be treated. Galen, in 150 B.C., reportedly performed the first experimental laminectomy and distinguished signs for the different levels of vertebral injury. These early classifications were later supplemented by Roentgen's discovery in 1895, which allowed the correlation of the site of the vertebral trauma to the clinical signs of neuronal dysfunction by cord segment level. Since that time, numerous clinical syndromes and classification systems have been introduced.

Certain descriptive terms of spinal cord injury are useful in understanding the pathophysiology, give some information as to the forces affecting the cord, and guide in decisions regarding therapy. These are listed in Table 27.1 and reflect damaged neuroanatomic areas.

Injuries are also divided according to bony level: cervical, thoracic, thoracolumbar, and lumbar, with the latter including lumbosacral. Spinal cord segmental anatomy is well defined and has readily identified myotomes and dermatomes that allow for accurate demarkation of the upper (cephalad) level of the cord lesion. After the level has been defined, the pathoanatomic type of lesion is named. Many of our current textbook data, including those of our own publications (1, 7), have classified cord injuries in this fashion. However, when it comes to recording recovery from cord injury, most authors speak of only complete lesions and partial lesions. This division was further divided by Guttman and Frankel (Table 27.4) into 2 types of complete and 2 type of partial injuries, this division being based more on motor than sensory abnormalities. Since observation of motor function is more objective, we confined our classification to motor findings for the purpose of calculating recovery (16, 17). Table 27.2 gives the distribution of nearly 500 spinal cord-injured patients, based on a motor classification.

Determination of the bony pathology of fractures, dislocations, and

TABLE 27.1

Spinal Cord Injury Classifications from 1950 to 1960

Complete lesions
Posterior cord syndrome (Crude sensation only)
Anterior cord syndrome
Central cord syndrome
Partial cord syndrome (Brown-Sequard)
Root syndrome

[a] In the 1950s and 1960s, spinal cord injury classification was (and still is) based on the intrinsic neuroanatomic damage that can be appreciated clinically.

TABLE 27.2

Distribution of Spinal Cord Injury with Either Cervical, Thoracic, and/or Lumbar Lesions

	Cervical (%)	Thoracolumbar (%)
Complete	40	64
Graded complete	21	12
Partial (severe)	9	5
Partial (caudal sparing)	21	4
Partial (uniform)	6	5
Root lesions	3	10

[a] The percent distribution from the 1973 to 1975 Spinal Cord Registry Study wherein the patients were divided based on a motor classification only (13). This chart is reproduced from that article.

combination injuries is dependent upon adequate x-rays. There are at least 6 different meaningful projections of the cervical spine (1, 7). The most important film is the lateral x-ray, which may require special x-ray techniques. After the lateral film, the anterioposterior view, open mouth view of the odontoid, and oblique views are necessary. Standard tomography and computerized tomography are further important adjuncts to accurate diagnosis of the bony pathology. The bone pathology can be divided into 5 different mechanisms of injury (1, 7). These five common states are: (a) flexion dislocation; (b) flexion compression; (c) compression burst; (d) extension, and (e) gunshot and penetrating injuries. In addition, there is the rare distraction injury, which we will discuss later, and there may be a rotational component to any of these injuries.

In the flexion dislocations there may be minimal bone pathology and maximal ligament damage, with unilateral or bilateral locked facets and a devastating neurologic deficit (3). In flexion compression injuries, the most anterior aspect of the vertebral body is invariably damaged and reduced in height, and there may be associated posterior ligamentous disruption. In the compression burst fracture due to axial loading, the vertebral bodies may be shattered, but the ligaments commonly are preserved. In severe extension injuries, there may be fractures of the spinous processes, intra-articular facets and lamina, and/or avulsion fractures from the anterior portions of the body. Less violent extension injuries may damage the cord in older patients with associated osteoarthritic spine degeneration; no fractures or acute findings are seen in such patients who have pre-existing cervical spondylosis with a resultant stenotic spinal canal, wherein extreme movements of the spine result in neurological deficits. In gunshot wounds and penetrating injuries, the spine may be properly aligned and stable, and the damage to the nervous system constitutes the most serious problem. The shock wave of a high velocity missle that misses the spinal cord entirely can result in a complete and permanent neurologic deficit. Not included in these 5 categories of bony pathology are distraction injuries. The cervical spine can indeed be distracted in acute injury, especially at the occipitoatlantial joint, and at the atlantoaxial joint. These hypermobile traumatic lesions occur in the ligaments of C_1, C_2, and the occipital bone and condyles.

While more standard neuropathologic terms are used in the American literature of neurosurgeons, the physical medicine and rehabilitation experts and the British literature report various numbers and letters to grade spinal cord injury and to assess recovery. Tables 27.3 and 27.4 lists two of these grading scemas.

The 0, or A, lesion is a complete lesion with no neurologic function below the level of cord trauma, and the 1, or B, lesion has no motor function but has some sensory sparing. The remaining grades are subdivided according to motor function: the deficit is listed as motor useless, motor useful, and normal motor or motor functional. These grading systems were the first ones sued in looking at recovery rates of patients with spinal cord injury.

TABLE 27.3

Standard Grading of Cord-Injured Patients Using a Number System

0—No neurologic function below lesion
1—Sensory function
2—Motor useless
3—Motor useful
4—Motor functional
5—Normal motor function

TABLE 27.4

Frankel's Classification[a]

A—Complete sensorimotor loss
B—Sensory only (complete motor loss)
C—Motor useless
D—Motor useful
E—Recovery

[a] Guttman's & Frankel's classification of cord-injured patients using a letter system (9, 11).

TABLE 27.5

Neurotrauma Motor Index[a]

Muscle	Right		Left
Diaphragm		2	
Deltoid	5		5
Biceps	5		5
Triceps	5		5
Flexor digitorim	5		5
Abductor digiti minimi	5		5
Intercostals		2	
Upper abdominals		2	
Lower abdominalis		2	
Iliopsoas	5		5
Quadriceps femoris	5		5
Extensors digiti	5		5
Gastrocnemius	5		5
Anal		2	
	Normal = 100 points		

[a] Major muscles are tested and indexed as follows: 0, there is no function whatsoever; 1, there is trace function; 2, the muscle can move a joint in a horizontal plane; 3, the distal part of limb pulled by a given muscle can function against gravity; 4, a muscle can work against some resistance; 5, the muscle is normal. Muscle function along the axis of the body can be graded only as 0, weak (1), and strong (2), without further subdivisions.

The most universal scale for grading muscle function is the 0–5 scale, with 0 representing no function, 1 trace, 2 poor, 3 fair (able to overcome gravity), 4 good, and 5 normal. Recovery of individual muscles or groups of muscles can be documented over a period of time. If one reviews patients' records in the United States, Canada, or most areas of the world, it can be seen that physical therapists and physicians alike commonly record the neurologic motor function using this system. The number of muscles tested may vary considerably, but there is at least a common language. Using 14 muscle groups initially and then reducing the data to 9 muscle groups, we established a neurotrauma motor index (Table 27.5). The total 100 points is readily summated and understood, as listed in Table 27.5.

A muscle, if found to be normal, is given a score of 5. When normal bilaterally, the score is 10. When all 9 muscles are found to be normal bilaterally, the score is 90. The remaining 10 points are alloted to 5 muscle groups, the diaphragm, intercostals, upper and lower abdominals, and anal muscles on the basis of 0 points for no function and 2 points for normal function.

Such a standardized motor examination aids in direct comparisons of patients and results from any treatment regimens. We have found it extremely useful in the day to day treatment of a patient and, as it will be demonstrated, we now use the same objective numbers to calculate recovery, but we cannot use our more detailed information in comparing our material to other reports, which use a simpler grading system. In the future we hope more and more professionals will adopt our system, but for this chapter we will simplify initially some of our material in order to compare our data with that of others. Once we have shown that the data is comparable, we then hope to show that more detailed subdivisions can lead to more useful conclusions.

Following the writings of Guttman (11), a comprehensive report in 1969 was presented by Frankel *et al*, regarding the value of postural reduction in the management of paraplegia and quadriplegia (9). This report represented a study of 682 patients admitted to the Stoke Mandeville Hospital over a 17-year period (1951–1968). The patients were grouped in two ways. The first used the level of initial skeletal injury—cervical fractures and fracture dislocations, dorsal (thoracic) fractures and fracture dislocations, dorsolumbar fractures and fracture dislocations (T_{11}, T_{12}, or L_1 vertebra), and lumbar fractures and fracture dislocations. The second used the type of bony injury: compression fracture, burst fractures, fracture dislocations displaced by less than 50% of the anteroposterior dimension of the vertebral body; and those bony fracture dislocations displaced by greater than 50%. The initial motor findings were compared to the motor status after 1 year.

Frankel *et al.* outlined what they considered the most interesting findings, utilizing their 5 degrees of neurological involvement (9). They felt that the causes of the accident influenced the degree of injury. They reported that large numbers of fractures and fracture dislocations were partially or completely reduced by postural methods alone, with a low incidence of late vertebral instability. They felt that as long as the patients had an adequate time in bed, there was no justification for early platings or fusions in order to prevent late instability. The time spent in bed was not wasted, as physiotherapy and occupational therapy prepare the patients both physically and mentally for the next stage of their rehabilitation.

We have analyzed the neurological results in as much detail as possible in relation to the bony lesions and the degree of reduction. In our series, a small number of initially complete neurological lesions became incomplete, and a larger number of incomplete lesions improved. There is, however, no clear correlation between the type and degree of the vertebral injury and the severity of the neurological lesion, nor is there any correlation between the degree of reduction achieved and the extent of neurological recovery. Whereas we consider it desirable to reduce the fractures and dislocations and essential to achieve vertebral stability, failure to reduce does not exclude the possibility of excellent neurological recovery in some cases.

Ten years after Frankel's report, Maynard *et al.* (19) presented the neurological prognosis of quadriplegia, based on a 3-year study of patients admitted to the California Regional Spinal Cord Care System (19). The results were presented only on the cervical cord injuries resulting from gunshot wounds, stab wounds, fracture dislocations, and neck injuries with no bone damage seen on x-ray. Neurologic examinations using the Frankel classification were reported 72 hours after admission and at 1 year.

A comparison of the population profiles of Maynard's series with that of Frankel's series reveal surprising similarities. The proportion of all patients with early complete injuries, with permanent complete injuries, and with injuries which improved is almost identical in both series. An interesting outcome of Maynard's review was the considerable interobserver variability in grading incomplete motor function into "motor useless" or "motor useful" Frankel categories. This prompted the development of a revised classification system: C, complete; S, sensory incomplete; M, motor incomplete; R, recovery; and W, walking in order to clarify and simplify the classification of these patients.

The influence of surgical intervention was included in Maynard's results. Forty-three percent of the patients in this series received early surgical intervention (up to 4 weeks after injury), while over 50% of the patients received nonoperative therapy. In comparing these two groups, few differences were noted. However, Maynard did state that no conclusion could be made about treatment from such a mixed group with operative procedures performed for a variety of reasons.

In 1979, we published an article on the motor classification of spinal cord injury (Tables 27.2 and 27.5). The system of classification is now used at the Neuro-Trauma Center associated with the Maryland Institute for Emergency Medical Services Systems (MIEMSS). The classification for patients with spinal cord injuries was based on the level of vertebral trauma (documented by x-ray) and the motor examination (16). This classification was used to evaluate over 500 patients in the 1973–1975 Spinal Cord Injury Registry. By reducing our more detailed information to that of the Frankel classification, comparative tables, at least on complete lesions, can be constructed in order to draw some conclusions (1, 6, 9, 11, 16, 19). Tables 27.6 and 27.7 present the comparative data on those quadriplegic patients.

These tables describe in general terms the current prognosis for persons with traumatic quadriplegia. Eighty-five percent of all patients who were initially complete will remain complete; a smaller percentage, between 11 and 17%, regain some motor function in their legs. Rarely will a patient who, on a very early initial examination was noted to be complete, regain sufficient motor strength to ambulate independently. These pa-

TABLE 27.6

Status of Initially Complete Cervical Spinal Cord-Injured Patient at 1 Year

Series (Initial Exam)	D/L at 24 hr (%)	M at 3 days (%)	F at 2–7 days (%)
Complete lesion	74	81	66
Sensory spared	11	6	17
Useless motor	5	5	8
Useful motor	7	6	9
Ambulatory	3	2	0

[a] Series D/L is that of Ducker and Lucas and consists of patients whose initial examination was within 24 hours and is based on 118 patients who could be followed. Series M is that of Maynard *et al.* and consists of 62 patients whose deficit was recorded at 3 days. Series F is that of Frankel *et al.* and consists of 123 patients admitted between 2 and 7 days, at which time their examinations were recorded.

TABLE 27.7

Status of Initially Complete Cervical Cord-Injured Patients at 1 Year

Inital Exam	24 hr (%)	3 days (%)	7 days (%)
Complete motor lesion	85	87	83
Partial motor recovery	12	11	17
Ambulatory	3	2	0

[a] The material in Table 27.6 can be condensed into these numbers for advice to the patient, family, etc.

TABLE 27.8

Status of Initially Complete Paraplegic Patients with Thoracic Injuries at 1 Year

Series	D/L (%)	F (%)
Complete motor lesion	95	92
Partial motor recovery	2	7
Ambulatory	3	1

[a] The D/L series is that from Ducker and Lucas in 1979 and consists of 55 patients. The F series is Frankel *et al.* and consists of 135 patients. Partial recovery in this table includes both motor useless and useful categories but does not include any patients with full motor recovery sufficient to ambulate independently.

tients (less than 3%) may improve because of aggressive therapy or because the first examination reflected a shock and/or concussive effect. Any patient who remains complete at 1 week essentially has no chance of walking independently.

Paraplegia similarly can be analyzed. There are only two series (9, 16) to compare, and the cord injury data can be reduced to thoracic (T_1-T_{10}) and thoracolumbar (T_{11}-T_{12}-L_1) lesions. In the pure thoracic lesions, the data is practically identical (Table 27.8). Once there is damage to that part of the spinal cord, the patients do poorly, wherein 92–95% never regain any motor power, and only 1–3% ever ambulate. In the thoracolumbar junction, where there is a mixture of cord and cauda equina, the results are less clear. Few patients recover to normal, but it appears that many (as much as 29%) regain some motor function. The time of examination may help to explain the differences in the thoracolumbar group. In the D/L series the initial examination was early (within 24 hours) while this was not the case in the F series.

Again, in all of these tables it must be noted that Lucas and Ducker's recovery rates include operative and nonoperative treatment while Frankel's data reflects only nonoperative with postural reduction. Furthermore, the mortality of traumatic quadriplegia has not been addressed in these tables. The first-year prognosis from our epidemiology data from the early 1970s indicates that of patients with cervical lesions and complete quadriplegia, 27–34% will die. For thoracic cord-injured complete paraplegic patients, 7–10% will die, and for complete thoracolumbar injuries 6–11% will die. The mortality was not always included in the articles; the numbers reflect information about those who survived.

The data presented thus far have shown rather uniform conclusions about complete lesions. When discussing motor incomplete lesions, comparisons are less accurate, and we find it nearly impossible to compare our observations with those of others. Simply dividing the incomplete motor lesions into the three categories of motor useless, motor useful, and recovered is not sufficient. Consequently, where there are sufficient data, we calculated the 1-year percentage of recoveries, a method we have described previously (17). Basically, we divide our patients according to Table 27.2. Then we calculate the percent recovery at 1 year as follows

$$\frac{MI_f - MI_i}{100 - MI_i} = \text{recovery}$$

recovery × 100 = % recovery, wherein MI is the summed motor index described in Table 27.5, where i means initial examination within a few hours of injury and where f is follow-up exam at 1 year (13, 16, 24).

Using these calculations, we can compare patient recovery after ensuring that the patients have similar MI_is. If one group has an initially higher average MI_i, their outcome is better (because they have less of a neurologic deficit). This has been shown in calculated pure motor recoveries (16) and in motor plus sensory recoveries (2). Both United States-based registries have come to similar conclusions (2, 16). Using patients with similar group MI_is, we have calculated percent recovery at 1 year for the cervical and thoracolumbar injured patients. The initial indices (mean) are listed in Table 27.10; Mean recoveries are recorded in Table 27.11.

Table 27.11 data can be applied clinically. Complete motor and sensory quadriplegics have only a 7–10% recovery of lost motor power. In complete motor quadriplegics, in whom the lesion is graded, the level is less defined and there is some sensory sparing, percent recovery is still low,

TABLE 27.9

Status of Initially Complete Paraplegic Patient with Thoracolumbar Injuries at 1 Year

Series	D/L (%)	F (%)
Complete motor lesion	68	91
Partial motor recovery	29	9
Ambulatory	3	0

[a] The D/L series is that of Ducker and Lucas, all of whom were examined within 24 hours. The Frankel *et al.* series had initial examinations after referral to their Rehabilitation Center and was usually days after injury.

TABLE 27.10

Initial Mean Motor Indices (MI_i, Mean) for Different Cord Injury Levels

	Levels				
	C_1-C_4	C_5-C_7	T_1-T_{10}	T_{11}-L_2	L_3-S_1
Complete	1	9	45	58	73
Graded (complete)	7	18	54	62	
Partial (severe)	32	21	61	82	89
Partial (caudal sparing)	50	57	65	81	
Partial (uniform)	65				

[a] Using the motor index as calculated according to Table 27.5, the average initial motor indices for the different spinal lesions with neurologic deficit have been calculated. A score of 100 would be normal. The above data is from more than 500 patients (14).

TABLE 27.11

Percent Recovery (at 1 Year) for Different Cord Injury Levels

	Levels				
	C_1-C_4 (%)	C_5-C_7 (%)	T_1-T_{10} (%)	T_{11}-L_2 (%)	L_3-S_1
Complete	7	10	7	14	
Graded (complete)	12	19	20	67	
Partial (severe)	8	24	61		
Partial (caudal sparing)	80	73		69	
Partial (uniform)	64	(65)			

[a] The 1-year recovery is calculated as a percent of lost motor function regained (14). Where there is a blank space, we did not have sufficient data to calculate an accurate mean determination.

only 12–19%. In severe partial lesions, the percent of recovery is 8–24%. In central cord partial lesions with fair function in the legs, recovery of lost motor power is 73–80% (15–21). In our patients with Brown-Sequard uniform lesions, 64% recover. These recoveries include a large number of patients and a variety of treatments.

Similar data can be obtained from Table 27.11 for paraplegic and paraparetic patients. Recovery from a complete motor sensory lesion is only 7%, but recovery from partial lesions exceeds 60%.

Using our data and that of others (2, 9, 11, 16, 21, 22), we find that a patient presenting with 25–30% of possible distal motor power will have a 1-year recovery of 80% (+/− 20%). Similar calculations, perhaps, can be used to determine the best treatment for a patient, but there is no uniform treatment protocol from which one can compare data across North America and Europe. Consequently, we can discuss our own data with reference to others but without actual comparisons being made.

Several treatment modalities have been studied in the last 3 decades. Conservative treatment consists of immobilization for all patients who are suspected of having a spinal injury. Various treatment regimens have been used as adjuncts to immobilization, including steroids, cord cooling, surgery, etc. The value of many of these adjuncts is still controversial, primarily because of the lack of a consistent approach toward instituting these therapies.

We feel that there are 6 steps in the care of the patient with a spinal injury and neurologic deficit (7). Each of these 6 steps must be carefully planned and instituted, as each phase of treatment may influence the final neurologic outcome. These 6 are: (a) splinting and immobilization; (b) medical stabilization, (c) alignment of the spine, (d) diagnostic procedures, (e) operative decompression if there is compression of the neural elements, and (f) stabilization of the spine.

Immobilization should be carried out as soon as possible, preferably at the scene of the accident. For cervical spine injuries, a soft collar or sandbags and spine board are used to immobilize the head and neck. A long spine board is used for the back. Movement of an injured spinal cord may accentuate the pathologic damage within the spinal cord (5). Immobilizing and splinting the injured spinal cord is just as important as immobilizing the fractured bones. There are instances of patients with partial deficits who have lost neural function because of continued movement of the damaged spine and spinal cord during transfer to or within a hospital. The training of emergency medical technicians should stress the initial immobilization and assessment of the clothed or unclothed patient, including movement of the arms, hands, legs, and feet, and voluntary anal contractions examined by means of rectal examination. All personnel should be educated to test for various patterns of arm and hand function associated with cervical spine and cord injuries. If the patient has not been splinted in the field, then it must be done upon his arrival at an emergency room. A uniform field medical program would greatly facilitate comparison of patient recoveries. How rapidly the cord injury is recognized and how rapidly treatment is initiated could well influence recovery.

The next important step in the initial treatment of spinal cord injuries is spinal alignment. Vertebral dislocations may compress the spinal cord. The performance of myelography or other specific studies in a malaligned spine is unnecessary prior to realignment. Spinal alignment of cervical fractures usually can be accomplished with skeletal traction. In the thoracic and lumbar area, closed manipulation may be attempted, together with skeletal traction. Each part of the spine will be discussed in other chapters. Again, a uniform protocol would vastly improve analysis of the patient recoveries. Without such data, dogmatic conclusions are not possible.

Next in our treatment protocol are diagnostic studies of the spinal canal to exclude compression. If traction produces spinal alignment, we proceed with either minimyelography or computerized tomography. In 1976, it was not possible to carry out computerized tomography or myelography with metrizamide, so we initiated our studies at that time with Pantopaque by cervical puncture. We found this to be quite successful and have performed this procedure in more than 150 patients. When we last reported on 100 consecutive minimyelograms after the patient was reduced, the most common cause of the myelographic defect was improper traction and alignment. These studies taught us not only how to use traction properly but also demonstrated a significant herniated disc within the canal in 5% of the patients with neurologic deficits. We do not know how common protruded disc material is in these patients who suffer a fracture dislocation without a neurological deficit, for myelograms are not performed in these patients. With the aid of the more sophisticated computerized tomography, more information is now available in many patients. The use of metrizamide for the minimyelogram is accepted in many centers, but it is not entirely hazard free, for on very rare occasions, seizures have occurred. If there is bone in the cervical canal, often this can be corrected by adjusting the traction and the patient's position. If there is disc in the cervical or thoracic canal and it makes contact with the spinal cord or deforms it, operative decompression may, on rare occasions, dramatically improve the patient (1); therefore, good diagnostic studies are of value when they can be obtained. Provided that the first evaluation of the patient is within 24 hours after injury, myelographic studies are usually not clouded by cord swelling, even in those patients with a marked deficit. Since we have seen marked swelling only occasionally, we often proceed with the study, but an equally strong argument could be made for delaying the study until the patient is stabilized further if, indeed, either the study or treatment could not be carried out in the first 6–12 hours. Diagnostic delays do occur, but as our entire emergency medical service systems improve, they should become less common.

Decompressive operative procedures should be carried out only if there is proven residual compression of neural elements following spinal alignment. In certain injuries, there may be bone fragments or foreign bodies (such as a bullet) in the spinal canal which require operative removal in order to achieve sufficient space for the injured cord. In the cervical area, less than 15% of our patients require anterior or posterior decompressive operations after there has been satisfactory spinal alignment. In the thoracic area, operations are more common. The operative decompression must be carefully planned to avoid further compromise of neurological function.

Recognizing that there are different philosophies and protocols and variations which limit data accuracy, nevertheless, we would like to present some comparisons. Laminectomy, anterior operations, and steroids are used commonly, and we have chosen these variables to analyze further. Also, we will briefly review our initial observations on how hyperbaric oxygen may influence recovery.

Discussions of laminectomy in the treatment of spinal cord injury has consumed many hours in our law courts and at our medical meetings. This procedure, initially advocated to "decompress" a swollen cord, has been found to benefit few patients and on occasion may have caused harm (1, 3, 11). As a result, the treatment of cord-damaged patients by laminectomy in Great Britain and many centers in this country has been abandoned (9, 11). Nonetheless, laminectomy may be indicated in a very select group of cord-damaged patients, in which there is proven cord compression (1, 8, 12, 18, 22).

Table 27.12 gives the mathematical analysis of the influence of laminectomy on spinal cord injury recovery in complete and partial lesions (1, 18). In complete injuries, improved recovery by laminectomy was not significant. Neither was laminectomy harmful, as certain experts have testified in the courtroom. In partially cord-damaged patients, in whom the neurologic loss was quite severe, laminectomy did not improve recovery when compared with treatment of patients who did not have surgery. In patients with a uniform partial loss, typically with high

TABLE 27.12

Laminectomy in Cord Trauma Lesion: Lesion Type and Percent Recovery

	No Laminectomy (%)	Laminectomy (%)
Complete (cervical)	11	13
Complete (thoracic)	9	14
Graded complete (cervical)	15	15
Graded complete (thoracic)	S	S
Partial (severe, C + T)	S	S
Partial (sparing, C + T)	65	71
Partial (uniform, C + T)	68	55

[a] If there were matched (roughly equal) initial motor indexes between the no laminectomy and laminectomy groups, then we listed the percent recovery at 1 year. If there was a sample basis in favor of one group of patients, then we listed only "S" to show that fair comparisons were not possible. G, graded; C, cervical; T, thoracic.

cervical cord injuries between the 1st and 4th cervical levels, laminectomy did not improve outcome and on occasion was harmful.

It appears that only one group of patients, those with the central cord syndrome and a narrow spinal canal, benefited from laminectomy. The patients with partial lesions and caudal sparing (central cord syndrome) without laminectomy had higher initial motor indices ($MI_i = 60$) than those treated with the operation ($MI_i = 49$) (18). Those treated with the operation had a slightly higher (6 percentage points) recovery, despite starting out with lower motor indices. The fact that the patients with lower motor indices initially (49.0 on a scale from 0 to 100) did better made us re-examine those patients who benefited from operation. If patients have continued cord compression after cord injury, specifically patients with cervical spondylosis and stenosis whose clinical condition quickly plateaus, then laminectomy may help. Laminectomy in these patients, in our institution, is now done with the patient in skeletal traction on a frame and with high-speed air drills, so that no instrument is placed underneath the lamina at the time that the bone is removed. Many patients who improved initially, again improved after operation. There was a 35% recovery in operated patients, compared with 25% in patients who had no operation (Table 27.13). However, laminectomy was not without a certain morbidity. In the series presented here, approximately 7% had a negative recovery, with an average of 12% loss of previous motor function.

Thus, from the data we conclude that patients with complete and certain partial lesions probably rarely benefit from decompressive laminectomy. In a series of patients of Bohlman *et al.*, laminectomy often produced a loss of function and a high mortality rate (1). A recent article by Wagner and Chehraz could not document usefulness of laminectomy. Epstein *et al.* (8), at New York University, have presented data similar to our own; laminectomy was not harmful, and it did help a few select patients. We feel that in the case of central cord syndrome, it is probably best to immobilize the patient initially until one demonstrates bony or soft tissue compression, and/or the patient deteriorates neurologically (12, 21). Medical stabilization improves the operative results in this

TABLE 27.13

Delayed Recovery in Delayed Operation Subgroup Population with Acquired Spondylitic Stenosis[a]

	MI_i	% Recovery
Treated with laminectomy	44	35%
Treated without laminectomy	30	25%

[a] With the delayed laminectomy for cervical stenosis and spondylosis, the delayed recovery is slightly enhanced from 25 to 35%.

group of patients. Delay of the operation for 10–19 days appears more helpful than harmful (Table 27.14).

Anterior spinal decompressive operations may be indicated if there is proven anterior compression of the spinal cord. In our experience, a rare quadriplegic patient may have improvement with early operation with the gain of one or two spinal cord segments (15). The patient with an anterior cord syndrome may improve following an anterior decompression with removal of the disc and bone fragments. We have witnessed treated patients with motor complete lesions in whom there was anterior compression on the spinal cord due to disc or bone and in whom an anterior decompressive operation resulted in definite improvement in the motor function, either segmentally or caudally in the lower extremities (1, 12, 15). While this is difficult to prove statistically, it is still worthy of consideration in the evaluation of the spinal cord-injured patient.

Table 27.15 shows our analysis of the influence of anterior spinal operations (1, 15). In patients with complete transverse traumatic myelitis with comparable initial motor indices, the recovery from injury was improved by 8% without surgery to 18% with anterior decompression and fusion. In all of the partial cord-injured patients, the improved recovery reflected primarily the better initial motor indices, but certain patients also may have benefited. In a series of 300 patients of Bohlman *et al.* (1) anterior decompression and fusion appeared to be beneficial in patients with incomplete cord syndromes, and their results favored that operation over laminectomy.

TABLE 27.14

Time of Laminectomy and Recovery

Time Postinjury	Mean MI_i	% Recovery
48 hours	47.4	22%
2–9 days	37.0	32%
10–19 days	37.8	35%
20 or more days	40.8	31%

[a] In basically similar patient groups, delay of laminectomy for 10–19 days appeared to be optimal in patients who are to have that procedure.

TABLE 27.15

Anterior Spinal Decompression-Fusion Operation in Acute Spinal Cord Injury

	No Operation	Anterior Spinal Operation (%)
Complete	8	18
Graded complete	14	15
Partial or all	60	72

[a] The influence of anterior spinal operations on the various groupings appears to be favorable. The initial MI for all patients groups is comparable. However, the variation in recovery is such that statistical comparisons are not possible.

The exact timing of the anterior operation is not clear, but some of our data with a small number of patients is helpful. Generally speaking, surgery is done as soon as we find anterior compression, within the first few days. The recovery was 29% in 9 patients with complete neurologic lesions and an acute anterior disc compression, as compared to the overall recovery rate of 8% in patients who had no surgery. Operating between days 5 and 10, when there is swelling of the cord, seems to be less beneficial, since surgery during that period lowered recovery to 5% when it was 8% without operation. However, surgery for anterior decompression 10–14 days following injury was associated with a recovery of 20% in selected patients. In the patients with graded complete anterior cord syndrome lesions that we were able to study, the recovery rate with early operation was no higher than that of the nonoperated patients, but there were some patients who did very well with a delayed anterior operation. Seven of these patients, who were operated on 10–19 days after initial injury, showed 23% recovery, as opposed to only 14% for the nonoperative group. Two patients with partial lesions and early removal of soft disc material within the canal showed an 88% recovery after anterior decompression and fusion. Six patients had delayed operation for anterior compression and had a 79% recovery. In summary, we feel that the anterior operation has its indications, namely, proven anterior compression of the spinal cord. The selection of a stabilization procedure is dependent on the osseous and ligamentous pathology, whereas a decompression procedure is dependent on the site of the spinal cord compression. Anterior operations are sometimes poor in achieving stability.

These data are derived retrospectively, with no attempt having been made to place patients in surgical or nonsurgical groups prospectively. Group size, specific bony abnormalities, neurological function, and frequency and severity of associated injuries make difficult the direct comparison of outcomes in surgical and nonsurgical groups. The data are presented as a summary of our experience and provide the basis for some of our management decisions.

In the handling of patients with gunshot wounds and penetrating wounds, we still believe that the spine should be immobilized. However, medical support becomes considerably more complex, for it is important to restore hemostasis, pulmonary function, and other vital organ function in the neck, chest, or abdomen. Immediate or delayed damage to the trachea, esophagus, lungs, etc. is an important consideration, and neurosurgical treatment has to be carried out after there has been full evaluation and stabilization of these structures. This general medical evaluation can be safely carried out in detail, for rarely is the spine unstable or malaligned in any of these injuries. Neurosurgical management is involved in ordering the appropriate diagnostic studies, in carrying out the rare decompression when necessary, in repairing the occasional persistent cerebral spinal fluid leak, and in following the patient to ensure that the lesion is indeed stable (14).

Diagnostic procedures for penetrating gunshot wounds utilize sophisticated x-ray equipment. Computerized tomography and laminographic tomography of the spine will give the physician a better definition of the status of the spinal canal. If, indeed, the missile fragment and/or penetrating object traveled completely through the spinal canal and disrupted its contents, no neurosurgical decompression is indicated initially. There is little to be gained from this exercise, for the neural elements are invariably disrupted beyond repair. However, if the missile and/or penetrating object stopped before entering the canal, or barely entered it, then removal of the compressing elements has been, on rare occasion, extremely helpful to the patient. Also, retained intraspinal metallic fragments can cause a delayed myopathy, and we (7) and other authors (14) have favored relatively early removal. Each case has to be handled individually, and routine laminectomy for gunshot wounds is not indicated (3, 7, 11). We cannot provide recovery figures for gunshot wounds other than those provided within our basic classification of cord-injured patients.

Steroids appear beneficial in the treatment of a few selected cord-damaged patients, but improvement is difficult to document (1, 4, 7, 12). The typical initial dose is 20 mg of dexamethasone or 125 mg of methylprednisolone. All of our patients are started on this regimen initially. The dosage is repeated every 6 hours for the first 3 days. If the patient has a partial lesion and is responding to our overall treatment with improvement, we tend to continue the steroids for approximately 1 week in high doses before we begin to taper them.

The effectiveness of steroids in the treatment of spinal cord injuries was evaluated using our data (15). Fifty-three patients received a therapeutic course of corticosteroids immediately postinjury. These patients were matched with a corresponding nonsteroid group of patients similar in age, sex, level of injury, neurologic deficit, and surgical procedures. We found no evidence that large doses of glucocorticoid steroids improved recovery in complete lesion patients (Table 27.16). On the other hand, partial cord-injured patients receiving corticosteroids did indeed have a higher recovery rate. With this information, we recommend that all patients should be started on steroids. If they do indeed have complete lesions, and do not respond after 3 days, the medication is discontinued. If they are improving, we think the drug should be continued.

The main thrust, however, of medical treatment for cord injuries is to optimize tissue oxygenation and perfusion (20). The use of hyperbaric

TABLE 27.16
The Influence of Steroids on Percent Recovery in Different Cord Injuries

	No Steroids (%)	Steroids (%)
Complete	11	11
Graded complete	13	15
Partial (severe)	34	45
Partial (caudal sparing)	68	83
Partial (uniform)		

[a] Steroids were used in more than 50 patients. The initial motor indices were matched in the nontreatment and treatment groups in all except the uniform partial lesions, in which the nonsteroid group started off better and consequently had a higher recovery. Except for that group, the steroid-treated groups, especially partial lesions, did slightly better.

oxygen is helpful experimentally (10). Hyperbaric treatments increase the amount of oxygen dissolved in blood. In order for the injured cord to benefit from this increased oxygen tension, it must be sufficiently decompressed to allow some blood flow to the site of injury. Accordingly, hyperbaric therapy should begin only after spinal alignment and cord decompression have been achieved.

In a preliminary study done on the effects of hyperbaric oxygen on the spinal cord-injured patients at our emergency trauma unit, the data revealed that patients receiving the hyperbaric oxygen therapy appeared to recover more quickly, although their final motor scores were approximately the same as those of patients receiving conventional therapy. Again, patients with partial injuries demonstrated these significant recoveries (10). All cord-injured patients should receive active pulmonary therapy, oxygen administration, and assisted ventilation when necessary. Measures to minimize infection are important also since, in addition to threatening the life of the patient, infection can lower oxygen delivery and interfere with cord recovery.

SUMMARY

There are many classifications of spinal cord injury. The anatomic definitions help in understanding the pathophysiology but are less useful in calculating recovery. Basic classifications, such as those by Guttman and Frankel, are useful for epidemiological studies, especially if one wishes to compare patients internationally or to compare data bases but this information, except in complete lesions, is too limited to allow more refined calculations as to the effectiveness of treatment modalities, especially in partial lesions. An accurate motor index, such as we have described, or such as the Yale index (2), is needed for more specific calculations of recovery if any prediction about the efficacy of various treatments are to be made. We have described our data from the mid-1970s in detail to explain our current treatment protocols.

While nothing can be done for the completely paralyzed patient, our treatment of the acute (transiently concussed) near complete lesion and partial lesion must be tailored to maximize recovery. The fact that patients with initially complete motor lesion show some motor recovery in 15% indicates that some lesions are reversible and that we should try to learn to identify these patients and treat them to maximize their recovery. Certain severe partial lesions show poor recovery; we must improve therapy for these patients. Patients with partial lesions and 25–30% motor power below the injury have an 80% (+/− 20%) recovery; we should strive to attain and improve on these good results by appropriate medical and surgical management.

In sharing with you our methods and data, we have provided these preliminary conclusions which influence our behavior as neurosurgeons, but it is equally clear that much work still needs to be done. This chapter should represent a reference source with which we can continue to work.

REFERENCES

1. Bohlman, H. H., Ducker, T. B., and Lucas, J. T. Spine and spinal cord injury. In: *The Spine*, edited by R. H. Rothman and F. Simeone, Ed. 2, pp. 661–756, W.B. Saunders, Philadelphia, 1982.
2. Chehrazi, B., Wagner, F. C., Collins, W. F., and Freeman, D. H. A scale for evaluation of spinal cord injury. J. Neurosurg., *54:* 310–315, 1981.
3. Comarr, A. E. Laminectomy in patients with injuries of the spinal cord. J. Int. Coll. Surg., *31:* 437, 1959.
4. Ducker, T. B., and Hamit, H. F. Experimental treatment of acute spinal cord injury. J. Neurosurg., *30:* 693, 1969.
5. Ducker, T. B., Salcman, M., and Daniell, H. B. Experimental spinal cord trauma. III. Therapeutic effect of immobilization and pharmacologic agents. Surg. Neurol., *10:* 71–76, 1978.
6. Ducker, T. B., Russo, G. L., Bellegarrigue, R., and Lucas, J. T. Complete sensorimotor paralysis after cord injury: Mortality, recovery, and therapeutic implications. J. Trauma, *19:* 837, 1979.
7. Ducker, T. B., and Bellegarrigue, R. The fractured cervical spine—How we do it. Contemp. Neurosurg., 1982.
8. Epstein, N., Epstein, J. A., Benjamin, V., and Ranshoff, J. Traumatic myelopathy in patients with cervical spinal stenosis without fracture dislocation. Spine, *5:* 489–495, 1980.
9. Frankel, H. L., Hancock, D. O., Hyslop, G. *et al.* The value of postural reduction in the initial management of closed injuries of the spine with paraplegia and tetraplegia. Paraplegia, *7:* 179–192, 1969.
10. Gamache, F. W., Myers, R. A. M., Ducker, T. B., and Cowley, R. A. The clinical application of hyperbaric oxygen therapy in spinal cord injury: A preliminary report. Surg. Neurol., *15*(2): 85–87, 1981.
11. Guttman, L. *Spinal Cord Injuries*. Blackwell Scientific Publications, London, 1973.
12. Hansebout, R. R. A comprehensive review of methods of improving cord recovery after acute spinal cord injury. In: *Early Management of Acute Spinal Cord Injury*, edited by C. H. Tator, Chap. 14, pp. 181–196. Raven Press, New York, 1982.
13. Huntsberger, D. V. *Statistical Inference in the Biomedical Sciences*. Allyn & Bacon, Rockleigh, N.J., 1970.

14. Jones, F. S., and Woslay, R. D. Delayed myelopathy secondary to retained intraspinal metallic fragment. *J. Neurosurg., 55:* 979–982, 1981.
15. Lucas, J. T., and Ducker, T. B. Morbidity, mortality, and recovery rates of spinal cord injuries undergoing anterior decompression and/or fusion procedures. Surg. Forum, *27:* 451–453, 1977.
16. Lucas, J. T., and Ducker, T. B. Recovery in spinal cord injuries. Adv. Neurosurg., *7:* 281–294, 1979.
17. Lucas, J. T., and Ducker, T. B. Motor classification of spinal cord injuries with mobility, morbidity, and recovery indices. Am. Surg., *45:* 151–158, 1979.
18. Lucas, J. T., and Ducker, T. B. Laminectomy in spinal cord trauma: Harmful or helpful? Neurosurgery, *6:* 688–689, 1980.
19. Maynard, F. M., Reynolds, G. G., Fountain, S., Wilmot, C., and Hamilton R. Neurological prognosis after traumatic quadriplegia: Regional spinal cord injury system. J. Neurosurg., *50:* 611–616, 1979.
20. Osterholm, J. L. The pathophysiological response to spinal cord injury. The current status of related research. J. Neurosurg., *40:* 5–34, 1974.
21. Schneider, R. C., Crosby, E. C., and Russo, R. H. *et al.* Traumatic spinal cord syndromes and their management. Clin. Neurosurg., *20:* 424–492, 1973.
22. Tator, C. H. Spine spinal cord relationships in spinal cord trauma. In: Clin. Neurosurg., *30:* 479–494, 1983.
23. Wagner, F. C., and Cherai, B. Early decompression and neurological outcome in acute cervical spinal cord injuries. J. Neurosurg., *56:* 699–705, 1982.
24. Weinberg, G. H., and Schumaker, J. A. *Statistics: An Intuitive Approach*, Ed. 3. Brooks Cole, 1974.

CHAPTER

28

Craniovertebral Junction Abnormalities

JOHN C. VANGILDER, M.D., and ARNOLD H. MENEZES, M.D.

The craniovertebral junction includes the occipital bone; its opening, the foramen magnum; and the atlas and axis vertebrae. The abnormalities of this area may be congenital, inflammatory, developmental, and/or traumatic in nature.

To understand craniovertebral anomalies it is necessary to understand the embryology and anatomy of this area. Patients present with a myriad of abnormal neurological signs and symptoms, and the surgical management of these disorders is dependent on precise radiographic identification of the underlying pathology. Operative treatment includes anterior and posterior operations at the craniovertebral junction with or without bony fusion. Our experience with over 60 patients at the University of Iowa is the basis for recommendations in the management of this entity.

EMBRYOLOGY-ANATOMY

The occipital bone is formed by fusion of the four sclerotomes corresponding to the three primary roots of the hypoglossal nerve. The most caudal of these sclerotomes is called the proatlas, and its neural arch divides into anterior and posterior segments (5). The occipital condyles arise from the anterior segment, and the posterior segment forms a portion of the rostral articular facets of the atlas. A rare anomaly with horizontal instability of the occipitoatlantial joint may occur if the posterior segment of the proatlas fails to fuse with the atlas, resulting in bipartite cranial articular facets. The dorsal portion of the atlas lateral masses and the distal ossification center of the dens also arise from the proatlas (14).

The body of the dens originates from the first cervical sclerotome and represents the body of the atlas. The anterior arch of the atlas has one and, occasionally, two ossification centers. The posterior arch of the atlas ossifies by 3–4 years of age, and failure of fusion results in a bifid arch.

The axis originates from four primary ossification centers. The top of the dens develops from the proatlas, the body of the dens from the first cervical sclerotome, and the body and two neural arches from the second cervical sclerotome. These centers ossify and fuse by 3 years of age, except for the proatlas, which fuses to the dens body by age 12.

A variety of congenital anomalies occurs in dysgenesis of the odontoid process. *Ossiculum terminale* is failure of fusion of the proatlas to the dens. *Os odontoideum* is a fusion failure between the odontoid process and the axis. Developmental failure of the distal odontoid ossification centers results in hypoplasia and agenesis of the dens. With these entities there is instability between the atlas and axis due to an incompetent cruciate ligament.

An occipital vertebra incorporating the occipital condyles is a bony anomaly forming separately from the foramen magnum. The anterior arch may be partially or completely fused to the anterior margin of the foramen magnum. If a transverse process is present, it does not have a foramen for the vertebral artery. An atlantooccipital fusion is characterized by ankylosis between the atlas and base of the skull, and the transverse processes have foramina for the vertebral arteries.

The occipitoatlantoaxial joints contain two occipitoatlantial articulations and four atlantoaxial joints. There is a common synovial lining between the dens and anterior atlas arch, between the dens and transverse ligament, and between the lateral masses. Inflammation of the lining of one joint may be transferred to the rest. $C_{1\text{-}2}$ subluxation may develop secondary to nasopharyngeal infections, and has been reported in children (7, 9, 16).

Multiple ligaments approximate the occipitoatlantoaxial joints and are responsible for their complex movement and stability (Figs. 28.1 and 28.2). The anterior atlantooccipital membrane is the rostral extension of

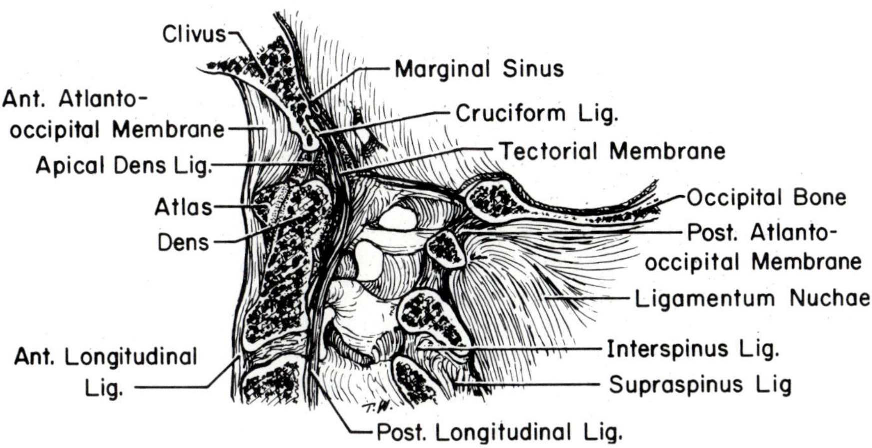

FIG. 28.1. Midsagittal drawing through the craniovertebral junction.

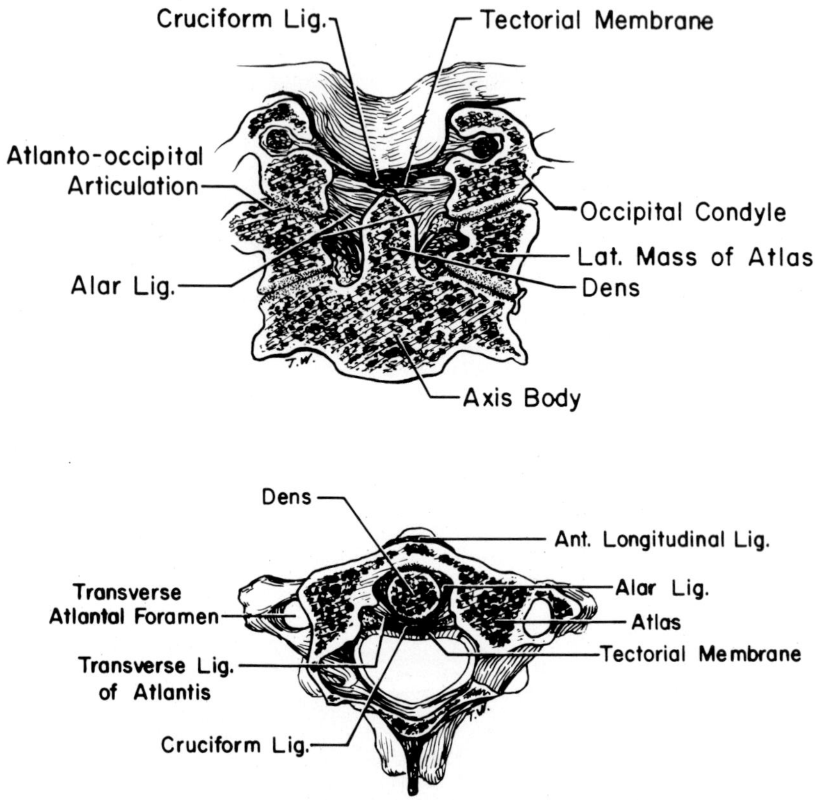

FIG. 28.2. Dorsal view of the cut surface drawing of the craniovertebral junction (*top*). Transverse drawing at the level of the atlas (*bottom*).

the anterior longitudinal ligament and inserts on the anterior portion of clivus. The transverse ligament approximates the dens to the atlas and inserts on the mesial aspect of each lateral mass of the atlas. This ligament is the principal stabilizer of the atlantoaxial joint. The axis is connected to the occiput by the apical dens ligament that arises from the top of the dens and inserts into the occipital bone ventral to the foramen magnum, and by the alar ligaments originating from the posterior lateral dens and inserting into the bone medial to the occipital condyles. The tectorial membrane, the rostral extension of the posterior longitudinal ligament, and the cruciate ligament insert on the posterior rim of the occipital bone anterior to the foramen magnum.

The posterior stabilizing structures include the ligamentum nuchae, interspinous ligaments, posterior atlantooccipital membrane, ligamentum flavum, supraspinal ligaments, and paracervical musculature. The neck muscle development is inadequate to supplement joint stability until 8 years of age (1, 10).

The atlantoaxial facet joint is horizontally oriented with convex articular surfaces and has limited movement. Rotation of the head produces a telescoping effect because these joint convex surfaces are not exactly reciprocal. The head spine motion is primarily between the axis and occipital condyles. There is potential instability, especially in children, because of laxity of the ligamentous tissue at the craniovertebral junction with extension, flexion, and rotation (6, 19). Hypermobility of the atlantooccipital joint may increase progressively in patients with congenital high cervical fusion, which may be the etiology of basilar invagination associated with the Klippel-Feil syndrome.

ETIOLOGY

The etiology of craniovertebral abnormalities is diverse and may be congenital, inflammatory, acquired, or traumatic in origin (Table 28.1). These etiologies may occur singularly or in combination resulting in neurological deficit from compression or ischemia at the cervicomedullary junction.

Dysgenesis of the odontoid process (os odontoideum and ossiculum terminale) is a congenital abnormality and is associated with displacement of the distal segment of the dens rostrally and/or instability of the atlantoaxial joint secondary to an incompetent cruciate ligament with compression at the cervicomedullary junction (20). Basilar invagination, when congenital, is often associated with atlantooccipital fusion. Five of the 16 patients with congenital basilar invagination had Down's syn-

TABLE 28.1

Etiology in 63 Patients with Craniocervical Junction Abnormalities

Odontoid dysgenesis	4
Basilar invagination	16
(Down's syndrome)	5
(Atlantooccipital fusion)	7
Abnormal condyles and occiput	7
(Achondroplasia)	1
Klippel-Feil syndrome	11
(Chiari malformation)	5
Fetal warfarin syndrome	1
Rickets	2
Osteomalacia	1
Rheumatoid arthritis	13
Postinfectious	1
Traumatic	7
(Unfused odontoid with upward migration)	2

drome. In those conditions associated with hypoplastic occipital condyles, there is a forward gliding of the skull in relation to the spine. This entity may be present in Morquio's disease, spondyloepiphyseal dysplasia, and Conradi's syndrome (4, 11, 19).

The acquired type of basilar invagination is frequently found in diseases such as osteogenesis imperfecta, osteomalacia, rickets, hyperparathyroidism, and Paget's disease. Eleven patients with cervicomedullary symptoms had the Klippel-Feil syndrome. Five had an associated Chiari malformation, and an associated anomaly which has been reported by several investigators (2, 11, 13, 15).

Rheumatoid arthritis with its associated osseo-ligamentous destruction may decrease the effective sagittal diameter of the foramen magnum and frequently is associated with instability. Atlantoaxial dislocation was the main cause of death in 8% and was contributory in 2% of patients in a consecutive series of 104 autopsies with rheumatoid arthritis (12). This disease was a common cause of basilar invagination in our series, and it accounted for 20% of patients undergoing surgical treatment for cervicomedullary compression. A single patient, age 5, had atlantooccipital subluxation associated with a nasopharyngeal infection. This entity has been reported exclusively in children (7, 9, 16).

Posttraumatic invagination of the unfused odontoid process into the posterior fossa occurred in two patients resulting in ventral cervicomedullary compromise. These congenital and acquired bone or ligamentous tissue defects may be associated with excessive motion and may become symptomatic following trauma.

SIGNS AND SYMPTOMS

The symptoms and signs of cervicomedullary pathology may present as myelopathy, brain stem, cranial and cervical nerve dysfunction, and/or vascular insufficiency. With one exception, all patients had evidence of myelopathy. The extent of motor deficit was variable, ranging between mild weakness and quadriplegia.

Motor and sensory abnormalities were often falsely localized. Myelopathy mimicking the "central cord" syndrome was common in patients with basilar invagination, probably secondary to the spinal cord gray matter vulnerability to compressive anoxic changes. The motor myelopathy has been attributed to repetitive trauma of pyramidal tracts secondary to compression, and the false localizing signs have been attributed to venous stasis of the cervical spinal cord (17).

Brain stem signs included downbeat nystagmus in 4 patients. This finding has been documented with caudal medullary pathology (3). Lateral nystagmus was a less common finding. Respiratory arrest occurred in two patients and sleep apnea in one. Respiratory signs occurred with both anterior and posterior cervicomedullary compression and reversed in each patient after decompression. Abnormal cranial nerve symptoms included in the trigeminal, glossopharyngeal, vagus, and accessory nerves, with no patient having hypoglossal nerve dysfunction. Tinnitus and/or decreased hearing was present in 22% of the patients, although this was an uncommon complaint. Cervical nerve symptoms, often associated with rheumatoid arthritis, were manifest by suboccipital headaches secondary to irritation of the second cervical nerve as it coursed through the atlantoaxial joint capsule.

Vascular symptoms included syncope, vertigo, altered level of consciousness, and transient visual field loss. These symptoms are attributed to intermittent compromise of the vertebral and anterior spinal arteries. This may occur from excessive mobility of an unstable atlantoaxial joint or with an abnormally placed atlas ring, resulting in excessive stretching or angulation of these vessels. Although 9 patients had vascular symptoms, only two patients demonstrated vertebral flow compromise at the atlantooccipital junction by means of angiography.

INVESTIGATIVE PROCEDURES

The diagnosis of craniovertebral junction abnormalities is made using roentgenographic studies. The two most important reference lines that can be evaluated by plain roentgenograms are Chamberlain's line and Wackenheim's clivus canal line (Fig. 28.3). Chamberlain's line is defined as a straight line drawn from the hard palate to the posterior margin of the foramen magnum. No greater than one-third of the odontoid process should be above this line. Wackenheim's clivus canal line is a basilar line drawn along the posterior surface of the clivus. The dens should lay anterior and caudal to the line, and any intersection of this tangent by the odontoid process is pathological. Other references include Fishgold's digastric line, which is a tangent connecting the digastric grooves. This line is 11 ± 4 mm above the atlantooccipital junction and is the upper limit of the odontoid tip. McRae's line is a line between the anterior posterior margin of the foramen magnum, which has an average sagittal diameter of 35 mm. In the Towne projection, the transverse diameter of the foramen magnum measures 35 ± 4 mm.

Gas or metrizamide myelography is usually combined with pleuridirectional tomography to demonstrate the site and nature of the pathology at the cervicomedullary junction. These studies will demonstrate the site and type of compression at the craniovertebral junction, will outline the brain stem, spinal cord, and subarachnoid space, and may demonstrate associated hydromyelia by the "collapsing" cord sign. The air myelogram lateral polytome in Figure 28.4 demonstrates basilar invagination. The tip of the odontoid process lies posterior to Wackenheim's clivus canal

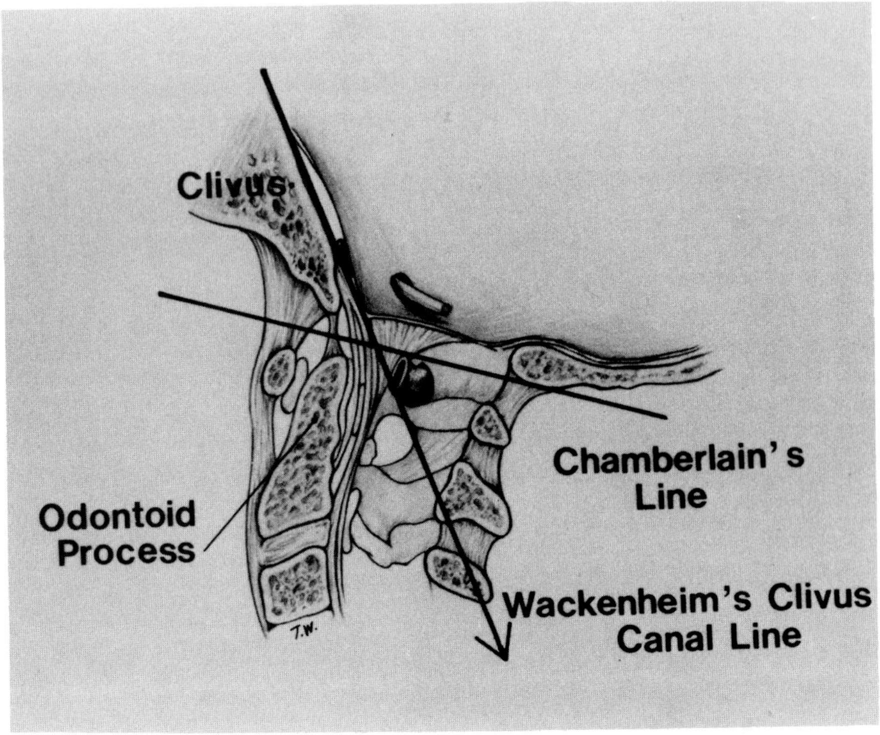

FIG. 28.3. Radiologic reference lines for the craniovertebral junction.

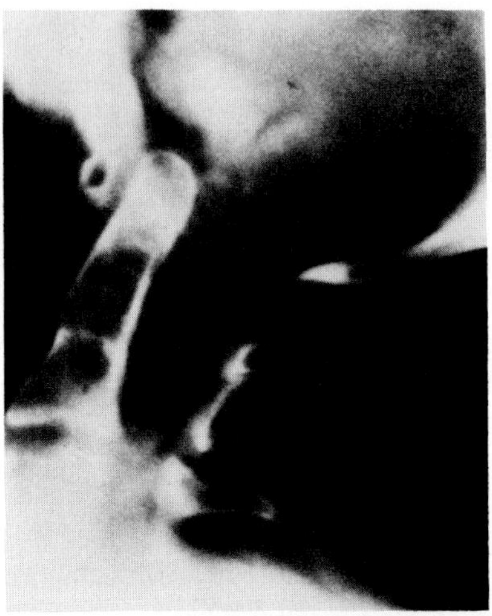

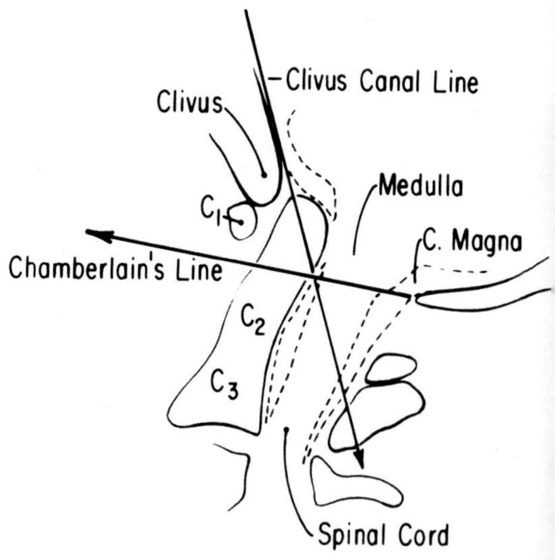

FIG. 28.4. Lateral polytome air myelogram of basilar invagination (*left*). Corresponding line drawing (*right*).

line, and greater than one-third of the odontoid process is above Chamberlain's line. There is ventral compression of the medulla by the dens with oblitaration of the subarachnoid space.

The lateral midline tomogram using Amipaque (metrizamide) contrast myelography in Figure 28.5 demonstrates posterior compression of the rostral spinal cord. The subarachnoid space is obliterated posteriorly by the atlas. The maximum sagittal diameter of the upper cervical canal and the foramen magnum should increase in a gradual arc in the caudal-rostral direction.

Radiological diagnostic studies of the craniovertebral junction should include flexion extension lateral polytomes in order to study the dynamic pathological process. This technique will determine the stability and/or reducibility of compressive pathology. Figure 28.6 is a lateral tomogram in a patient with juvenile rheumatoid arthritis and ossiculum terminale, using metrizamide myelography. There is both anterior and posterior cervicomedullary compression in flexion. When the head is extended, the ventral compromise is reduced, and only posterior compression is present (Figure 28.7).

Vertebral angiography was done in 9 patients who had ischemic symptoms. Only two patients demonstrated vertebral artery vascular compromise at the craniovertebral junction. Angiography also has been helpful in confirming tonsillar herniation in the Chiari malformation.

Computerized axial tomograms in the horizontal and sagittal reconstructions have been used to identify bony abnormalities as well as the position of neural structures in relation to bone and soft tissue. This axial CT scan in a patient with basilar invagination demonstrates the

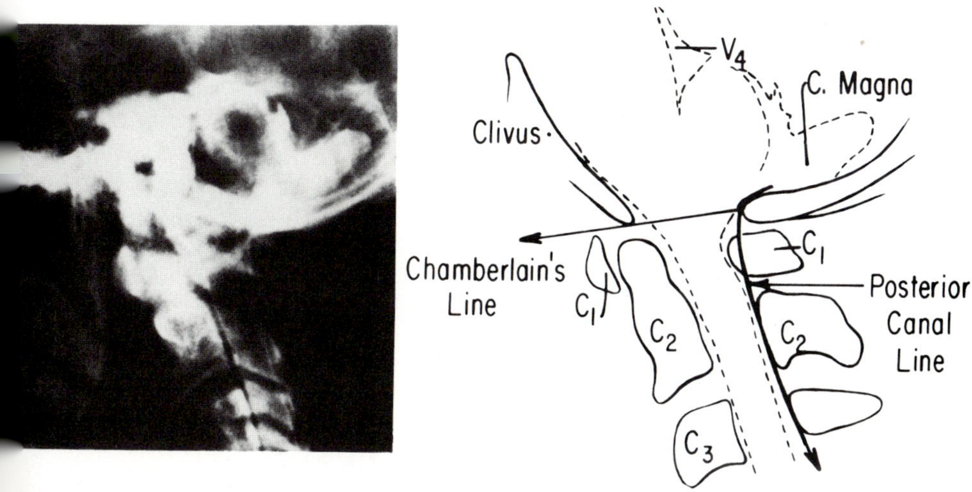

FIG. 28.5. Lateral midline polytome metrizamide myelogram (*left*). Corresponding line drawing (*right*).

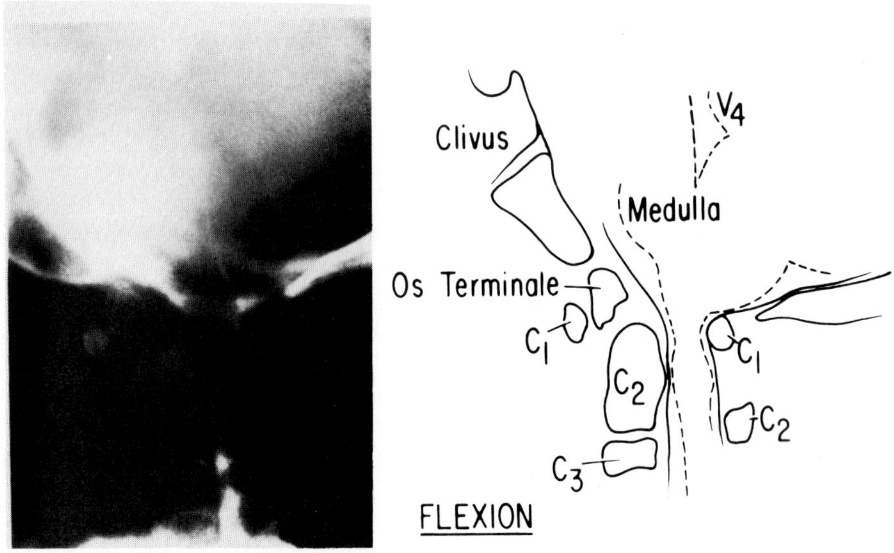

OSSICULUM TERMINALE

FIG. 28.6. Midline tomogram in flexion illustrating anterior and posterior compression (*left*) with a corresponding line drawing (*right*).

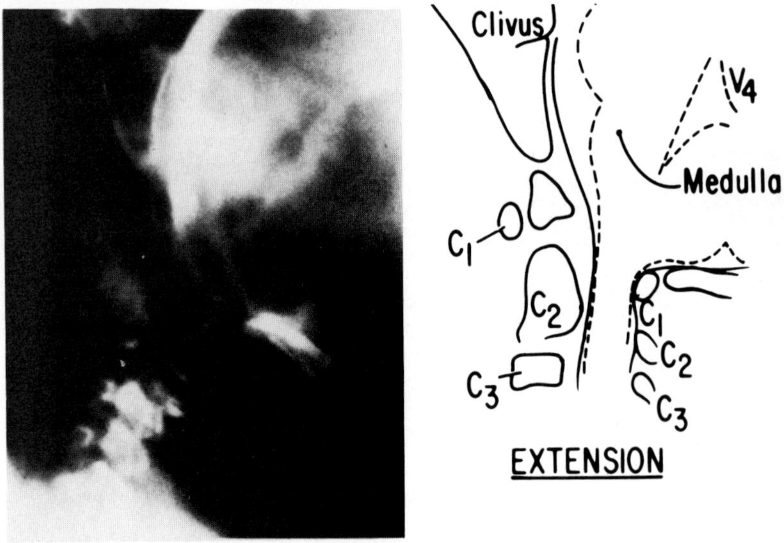

OSSICULUM TERMINALE

FIG. 28.7. Midline tomogram in extension illustrating posterior compression only (*left*) with a corresponding line drawing (*right*).

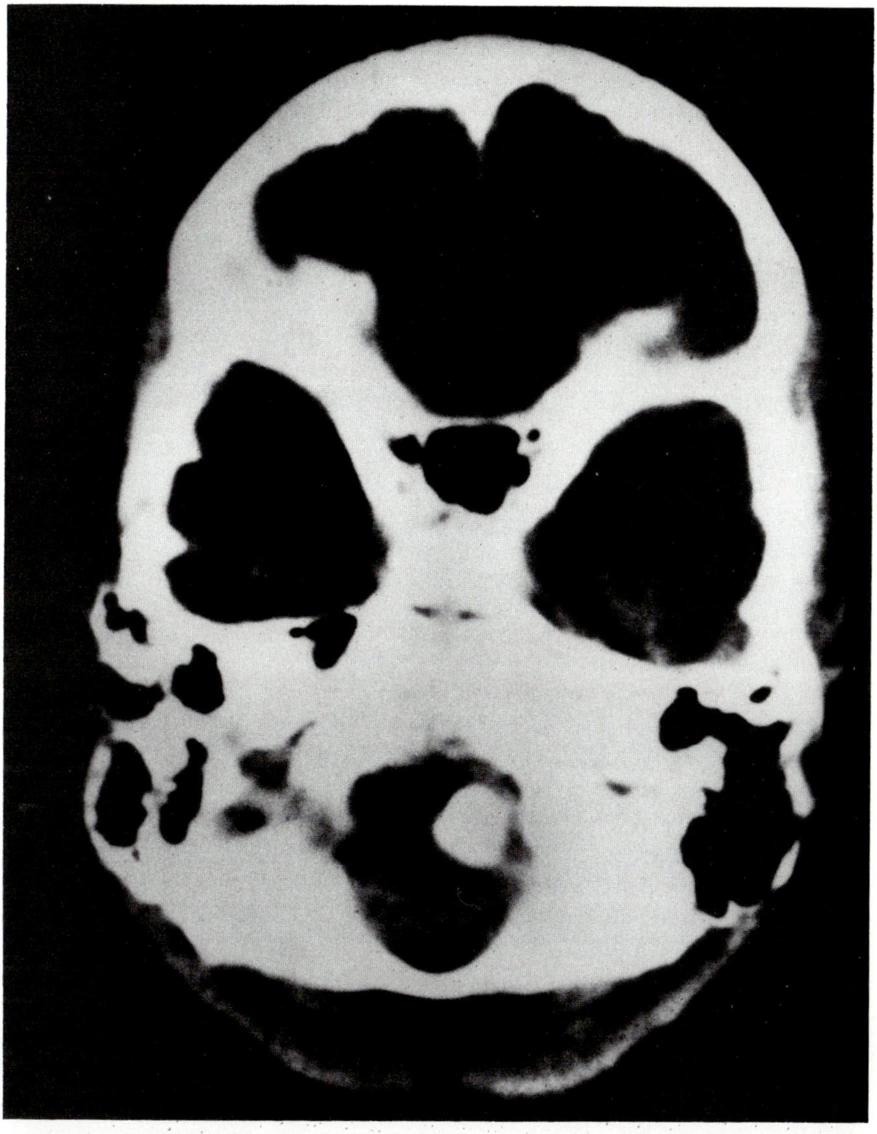

FIG. 28.8. Base CT scan without contrast demonstrating dens invagination into foramen magnum.

dens protruding ventrally through the foramen magnum eccentrically to the left (Fig. 28.8).

TREATMENT

The treatment of craniovertebral junction abnormalities can be divided into those patients whose spinal-cranial deformity can be realigned and require only stabilization, and those whose deformity cannot be realigned and thus require decompression (Table 28.2). Detailed descriptions of our operative technique have been published previously (18).

In those patients who can be reduced with craniovertebral junction instability secondary to inflammatory disease, halo brace immobilization is initially attempted. A 5-year-old child was admitted 2 weeks after a severe nasopharyngeal infection with signs of increased muscle tone and progressive arm weakness. Polytomes of the craniovertebral junction demonstrated invagination of the dens into the foramen magnum, implying ligamentous instability (Fig. 28.9). Following traction, a lateral tomogram shows reduction of the invagination and a normal dens-clivus alignment (Fig. 28.9). She was immobilized in a halo cast for 4 months and 5 months after discontinuing immobilization; the lateral tomogram

TABLE 28.2
Craniocervical Junction Abnormalities

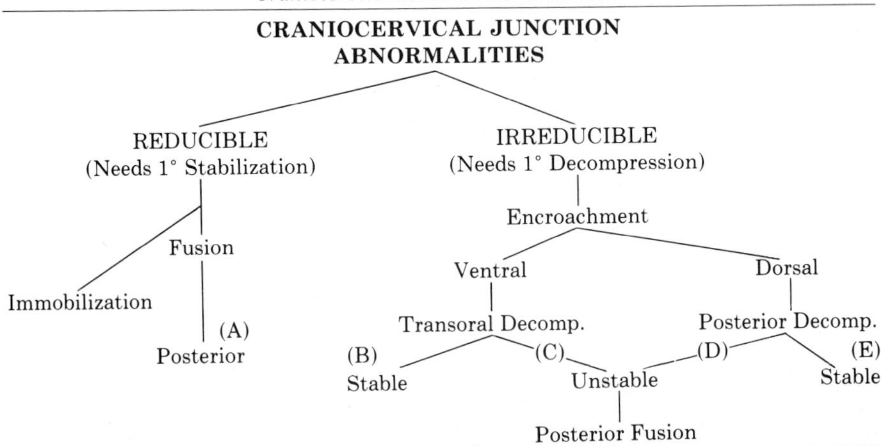

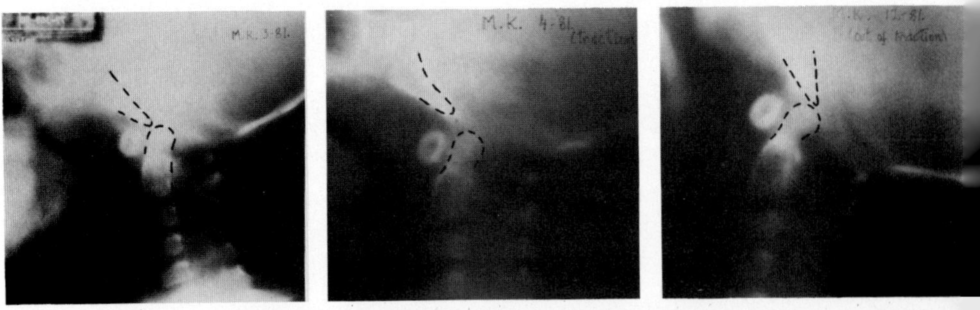

FIG. 28.9. Lateral tomograms illustrating basilar invagination pretraction (*left*), after traction (*middle*), and 5 months after removal of the halo brace (*right*).

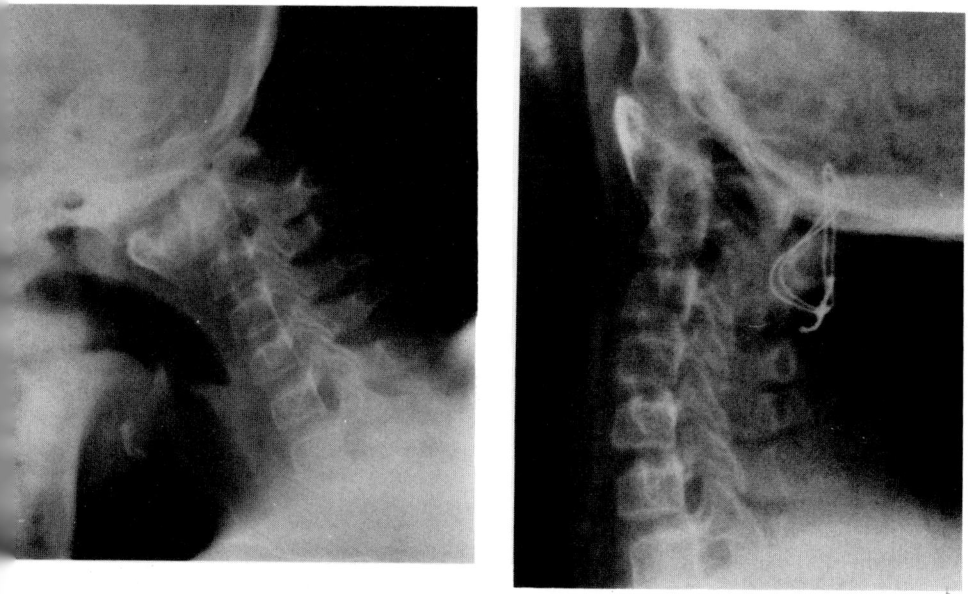

FIG. 28.10. (*Left*) Preoperative lateral roentgenogram showing craniovertebral junction compression. (*Right*) After reduction and posterior occiput-C_2 fusion.

shows normal alignment and no instability at the craniovertebral junction (Fig. 28.9). Her neurological deficit cleared in 2 weeks following treatment, and she has remained asymptomatic.

In those patients with unstable reducible lesions, a posterior bony fusion is necessary. The fusion extends from C_1-C_3 when reducible atlantoaxial instability is present and from the occiput to C_2 for occipitoaxial instability. Twisted No. 24 wire is placed under the lamina and through holes placed in the squamooccipital bone to anchor the grafts. An example of this technique is a 12-year-old child with Down's syndrome and rheumatoid disease who developed quadriparesis with occipitoatlantoaxial instability (Fig. 28.10).

Realignment was successful with cervical traction in extension, and the child was fused posteriorly, followed by full neurological recovery (Fig. 28.10). She was immobilized for 9 months in a halo cast. Lateral flexion-extension roentgenograms 1 year later demonstrated spontaneous anterior fusion between the clivus, the anterior arch of the atlas, and the odontoid process as well as posterior fusion (Fig. 28.11).

The ventral transoral transpalatine operation to the clivus atlantoaxial region is used in patients with irreducible ventral encroachment. Skeletal traction between 5 and 7 lbs is applied, and tracheostomy is performed prior to transoral odontoidectomy to permit adequate airway and opera-

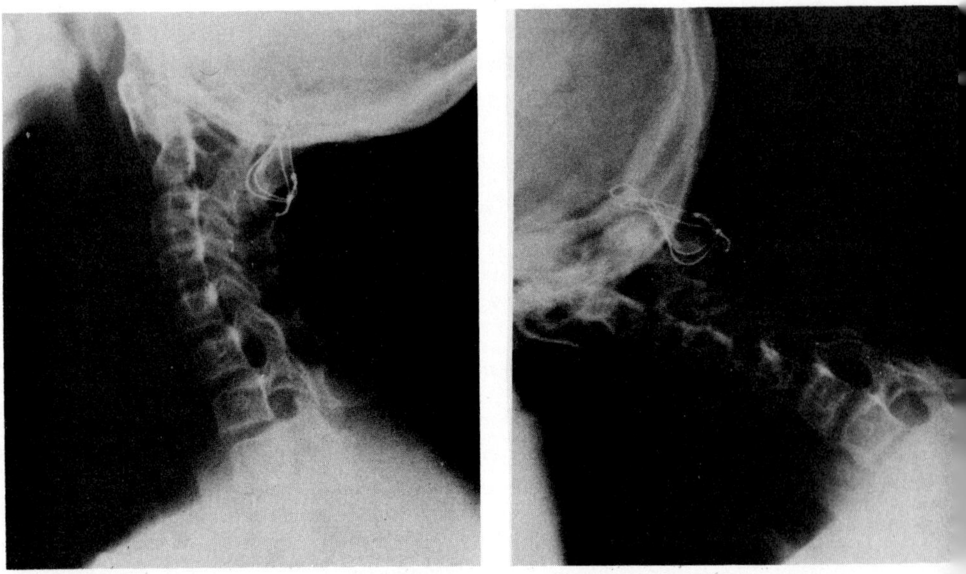

FIG. 28.11. One-year postfusion extension (*left*) and flexion (*right*). Roentgenograms showing posterior fusion and spontaneous anterior fusion.

tive exposure. A spft palate midline incision is made from the hard palate, diverting to one side at the base of the uvula. This incision exposes the pharynx rostral to the clivus, and the operating microscope is used throughout the operation for illumination and magnification. A linear midline incision in the posterior pharyngeal wall will expose the caudal clivus, anterior arch of C_1, and body of C_2. Soft tissue retraction is maintained with stay sutures.

The anterior arch of the atlas and adjacent clivus is resected with rongeurs and diamond drill. Removal of granulation tissue anterior to the dens exposes the odontoid process, and the odontoid tip is identified prior to resection of the dens. Removal of the odontoid process is then done in a rostral-caudal direction, using a high speed diamond tip burr and small Smith-Lee rongeurs. In entities like rheumatoid arthritis and chronic dislocation, there is usually hypertrophic tissue dorsal to the odontoid process. It is necessary to remove this tissue in order to achieve complete decompression of neural elements. The soft tissue closure is done in layers with absorbable sutures. Seven to 10 days after surgery, flexion-extension polytomes are obtained to determine stability. If instability is present, a posterior fusion is necessary. Illustrated in Figure 28.12 is a lateral polytomogram preoperative and postoperative following odontoid resection for basilar invagination.

In those patients with dorsal compression and no instability, a standard

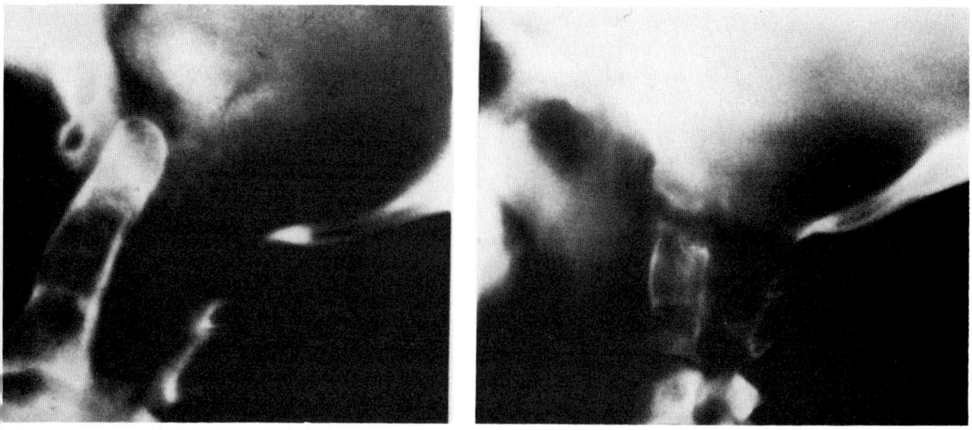

FIG. 28.12. (*Left*) Preoperative lateral polytomes illustrating basilar invagination. (*Right*) After dens resection. Note the C_2-C_3 ventral congenital fusion.

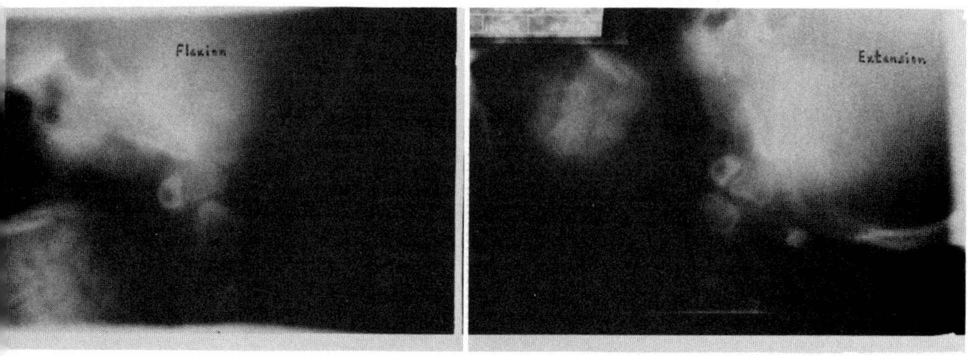

FIG. 28.13. Lateral midline polytome in flexion (*left*) and in extension (*right*).

laminectomy and/or resection of the posterior rim of the foramen magnum is done. It is important to excise all compressive soft tissue, with particular attention to contstricting dural and arachnoid bands. These bands are frequently present in the Chiari malformation, and opening the dura with insertion of a dural graft is often necessary.

If instability is present associated with posterior decompression, a lateral interfacet fusion is done. Twisted No. 24 or No. 26 wire is passed through holes made in the inferior facets in the involved cervical vertebrae and the occipital bone if needed for fixation of the donor grafts. The donor graft is obtained from either iliac crest or rib. Figure 28.13 demonstrates occipitoatlantoaxial instability secondary to os odontoideum in a 14-year-old male with quadriparesis and a central cord syndrome. Flexion-extension midline polytomes demonstrated both ventral and

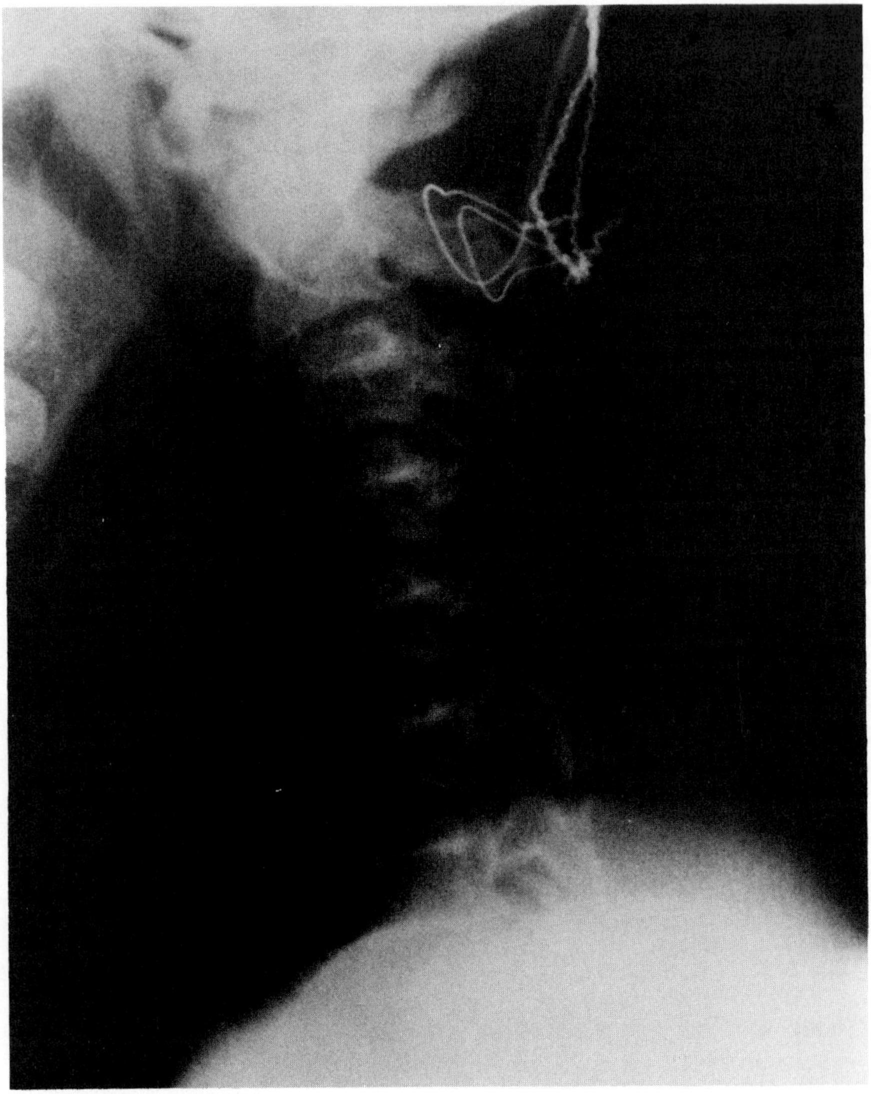

FIG. 28.14. Lateral postoperative roentgenogram after C_1 laminectomy illustrating occiput to C_2 lateral fusion.

dorsal compression of the craniovertebral junction by the unfused odontoid segment and the posterior arch of the atlas. In the neutral position there was only dorsal compression. A posterior decompression of the foramen magnum and C_1 was followed by a posterior lateral fusion of the occiput to C_2 with complete resolution of symptoms (Fig. 28.14).

The incidence and type of procedure in our series of 63 consecutive patients with symptomatic craniovertebral junction abnormalities is outlined in Table 28.3. Sixty-one of the patients recovered or are improved neurologically after surgery.

COMPLICATIONS

A 66-year-old female presenting with a rapidly progressive quadriparesis and respiratory arrest was the only fatality in this series. The patient had basilar invagination, and the odontoid was removed by the transoral operation. A posterior C_1-C_3 fusion was done 10 days later because of instability. The patient was ambulatory after surgery, but died from sepsis secondary to a urinary tract infection.

One patient developed a cerebrospinal fluid fistula following a ventral transoral operation. This required a second operation in which a fascial graft was used to seal the fistula without complications.

One patient with spondyloepiphyseal dysplasia associated with ossiculum terminale had posterior decompression with occipital-C_2 fusion. She had resorption of the bone graft, and a second operation was required because of fusion failure.

An 11-year-old male with basilar invagination associated with the Klippel-Feil deformity underwent anterior odontoidectomy with complete resolution of his neurological symptomatology. Fifteen months postoperatively he developed a left hemiparesis, and there was instability of the atlantooccipital joint. A posterior occiput-C_2 fusion was followed with resolution of his neurological symptoms.

TABLE 28.3
Operative Treatment 63 Patients

Stability	Compression	Operative Approach	Postoperative Stability	Posterior Fusion
Reducible 15[a]				14
Nonreducible	Ventral 18	Anterior	Stable 11	
			Unstable 7	7
	Dorsal 30	Posterior	Stable 12	
			Unstable 18	18

[a] One patient required halo brace immobilization only.

REFERENCES

1. Alexander, E., Jr., Forsyth, H. F., Davis, C. H., Jr., *et al.* Dislocation of the atlas on the axis. J. Neurosurg., *15:* 353–371, 1958.
2. Bharucha, E. P., and Dastur, H. M. Craniovertebral anomalies. A report on 40 cases. Brain, *87:* 469–480, 1964.
3. Cogan, D. G., and Barrows, L. J. Platybasia and Arnold-Chiari malformation. Arch. Ophthalmol., *52:* 13–29, 1954.
4. Dolan, K. D. Cervicobasilar relationships. *Radiol. Clin. North Am., 15*(2): 155–166, 1977.
5. Ganguly, D. N., and Roy, K. K. A study on the cranio-vertebral joint in the man. Anat. Anz., *114:* 433–452, 1964.
6. Gilles, R. H., Bina, M., and Sotrel, A. Infantile atlanto-occipital instability. The potential danger of extreme extension. Am. J. Dis. Child., *133:* 30–37, 1979.
7. Hess, J. H., Bronstein, I. P., and Abelson, S. M. Atlanto-axial dislocations. Unassociated with trauma and secondary to inflammatory foci in the neck. Am. J. Dis. Child., *49:* 1137–1147, 1935.
8. Kopits, S. E., Perovic, M. N., McKusick, V., *et al.* Congenital atlantoaxial dislocations in various forms of dwarfism. J. Bone Joint Surg. (Am.), *54:* 1349–1350, 1972.
9. Lippmann, R. K. Arthropathy due to adjacent inflammation. J. Bone Joint Surg. (Am.), *35:* 967–979, 1953.
10. Menezes, A. H., Graf, C. J., and Hibri, N. Abnormalities of the cranio-vertebral junction with cervicomedullary compression. Child's Brain, *7:* 15–30, 1980.
11. Menezes, A. H., VanGilder, J. C., Graf, C. J., *et al.* Craniocervical abnormalities. A comprehensive surgical approach. J. Neurosurg., *53:* 444–455, 1980.
12. Mikulowski, P., Wollheim, F. A., Rotmil, P., *et al.* Sudden death in rheumatoid arthritis with atlanto-axial dislocation. Acta Med. Scand., *198:* 445–451, 1975.
13. Saez, R. J., Onofrio, B. M., and Yanaghihara, T. Experience with Arnold-Chiari malformation, 1960–1970. J. Neurosurg., *45:* 416–422, 1976.
14. Shapiro, R., Youngberg, A. S., and Rothman, S. L. G. The differential diagnosis of traumatic lesions of the occipito-atlanto-axial segment. Radiol. Clin. North Am., *11*(3): 505–526, 1973.
15. Spillane, J. D., Pallis, C., and Jones, A. M. Developmental abnormalities in the region of the foramen magnum. Brain, *80:* 11–48, 1957.
16. Sullivan, A. W. Subluxation of the atlanto-axial joint: Sequel to inflammatory processes of the neck. J. Pediatr., *35:* 451–464, 1949.
17. Taylor, A. R., and Byrnes, D. P. Foramen magnum and high cervical cord compression. Brain, *97:* 473–480, 1974.
18. VanGilder, J. C., and Menezes, A. H. Craniovertebral abnormalities and their treatment. In: *Current Techniques in Operative Neurosurgery*, Ed. 2, Chap. 79, H. H. Schmidek and W. H. Sweet. New York, Grune & Stratton, 1982.
19. White, A. A., III, and Panjabi, M. M. The clinical biomechanics of the occipitoatlantoaxial complex. Orthop. Clin. North Am., *9:* 867–878, 1978.
20. Wollin, D. G. The os odontoideum. Separate odontoid process. J. Bone Joint Surg. (Am.), *45:* 1459–1471, 1963.

CHAPTER

29

Management of Syringomyelia: A Pathophysiological Approach

S. J. PEERLESS, M.D., F.R.C.S.(C), and
QUENTIN J. DURWARD, M.B., Ch.B.

INTRODUCTION

It is increasingly clear that syringomyelia can no longer be regarded as a single entity. From the surgeon's vantage point, the disorders commonly defined as syringomyelia are not a hopeless, chronic, relentlessly progressive, degenerative disorder. Destructive central cord cavitation and gliosis are common to all forms, often gradually resulting in pain, amyotrophy, dissociated anesthesia, paraparesis, scoliosis, and eventually the development of trophic lesions in the limbs. Nevertheless, the clinical presentation, pathogenesis, and most importantly rational therapy is necessarily diverse.

The management of syringomyelia remains controversial. Arising from the many conflicting theories postulated to explain its etiology, syringomyelia has been treated in the past by a variety of methods, including irradiation, decompressive laminectomy, myelotomy, syrinx drainage, and terminal ventriculostomy (6, 7, 9, 15, 20, 28, 31, 38, 41–43, 45). More recently, recognition of the frequent association of syringomyelia with developmental or acquired anomalies of the posterior fossa has led to the operation of foramen magnum decompression (FMD) with CSF diversion from a patent central canal. This "Gardner procedure" has been proposed as the primary and at times the only treatment for syringomyelia (4, 14, 18, 19, 30, 33, 46). However, efficacy of each of these diverse procedures has been variable, but well documented cases of patient improvement have been recorded following each of them. Even so, the failure of these procedures to halt deterioration or produce improvement in a significant proportion of cases is not uncommon (1, 6, 10, 15, 18, 30, 39, 43, 46).

Two major types of syringomyelia, communicating and noncommunicating, have been described (6, 8, 30, 47). In communicating syringomyelia, a direct communication of the syrinx with the ventricular system, usually via a patent central canal, is at least in part responsible for maintenance of the syrinx. A developmental or acquired anomaly of the posterior fossa and foramen magnum region may promote the persistence and expansion of the syrinx by directing the force of pulsatile CSF from the IVth ventricle into a patent central canal via the obex (6, 11, 12, 19, 29, 33). Using the same pathology, others have suggested a pressure differential between the intracranial and spinal compartments produced by the hindbrain malformation impacted into the foramen magnum and acting as a ball valve to promote the entry of CSF into the central canal by suction (48).

In noncommunicating syringomyelia, the posterior fossa and foramen magnum region are normal, and a direct communication of the syrinx with the ventricular system is not evident (6, 16, 23, 24, 27, 30, 34, 38, 44, 47). The pathogenesis of this type of syringomyelia is less clear, but the source of the fluid in the syrinx is probably from one of two sources. Fluid may enter the syrinx from the spinal subarachnoid space either via enlarged Virchow-Robin spaces communicating between the subarachnoid space and the syrinx (3, 13) or rarely by passing through macroscopic connections (32, 38). Furthermore, pulsations from the small arteries within the Virchow-Robin spaces and the transient increases in the pressure within the spinal subarachnoid space produced by a Valsalva maneuver may both act to direct fluid into the syrinx (45). This mechanism would account for the syrinx fluid to be similar if not identical with CSF in many cases of noncommunicating syringomyelia which are not secondary to a spinal cord tumor. The second possible mechanism of fluid entry into the syrinx in noncommunicating syringomyelia is secretion of fluid by glial cells lining the syrinx (6) or by a tumor.

A syrinx is associated with 25–58% of intramedullary spinal cord tumors (6, 36, 50). Secretion of fluid by the neoplastic cells is probably responsible for maintenance of the syrinx in most of these cases, although necrosis and cavitation within the tumor may also be factors.

Four varieties of noncommunicating syringomyelia may be identified. These include posttraumatic, those associated with spinal arachnoiditis and spinal cord tumor, and an idiopathic variety (6, 8, 43, 47). Because different mechanisms are responsible for the formation, maintenance, and expansion of the syrinx in noncommunicating and communicating syringomyelia, a different surgical approach is required for each. Our experience with the treatment of 90 patients with syringomyelia representing both the communicating and the 4 varieties of noncommunicating syringomyelia is reviewed.

PATIENT SELECTION

Ninety patients with syringomyelia have been surgically treated by the authors and their associates over the past 20 years (Table 29.1). Average follow-up has been 7 years.

TABLE 29.1
Etiology of Syringomyelia in 90 Cases

	No. of Cases	Total
Communicating		33
Arnold-Chiari malformation	28	
Foramen of Magendie cyst	2	
Basal arachnoiditis	1	
No cause	2	
Noncommunicating		
Nontumorous		44
Posttraumatic	28	
Idiopathic	9	
Spinal arachnoiditis	7	
Tumor		13

TABLE 29.2
Indication for Operation (154 Procedures)

	PND	Pain	Pain & PND	Other
Communicating	32	2	22	0
Posttraumatic	13	7	27	2
Idiopathic	5	0	14	0
Spinal arachnoiditis	5	0	5	0
Tumor	6	0	13	1
Total	61	9	81	3

[a] PND, progressive neurological deterioration.

Thirty-three patients had communicating syringomyelia. In 30 of these patients the presence of a patent central canal communicating with the IVth ventricle at the level of the obex was demonstrated radiologically or at operation. In the other 3 patients with communicating syringomyelia, a Chiari malformation was demonstrated myelographically, but it was treated by syrinx drainage (2 patients) and a ventriculoperitoneal shunt (1 patient) without exposure of the foramen magnum region.

In 31 instances of communicating syringomyelia, a Chiari malformation, basal arachnoiditis, or a foramen of Magendie cyst was identified. Two patients had communicating syringomyelia unassociated with any other posterior fossa abnormality, but a patent central canal communicating with the obex was confirmed at surgery. Thirteen patients had a syrinx associated with an intramedullary spinal cord tumor, and 28 had a posttraumatic syrinx. In 7 the syrinx was associated with spinal arachnoiditis, and 9 patients had the idiopathic variety with no discernible cause for the cavitation found. The indication for surgery in each case was progressive neurological deterioration caused by the syrinx, pain, or in the majority of patients both neurological deterioration and pain (Table 29.2). Patients were assessed as improved if their neurological examination was improved and they were pain-free or markedly improved following a procedure. If the patient had ceased deteriorating neurologically and the pain was less, he was considered stable. If no difference was made in the patient's neurological course or pain he was considered deteriorated.

Each patient had undergone complete myelography with visualization of the foramen magnum region to confirm or exclude congenital anomalies. Initially in our experience pantopaque and air myelography, supplemented frequently by direct puncture of the syrinx, were used to confirm the clinical diagnosis. Over the last 36 months, metrizamide myelography with delayed computerized tomographic (CT) imaging of the spinal canal to visualize the syrinx has been the standard initial radiological investigation (2, 17, 25, 26, 49). This technique is an important adjunct to the diagnosis of syringomyelia and deserves emphasis (Fig. 29.1). The purposes of this examination are: (a) to identify spinal cord enlargement, (b) to demonstrate the phenomenon of cord collapse, and (c) to image the uptake of the water-soluble contrast into the syrinx. Additionally the technique permits visualization of the spinomedullary junction for evidence of hind brain anomalies and the negative imaging of an intramedullary (usually neoplastic) mass. In 50 cases of syringomyelia thus studied (including 6 tumor-associated cases), the syrinx has been identified. In two cases of communicating syringomyelia, however, metrizamide myelography with delayed CT has failed to identify the syrinx, and additional

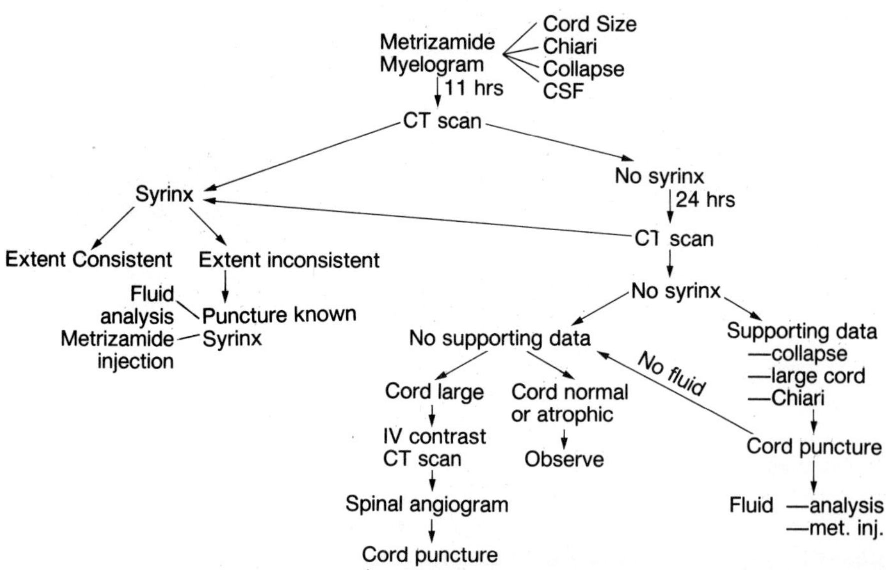

FIG. 29.1. Syringomyelia: Diagnostic Decision Tree.

studies were required. When the extent of the cord enlargement is greater than the extent of the syrinx seen on the delayed CT scan, we recommend direct puncture of the syrinx, fluid analysis for protein and cytology, and a Metrizamide injection into the syrinx to rule out the presence of tumor (see Fig. 29.9*D*). In approximately one half of the patients with syringomyelia who have been studied with metrizamide myelography, a reduction in cord diameter, or "collapse" of the cord when changing position from prone to supine, supine to erect, or erect to Trendelenburg can be seen and suggested the diagnosis in those instances where the syrinx is not imaged clearly on the delayed CT scan. This phenomenon of "cord collapse" has been seen in both communicating and noncommunicating syringomyelia (25). Confirmation of a tumor may also be obtained in some cases by enhancement of the tumor after intravenous infusion of contrast (26). Occasionally, angiography may be helpful to rule out the presence of a vascular tumor in the region before cord puncture is carried out.

SURGICAL PROCEDURES

One hundred and fifty-four surgical procedures have been performed in the 90 patients in this study (Table 29.3). Thirty-nine patients have required more than one procedure. Figure 29.2 summarizes the surgical procedures.

Foramen Magnum Decompression

Thirty-three procedures for foramen magnum decompression (FMD) were performed in 30 patients with communicating syringomyelia. One FMD procedure was performed in one patient with idiopathic syringomyelia. There have been 3 variations to this procedure performed in the 31 patients. Initially, FMD alone was advocated (Fig. 29.3*A* and *B*). Herniated cerebellar tissue is disimpacted from the foramen magnum region with decompression of the upper cervical cord and medulla. Lysis of adhesions and membranes, which occasionally may be dense, overlying the foramen of Magendie and impairing CSF outflow may be performed

TABLE 29.3

Operative Procedures Performed

	No. of Procedures
Foramen magnum decompression	34
Syrinx drainage	87
Tumor removal	17
Ventriculoperitoneal shunt	5
Decompressive laminectomy	7
Other	4
Total	154

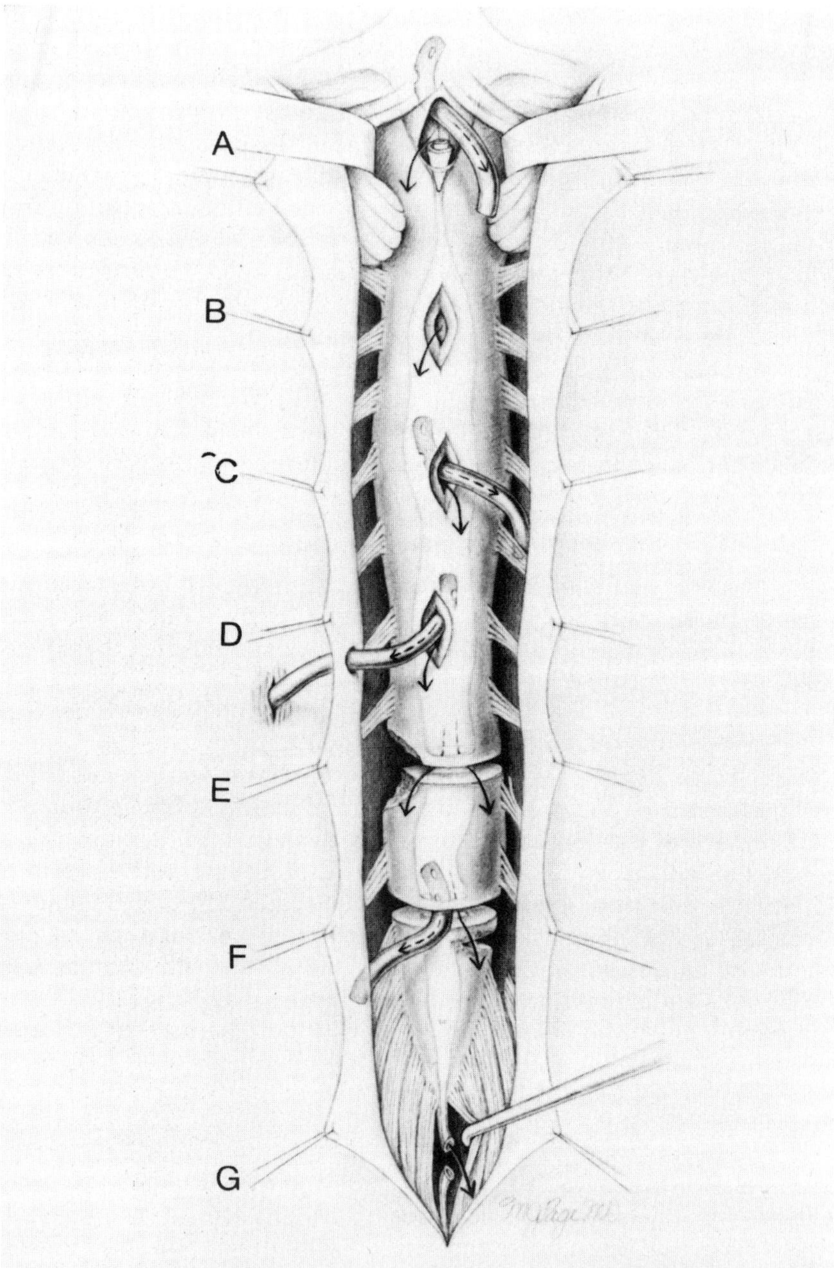

FIG. 29.2. Composite drawing summarizing the various surgical procedures. (*A*) FMD with drainage of IVth ventricle and plugging of central canal. (*B*) Myelotomy. (*C*) Syringosubarachnoid shunt. (*D*) Syringoperitoneal shunt. (*E*) Cordectomy. (*F*) Cordectomy with tube drainage. (*G*) Terminal ventriculostomy.

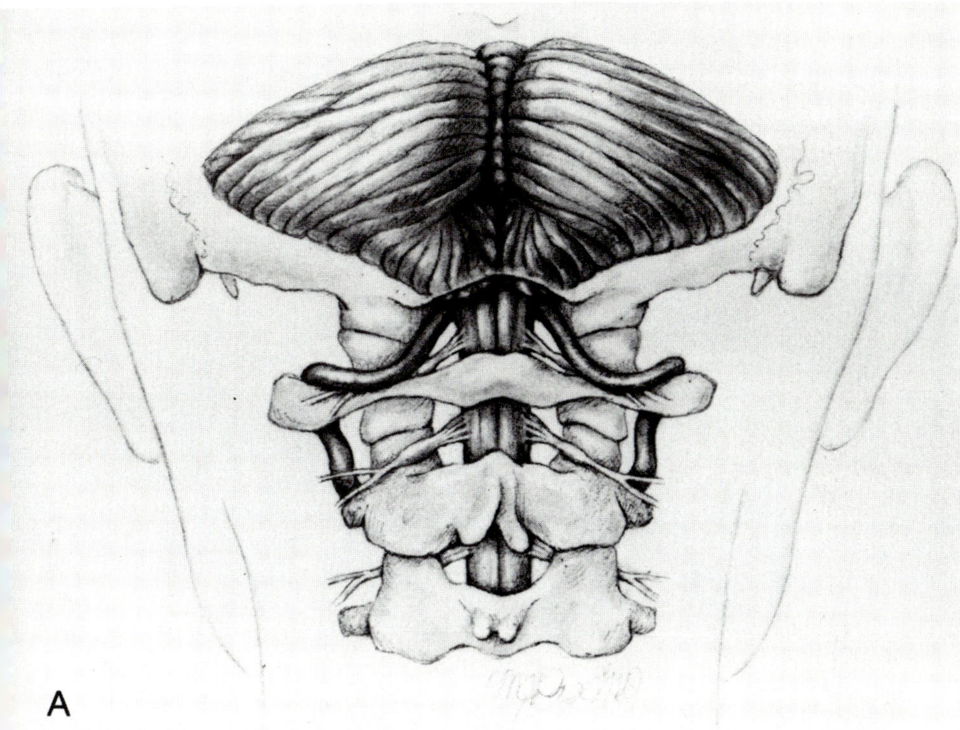

A

FIG. 29.3. (*A*) Normal anatomical relationships of the posterior fossa and spinomedullary junction. Note the cerebellar tonsils just reaching the foramen magnum and the downward and lateral course of the upper cervical roots.

to promote free CSF drainage from the IVth ventricle (Fig. 29.3*C*). Secondly, if an enlarged patent central canal communicating with the obex is encountered, it may be plugged with a cone-shaped Dacron or muscle plug. Finally, a combination of obex plug and tube drainage of CSF from the IVth ventricle can be performed (Fig. 29.3*D*). Magnification and microsurgical technique facilitates these manipulations. In most instances the authors believe post fossa duraplasty using Dacron or pericranium is of value to enlarge the volume of the posterior fossa (Fig. 29.3*E*). In this series, 10 patients have undergone foramen magnum decompression alone with or without tube drainage of CSF from the IVth ventricle into the subarachnoid space. Sixteen patients have undergone foramen magnum decompression and plugging of the obex with muscle or Dacron. Eight patients underwent both plugging of the obex and tube drainage of the IVth ventricle (Table 29.4). This latter procedure has been used only recently and consequently follow-up is shorter than for the other two types of procedure. Several details of the surgical technique

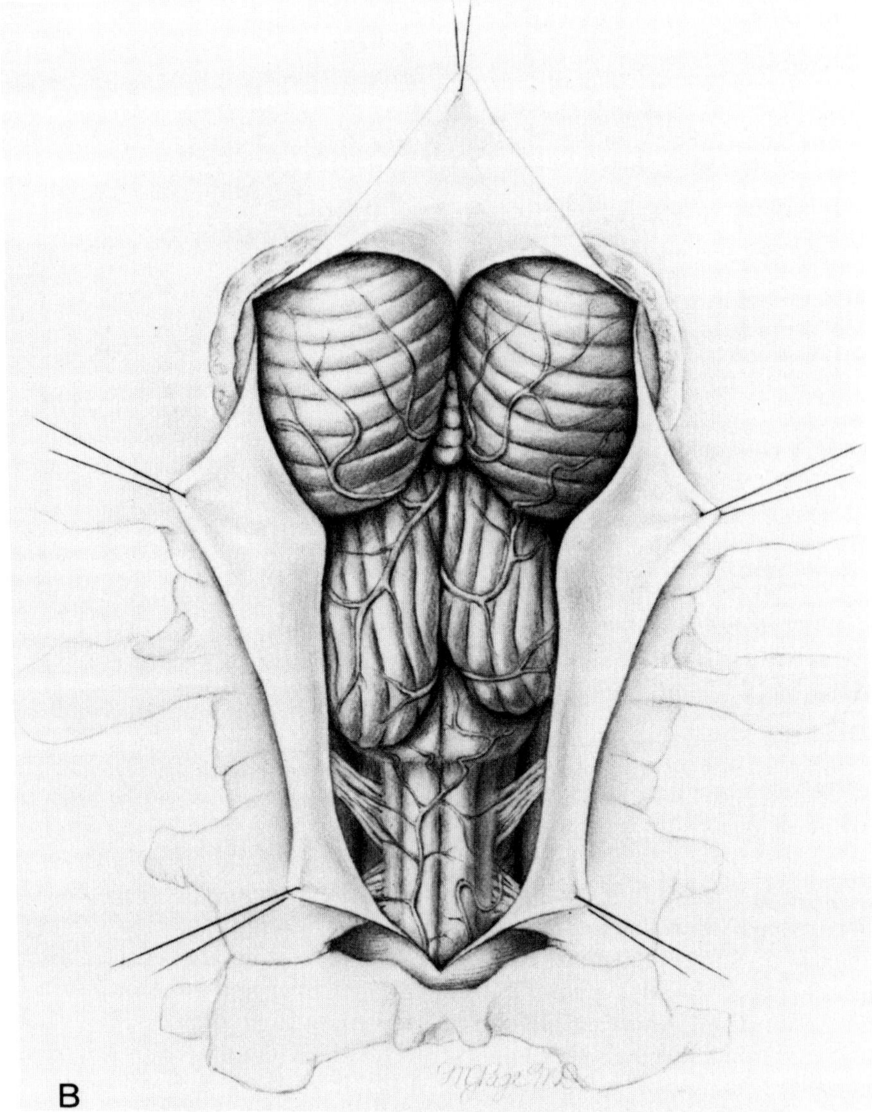

FIG. 29.3. (*B*) Chiari malformation commonly associated with communicating syringomyelia. Note hindbrain herniation into the upper spinal canal, upward and lateral course of roots, and elongated and often degenerated cerebellar tonsils.

deserve emphasis. On more than one occasion we have observed that the muscle plug has disappeared from the upper central canal either by absorption or by simply falling out. As a consequence we have turned to use a tiny cone of rolled Dacron inserted into the canal and fixed with a

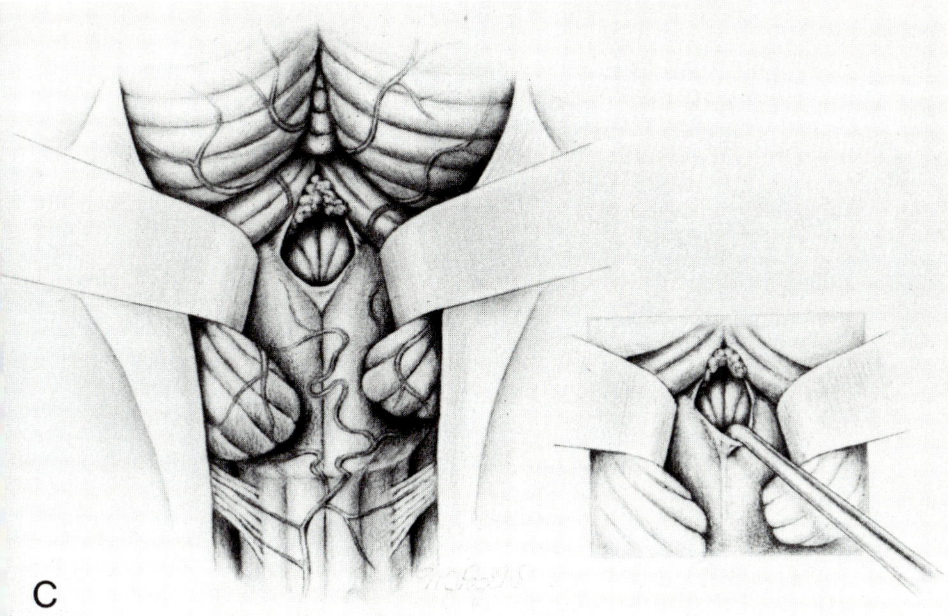

C

FIG. 29.3. (*C*) Cerebellar tonsils are separated after lysis of arachnoidal adhesions exposing caudally displaced IVth ventricle and distended cervicomedullary junction. (*Inset*) Probe in patent central canal deforming the obex.

minute drop of tissue adhesive. This alternative, we believe, is more secure and less likely to promote reactive scarring. Extensive surgical lysis of the often dense arachnoidal scar encountered is unnecessary and potentially hazardous by inadvertant damage to vital vascular structures and by promoting further scar. The ultimate purpose of these procedures is decompression of the spinal-medullary junction and the promotion of free drainage of CSF from the ventricular system into the basal cisterns and away from the syringomyelic cavity.

Syrinx Drainage

Eighty-seven syrinx drainage procedures were performed (Table 29.5). These included needle aspiration (7 operations), myelotomy with syringostomy (5 operations), placement of a syringosubarachnoid (32 operations) or syringoperitoneal (33 operations) drain using silastic or barium-impregnated shunt tubing, selective spinal cordectomy (5 operations), and terminal ventriculostomy (5 operations). Syringoperitoneal shunts are now the most frequent drainage procedures performed. The drain should be placed in the lower most extent of the syrinx. Multiple entrance holes are placed in the tubing which is anchored to the arachnoid and/

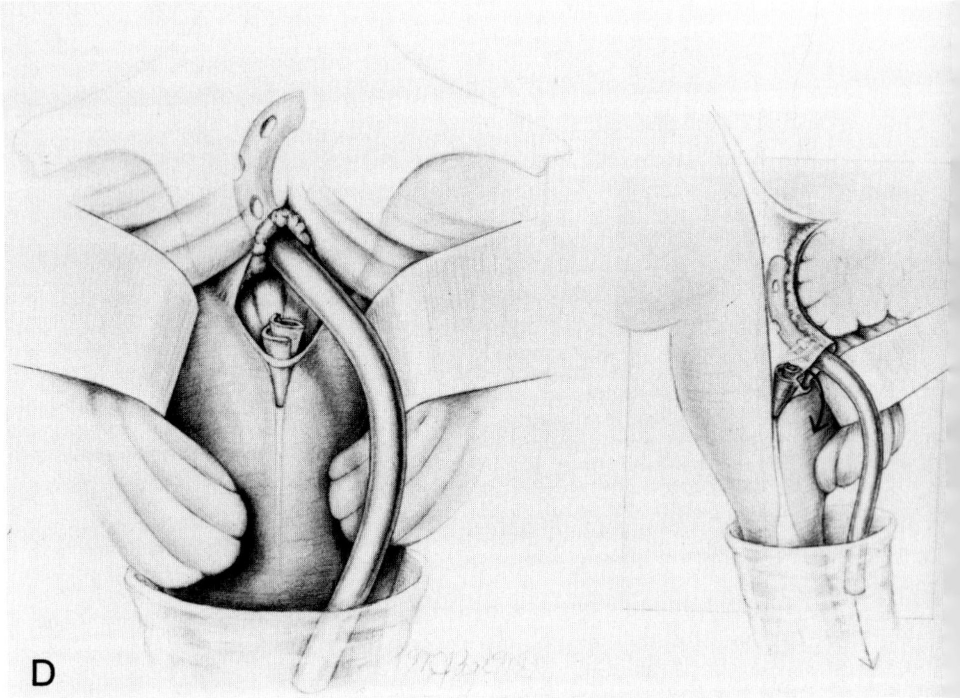

D

FIG. 29.3. (*D*) Final microsurgical exposure showing rolled cone of Dacron felt plugging communication between central canal and IVth ventricle, with silastic tubing providing free drainage between IVth ventricle and upper cervical subarachnoid space. (*Inset*) Stylized lateral view to emphasize fluid flow around as well as through the tubing.

or pia mater by fine sutures. With the syringosubarachnoid drain, great care must be taken not to place the subarachnoid end into the subdural space, but clearly beneath a well defined layer of arachnoid. Selective spinal cordectomy at or just above the area of spinal cord trauma has been used in 5 cases of complete spinal cord injury with posttraumatic syringomyelia. A tube is usually placed into the syrinx to maintain patency of the drain. Drainage via terminal ventriculostomy or division of the filum terminale is indicated when the syrinx is demonstrated to extend into the conus medullaris. Needle aspiration and myelotomy without tube drainage only transiently decompress the cavity and are no longer performed.

Syrinx drainage has been the primary treatment employed for noncommunicating nontumorous syringomyelia. However, 12 of the patients with communicating syringomyelia have also undergone a syrinx drainage procedure. In 10 of these patients the drainage procedure was in addition

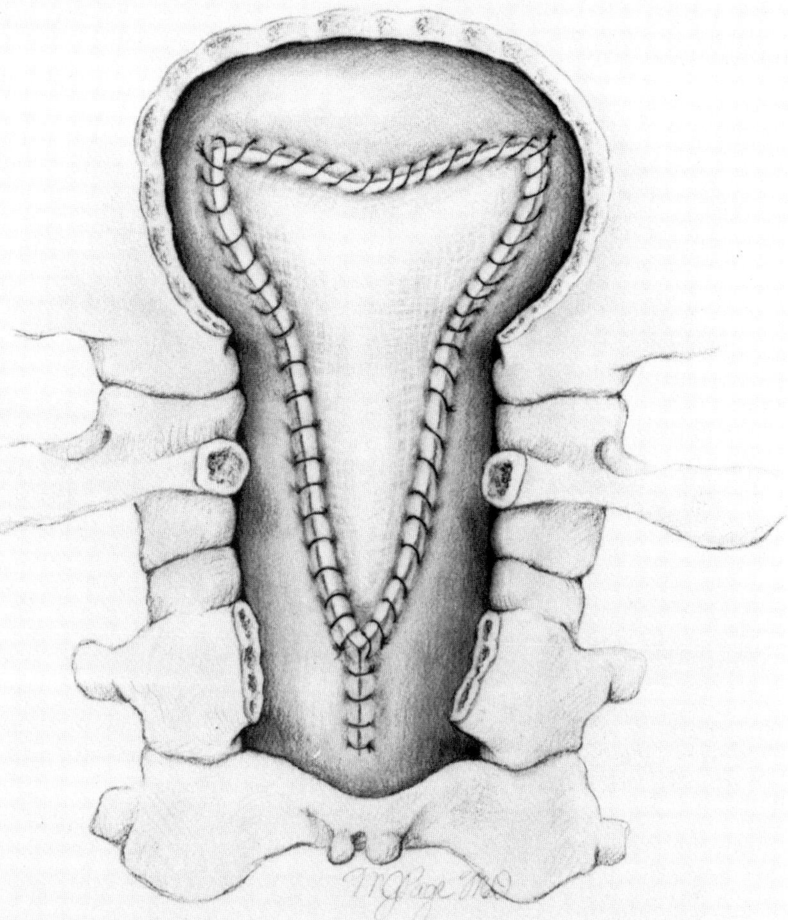

E

FIG. 29.3. (*E*) Duroplasty to enlarge volume of posterior fossa.

TABLE 29.4

Results of 34 Foramen Magnum Decompression (FMD) Procedures in 31 Patients

	No. of Procedures	Improved	Stable	Deteriorated
FMD	10	3 (0)	5 (5)	2 (5)
FMD + obex plug	16	10 (4)	4 (2)	2 (10)
FMD + obex plug + IV ventricle drain	8	8 (8)	0 (0)	0 (0)
Total	34	21 (12)	9 (7)	4 (15)

TABLE 29.5

Results of 87 Syrinx Drainage Procedures in 60 Patients

Syringosubarachnoid drain	32	20 (12)	4 (4)	8 (16)
Syringoperitoneal drain	33	20 (13)	8 (8)	5 (12)
Spinal cordectomy	5	3 (2)	1 (1)	1 (2)
Needle aspiration	7	4 (1)	1 (0)	2 (6)
Myelotomy and syringostomy	5	1 (1)	2 (0)	2 (4)
Terminal ventriculostomy	5	3 (3)	1 (1)	1 (1)
Total	87	51 (32)	17 (14)	19 (41)

to foramen magnum decompression when the latter procedure failed to halt the progression of the clinical picture.

Spinal Cord Tumor Removal

Seventeen procedures for spinal cord tumor removal have been performed in the 13 patients with syringomyelia associated with a spinal cord tumor. Drainage of the syrinx into the subarachnoid space was also carried out in 11 of these cases.

Other

One patient with a proven cervical syrinx, but with significant cord compression from a sequestrated cervical disc has undergone only laminectomy and discectomy with no further progression of his cord syndrome. Five patients have undergone a ventriculoperitoneal shunt and 7 a decompressive laminectomy. There were 2 procedures for drainage of an extramedullary arachnoid cyst in one patient, and one early patient underwent drainage of the syrinx via a tube into the IVth ventricle.

Several cases are presented as examples of the various clinical entities to illustrate not only triumphs, but some of the pitfalls of diagnosis and surgical management.

CASE REPORTS

Case 1 (Communicating, Chiari Malformation). This 33-year-old fireman presented with a 3-year history of progressive gait difficulty. Physical examination demonstrated a spastic paraparesis involving his left leg more than his right and early wasting and areflexia in his left arm. The only sensory change was a small patch of diminished pin appreciation over his left shoulder. Metrizamide myelography (Fig. 29.4*A*) demonstrated a wide cord from the foramen magnum to the conus, with collapse of the cervical cord when turned supine from the prone position. Views of the foramen magnum region showed the cerebellar tonsils at the level of C_1. 11-hour delayed CT scan showed a central "bull's eye" within the cord (Fig. 29.4*B*). This classic example of com-

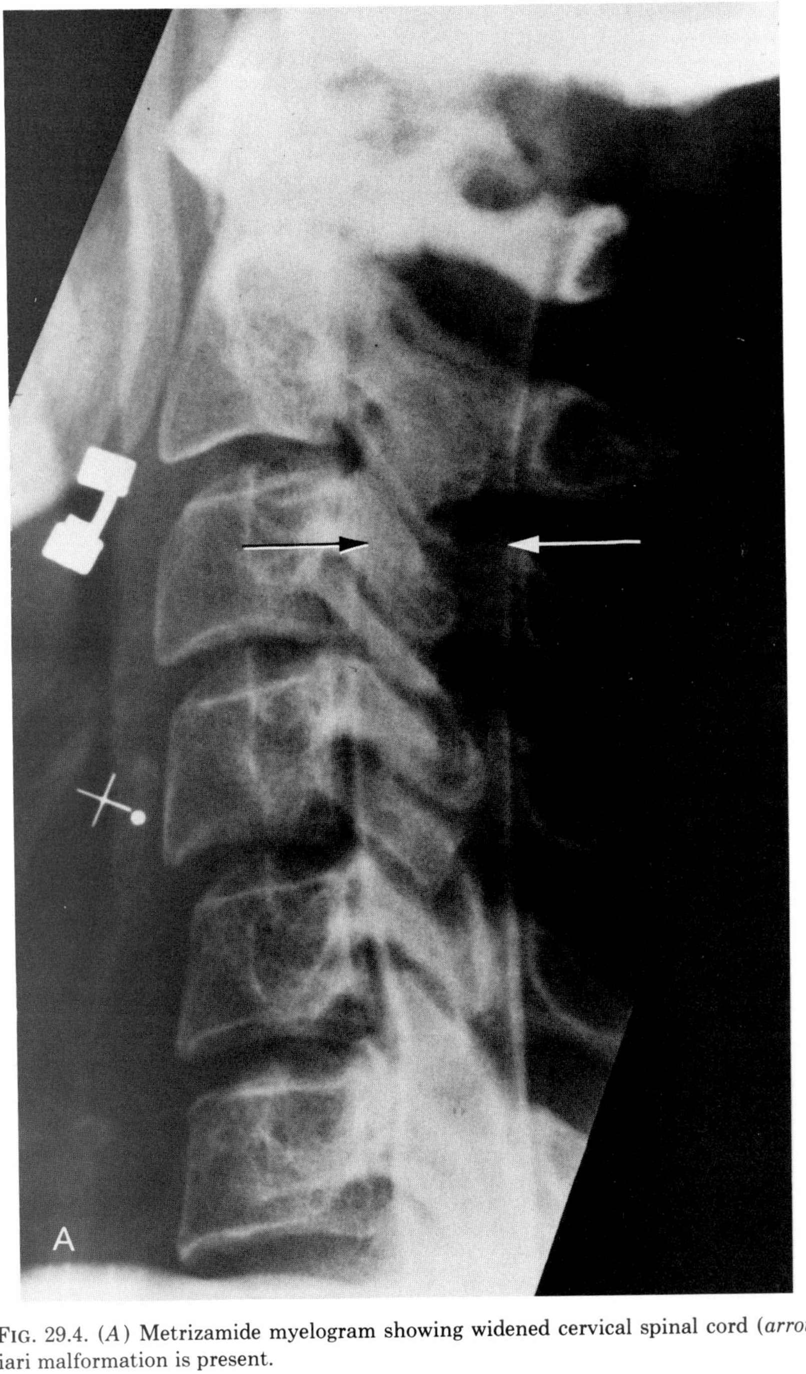

FIG. 29.4. (*A*) Metrizamide myelogram showing widened cervical spinal cord (*arrows*). Chiari malformation is present.

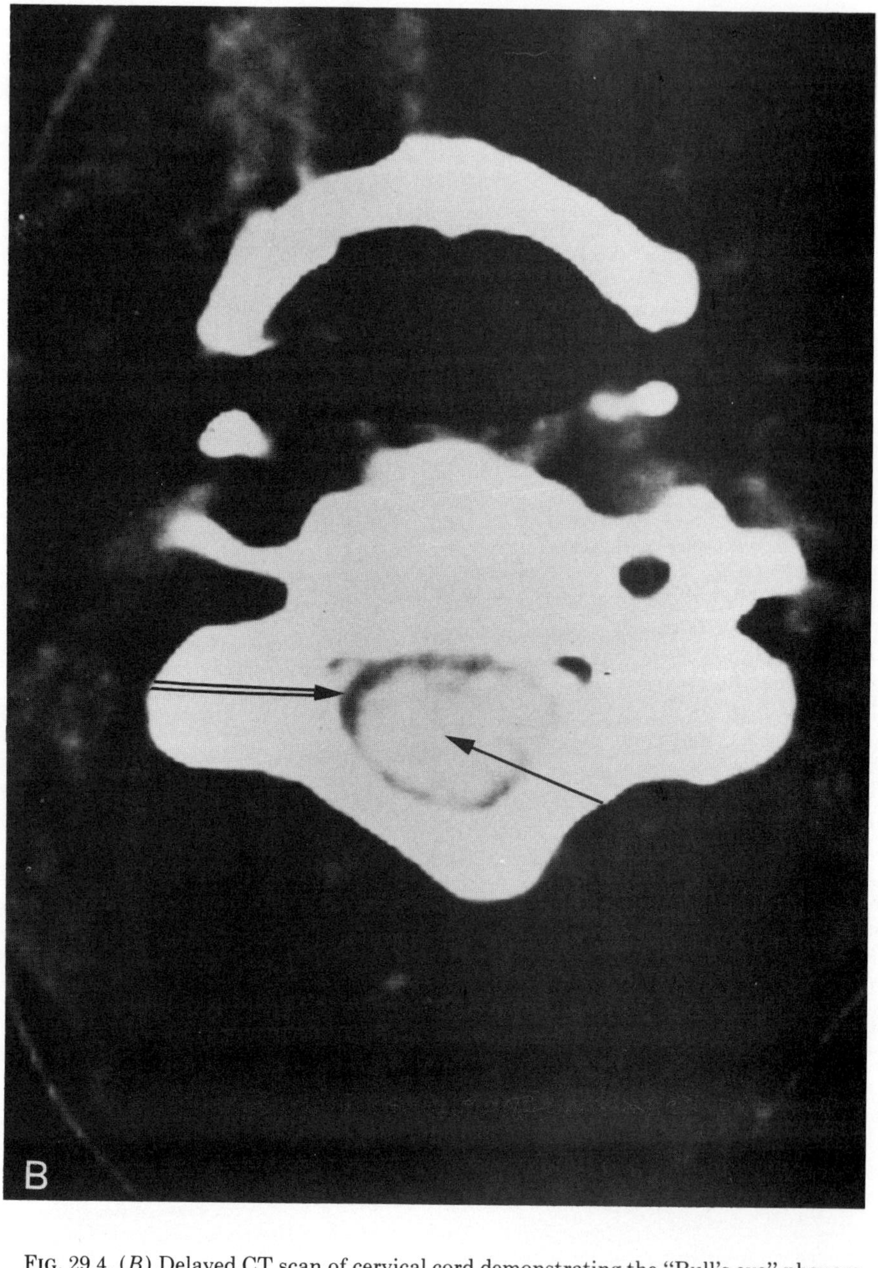

FIG. 29.4. (*B*) Delayed CT scan of cervical cord demonstrating the "Bull's eye" phenomena of imaged contrast within the syrinx and the thin rim of residual cord around the periphery.

municating syringomyelia underwent foramen magnum decompression, at which time the Chiari malformation was confirmed and a large patent central canal communicating with the IVth ventricle was found. The communication was plugged with a Dacron cone, and a silastic tube was placed into the IVth ventricle to improve drainage through the Foramen of Magendie. Postoperatively, the patient's neurologic condition dramatically improved, and he has remained well for 2 years. His repeat CT scan 6 months postoperatively shows the cord to be collapsed (Figs. 29.4*C* and *D*). A small syrinx is still present in the thoracic cord (Fig. 29.4*E*).

Case 2 (Communicating, Foramen of Magendie Cyst). This 36-year-old pharmacist presented with a 6-year history of intermittent left chest pain. For the previous year his left hand had become numb and weak, and his gait had deteriorated. Initial investigation and cervical laminectomy at a peripheral hospital showed an enlarged cerivcal cord harboring a syrinx which was drained into the subarachnoid space. His neurological condition was worse postoperatively but returned to his preoperative state over 8 months only to begin deteriorating again. Examination at that time demonstrated a loss of pain and temperature sensation on the left side from C2 to T1, a spastic gait, and wasting and areflexia in the left arm. His repeat myelogram and delayed CT scan showed the large cord from C2 to the midthoracic region, but the foramen magnum region appeared normal (Fig. 29.5*A*). He was thought to have idiopathic syringomyelia, and an upper thoracic syringoperitoneal shunt was performed. Postoperatively his neurologic condition was no better. Repeat myelography showed the lower cervical cord to be slightly smaller, but the upper cervical cord was unchanged (Fig. 29.5*B*). He was consequently returned to the operating room where upper cervical and foramen magnum exploration revealed atrophic tonsils without hindbrain herniation, but a thickened arachnoid membrane occluding the foramen of Magendie. The membrane was opened, and a patent central canal communicating with the IV ventricle was identified. This was plugged with Dacron, and the IVth venttricle was drained with a silastic tube. Postoperatively, the patient improved. Repeat myelography has confirmed collapse of the syrinx (Fig. 29.5*C*).

We suspect this patient had at least 2 loculations of his syrinx cavity, each of which communicated with a patent central canal but communicated poorly with each other. Syringoperitoneal drainage of one loculation did not drain fluid from the other. Prevention of fluid entering each loculation via the patient central canal and IVth ventricle was achieved by foramen magnum decompression with plugging of the communication.

Case 3 (Noncommunicating, Posttraumatic). This 18-year-old boy suffered a $C_{4,5}$ fracture dislocation with a complete C_4 quadriplegia.

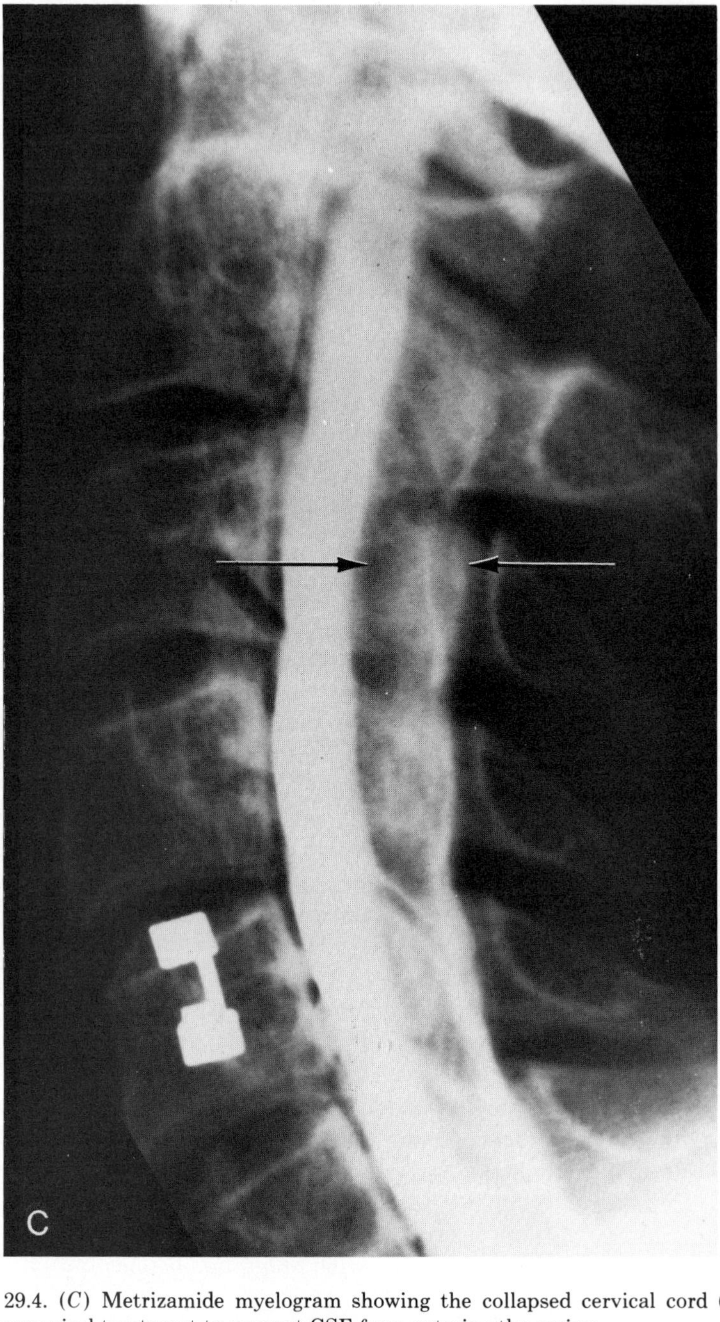

FIG. 29.4. (*C*) Metrizamide myelogram showing the collapsed cervical cord (*arrows*) following surgical treatment to prevent CSF from entering the syrinx.

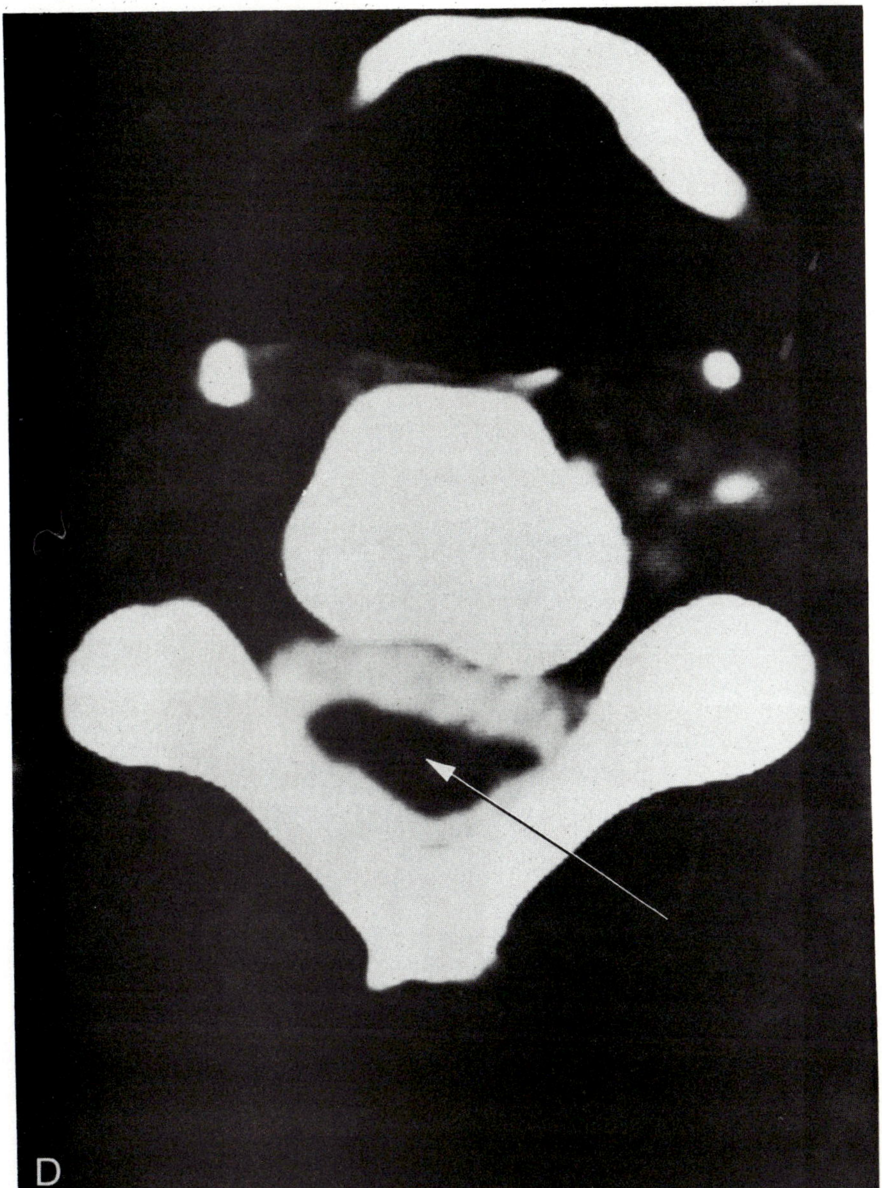

FIG. 29.4. (*D*) Postoperative delayed CT scan showing collapsed cervical cord and absence of contrast in syrinx (*arrow*).

Following reduction and $C_{4,5}$ posterior wire and acrylic fusion, he gradually (over 6 months) recovered function in C_5 innervated muscles to grade 4 in the right and left deltoid and biceps. Six months following the injury he rapidly (over 1 week) developed complete loss of power in his

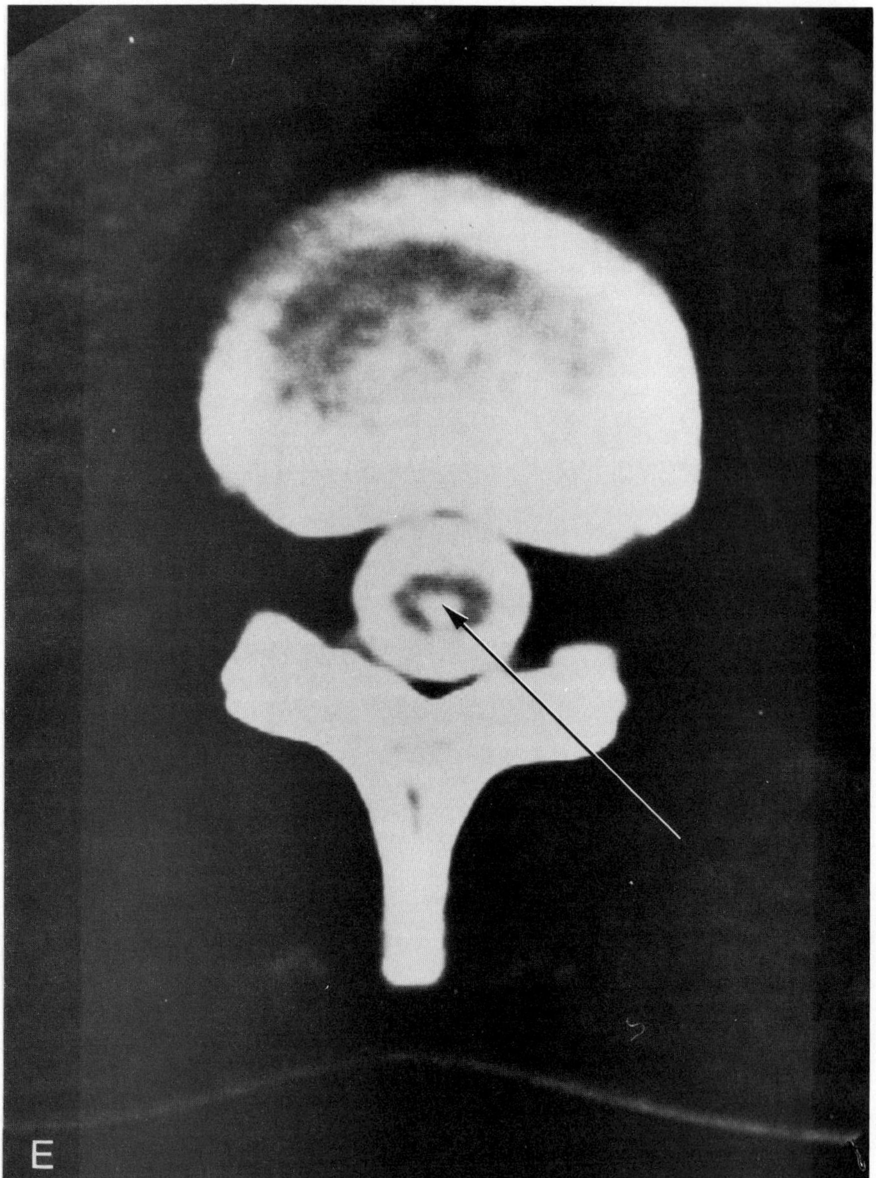

FIG. 29.4. (*E*) Postoperative delayed CT scan showing residual small syrinx in thoracic cord (*arrow*).

right deltoid and biceps. Myelography demonstrated an incomplete block at $C_{4,5}$, with widening of the cord from C_4 to T_1. The delayed (11 hour) CT scan demonstrated the syrinx from C_3 to T_3 (Fig. 29.6*A*).

A C_6 laminectomy was performed, and via a midline myelotomy the

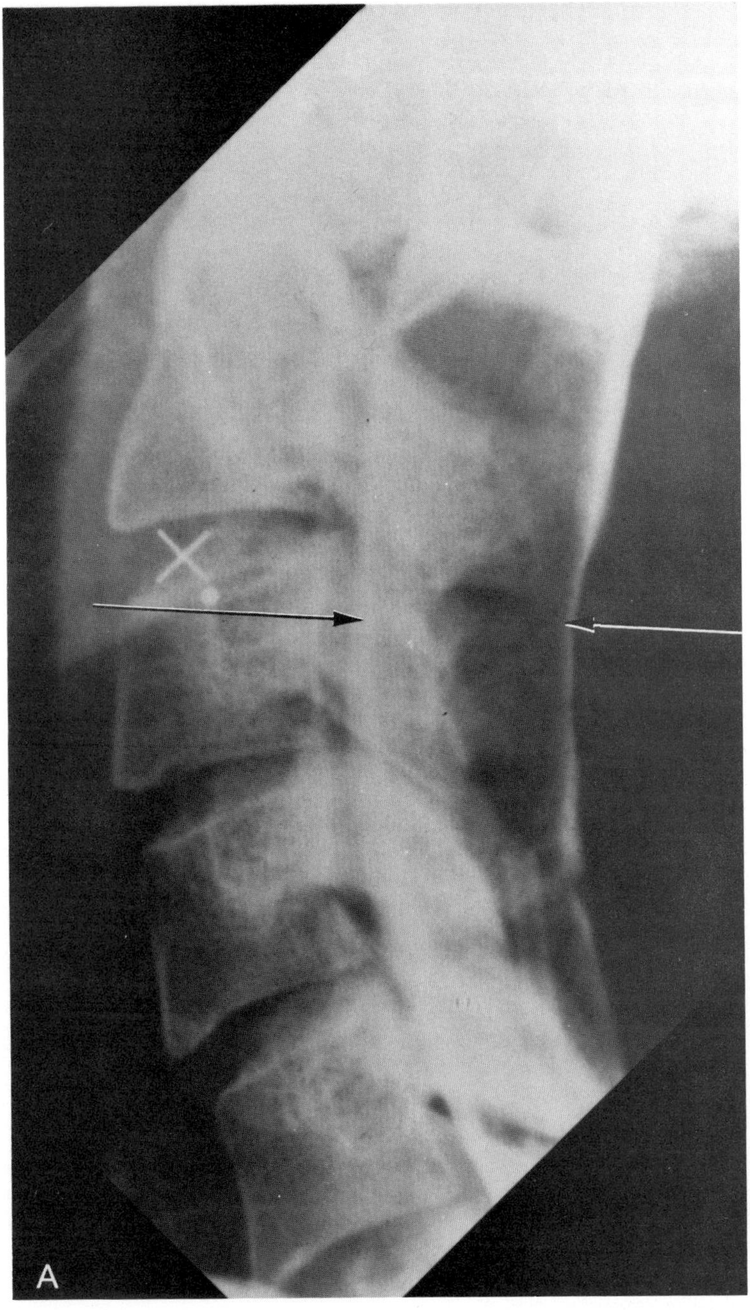

FIG. 29.5. (*A*) Metrizamide cervical myelogram showing enlarged spinal cord (*arrows*).

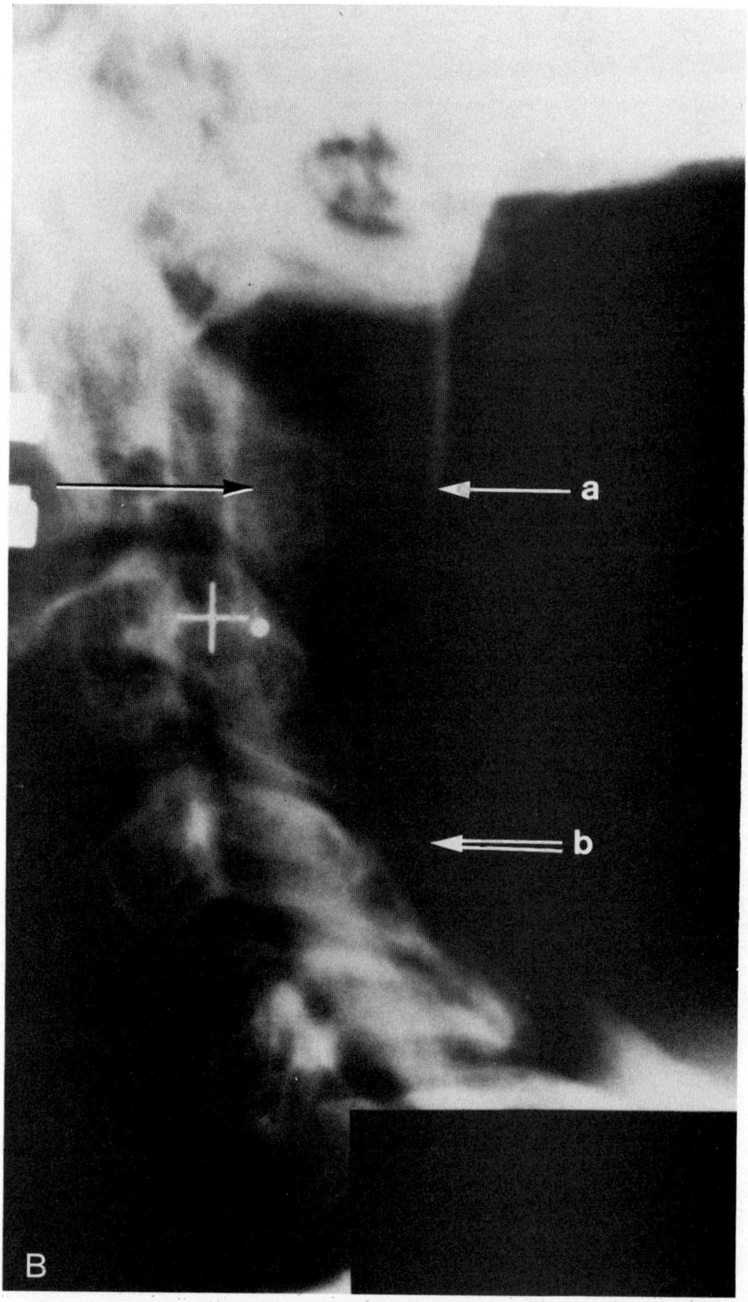

FIG. 29.5. (*B*) Metrizamide cervical myelogram following syringoperitoneal shunt. Lower cervical cord is smaller (*b*), but upper cervical cord is unchanged (*a*).

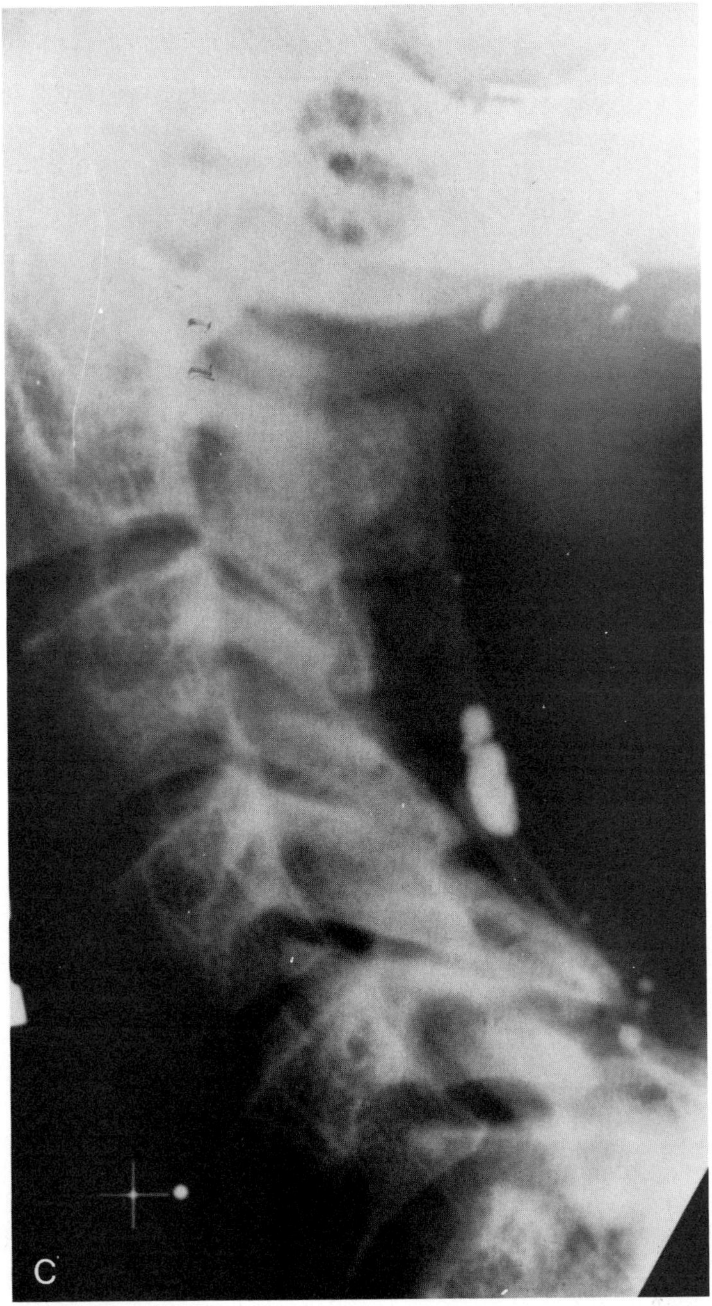

FIG. 29.5. (*C*) Metrizamide cervical myelogram following posterior fossa decompression and plugging of the central canal. Cord is now collapsed.

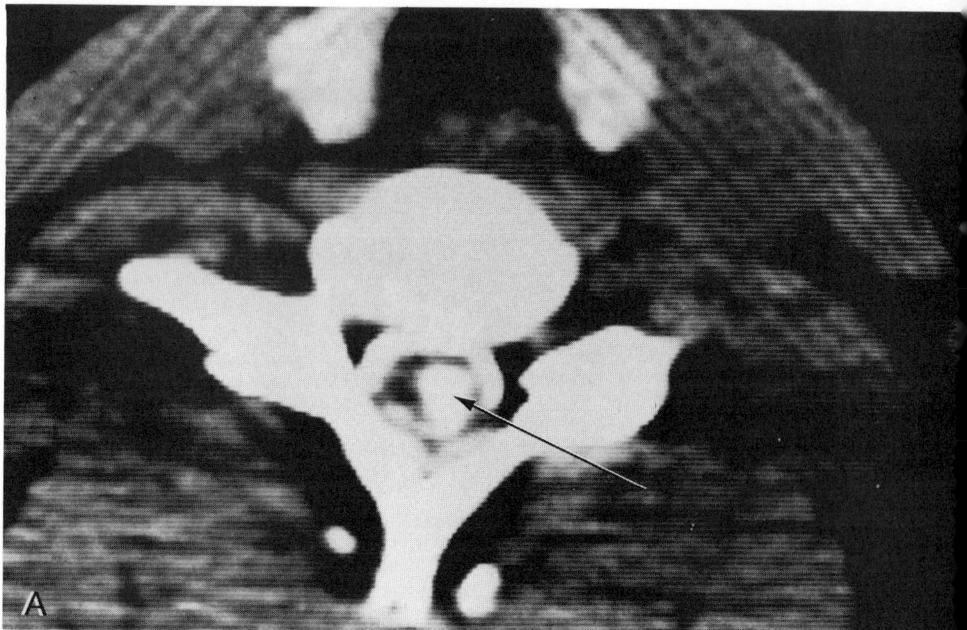

FIG. 29.6. (*A*) Delayed CT scan demonstrating large cavity within cervical spinal cord (*arrow*).

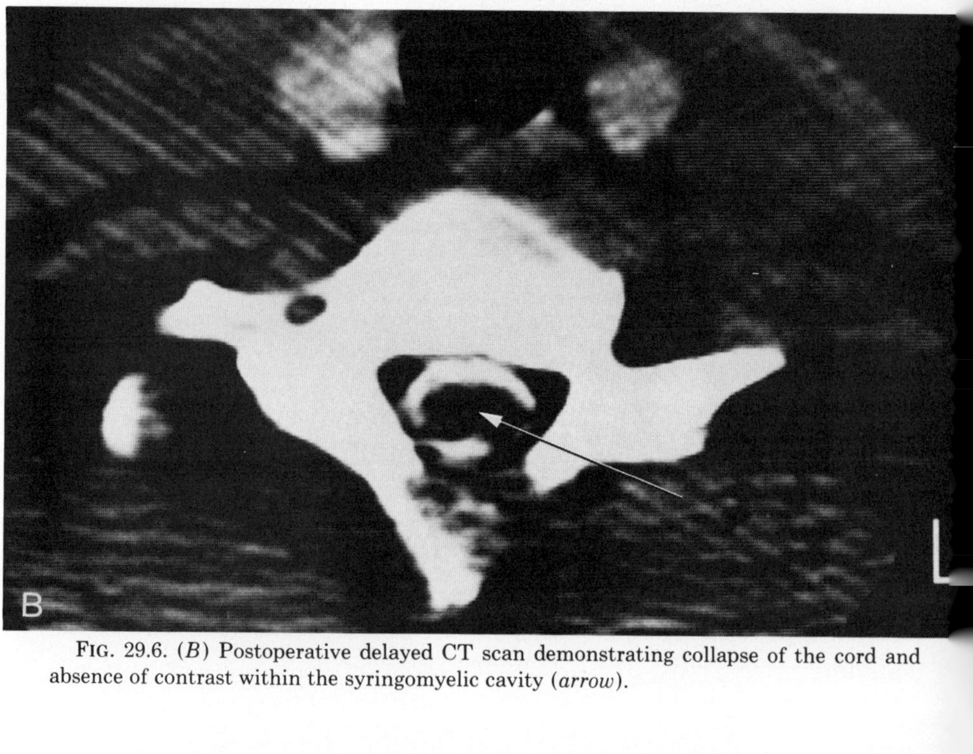

FIG. 29.6. (*B*) Postoperative delayed CT scan demonstrating collapse of the cord and absence of contrast within the syringomyelic cavity (*arrow*).

syrinx was encountered extending proximally and distally for at least 2 cm. A silastic drain was placed from the syrinx to the subarachnoid space. Postoperatively, the power in the C_5 innervated muscles on the right was immediately improved to grade 4. Repeat myelogram and delayed CT scan 2 weeks postoperatively demonstrated collapse of the cord and syrinx (Fig. 29.6*B*). He has had no further deterioration. This case illustrates a somewhat atypical course of posttraumatic syringomyelia. The neurologic deterioration was abrupt and disabling and resulted in an early diagnosis. Pain is, however, more commonly the first symptom of central cavitation following spinal cord injury.

Case 4 (Noncommunicating, Idiopathic). This 50-year-old laborer presented with a 2-year history of a gradual onset of right upper arm aching and numbness and weakness of the right hand. Over the 3 months before admission he had developed weakness in the left hand. Physical examination revealed wasting of both hands, right arm areflexia, and decreased pain and temperature sensation of the right arm. Metrizamide myelography demonstrated a normal sized cord which did not collapse with change in position, and a normal posterior fossa at the foramen magnum region. The 11-hour delayed CT scan, however, showed a syrinx extending from C_2 to C_7 (Fig. 29.7*A*). Of note, the cord above C_2 showed no syrinx (Fig. 29.7*B*). Diagnosis of idiopathic syringomyelia was made, and he underwent a C_5 to C_7 laminectomy and a syringosubarachnoid shunt. Immediately, postoperatively he had much more pain in the right shoulder and increased weakness in both arms. Within 3 weeks this pain had disappeared, and his strength was improved. At 3 month's follow-up, upper limb strength appeared normal although the hand wasting was still obvious. He remains improved 2 years following his operation.

Case 5 (Noncommunicating, Spinal Arachnoiditis). This 49-year-old man presented with a 10-year history of progressive spastic paraparesis. Over the previous 2 years he had become impotent and developed numbness in both legs. There was a family history of spinal arachnoiditis. Physical examination revealed a severe spastic paraparesis, worse on the left, although he could still walk. He had decreased sensation below T_9 to all modalities. Metrizamide myelography demonstrated an incomplete block from what appeared to be extradural compression at T_8 (Fig. 29.8*A*). The thoracic cord was large, although the cervical was normal in size. A delayed CT scan showed that a cavity extending from C_6 to T_9 was largest in the thoracic cord (Fig. 29.8*B*).

The patient was taken to the operating room where a T_8 to T_{10} laminectomy was performed. At the operation severe arachnoiditis was found completely encasing the cord and obliterating the subarachnoid space. The syrinx containing clear fluid was encountered through a midline myelotomy. The cavity was drained with a syringoperitoneal shunt.

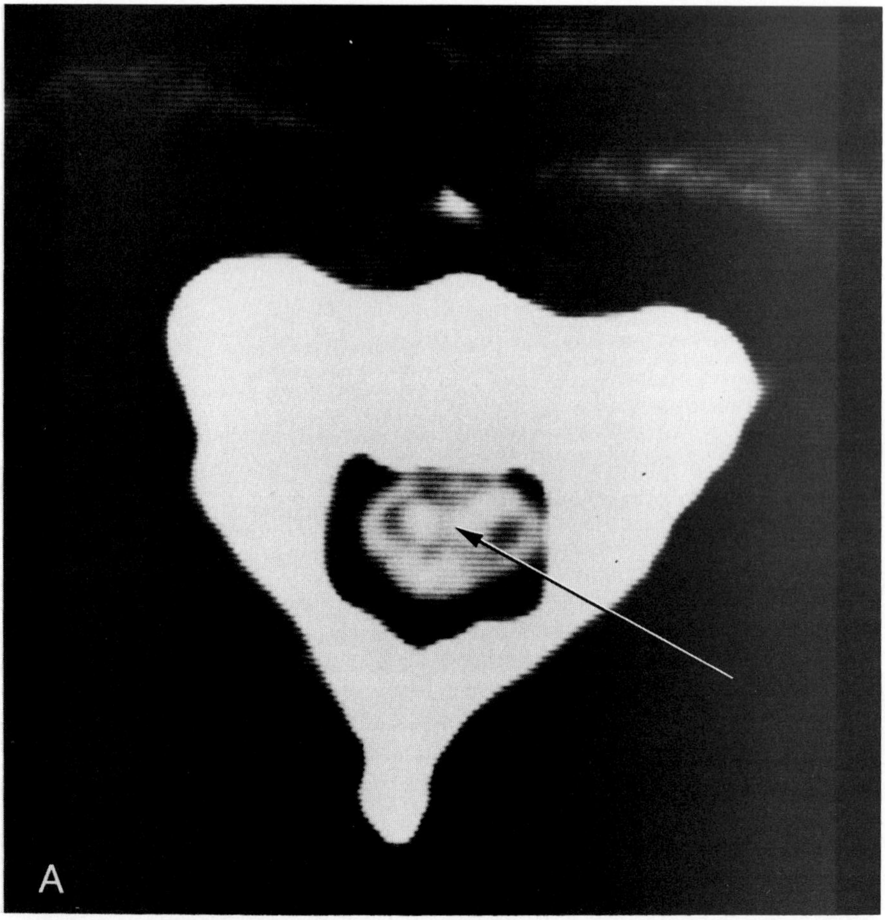

FIG. 29.7. (*A*) Delayed metrizamide CT scan demonstrating syringomyelic cavity (*arrow*) in midcervical cord.

Histologic examination of the arachnoid scar tissue showed chronic arachnoidal thickening consistent with long-standing idiopathic spinal arachnoiditis.

At last follow-up, 12 months following the surgical procedure, the patient is much improved. His gait is better, although his legs are still somewhat spastic. He is pleased with his erections. Pin prick sensation is now normal, but posterior column-mediated sensibility remains impaired. A postoperative myelogram has not been done.

Case 6 (Noncommunicating, Secondary to Spinal Cord Tumor). This 24-year-old woman presented with a 1-year history of progressive clumsiness and weakness of the left hand, decreased temperature sensation in both hands, and pain between her shoulders. Physical examination

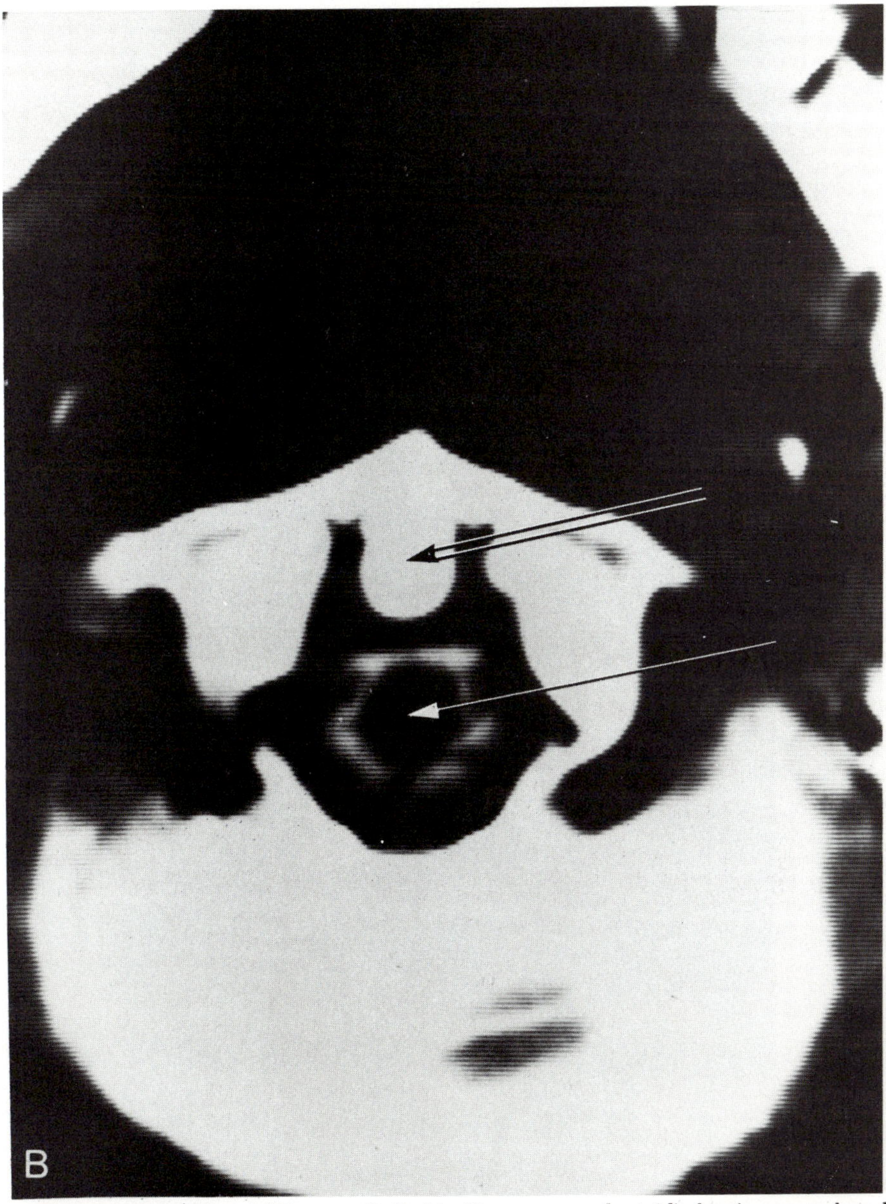

FIG. 29.7. (*B*) Delayed CT cut at C_1-C_2 (*double arrow* on odontoid) showing normal cord without a cavity (*single arrow*).

demonstrated nystagmus on lateral gaze, wasting of the left hand intrinsic muscles, mild leg spasticity, and a dissociated sensory loss for pain and temperature from C_6 to T_{12} on the left and C_6 to T_8 on the right. Vibration sensibility in the legs was markedly impaired. Metrizamide myelography

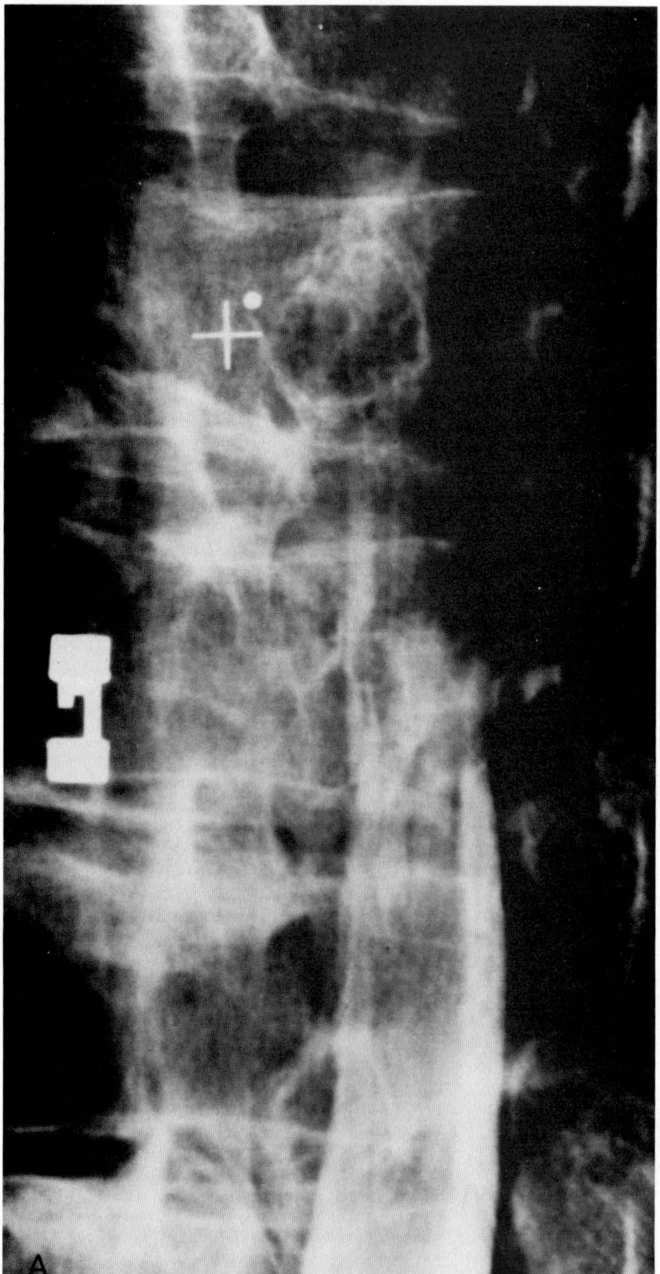

FIG. 29.8. (*A*) Metrizamide myelogram showing incomplete block at T_8.

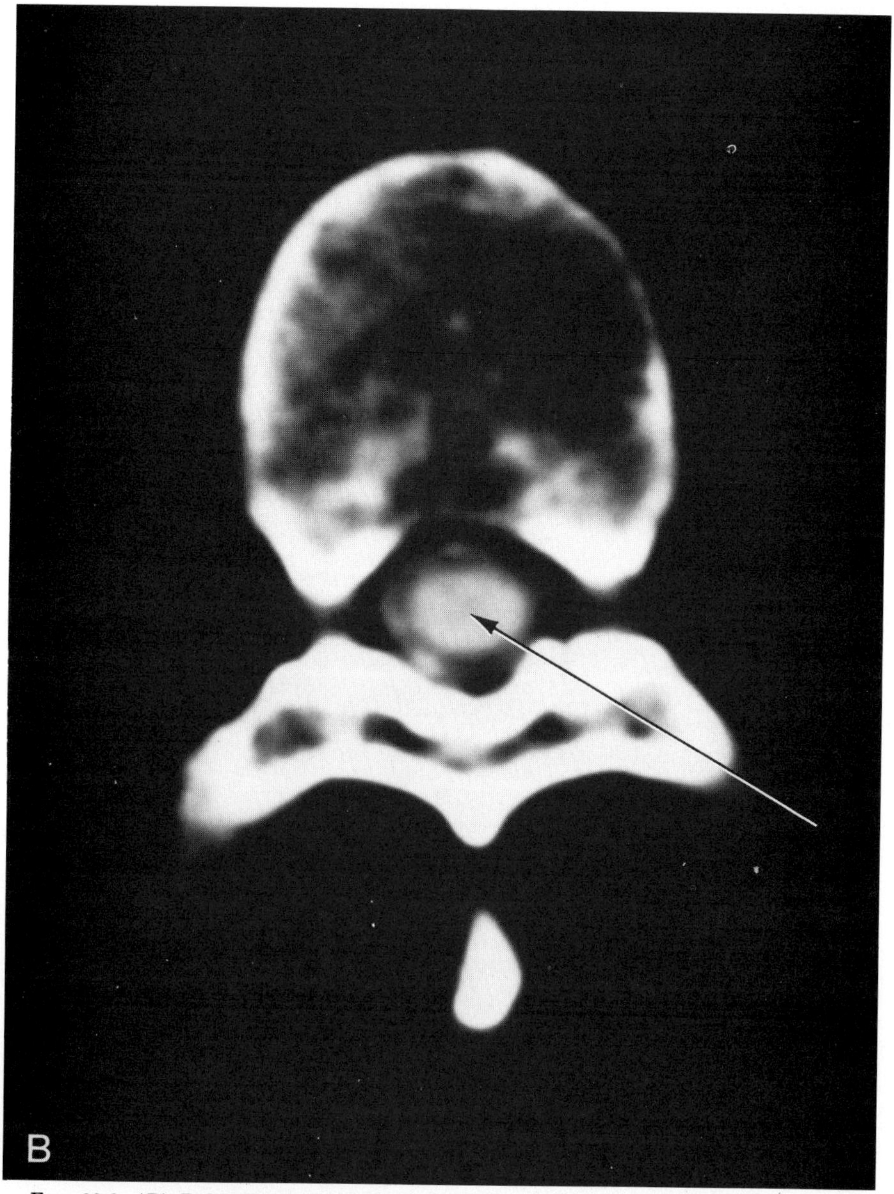

FIG. 29.8. (*B*) Delayed CT scan demonstrating "Bull's eye" phenomena of contrast within syrinx at T_5 (*arrow*) and thin rim of residual cord.

demonstrated an enlarged cervicothoracic cord with incomplete block at C_5 (Fig. 29.9*A*). Cerebrospinal fluid protein was 1 gm%. The 11-hour delayed CT scan showed a wide cord but no syrinx. A 24-hour delayed CT scan showed the presence of a syrinx from the midthoracic to the

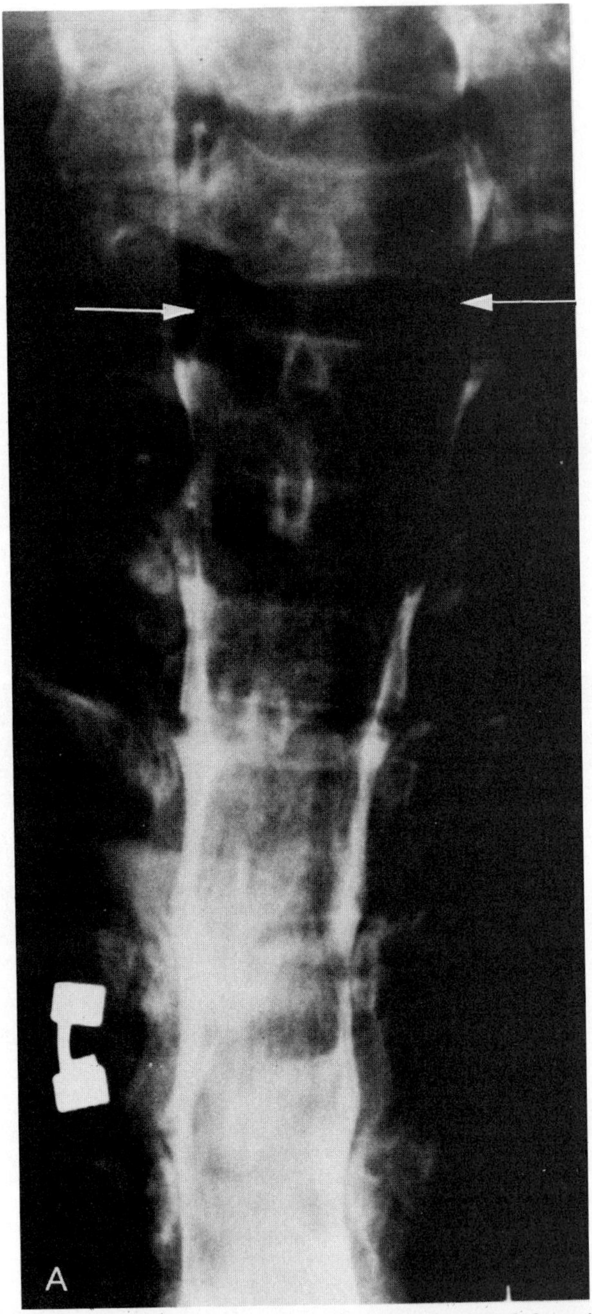

FIG. 29.9. (*A*) Metrizamide myelogram showing enlarged cervical thoracic cord (*arrows*) with an incomplete block at C_5.

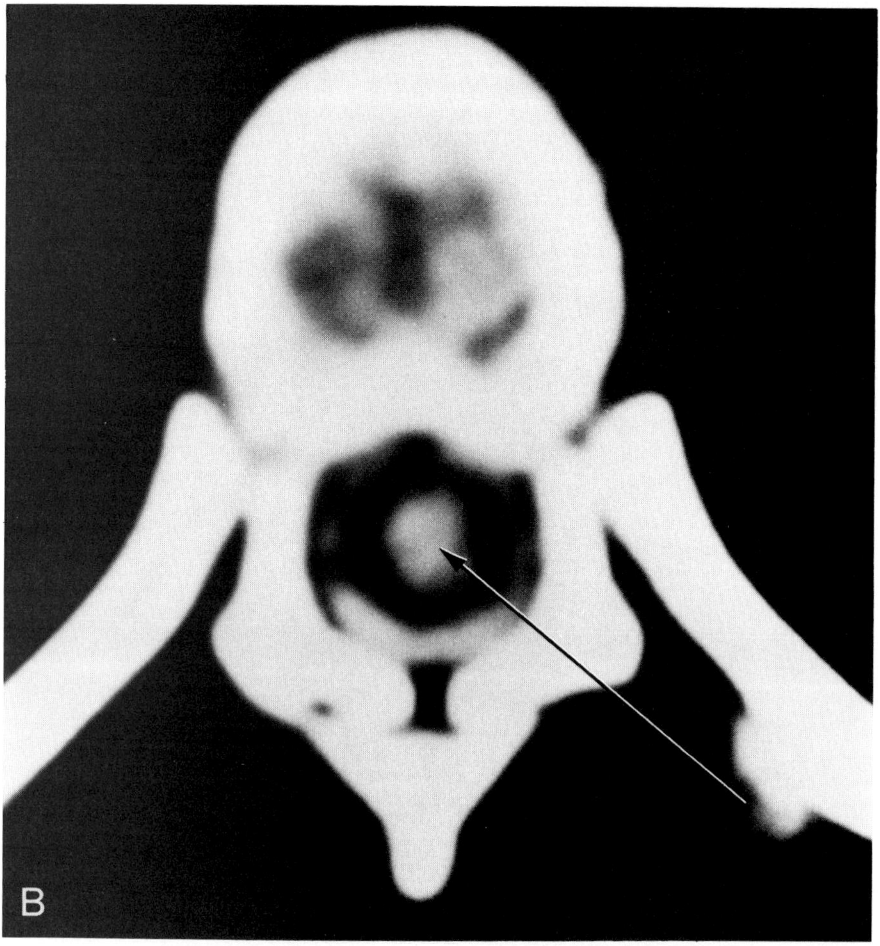

FIG. 29.9. (*B*) Delayed CT scan (24 hours) demonstrating the syringomyelic cavity (*arrow*) in the thoracic cord.

lower cervical cord (Fig. 29.9*B*), but the wide midcervical cord showed no syrinx (Fig. 29.9*C*). A tumor was suspected, and confirmation was obtained by a direct puncture at T_6 and a syringogram. The syrinx fluid protein was 2 gm%, and the tumor could be seen invaginating into the upper syrinx following metrizamide injection (Fig. 29.9*D*).

An intramedullary ependymoma extending from C_1 to T_1 was found at operation and completely removed. Postoperatively, the patient was markedly improved in strength and sensation, and has remained so now for 1½ yr.

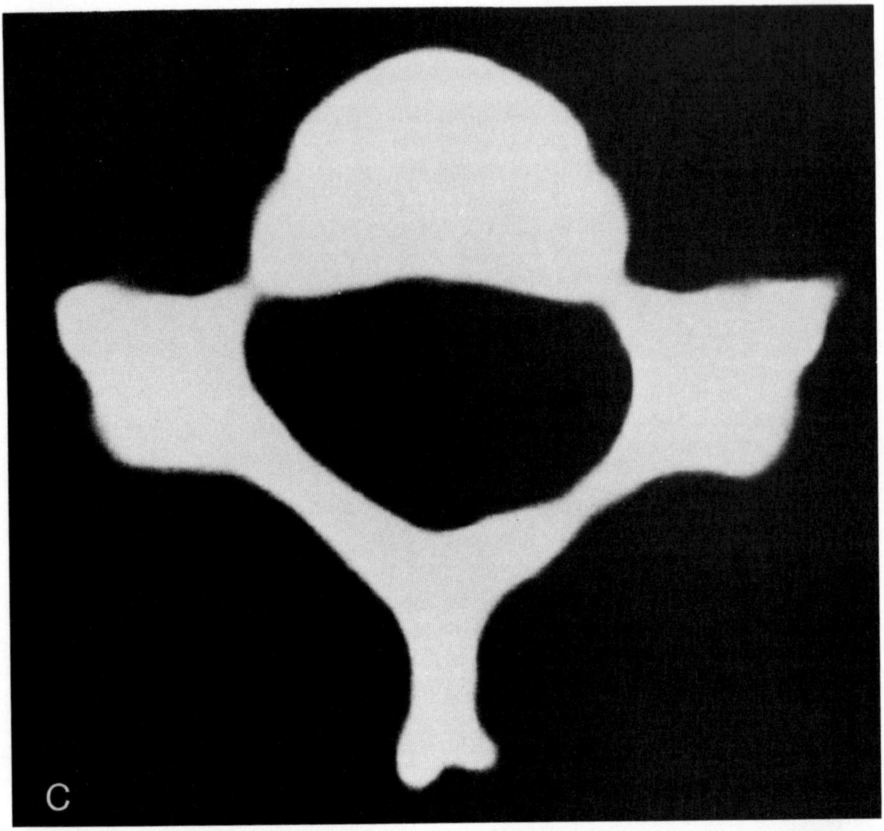

FIG. 29.9. (*C*) Delayed CT scan (24 hours) demonstrating the absence of a syrinx in the midcervical cord.

RESULTS

Although modern diagnostic and microsurgical techniques have been diligently employed in our unit for the past decade and for more than 75% of our cases, we have been unable to achieve the uniformly good results reported by some other surgeons. Because of the variable pathogenesis, natural history, and significant long-standing neurologic injury in some patients, follow-up must be long and repeated neurologic examination diligent. The relief of pain and improvement of neurologic dysfunction in the immediate postoperative period only too often has disappeared months or years later. The recovery of a C_5 segment in a traumatic quadriplegic following drainage of a rostral cavitation can be dramatic and gratifying and long-lasting. By contrast, these are patients who, despite enormous effort and every surgical trick, inexorably deteri-

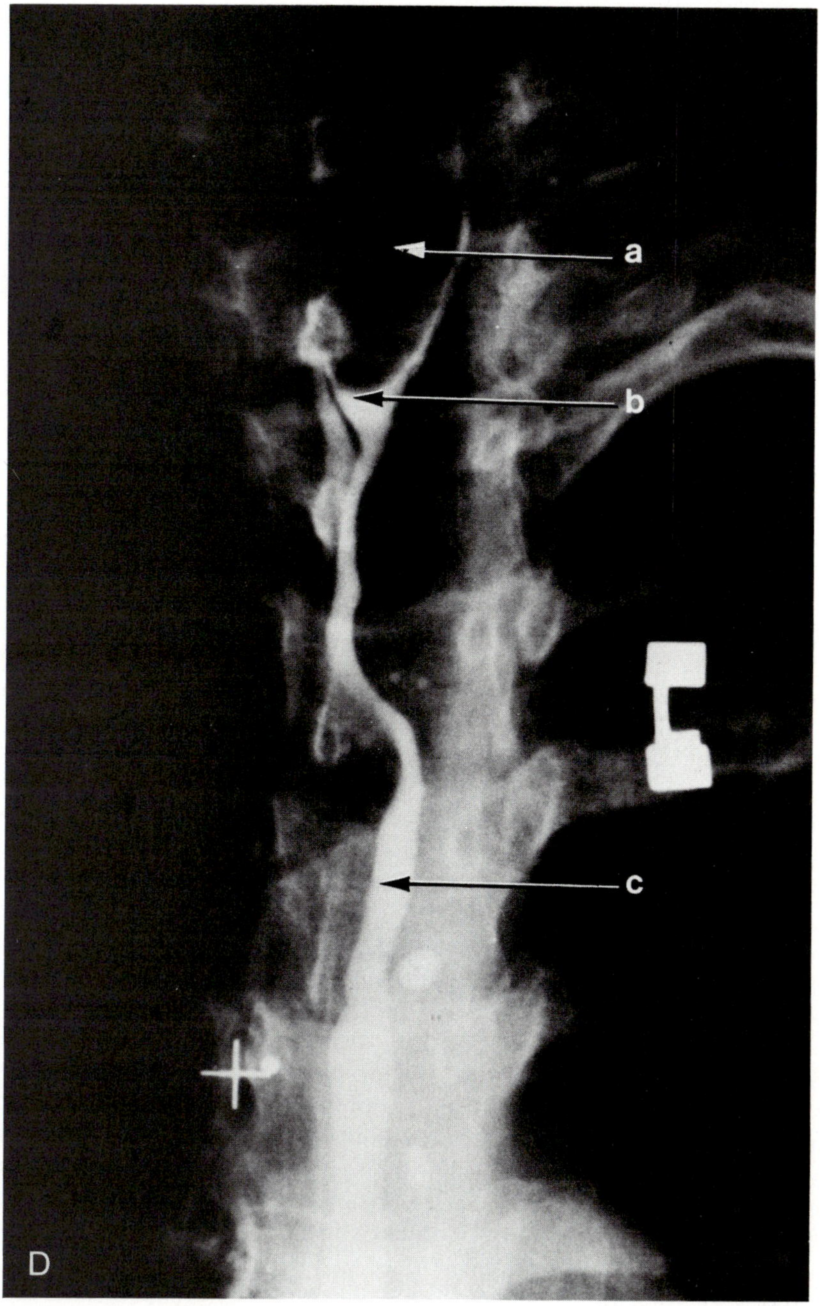

FIG. 29.9. (*D*) Syringogram following injection of metrizamide into the syrinx (*c*) at T_6. Note lower pole (*b*) of tumor (*a*) invaginating into the syrinx at T_1.

orate. Notwithstanding the enthusiasm with which some surgeons view syringomyelia we continue to be occasionally disappointed and frustrated by this disorder.

Syringomyelia and its surgical treatment are not situations that lend themselves to evaluation by the methodology of a clinical trial. Our experience, a series of surgical anecdotes with all of the inherent shortcomings of such an analysis, has been reviewed in 2 ways. An attempt has been made to look at our results in terms of the procedure done with a view to discern if any one procedure has an ovbious advantage over another. We have then reviewed the material to look at treatment as related to the etiology and pathogenesis of the cavitation.

Results of 121 FMD and Syrinx Drainage Procedures

The results at 3 months and long-term follow-up of the 34 foramen magnum decompression (FMD) procedures, all but one of which was performed on patients with communicating syringomyelia, are summarized in Table 29.4. Ten patients underwent foramen magnum decompression alone. None of these patients were improved on long-term follow-up, although 5 were stable. This was the earliest procedure performed, however, and the patients have been under scrutiny for the longest time. Sixteen patients underwent foramen magnum decompression, with plugging of the obex with either muscle or Dacron. Although 14 patients initially improved, long-term follow-up showed only 4 to be improved and 2 stable. The remaining 10 had deteriorated, and most went on to other procedures. More recently 8 patients have undergone foramen magnum decompression with plugging of the obex combined with a IVth ventricle to subarachnoid drain. These 8 patients remain improved, although follow-up is limited and we therefore would caution against enthusiastic endorsement of these microsurgical procedures until tested by the fullness of time. Table 29.5 indicates the 3-month and long-term follow-up results of the 87 syrinx drainage procedures performed in the 60 patients with all varieties of syringomyelia. These results indicate that the syringoperitoneal drain may have slightly better results than the syringosubarachnoid drain (21 of 33 long-term improvement or stability for the former, *vs.* 16 of 32 for the latter). Spinal cordectomy and terminal ventriculostomy had similarly good results, although indications for these procedures are limited to a complete spinal cord injury and a syrinx extending to the conus, respectively. As might be expected, needle aspiration or myelotomy and syringostomy without true drainage were ineffectual procedures. Closure of the myelotomy by pia and arachnoidal scar in 2 of these cases was confirmed at reoperation. Seven patients underwent laminectomy early in the series, usually for diagnosis when initial radiologic techniques demonstrated a spinal block in the face of progressive myelopathy. All of these patients subsequently had definitive drainage procedures.

Results of 90 Patients Treated by Diagnosis and Surgical Procedure

COMMUNICATING SYRINGOMYELIA

The procedures performed for the 33 patients with communicating syringomyelia are summarized in Table 29.6. Thirty patients have undergone 33 foramen magnum decompression procedures. For 26 of these patients, the foramen magnum decompression was the initial procedure performed to treat the syrinx. Following the 33 FMD procedures, 30 of the patients were improved or made stable for at least 3 months postoperatively (Table 29.4). Late deterioration, however (more than 3 months postoperatively), occurred in 8 of the 26 patients who underwent foramen magnum decompression as the initial treatment of the communicating syringomyelia and 2 of the 4 patients who underwent FMD as a second procedure. This necessitated the performance of a syrinx drainage procedure (in 7) or a repeat foramen magnum decompression (in 3) at some time after the foramen magnum decompression in these 10 patients.

Five patients underwent a syrinx drainage procedure as the initial treatment for the communicating syringomyelia. Continued deterioration postoperatively in 3 led to foramen magnum decompression. Two patients underwent a ventriculoperitoneal shunt as the initial treament for both syringomyelia and hydrocephalus. One, a 29-year-old woman, had presented with complaints of progressive headache and myelopathy. Hydrocephalus and syringomyelia, both related to a Chiari malformation, were diagnosed. A ventriculoperitoneal shunt was placed which improved both her hydrocephalus and syringomyelic syndrome. Pre- and postoperative myelograms confirmed the size reduction of the cervical cord postopera-

TABLE 29.6
Communicating Syringomyelia: Incidence of Procedures[a]

	No. of Patients
FMD (incl. 2 with VPS)	17
FMD → VPS	2
FMD → Syrinx drainage	7
Syrinx drainage alone	2
Syrinx drainage → FMD	3
VPS alone	1
VPS → FMD	1
Total	33

[a] FMD, foramen magnum decompression; VPS, ventriculoperitoneal shunt.

tively. The patient remains improved 5 years later. The other patient initially treated with a ventriculoperitoneal shunt had continued deterioration in his syringomyelic syndrome and required a foramen magnum decompression. Two patients had hydrocephalus precipitated after the foramen magnum decompression, and then underwent a ventriculoperitoneal shunt.

The clinical state of the patients at last follow-up are summarized in Table 29.11. Twenty-seven of the patients remain stable or improved when compared to their initial condition. Four patients have continued to deteriorate. One of these, a patient who had syringobulbia and syringomyelia, has since died of respiratory failure after his refusal of further treatment. The other 3 patients had undergone both foramen magnum decompression and syrinx drainage. In each, the spinal cord has been shown by delayed CT scan to be completely collapsed and containing a tiny syrinx. There is nothing more to be done for these 3 patients. Two patients have been lost to current follow-up.

NONCOMMUNICATING SYRINGOMYELIA

Nontumorous. *Posttraumatic Syringomyelia.* The 28 patients with posttraumatic syringomyelia underwent 49 surgical procedures, 44 of which were for syrinx drainage (Table 29.7). Two of the procedures were for laminectomy alone, 2 for drainage of an extramedullary arachnoid cyst associated with the syrinx, and 1 for an anterior cervical discectomy.

At follow-up to date, 12 of the 28 patients with posttraumatic syringomyelia are improved, 8 are stable, and 2 have been lost to follow-up. Six patients have deteriorated, and 3 of these have died, 1 from respiratory failure, 1 committed suicide, and 1 from unknown causes. The other 3 deteriorated patients have all undergone a formal drainage procedure.

TABLE 29.7

Procedures for 44 Patients with Noncommunicating Nontumorous Syringomyelia

	Post traumatic	Idiopathic	Post arachnoiditis
Syringosubarachnoid drain	17	5	0
Syringoperitoneal drain	17	3	7
Spinal cordectomy	5	0	0
Needle aspiration	3	2	1
Myelotomy and syringostomy	2	1	0
Terminal ventriculostomy	0	3	0
Laminectomy	2	3	2
Drainage extramedullary cyst	2	0	0
Discectomy	1	0	0
Foramen magnum decompression	0	1	0
Ventriculoperitoneal shunt	0	1	0

Metrizamide myelography and delayed CT scan have shown in 2 that the cord is atrophic and contains a tiny syrinx. Spinal arachnoiditis has developed in association with one of these. The third patient developed low pressure headaches with a syringoperitoneal drain he received after failure of a syringosubarachnoid shunt to relieve his pain. The syringoperitoneal shunt has since been removed as a consequence of the headaches.

Idiopathic Syringomyelia. Nine patients with no discernible cause for their syringomyelia were treated with 19 procedures (Table 29.7). In each case, myelography had shown a normal posterior fossa, and the one patient who underwent exploration of the foramen magnum region was found not to have a patent central cord. At current follow-up (Table 29.11), 7 patients are improved, 1 is stable, and 1 deteriorated following needle aspiration. This last patient has refused further investigation and treatment, but at current follow-up 2½ years postoperative she continues to show slight neurologic deterioration.

Syringomyelia with Spinal Arachnoiditis. The etiology of the 7 cases of arachnoiditis with syringomyelia were meningitis in 4 (tuberculosis, 2; pneumococcus, 1; unknown 1) pantopaque myelography in 1, a strong family history of arachnoiditis was present in 1, and in 1 no cause was found. Although 2 patients required more than one procedure, at final follow-up, 4 patients are improved, 2 are stable, and 1 has deteriorated (Table 29.11). Deterioration in the latter case is thought to be from the spinal arachnoiditis secondary to intrathecal penicillin and not the syrinx. One of the improved patients died of an unknown cause.

Syringomyelia Associated with Tumor. In 7 of the 13 patients who had syringomyelia associated with a tumor, the tumor was located within the cervical cord (Table 29.8). In 3 the tumor was in the thoracic cord and in 2 the thoracolumbar cord. One patient had an epidermoid tumor of the IVth ventricle associated with the syrinx which may represent a variant of communicating syringomyelia. Pathological examination revealed an ependymoma in 7 cases, a hemangioblastoma in 2, an

TABLE 29.8

Histological Classification and Location of 13 Tumors Associated with Syringomyelia

Type of Tumor	Anatomical Localization Tumor			
	IV Ventricle	Cervical	Thoracic	Thoraco-lumbar
Ependymoma	0	5	1	1
Hemangioblastoma	0	1	0	1
Astrocytoma	0	1	1	0
Vascular malformation	0	0	1	0
Epidermoid	1	0	0	0

TABLE 29.9

Operative Procedures Performed in 13 Patients with Tumor-Associated Syringomyelia

	No. of Procedures
Complete removal	9
Subtotal removal	6
Syrinx drainage	3
Biopsy	1
Feeding vessels clipped	1

astrocytoma in 2, an epidermoid in 1, and a vascular malformation in 1. Twenty surgical procedures were performed for the 13 patients (Table 29.9). Nine patients have had complete removal of the tumor.

Drainage of the syrinx prior to the tumor removal was performed in 3 cases, and in each immediate improvement in the patient's condition following the drainage was noted. One was a 24-year-old woman with progressive paraparesis who had a wide cord producing a complete block at T_{12}. Exploration of the thoracolumbar region was performed, and a syrinx with fluid containing a protein level of 2.6 gm% was found and drained by a syringosubarachnoid drain. Her paraparesis was markedly improved postoperatively, but she then developed symptoms in her arms. Repeat myelography showed the presence of a cervical intramedullary tumor. At operation, an astrocytoma was completely removed from the cervical cord, and she has remained improved and stable to date. Exploration with biopsy of an ependymoma (1 case) and clipping of feeding vessels to a hemangioblastoma (1 case) were performed in a peripheral hospital prior to referral to our unit. In both instances complete removal of the offending tumor was accomplished.

The 13 patients with tumor-associated syringomyelia have done well, with 11 currently improved or stable (Table 29.11). Two of the 4 patients with incomplete tumor removal have deteriorated, and 1 has since died following anaplastic evolution of an astrocytoma to a glioblastoma. The other patient has gradually deteriorated following incomplete removal of an ependymoma.

COMPLICATIONS

A frequent complication of the patient who has undergone syrinx drainage has been the development of a transient worsening of the neurological deficit and arm pain (Table 29.10). We have demonstrated collapse of the syrinx on postoperative myelography in one of these individuals. This distressing complication has been seen particularly frequently after drainage of a posttraumatic syrinx. Fortunately, recovery to the previous neurological state has occurred within 3 to 4 weeks in all

TABLE 29.10

Complications of the Treatment of 90 Patients with Syringomyelia[a]

	FMD (34 Procedures)	Syrinx Drainage (87 Procedures)	Tumor Removal (15 Procedures)	VPS (5 Procedures)
Postoperative neurologic deterioration				
Transient	0	5	4	0
Permanent	0	0	2	0
Increased pain	0	5	0	0
Nausea/vomiting	5	1	0	0
Hydrocephalus	1	2	0	0
Unable to locate syrinx	NA	6	0	NA
Wound infection	0	3	0	0
CSF leak	1	2	0	0
Disappeared muscle plug	1	NA	NA	NA
Drain/shunt blockage	NA	6	NA	2

[a] FMD, foramen magnum decompression; VPS; ventriculoperitoneal shunt; NA, not applicable.

TABLE 29.11

Results of Treatment of 90 Patients with Syringomyelia

Type of Syringomyelia	Improved	Stable	Deteriorated	Unknown
Communicating	18	9	4	2
Noncommunicating				
Nontumorous				
Posttraumatic	12	8	6	2
Idiopathic	7	1	1	0
Spinal arachnoiditis	4	2	1	0
Tumor-associated	9	2	2	0
Total	50	22	14	4

patients. The increased postoperative pain appeared to be neurogenic in origin, was associated with hyperpathia, and responded well to carbamazepine (Tegretol, Geigy Pharmaceuticals, Summit, N.J.) in 2 patients. The cause of this transient deterioration is unknown, but may be the result of increased tension in the nerve roots or increased stress on long tracts or microvasculature within the suddenly collapsed cord following drainage of the cavity.

The problem of negative cord exploration, which occurred with 6 of the syrinx drainage procedures, will, hopefully, become less frequent with the wider use of modern diagnostic techniques to demonstrate the extent and position of the syrinx within the cord.

Complications of the foramen magnum decompression procedures have included 5 patients who suffered troublesome postoperative nausea and vomiting. In 3 patients these troublesome symptoms subsided spontaneously, and one obtained relief from a short course of clomipramine (Anafranil HCL, Geigy Pharmaceuticals, Summit, N.J.). One other patient was demonstrated to have marginal hydrocephalus, and relief from her nausea and vomiting was achieved immediately following placement of a ventriculoperitoneal shunt.

Three patients developed symptomatic hydrocephalus requiring a V-P shunt. In each a foramen magnum decompression had been done previously, but in 2 of the patients, the hydrocephalus was precipitated following a drainage procedure done after the foramen magnum decompression had failed.

Over the period of review 6 patients have died. In 2 cases this was from respiratory failure, 1 case died from a spinal cord tumor, 1 committed suicide, and 2 patients died of unknown causes and no autopsy was obtained.

DISCUSSION

Over the last 20 years our understanding of the pathophysiology of syringomyelia has evolved dramatically (2, 5, 8, 11, 14, 19, 48). This has led in turn to many different treatments for the condition, including observation alone, radiotherapy, laminectomy, and various syrinx drainage procedures designed to eradicate the syrinx or decompress the cord (6, 7, 9, 15, 20, 31, 41–43, 45). More recently, foramen magnum decompression designed to correct the presumed disordered hydrodynamics responsible for development of the syrinx has been recommended (6, 19, 22, 33, 46).

Many theories have been proposed to explain the development of syringomyelia. Methods of treatment have largely depended upon the surgeon's understanding of the cause of the syrinx. Belief that syringomyelia was caused by neoplastic glial tissue secreting fluid led to radiotherapy of the spinal cord (9, 41). Recognition that fluid within the syrinx frequently has a composition similar to cerebrospinal fluid led to a search for mechanisms which would allow entry of CSF into the cord. Gardner's observation of the frequent association of syringomyelia with the Chiari malformation led to his theory that syringomyelia was a manifestation of spinal dysraphism, with maintenance and expansion of the syrinx being due to pulsating cerebrospinal fluid entering from the IVth ventricle obex usually via a patent central canal (19). Gardner has since stated that all cases of syringomyelia have an associated hindbrain anomaly and that operation directed at decompressing the foramen magnum region and plugging the patent central canal is the recommended treatment (21). Others have supported his theory at least in part (5, 6, 10, 22, 33, 37), although Williams felt a negative pressure in the spinal cord induced by the hindbrain malformation acting at the foramen magnum region as a ball valve following a Valsalva maneuver may cause fluid to be "sucked" into the syrinx through the central canal (46).

It was clear, however, from autopsy cases of syringomyelia (6, 16, 24, 27, 30) and observations at operations for foramen magnum decompression (33, 34, and 1 patient in this series) that not all cases of syringomyelia have a communication of the syrinx with the IVth ventricle. Other possible mechanisms for entry of fluid into the syrinx have been postulated. Ball and Dayan (3) and Durward *et al.* (13) observed in cases of syringomyelia large Virchow-Robin spaces communicating between the subarachnoid space and syrinx through which a marker dye could pass. Macroscopic connections between the subarachnoid space and syrinx have occasionally also been demonstrated (32, 38). More recently, water-soluble iodinated contrast material injected into the subarachnoid space for myelography has been demonstrated to enter syrinx cavities when no IVth ventricular or macroscopic connection was present (2, 26; cases 1 (postop) and 6 this chapter). This evidence strongly supports a concept that "noncommunicating" syringomyelia does exist where no communication with the IVth ventricle is present, in contrast to "communicating" syringomyelia, where the communication to the ventricular system does exist (6, 30, 47).

Four varieties of noncommunicating syringomyelia have been described (6, 8, 47). Three have a demonstrated pathological association—the posttraumatic and tumor-associated varieties and those occurring in association with spinal arachnoiditis. An idiopathic or "fifth variety" with no known associated pathology has also been described (6, 43). Surgery to the foramen magnum region is obviously not warranted for these varieties of syringomyelia. Treatment must be either directed at the causative lesion (e.g., tumor), or adequate drainage of the syrinx must be achieved.

The results of surgery for syringomyelia must be viewed with the knowledge that 50% of patients with syringomyelia may remain stable if left untreated over the 10-year period following diagnosis of the syrinx (9). In addition, Scher (40) and Barnett *et al.* (6) recently reported 4 patients with posttraumatic syringomyelia who improved spontaneously. Because not all patients with syringomyelia will deteriorate, and the best that can be hoped for in a significant proportion of treated cases (22 of 90 in this series) is a stable condition, we recommend operative treatment only for patients who are deteriorating. However, we concur with Tator's observation that the shorter the duration of presenting symptoms the better are the results from surgery in noncommunicating syringomyelia (43).

For communicating syringomyelia, we recommend that a foramen magnum decompression procedure be performed first. In this series, 3 of the 5 patients who underwent a drainage procedure (Case 2) and 1 of the 2 patients who underwent a ventriculoperitoneal shunt required a foramen magnum decompression procedure at a later date. Despite having had a foramen magnum decompression, however, a significant proportion of patients (11 of 30) have required a repeat foramen magnum decompression, syrinx drainage, or ventriculoperitoneal shunt at a later date. In one of the repeat foramen magnum decompression procedures, the initially placed muscle plug had disappeared. The precise type of FMD procedure that should be performed is controversial. In this series, the combination of FMD with plugging of the communication between the IVth ventricle and the syrinx and drainage of the IVth ventricle would appear to be the best procedure and superior to foramen magnum decompression alone or simple IVth ventricle drainage or obex plug. Logue and Edwards (30), however, reported that FMD alone had the same success rate as FMD with plugging of the obex in communicating syringomyelia. They felt the major benefit of the operation was decompressing the medulla with the possible benefit of preventing enlargement of the syrinx. Cahan and Bentson (10) reported no difference in patients undergoing the "Gardner" procedure who did or did not have a IVth ventricle to subarachnoid drain placed in addition to the muscle plug. Using postoperative myelography, we have now demonstrated cord and syrinx collapse in 6 of 7 patients who have had foramen magnum decompression with plugging of the obex (Figs. 29.4 and 29.5). Length of follow-up in the patients who have undergone FMD with both obex plugging and IVth ventricular drainage has, however, been less than for the other foramen magnum decompression procedures in this series. Aboulker (1) has reported an increasing number of deteriorating patients with longer follow-up, and in his series, more than half the patients had deteriorated 5 years after treatment.

The cause of late deterioration is unknown. In occasional cases, it may be from a dislocated or dissolved plug, but we suspect further scarring and other mechanisms for entry of fluid into the cord, as in noncommunicating syringomyelia, may account for enlargement of the cavity with time (Fig. 29.4*E*).

For noncommunicating syringomyelia not secondary to a tumor, drainage of the syrinx with a permanent silastic drain is recommended (6, 35, 43, 45). Previous reported attempts to maintain drainage by needle aspiration with myelotomy alone or placement of a seton have had poor results because of inability to maintain drainage. Placement of the drain into the lowermost extent of the syrinx would seem most logical, and this is the procedure followed in the current series. If the syrinx extends to the conus, then terminal ventriculostomy may achieve excellent permanent syringosubarachnoid drainage. Williams *et al.* (45) postulated that fluid from the subarachnoid space may be forced back into the syrinx during a Valsalva maneuver, and drainage into the peritoneum may be better. Our results indicate, however, only a marginal benefit of the syringoperitoneal drain over the syringosubarachnoid drain. Drainage of the syrinx by spinal cordectomy in the patient with posttraumatic syringomyelia and a complete spinal cord injury has provided satisfactory results (6, 13).

In this series, 9 patients had syringomyelia without any identifiable associated pathology. This included one patient who was shown at operation to have a nonpatent central canal at the obex. We recommend treatment of this "idiopathic" variety by syrinx drainage. However, in our series of 33 patients with communicating syringomyelia, 3 had initially been diagnosed as having idiopathic syringomyelia. All had normal posterior fossa anatomy on myelography. One underwent 2 drainage procedures which both failed before having foramen magnum decompression (case 2). The other 2 were initially treated by foramen magnum decompression because in one, the patient had evidence of syringobulbia and in the other, the syrinx as seen on the delayed CT scan appeared to extend to the foramen magnum. In each of these 3 cases, a patent central canal communicating with the obex was found, although in one obstruction of the foramen of Magendie by an arachnoidal membrane was also found. These troublesome recollections will hopefully be few in the future, but have led us to recommend exploration of the foramen magnum region when a patient with idiopathic syringomyelia fails to improve or stabilize following simple drainage of the syrinx.

Syringomyelia associated with spinal arachnoiditis has been well described and most often has been reported to have a poor prognosis (6, 16, 38, 43). Spinal arachnoiditis may produce symptoms in 3 ways (6): (a) From the arachnoiditis itself by a constricting effect on the cord roots and possibly on the blood vessels. (b) From loculation of an arachnoid cyst under pressure within the area of arachnoiditis. (c) From formation of a syrinx. No cases of extramedullary cyst were encountered in the 7 cases of syringomyelia associated with spinal arachnoiditis in this series. Following drainage procedures, however, 4 improved (one has since died), 2 have ceased deteriorating, and one has continued to deteriorate. Because of the obliteration of part of the subarachnoid space in patients with this disease, we strongly recommend drainage from the syrinx into the peritoneal cavity. This practice may in part account for the better results in this series when compared to earlier reports (6).

A number of factors may be responsible for the late failure of a drainage procedure for noncommunicating, nontumorous syringomyelia. The tube of a syringosubarachnoid drain may have been placed in the subdural space instead of the subarachnoid space, it may have fallen out of the syrinx, or arachnoidal scarring may have occluded its end. We emphasize the need for meticulous placement into the subarachnoid space, anchoring of the drain to the pia-arachnoid, and the placement of multiple holes into the tubing to facilitate drainage. Septation and loculation of the syrinx (case 2 of this report) may also prevent complete drainage of the entire syrinx.

The presenting symptoms and signs of the 13 patients with the syrinx associated with a tumor (spinal cord in 12, IVth ventricle in 1) were at least in part secondary to the syrinx. This was borne out by the clinical improvement achieved in 3, with only drainage of the cyst prior to tumor removal. Undoubtedly, the surgical removal of the tumor may provide permanent drainage of the syrinx, as well as removing the source of the syrinx fluid. In the 13 patients in this series, tumor removal has produced cessation of deterioration in 11. In the patient with incomplete tumor removal, improvement may in part be related to syrinx drainage. Obviously, further neurologic deterioration in these patients may result from tumor regrowth.

Thirty-nine of the 90 patients have required more than one procedure to treat the syringomyelia (Table 29.12). The results of this aggressive approach based upon understanding of the pathophysiology of the different varieties of syringomyelia with appropriate treatment directed accordingly have been a stable or improved condition in 72 of the patients with an average follow-up of 7 years.

The investigation and treatment of syringomyelia are not without complications. Although there were no deaths related to surgery, 11 patients were worse immediately following the procedure, but fortunately only transiently in all but 3. The inability to locate the syrinx will undoubtedly occur less frequently in the future, with the more accurate delineation of the extent and position of the cavity within the cord allowed by the modern neuroradiological techniques. Neurologic deteri-

TABLE 29.12

Incidence of Multiple Procedures

Type of Syringomyelia	No. of Procedures				
	1	2	3	4	5
Communicating	19	7	5	2	0
Posttraumatic	15	6	6	1	0
Idiopathic	4	3	0	1	1
Spinal arachnoiditis	5	1	1	0	0
Tumor	8	3	2	0	0
Total	51	20	14	4	1

oration after appropriate surgical therapy, whether occurring soon after surgery or as a late development, does warrant further investigation and consideration of another procedure. Reasons for failure of the first procedure are incorrect diagnosis of the types and pathogenesis of syringomyelia, the presence of anatomically separate cavities within the cord, and technical failure of the original procedure. Excellent long-term results can be obtained if this aggressive approach is thoughtfully applied.

CONCLUSIONS

Modern neuroradiological investigation, including metrizamide myelography, delayed computerized spinal tomography, and occasionally direct puncture of the syrinx for fluid analysis and contrast injection has remarkably improved our ability to diagnose and understand the hydrodynamics of syringomyelia.

Using these techniques, syringomyelia may be divided into 2 major types: *communicating*, in which the syrinx is directly connected to the ventricular system and *noncommunicating*, in which there is no connection. The noncommunicating type may be subdivided into a posttraumatic variety, those associated with spinal arachnoiditis and neoplasia, and an idiopathic variety.

Ninety patients representing all varieties of syringomyelia have been treated with 154 surgical procedures aimed at producing a stable or improved neurological state. Thirty-nine patients required 2 or more procedures.

Of 33 patients with communicating syringomyelia, foramen magnum decompression with IVth ventricular CSF diversion was performed in 30. Thirteen of these patients required an additional procedure, either repeat foramen magnum decompression, syrinx cavity drainage, or a ventriculoperitoneal shunt. Improvement or cessation of neurological deterioration has been achieved in 27 of the 33.

Forty-four patients had posttraumatic, idiopathic, or syringomyelia associated with spinal arachnoiditis. Improvement or clinical stability has resulted from drainage procedures (including spinal cordectomy, syringosubarachnoid and syringoperitoneal shunts) in 34 of these 44 patients. Eleven of 13 patients with tumor-associated syringomyelia have had improvement in their syringomyelic syndromes following resection (total in 8, partial in 4) of the tumor and drainage of the syrinx.

Significant complications of the 154 procedures included severe nausea and vomiting (5 cases) and hydrocephalus (3 cases) after a foramen magnum decompression procedure, transient neurological deterioration (5 cases), increased upper limb pain (5 cases), and inability to locate the syrinx (6 cases) with drainage procedures. Six patients were clinically worse after tumor removal (4 transient, 2 permanent).

Based on this experience we recommend appropriate radiological investigation and surgical treatment in the presence of a progressive neurological condition with a syrinx of moderate to large size. The operative approach to each patient must be based on a clear understanding of the etiology and pathogenesis of the particular syrinx. We see no benefit in operating on the patient with a small syrinx in a collapsed cord or on the patient who is clinically stable. Deterioration in the patient's condition at any time following surgery warrants reinvestigation and reconsideration of further operative treatment.

ACKNOWLEDGMENTS

The authors are indebted to their surgical colleagues Dr. H. W. K. Barr, Dr. C. G. Drake, Dr. G. G. Ferguson, and Dr. J. G. Girvin for permission to include their cases in this review and for their thoughtful care of these patients. We are also particularly fortunate to have been associated with Dr. H. J. M. Barnett whose neurologic expertise and long time interest and enthusiasm for the aggressive investigation and surgical treatment of syringomyelia has attracted many patients to our department. Dr. Alan Fox and his neuroradiological colleagues at the University Hospital, London, have pioneered the development of the modern imaging techniques for syringomyelia which has been invaluable. Finally, we are grateful to Dr. Mary Jean Page for her skillful drawings and to Miss Robin Affleck for preparing the manuscript.

REFERENCES

1. Aboulker, J. La syringomyelie et les liquides intrarachidiens. Neurochirurgie, *25*(Suppl. 1): 1–144, 1979.
2. Aubin, M. L., Vignaud, J., Jardin, C., and Bar, D. Computed tomography in 75 clinical cases of syringomyelia. Am. J. Neuroradiol., *2:* 199–204, 1981.
3. Ball, M. J., and Dayan, A. D. Pathogenesis of syringomyelia. Lancet, *2:* 799–801, 1972.
4. Ballantine, H. T., Ojemann, R. G., and Drew, J. H. Syringohydromyelia. Prog. Neurol. Surg., *4:* 227–245, 1971.
5. Banerji, N. K., and Millar, J. H. D. Chiari malformation presenting in adult life. Its relationship to syringomyelia. Brain, *97:* 157–168, 1974.
6. Barnett, H. J. M., Foster, J. B., and Hudgson, P. Syringomyelia. In *Major Problems in Neurology*, Vol. I, edited by J. N. Walton. W.B. Saunders, Philadelphia, 1973.
7. Barnett, H. J. M., and Jousse, A. T. Post-traumatic syringomyelia (cystic myelopathy) In: *Handbook of Clinical Neurology*, Vol. 26, edited by P. J. Vinken and G. W. Bruyn, pp. 113–157. Elsevier/North-Holland, New York, 1976.
8. Barnett, H. J. M., Jousse, A. T., and Wortzmann, G. W. Four distinct varieties of the syringomyelic syndrome. Trans. Am. Neurol. Assoc., *97:* 171–174, 1972.
9. Boman, K., and Iivanainen, M. Prognosis of syringomyelia. Acta Neurol. Scand., *43:* 61–68, 1967.
10. Cahan, L. D., and Bentson, J. R. Considerations in the diagnosis and treatment of syringomyelia and the Chiari malformation. J. Neurosurg., *57:* 24–31, 1982.
11. Conway, L. W. Hydrodynamic studies in syringomyelia. J. Neurosurg., *27:* 501–514, 1967.
12. duBoulay, G., Shah, S. H., Currie, J. C., and Logue, V. The mechanism of hydromyelia in Chiari type I malformations. Br. J. Radiol., *47:* 579–587, 1974.
13. Durward, Q. J., Rice, G. P., Ball, M. J., Gilbert, J. J., and Kaufmann, J. C. E. Selective spinal cordectomy: Clinicopathological correlation. J. Neurosurg., *56:* 359–367, 1982.

14. Ellestsson, A. B., and Greitz, T. Myelocystographic and fluorescein studies to demonstrate communication between intramedullary cysts and the cerebrospinal fluid space. Acta Neurol. Scand., *45:* 418–430, 1969.
15. Faulhauer, K., Loew, K. The surgical treatment of syringomyelia. Long term results. Acta Neurochir. (Wien) *44:* 215–222, 1978.
16. Feigin, I., Ogota, J., and Budzilovich, J. Syringomyelia: The role of edema in its pathogenesis. J. Neuropathol. Exp. Neurol., *30:* 216–232, 1971.
17. Fox, A. J., Vinuela, F., and Debrun, G. Complete myelography with metrizamide. Am. J. Neuroradiol., *2:* 79–84, 1981.
18. Garcia-Uria, J., Leunda, G., Carrillo, R., and Bravo, G. Syringomyelia: Long-term results after posterior fossa decompression. J. Neurosurg., *54:* 380–383, 1981.
19. Gardner, W. J. Hydrodynamic mechanism of syringomyelia: Its relationship to myelocele. J. Neurol. Neurosurg. Psychiatry, *28:* 247–259, 1965.
20. Gardner, W. J., Bell, H. S., Pooloos, P. N., Dohn, D. F., and Steinberg, M. Terminal ventriculostomy for syringomyelia. J. Neurosurg., *46:* 609–617, 1977.
21. Gardner, W. J., and McMurry, F. G. "Non-communicating syringomyelia": A nonexistent entity. Surg. Neurol., *6:* 251–256, 1976.
22. Hankinson, J. Syringomyelia and the surgeon. Mod. Trends. Neurol., *5:* 127–148, 1970.
23. Jensen, F., and Reske-Nielsen, E. Post-traumatic syringomyelia. Review of the literature and two new autopsy cases. Scand. J. Rehabil. Med., *9:* 35–43, 1977.
24. Jung, E. Syringomyelie in Kombination mit Entwicklungsstorung der Nieren und mit schwerer Wirbelsaulenvertetzung. Med. Klin. *55:* 1678–1689, 1960.
25. Kan, S., Fox, A. J., Vinuela, F., and Debrun, G. Water soluble myelography in syringomyelia: Positional change in cord size. Radiology, *146:* 409–414, 1983.
26. Kan, S., Fox, A. J., Vinuela, F., Barnett, H. J. M., and Peerless, S. J. Delayed CT metrizamide enhancement of syringomyelia secondary to tumor. Am. J. Neuroradiol., *4:* 73–78, 1983.
27. Klawans, H. L., Jr. Delayed traumatic syringomyelia. Dis. Nerv. Syst., *29:* 525–528, 1968.
28. Krayenbuhl, H. Evaluation of the different surgical approaches in the treatment of syringomyelia. Clin. Neurol. Neurosurg., *77:* 110–128, 1975.
29. Krayenbuhl, H., and Benini, A. A new surgical approach in the treatment of hydromyelia and syringomyelia. The embryological basis and first results. J. R. Coll. Surg. Edinb., *16:* 147–161, 1971.
30. Logue, V., and Edwards, M. R. Syringomyelia and its surgical treatment—an analysis of 75 patients. J. Neurol. Neurosurg. Psychiatry, *44:* 273–284, 1981.
31. Love, J. G., Olafson, R. A. Syringomyelia: A look at surgical therapy. J. Neurosurg., *24:* 714–718, 1966.
32. McLean, D. R., Miller, J. D. R., Allen, P. B. R., and Ezzeddin, S. A. Post-traumatic syringomyelia. J. Neurosurg., *39:* 485–492, 1973.
33. Newton, E. J. Syringomyelia as a manifestation of defective fourth ventricular drainage. Ann. R. Coll. Surg. Engl., *44:* 194–213, 1969.
34. Nurick, S., Russell, J. A., and Deck, M. D. A. Cystic degeneration of the spinal cord following spinal cord injury. Brain, *93:* 211–222, 1970.
35. Pitts, F. W., and Groff, R. A. Syringomyelia: Current status of surgical therapy. Surgery, *56:* 806–809, 1964.
36. Poser, C. M. The Relationship between Syringomyelia and Neoplasm. Charles C Thomas, Springfield, Ill., 1956.
37. Rhoton, A. L., Jr. Microsurgery of Arnold-Chiari malformation and hydromyelia in adults. In: *Microneurosurgery*, Ed. 2, edited by R. W. Rand, C.V. Mosby, St. Louis, 1978.

38. Savoiardo, M. Syringomyelia associated with post-meningitis spinal arachnoiditis. Filling of the syrinx through a communication with the subarachnoid space. Neurology, *26:* 551–554, 1976.
39. Saez, R. J., Onofrio, B. M., and Yanaghihara, T. Experience with Arnold-Chiari malformation, 1960–1970. J. Neurosurg., *45:* 416–422, 1976.
40. Scher, A. T. Syringomyelia secondary to paraplegia due to fracture of the thoracic spine. South African Med. J., *50:* 1406–1408, 1976.
41. Schliep, G. Syringomyelia and syringobulbia. In: *Handbook of Clinical Neurology*, Vol. 32, edited by P. J. Vinken, and G. W. Bruyn, pp. 255–327. Elsevier/North Holland, New York, 1978.
42. Shannon, N., Symon, L., Logue, V., Cull, D., Kang, J., and Kendall, B. Clinical features, investigation and treatment of post-traumatic syringomyelia. J. Neurol. Neurosurg. Psychiatry, *44:* 35–42, 1981.
43. Tator, C. H., Meguro, K., and Rowed, D. W. Favourable results with syringosubarachnoid shunts for treatment of syringomyelia. J. Neurosurg., *56:* 517–523, 1982.
44. Werner, A., Rossier, A., Berney, J., and Zdojewski, B. A propos de quatre observations de syringomyelie cervicale tardive apres traumatisme medullaire. Arch. Suisse Neurol. Neurochir. Psychiatr., *104:* 77–86, 1969.
45. Williams, B., Terry, A. F., Jones, F., and McSweeney, T. Syringomyelia as a sequel to traumatic paraplegia. Paraplegia, *19:* 67–80, 1981.
46. Williams, B. A critical appraisal of posterior fossa surgery for communicating syringomyelia. Brain, *101:* 223–250, 1978.
47. Williams, B. Current concepts of syringomyelia. Br. J. Hosp. Med., *4:* 331–342, 1970.
48. Williams, B. On the pathogenesis of syringomyelia: A review. J. R. Soc. Med., *73:* 798–806, 1980.
49. Woosley, R. E., and Whaley, R. A. Use of metrizamide in computerized tomography to diagnose the Chiari I malformation. J. Neurosurg., *56:* 373–376, 1982.
50. Wyburn-Mason, R. The vascular abnormalities and tumours of the spinal cord and its membranes. H. Kimptom, London, 1943.

CHAPTER

30

Diagnosis and Management of Thoracic Disc Disease

VALLO BENJAMIN, M.D.

Since the first report by Middleton and Teacher (19) in 1911 of a ruptured thoracic disc, resulting in paraplegia and subsequent death, the rarity as well as the extreme difficulty in diagnosis and management of thoracic disc protrusions has been documented in numerous publications (2, 11, 15, 16, 20, 21, 26).

In this report we shall review recent developments in the methods of diagnosis and surgical treatment of symptomatic protrusions of thoracic discs.

DIAGNOSIS

Clinical Diagnosis

An accurate diagnosis of this disease based on clinical features is, for all practical intents and purposes, impossible. *Pain* or Myelopathy, either alone or in combination, are the two modes of clinical presentation seen in this disease. A "high index of suspicion" in thoracic myelopathies may steer the clinician's attention to the appropriate investigations leading to a definitive diagnosis.

PAIN

An overwhelming majority of patients will describe a dull dorsal, deep retrosternal, or retrogastric pain which may have been present for many years. Others may complain of unilateral or bilateral radicular pain, but it is rare that the pain is "unbearable in nature."

MYELOPATHY

Most patients seen by neurological surgeons have some evidence of spinal cord dysfunction. Although a typical or classical clinical picture of myelopathy has not been established throughout the literature, the motor signs and symptoms predominate. It is extremely unusual that a patient will have sensory manifestations without any motor component. Problems of sexual and sphincteric malfunctions are uncommon, and are seen mostly in the latter stages of this disease.

Radiological Diagnosis

In the literature it is agreed that a definitive diagnosis can only be made based on radiological examinations, *i.e.*, conventional radiography, tomography, positive contrast myelography, and CT scan.

CONVENTIONAL RADIOGRAPHY

It is certainly unusual that the initial diagnosis is suspected or made from routine radiological examination of the thoracic spine. This difficulty is in part related to the generally poor technical quality of most radiographs of this area and to some extent to inattention to the posterior margins of the disc spaces in multiple segments of the thoracic spine (Fig. 30.1).

It should be noted that conventional x-ray is valuable only in the presence of calcified protrusions or spondylosis of the spine. A retrospective review of the radiographs of our 24 cases with hard protrusions has shown that in 10 patients the calcified protrusion could be seen within the spinal canal (Fig. 30.2).

TOMOGRAPHY

This examination is similarly useful only in patients with calcified protrusions and spondylosis. Its value is generally in the initial screening of multiple levels of the spinal column (Fig. 30.3). For a more definitive diagnosis, however, the high resolution CT scan is rapidly replacing the need for tomography.

POSITIVE CONTRAST MYELOGRAPHY

The diagnosis of thoracic disc protrusion can be accurately established by myelography. With oil myelography (Pantopaque), at least 30–40 ml of contrast are required for visualization of the thoracic segment. The advantage of Pantopaque is in its high contrast *vs.* the low contrast of the water-soluble mediums, caused partially by dilution factors. The disadvantages of Pantopaque are problems related to its high viscosity and its permanent retention within the subarachnoid space. Due to the high viscosity of the oil in cases of complete subarachnoid block, thoracic disc protrusions have been mistaken for intra- or extramedullary tumors (Figs. 30.4–30.6). The problem of retention of contrast can be troublesome in patients with congenital narrowing of the spinal canal, in those requiring repeated examinations, or in the presence of arachnoiditis. Finally, retention of oil contrast around the area of pathology may render CT scanning very difficult.

The advantages of water-soluble contrast are in its lower viscosity, which generally allows the medium to pass the area of blockage and encircle the lesion. There is no possibility of retention, and multiple

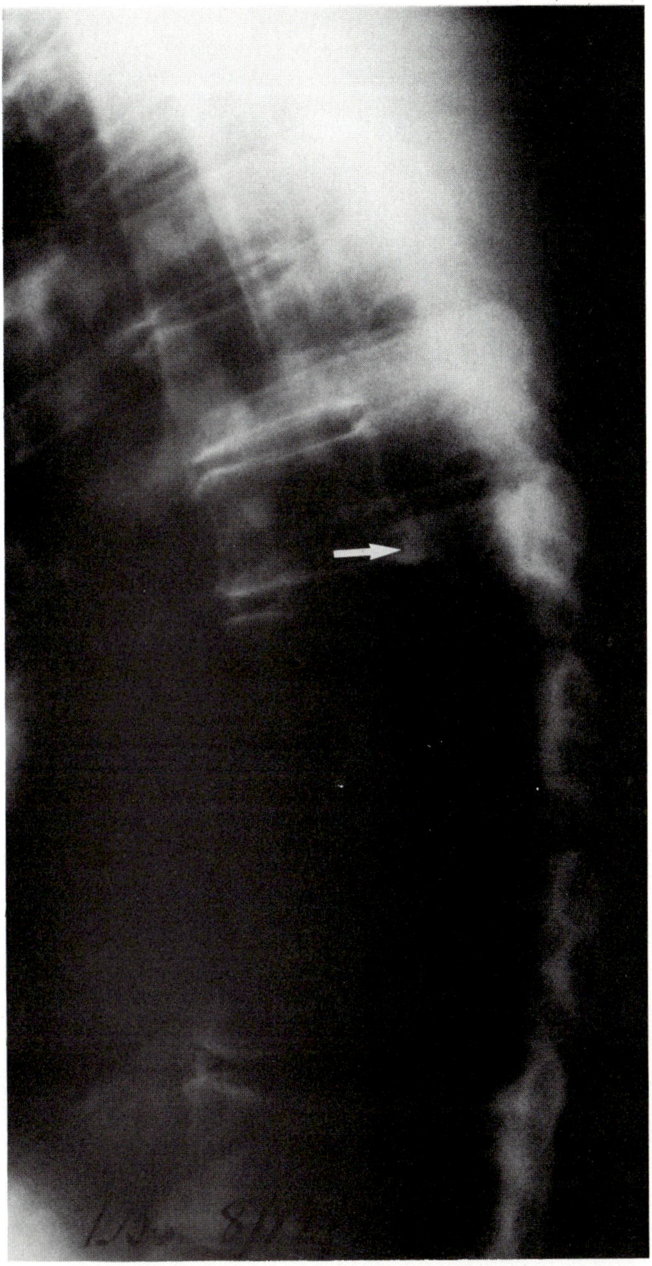

FIG. 30.1. Despite an inadequate lateral view of the thoracic spine, with careful attention to the posterior margin of the T_6 vertebra, a protruding calcified disc can be seen (*arrow*).

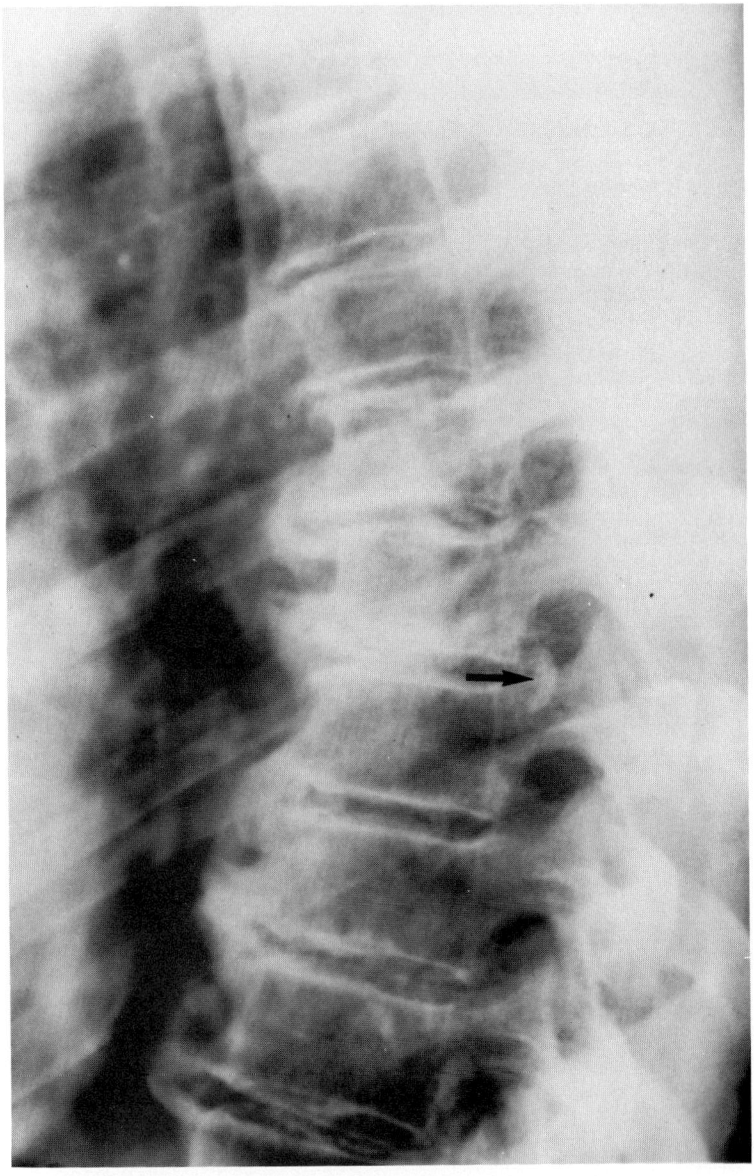

FIG. 30.2. A retrospective review of the lateral thoracic spine showing a calcified thoracic disc protrusion within the spinal canal (*arrow*).

examinations can be done without any difficulty. However, the main advantage is that it can be used in conjunction with a CT scan (Fig. 30.7). In the light of recent experience water soluble mediums are the agents of choice for myelography.

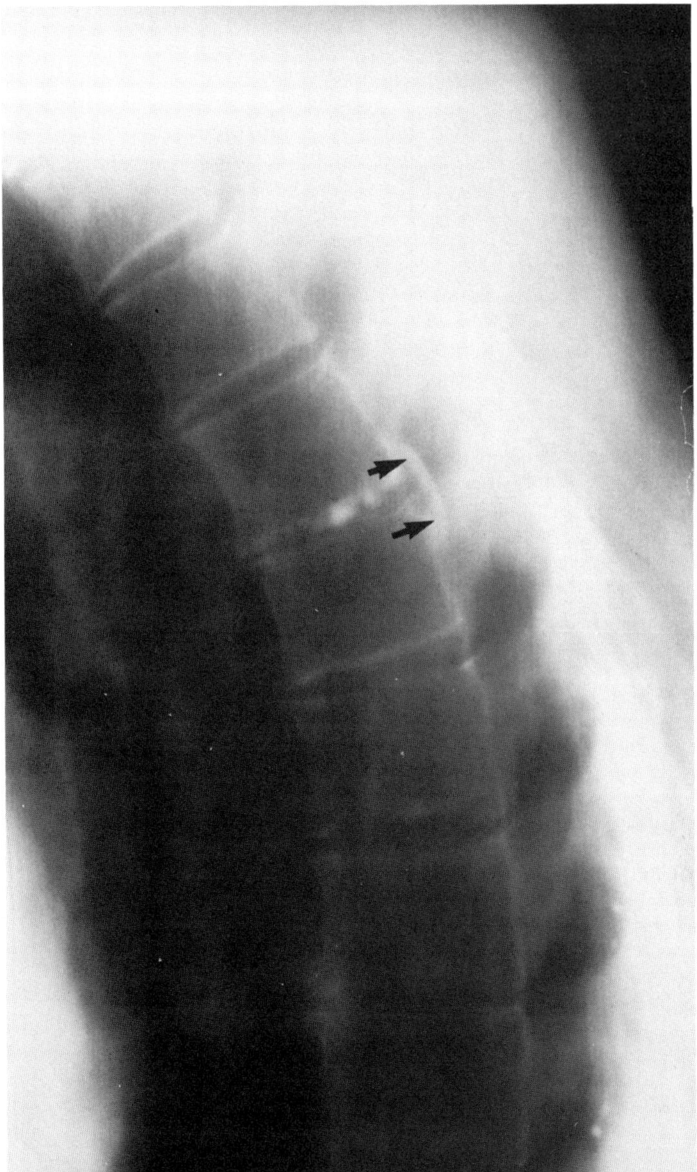

FIG. 30.3. Tomography of the thoracic spine, used for initial screening, indicating a calcified thoracic disc protrusion (*arrows*).

CT SCANNING

It is obvious that a CT scan is done only when the level of the involved disc is either suspected or the diagnosis is firmly established by conventional x-rays, tomography, or myelography. Although the entire thoracic

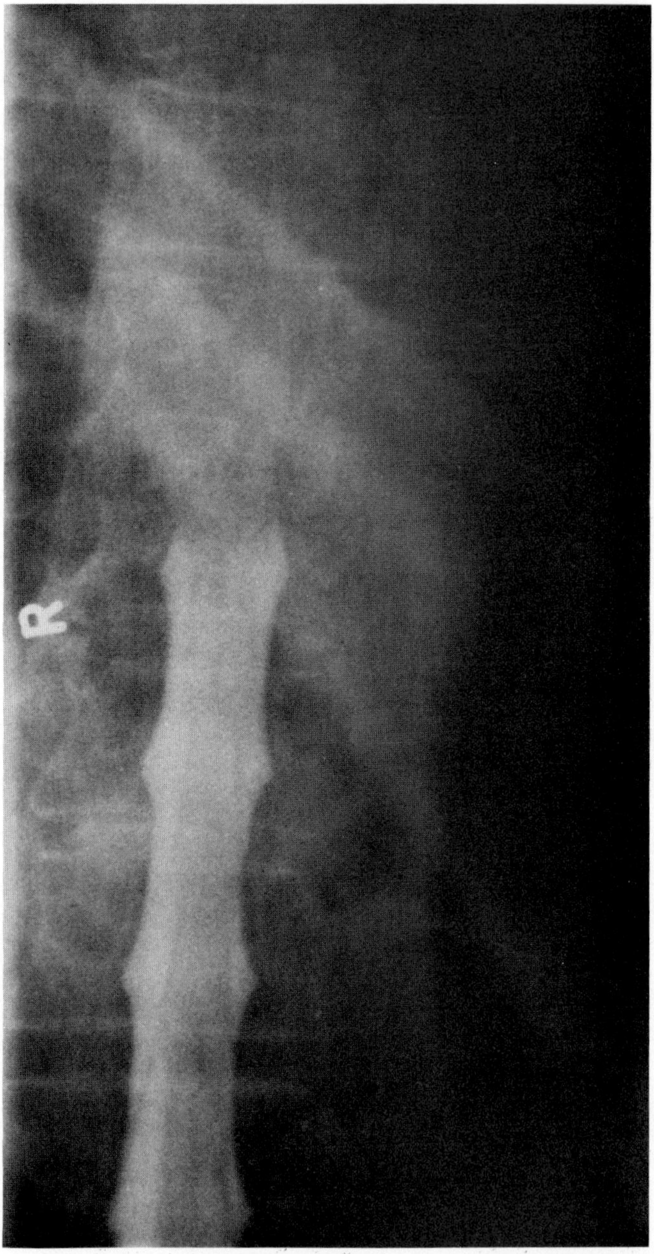

FIG. 30.4. AP view of a Pantopaque myelogram with complete block at $T_{8\text{-}9}$, initially interpreted as an intradural extramedullary tumor.

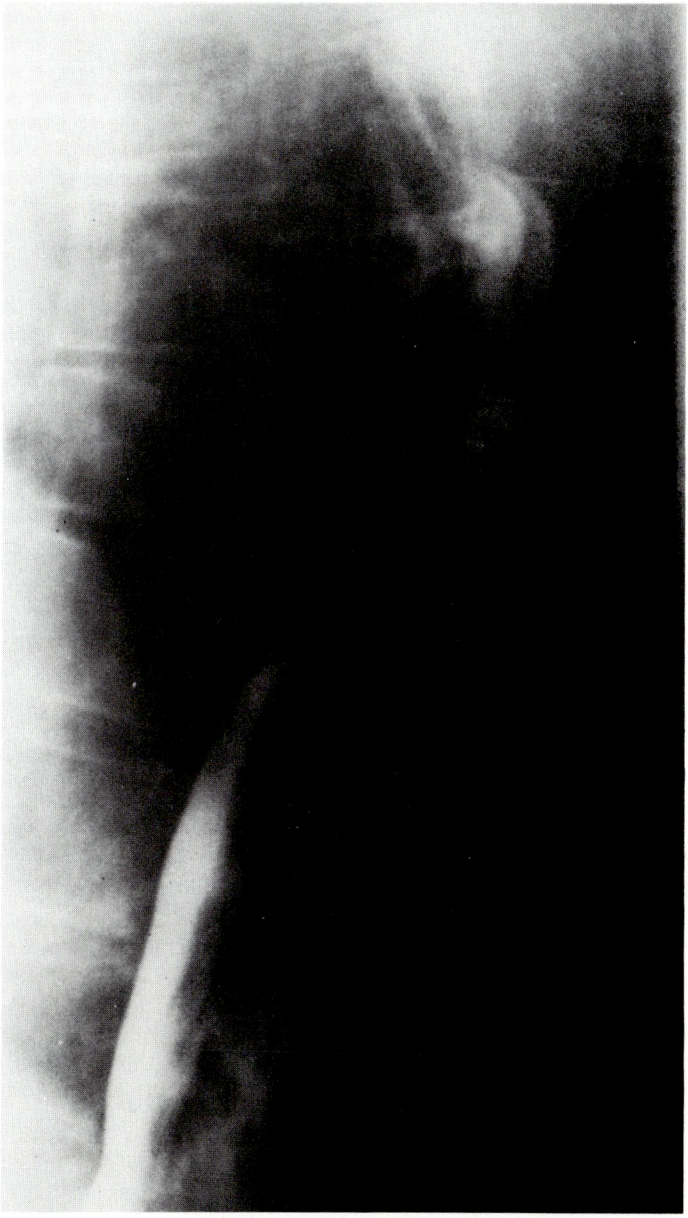

FIG. 30.5. Lateral view of the Pantopaque myelogram in the same patient as Figure 30.4

spine can as a routine be evaluated by CT scan, using the CT scan increases significantly the patient's exposure to radiation.

Since 1976, 12 patients with thoracic disc disease have been studied with CT scan, and the information gained has been invaluable. In the

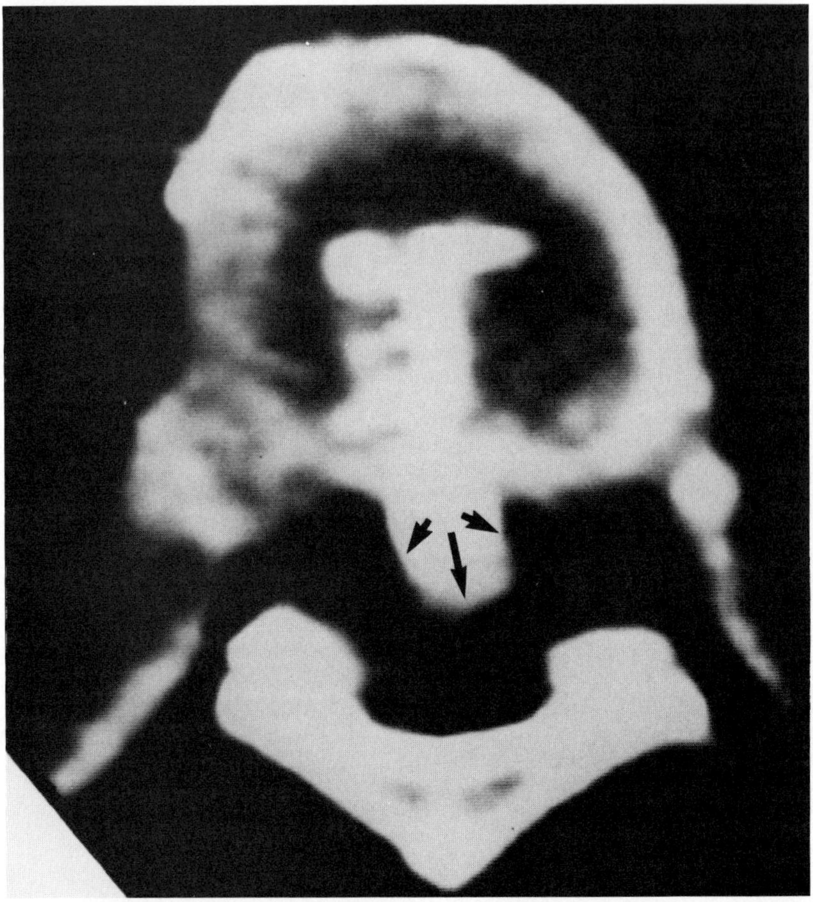

FIG. 30.6. Postmyelographic CT scan of the same patient as in Figures 30.4 and 30.5, showing a large calcified protrusion of the thoracic disc within the spinal canal (*arrows*).

latest patient in whom a calcified T_{7-8} disc protrusion was suspected from conventional radiographs, CT examination of the lesion with sagittal reconstruction gave sufficient information to preclude the need for myelography (Figs. 30.8–30.11). CT examination without subarachnoid contrast is mainly valuable in the presence of calcifications, *i.e.*, anterior calcified discs, spondylosis of the vertebrae or joints, and ossification of the ligamentous structures. In all of these lesions the sagittal reconstruction of the spine will show the longitudinal and transverse extent of the pathology.

Combined CT scan with water-soluble contrast myelography is particularly useful in patients with soft herniations of the disc.

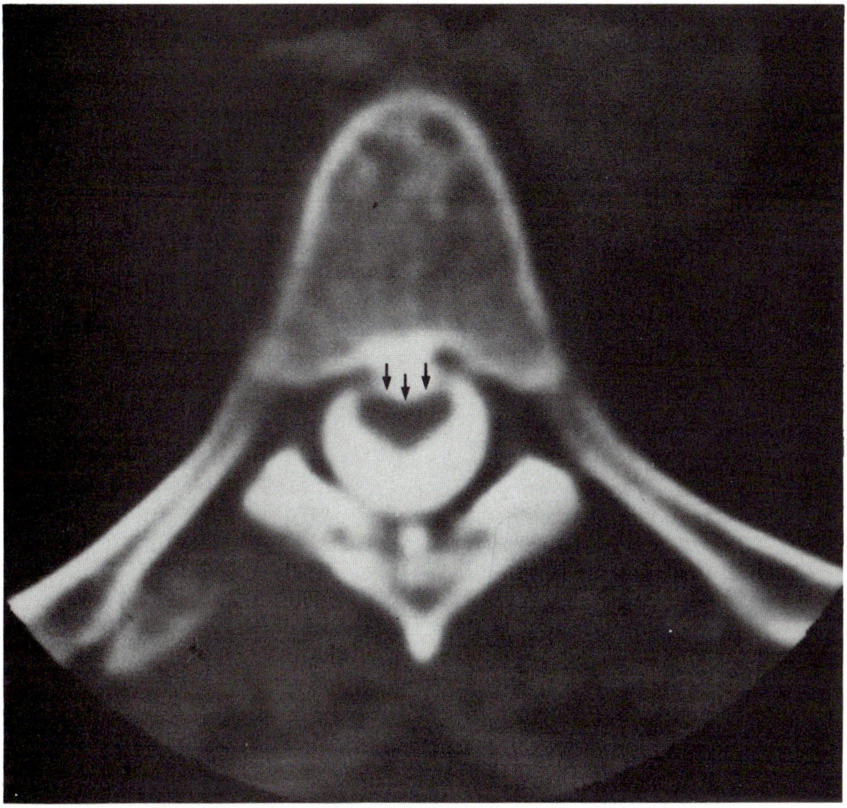

FIG. 30.7. Combined water-soluble myelography and CT scan showing a calcified disc protrusion with ventral compression of the spinal cord (*arrows*).

High resolution CT scan has significantly improved the diagnosis and aided immeasurably in planning the surgical treatment of these difficult lesions.

MANAGEMENT

Pain

Patients suffering from midline or radicular pain without neurological deficits rarely require surgical intervention. Only one patient in our series of 30 operated thoracic discs presented with pain alone. However, if the pain is intractable, there may be no other alternative but surgical excision of the lesion.

Myelopathy

Progressive signs and symptoms of spinal cord dysfunction due to a thoracic disc protrusion are absolute indications for surgical treatment.

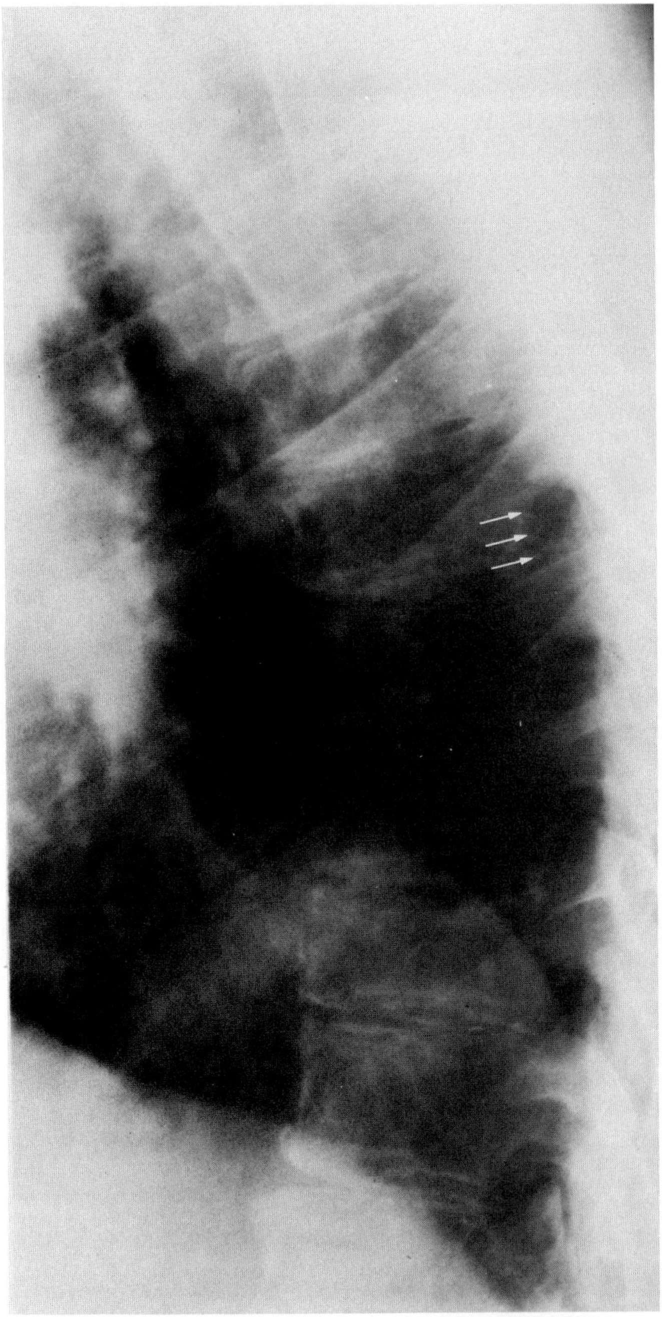

FIG. 30.8. A calcified thoracic disc protrusion at $T_{7\text{-}8}$ (*arrows*) was suspected on a lateral x-ray taken 2 years prior to the patient's evaluation at NYU Medical Center.

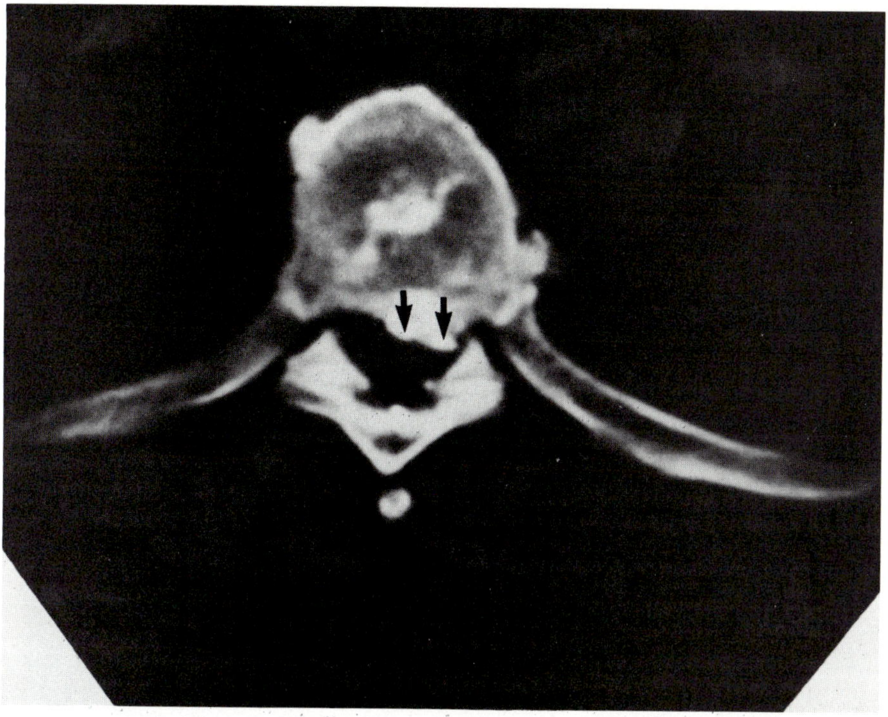

FIG. 30.9. CT scan of the same patient as in Figure 30.8, showing a left paramedian calcified disc protrusion (*arrows*).

The results of surgical decompression are best in those patients with shorter clinical histories, a result similar to observations reported in patients with cervical spondylotic myelopathy.

SURGERY OF THORACIC DISC DISEASE

From early experiences of surgical assault on thoracic discs by Mixter and Barr (20), Hawk (11), Love and Kiefer (16), Müller (21), and Logue (15), it was abundantly clear that laminectomy resulted in an unacceptably high incidence of severe neurological deterioration or paraplegia. In the 206 reported cases collected from the literature, 23 presented with radicular pain and 183 with myelopathy. After laminectomy 107 patients improved, 29 were unchanged, and 68 were made worse, paraplegic, or subsequently died, a poor result amounting to 47% (Table 30.1) (3).

Since the first report of Crafoord *et. al.* in 1958 (10) of a transthoracic approach, and that of Hulme in 1960 (12) of 6 patients with anterior-lateral approaches for thoracic discs, it is generally agreed that some form of an anterior or lateral approach carries the least risk of injury to the cord during surgery and produces the best neurological results.

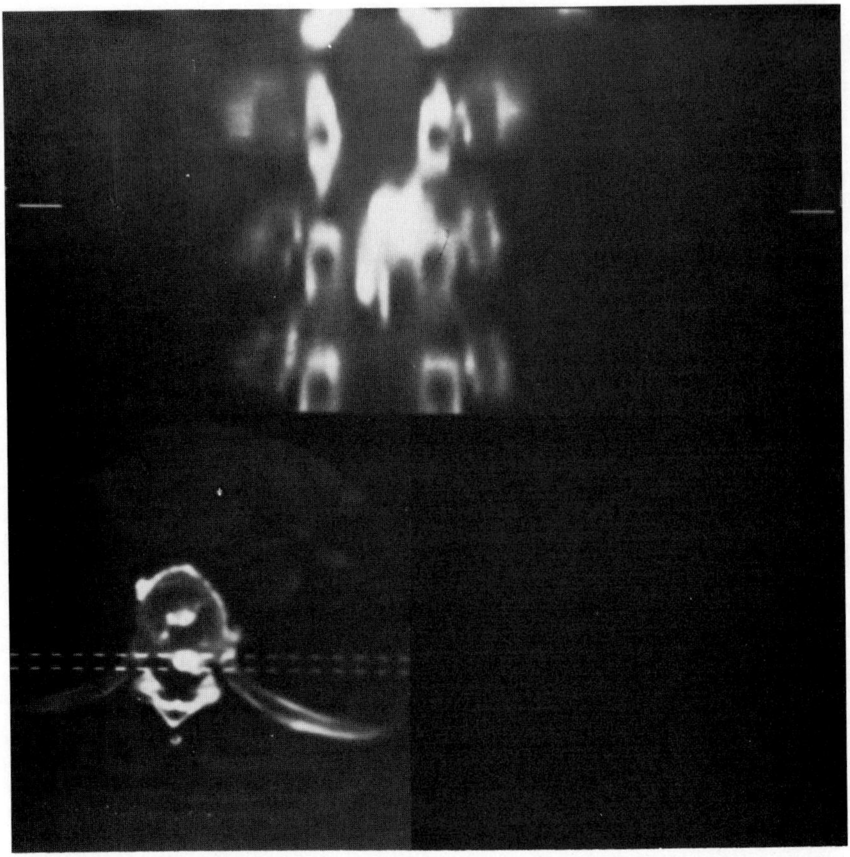

FIG. 30.10. AP reconstruction of CT scan of the same patient as in Figures 30.8 and 30.9, showing the predominantly left-sided location, and the transverse and the inferior extensions of the lesion.

At present there are 3 types of anterior or lateral approaches used for removal of thoracic disc protrusion:

1. Transthoracic transpleural (10)
2. Anterior-lateral extrapleural approach (or modified costotransversectomy) (12)
3. Posterior-lateral approach (through laminectomy, facetectomy, and pediculectomy) (13)

In the literature there is no consensus of opinion as to which of these approaches incurs the least risk of injury to the cord and results in maximum neurological improvement. This is in part related to the small number of reported cases (40 of them) and their relatively short follow-up (3). In our series of 29 patients, the transthoracic transpleural ap-

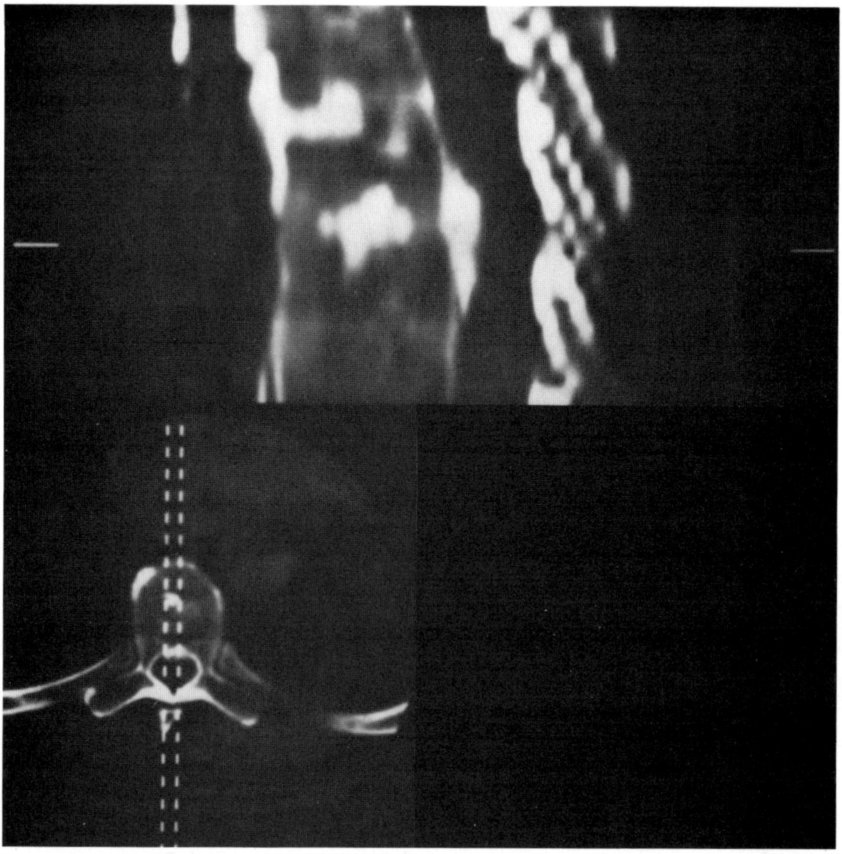

FIG. 30.11. Lateral reconstruction of the CT scan of the same patient as in Figures 30.8–30.10, showing the superior, inferior, and posterior protrusions of the calcification within the spinal canal.

TABLE 30.1
Literature (1922–1982): Results of Laminectomy[a]

Improved	Unchanged	Worse, Paraplegic, or Dead
107 (51.9%)	29 (14%)	68 (33%)

[a] A total of 206 cases were studied, 23 of them involving radiculopathy.

proach was clearly a superior procedure in 25 cases. Of the 4 patients operated by the anterior-lateral (extrapleural operation), 3 required re-operations via the transthoracic transpleural approach at a later date, due to inadequate removal of the calcified disc (3).

One should keep in mind that the procedure of choice should be capable of resulting in total removal of all the protruding disc material within the spinal canal, without the slightest manipulation of the spinal cord. Therefore, an accurate preoperative assessment and knowledge of the gross pathological anatomy of the lesion is essential, prior to selection of the best surgical method.

GROSS PATHOLOGICAL ANATOMY AND SELECTION OF SURGICAL APPROACH

For *surgical* purposes a diseased thoracic disc resulting in root or cord compression can be divided into *soft* and *hard* protrusion; 30 patients operated for thoracic disc problems have shown the following pathological varieties, as illustrated in Table 30.2.

Soft Herniations

For *lateral soft* disc herniations a posterior-lateral appraoch through resection of the lamina, facet, and pedicle, as described by Jefferson (13) and Patterson and Arbit (25), is sufficient for safe removal of these lesions; however, the anterior-lateral extrapleural approach of Hulme (12) is as good, if not better. The transthoracic transpleural approach, despite affording the most direct and best exposure of the anterior aspect of the dura, may be too major a procedure for this variety.

Paramedian soft herniations can safely be removed with either an anterior-lateral (extrapleural) or transthoracic transpleural approach. The posterior-lateral approach is the least desirable method of surgery.

In *central soft* herniations, the best approach for this pathology, which may on occasion lie under the posterior longitudinal ligament, or rarely penetrate through the dura, is the transthoracic transpleural approach. The anterior-lateral extrapleural approach is less, and the posterior-lateral certainly is the least suitable of the three.

TABLE 30.2

Results of Surgery for 30 Patients with Thoracic Disc Problems

Soft Protrusions	6	1 Lateral
		4 Paramedian
		1 Central
Hard Protrusions	24	0 Lateral
		5 Paramedian
		11 Central
		6 Transverse bars
		2 Posterior-lateral spondylosis
Total	30	

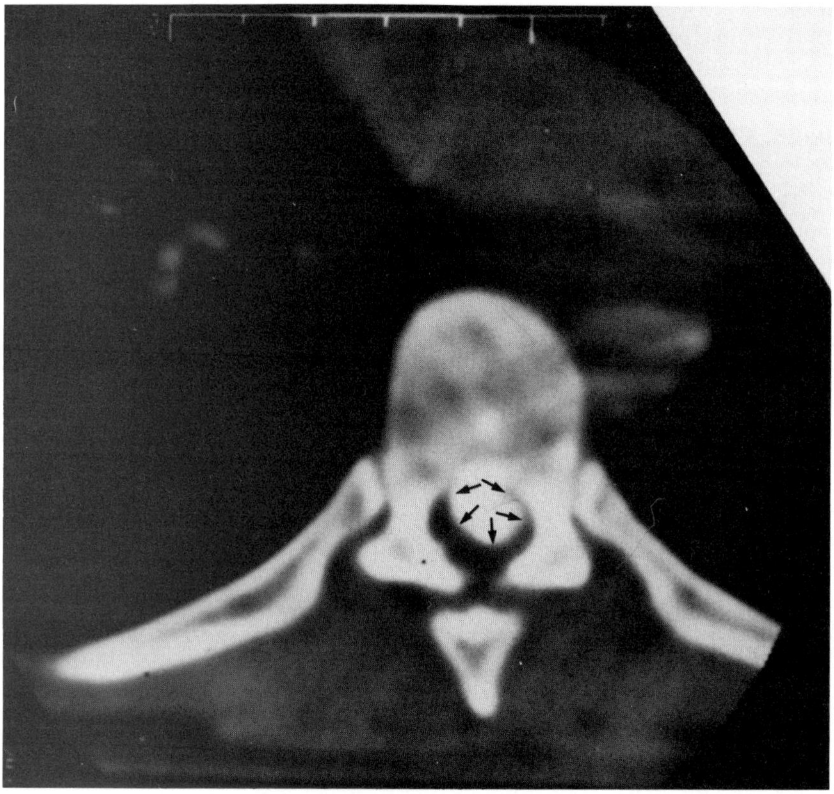

FIG. 30.12. CT scan showing a very large calcified disc protrusion occupying most of the spinal canal (*arrows*) which, in the author's opinion, could not be safely removed, except through a transthoracic transpleural approach.

Hard Protrusions

In all hard varieites of disc protrusion, the operation of choice, with the exception of posterior-lateral spondylosis, is undoubtedly the transthoracic transpleural. This method affords the most direct exposure of the anterior dura and permits removal of the calcified protruding lesion without the least manipulation of the cord (Figs. 30.12 and 30.13). In addition, multiple levels can be approached with ease, and if fusion is deemed necessary, it can be readily performed.

Posterior-lateral spondylosis with cord compression is an extremely rare pathological entity, as verified by a few reported cases (14, 18, 22), and in our own series of 30 patients, only 2 presented with such pathology (Figs. 30.14–30.17). The best operation for these lesions is a posterior-lateral approach, with bilateral removal of the lamina, the medial half of

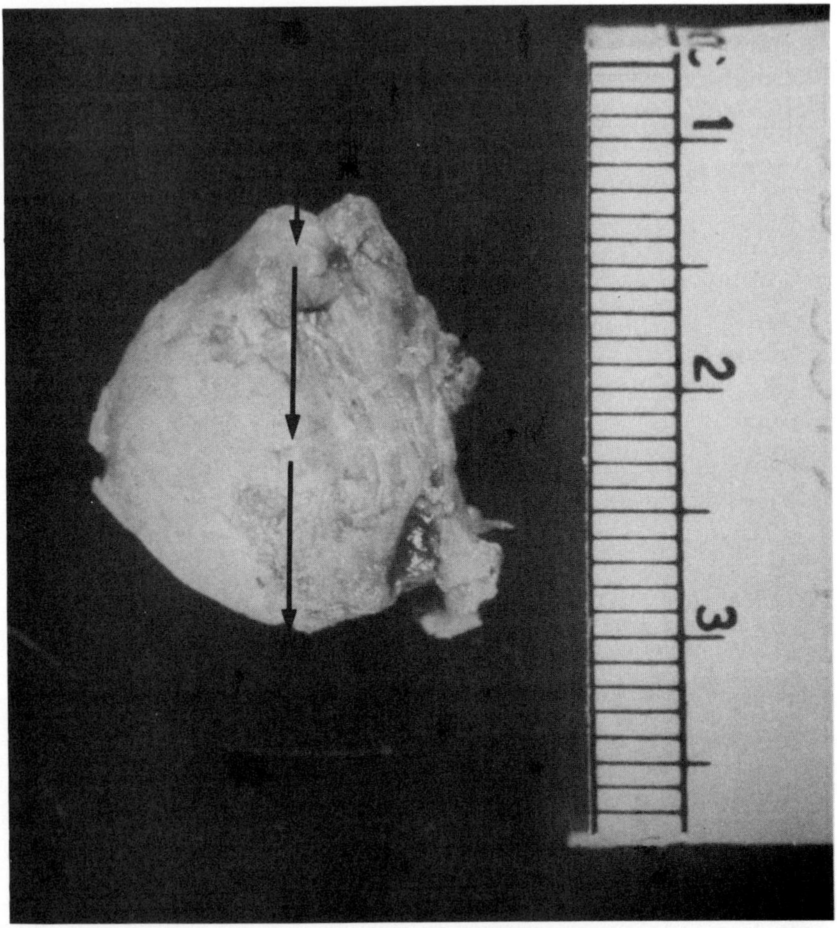

FIG. 30.13. Operative specimen of a large calcified disc with 8 mm of protrusion into the spinal canal (to the *left* of the *arrows*), removed through a transthoracic transpleural approach.

the diseased facet, and the buckled ligamentum flavum. Since by definition in this variety the anterior protrusion of the disc does not exist, manipulation of the cord is unnecessary. In rare cases which present with a significant protrusion of the disc anteriorly, in conjunction with posterior-lateral spondylosis, the transthoracic transpleural operation with fusion should be done first, and at a later date a posterior laminectomy and facetectomy should result in decompression of the spinal cord circumferentially.

Although these given categories may be somewhat arbitrary, and patients may present with other varieties and/or multiple levels, the

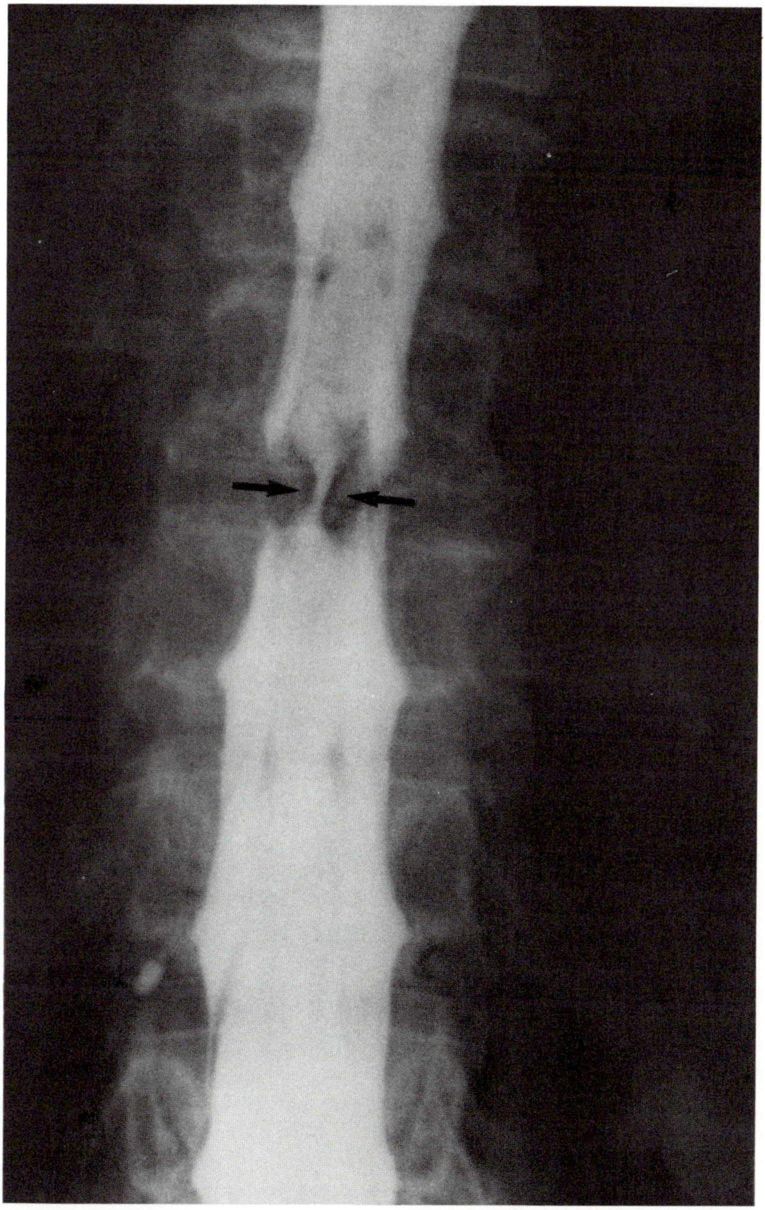

FIG. 30.14. AP view of a Pantopaque myelogram showing bilateral defects (*arrows*) related to lateral spondylosis with a consequent cord compression.

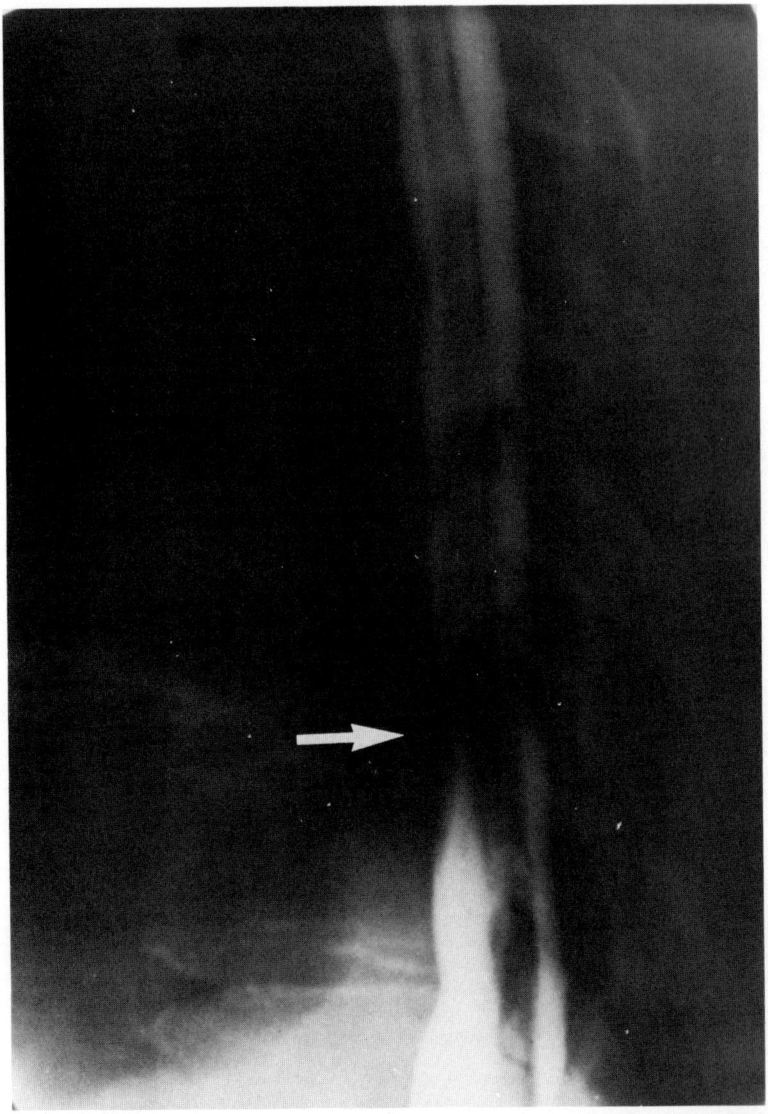

FIG. 30.15. Lateral view of the myelogram in the same patient showing no evidence of a ventral disc protrusion (*arrow*).

point to be made is that the selection of the appropriate operation must be tailored to the 3-dimensional configuration of the pathology.

RECENT DEVELOPMENTS

Water-soluble myelography and high resolution CT scanning of the spine with sagittal and coronal reconstruction have been important

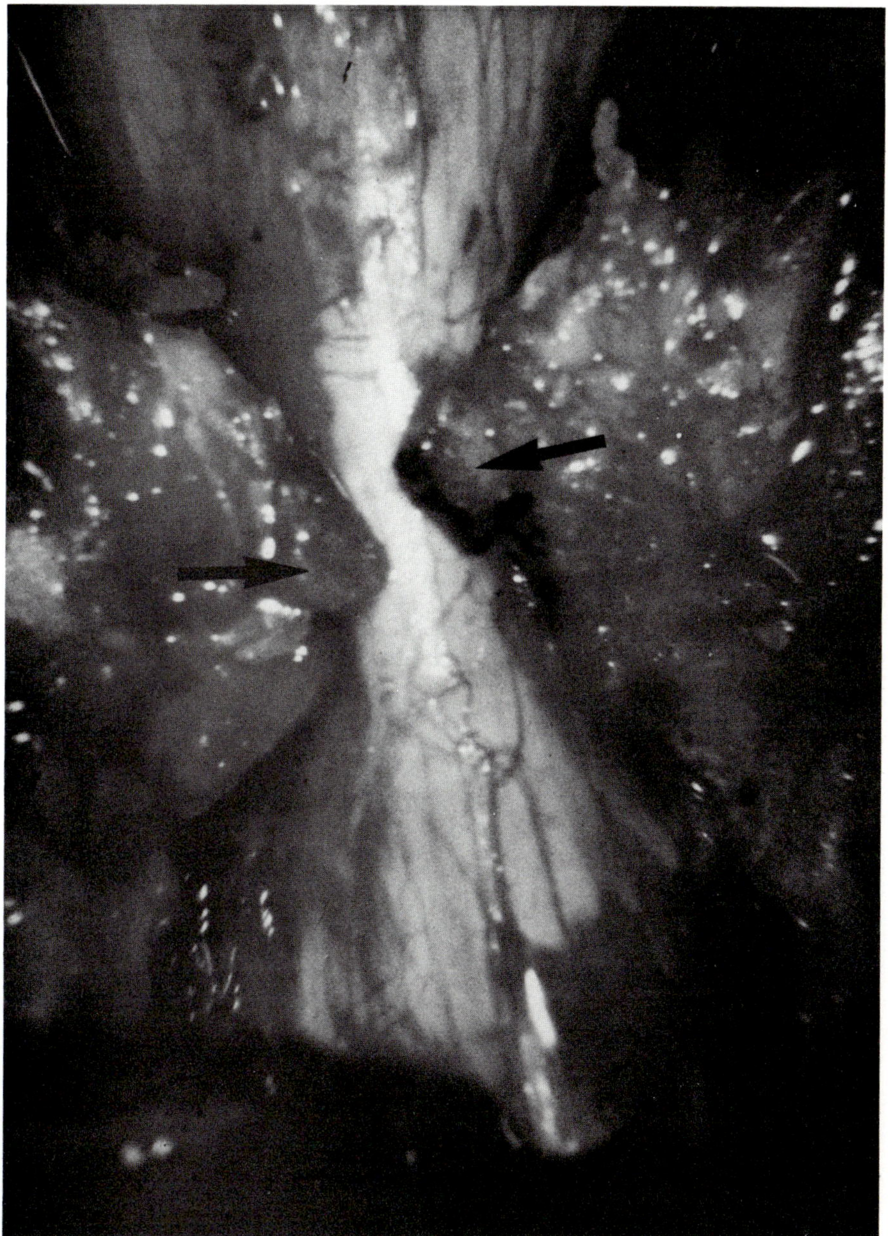

FIG. 30.16. Intraoperative dorsal view of the lateral spondylosis (*arrows*), with dural compression corresponding to AP myelographic defects in Figure 30.14.

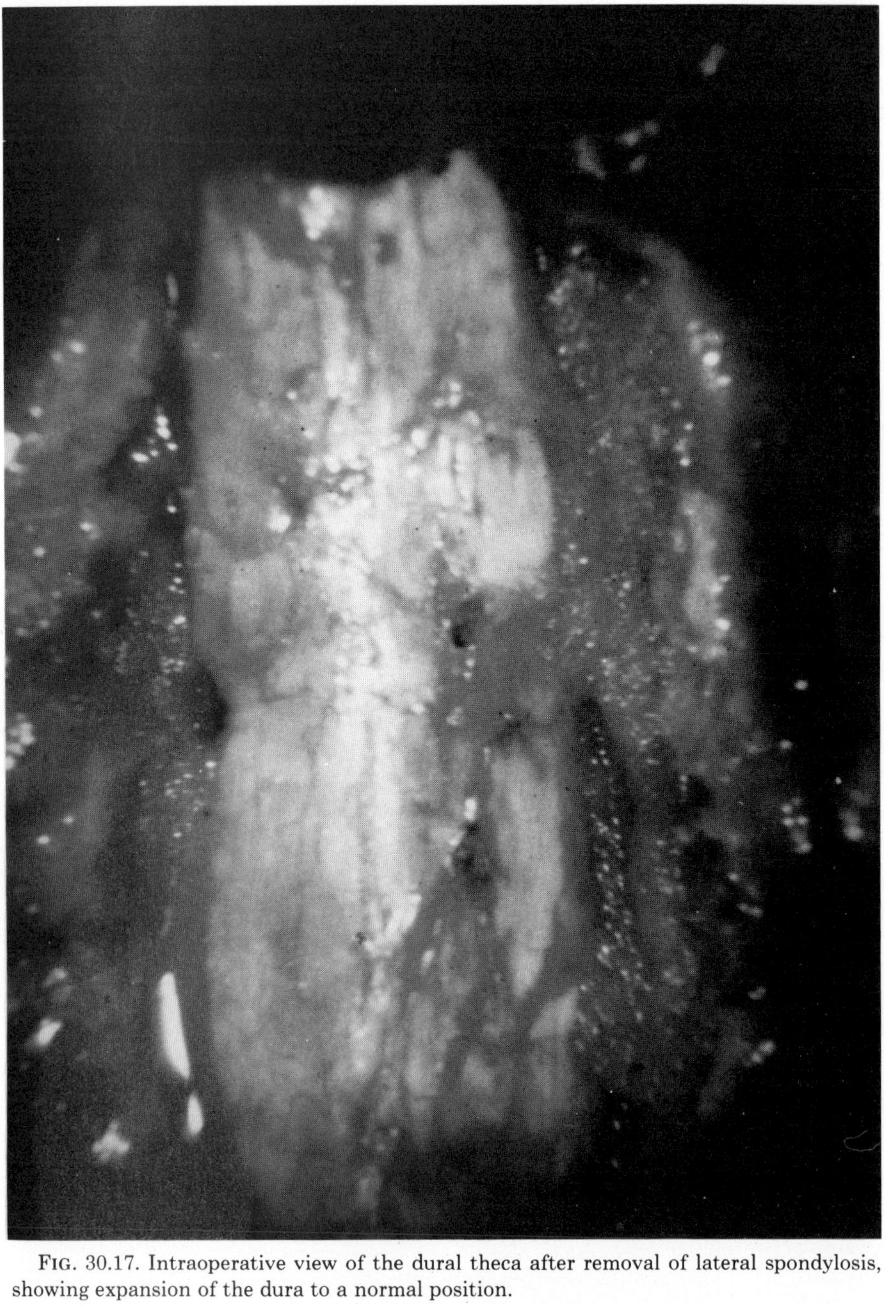

FIG. 30.17. Intraoperative view of the dural theca after removal of lateral spondylosis, showing expansion of the dura to a normal position.

advances in understanding the surgical anatomy of these lesions. The CT may also show whether the lesion is eccentric and thus enables one to change appropriately the side of operation, either to the right or left (Fig. 30.9). In some patients with large calcified discs, the protrusion appears to occupy almost the entire spinal canal (Fig. 30.12). Clearly, in such cases the slightest manipulation of the cord could have disastrous consequences; therefore, this leaves one with very little margin for error.

In the surgical field, development of high speed drills, bipolar coagulation, and magnification have made it possible to excise these lesions with excellent results. The numbers are admittedly small, but they have been consistent, both in the literature and in our own series (Table 30.3 and 30.4). Regardless of which of the three basic approaches is utilized, usage of the high speed drill is imperative in removal of the lamina, facet, pedicle, rib, or vertebra. The advantages of bipolar coagulation and magnification are self evident.

Anterior Approaches

Detailed techniques for the various lateral and anterior approaches and their modficiations have already been described in the literature (4, 5, 9, 10, 12, 13, 25–27). In the anterior intra- or extrapleural approaches, the following steps should be kept in mind.

VASCULAR BUNDLE

The radicular arteries and veins traverse the midsection of the vertebra and enter the neural foramina below each pedicle of the respective vertebra. These vessels can be dissected from their adipose and vertebral attachments, retracted by a suture, and secured to the pleura above and below, thus exposing half of each vertebra adjacent to the affected disc.

TABLE 30.3

Literature (1958–1982) Results of Anterior Approach[a]

Improved	Unchanged	Paraplegic
37 (90.2%)	3 (7.3%)	1 (2.4%)

[a] A total of 41 cases were studied.

TABLE 30.4

Author's Surgical Results[a]

Immediate Neurological Improvement	Unchanged	Worse
25 (92.6%)	2 (7.4%)	0

[a] Data from total of 27 patients.

Section of one or more of these vessels during operations for kyphosis, tumors, and infections has not resulted in injury to the spinal cord.

RIB RESECTION

One must remove the head of the rib overlying the posterior-lateral anulus and the adjacent vertebral bodies. In the transthoracic transpleural approach, the neck of the rib does not need to be excised; on the other hand, in the anterior-lateral extrapleural operation, the head, neck, and angle of one or more ribs should be removed, for a more anterior visualization of the dural theca. Another reason for the removal of rib is exposure of the pedicle of the inferior vertebrae, which underlies the head of the rib.

DRILLING OF VERTEBRAE

Drilling is begun at the posterior margin of the two vertebrae adjacent to the disc. A cavity 2.5 to 3 cm deep is made in the posterior half of the vertebrae, and a thin layer of bone is left overlying the anterior bony canal (Fig. 30.18).

PEDICLE

The pedicle of the inferior vertebra should be removed with the drill, as this results in exposure of the lateral spinal canal. The dura underlying the pedicle is virtually free of venous structures (Fig. 30.19). Removal of the pedicle also facilitates the exposure of the posterior longitudinal ligament. Since most large calcified discs extend below the pedicle, complete and safe removal depends on adequate exposure beyond the protrusion.

EPIDURAL VENOUS PLEXUS

Anatomically, most of the venous drainage exits through a venous plexus firmly attached to the root sleeve, which can be troublesome during surgery, but the use of bipolar coagulation and Gelfoam should be sufficient to stop the bleeding.

REMOVAL OF DISC COMPLEX

Since in all calcified discs and in spondylotic bars some portion of the vertebra is involved in the protrusion, the entire complex should be removed in one piece (Figs. 30.20–30.22).

If the posterior longitudinal ligament and the disc complex are found to be firmly attached to the dura (in our series, this occurred in 4 of 30

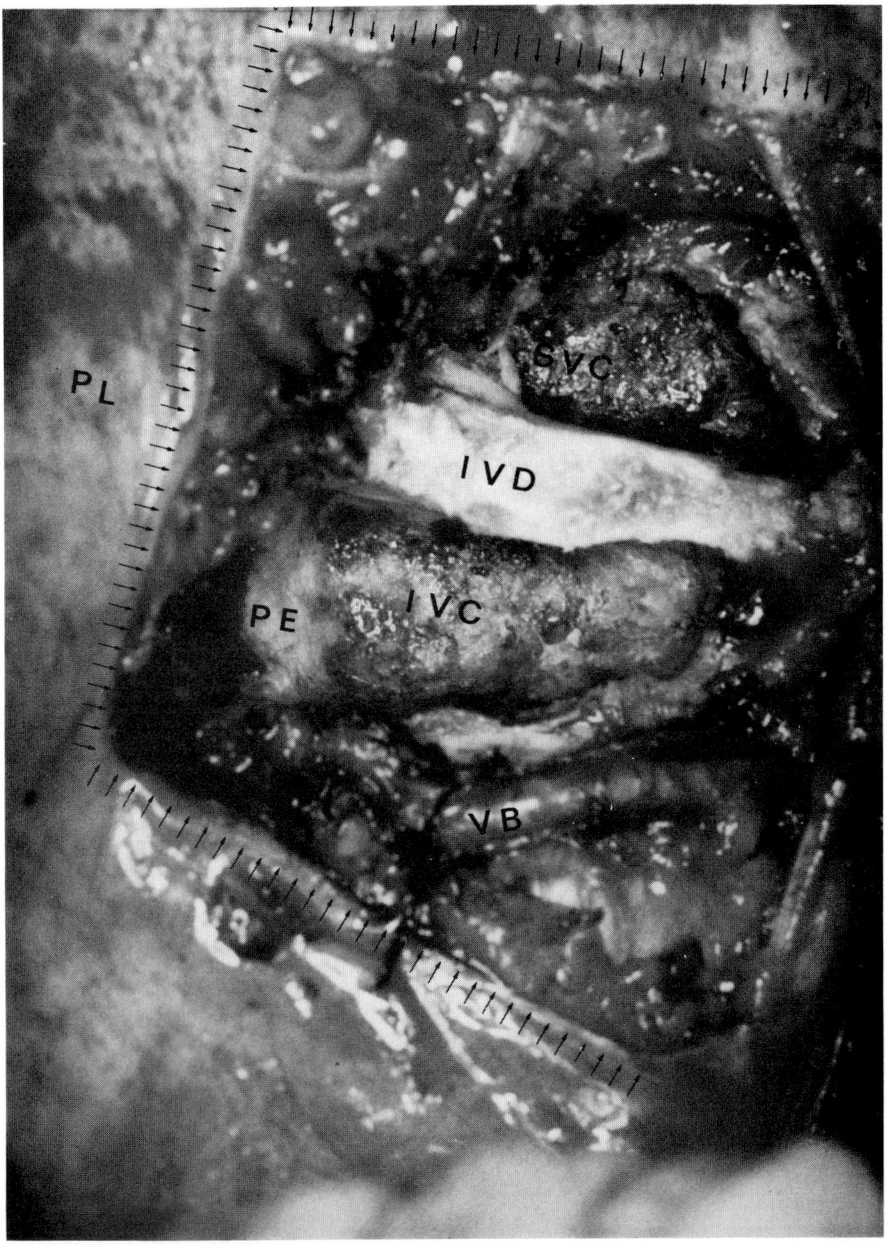

FIG. 30.18. Intraoperative view through a right transthoracic transpleural approach showing the surgical anatomy. *PL*, Margins of pleural flap (*arrows*); *SVC*, superior vertebral cavity; *IVC*, inferior vertebral cavity; *IVD*, intervertebral disc; *VB*, vascular bundle; *PE*, region of inferior pedicle.

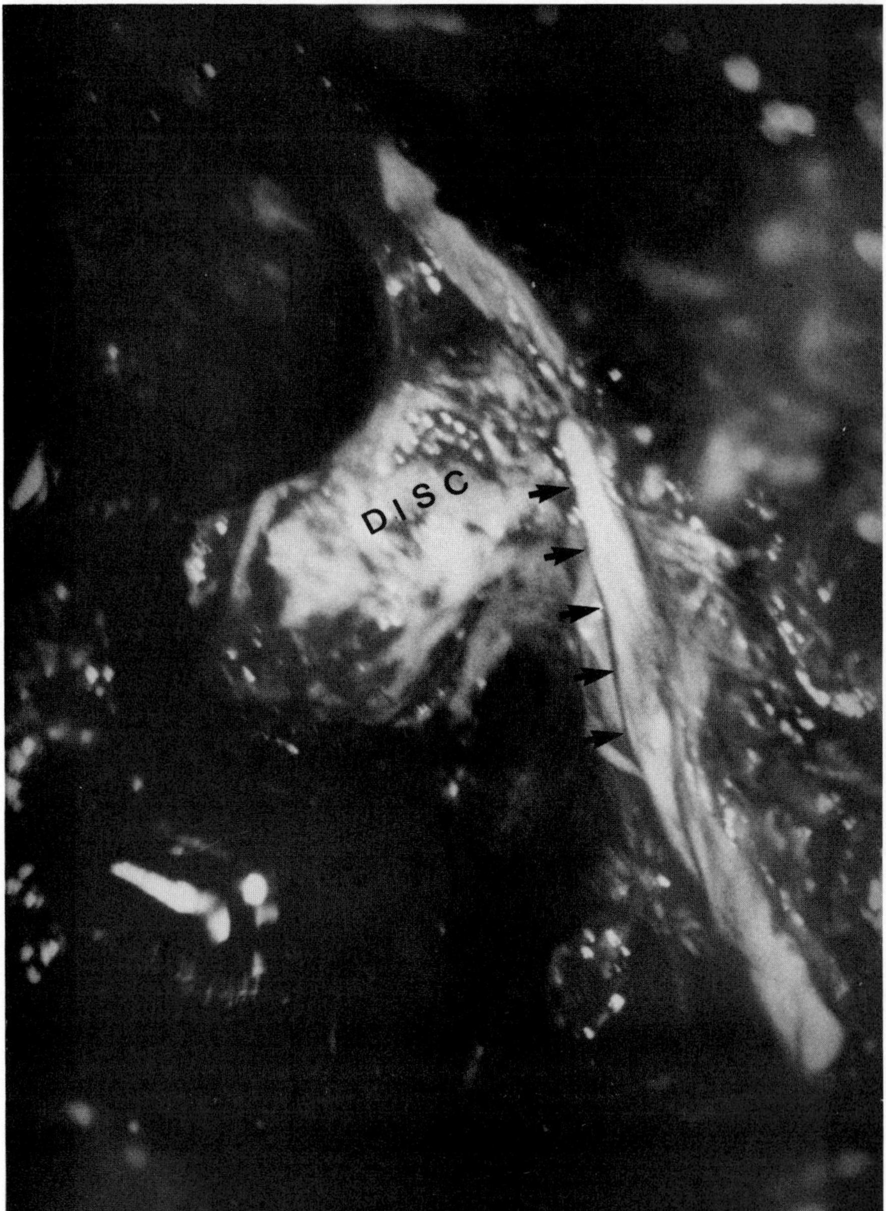

FIG. 30.19. Intraoperative view through a left transthoracic transpleural approach. After removal of the inferior pedicle, the lateral aspect of the dura is visualized (*arrows*).

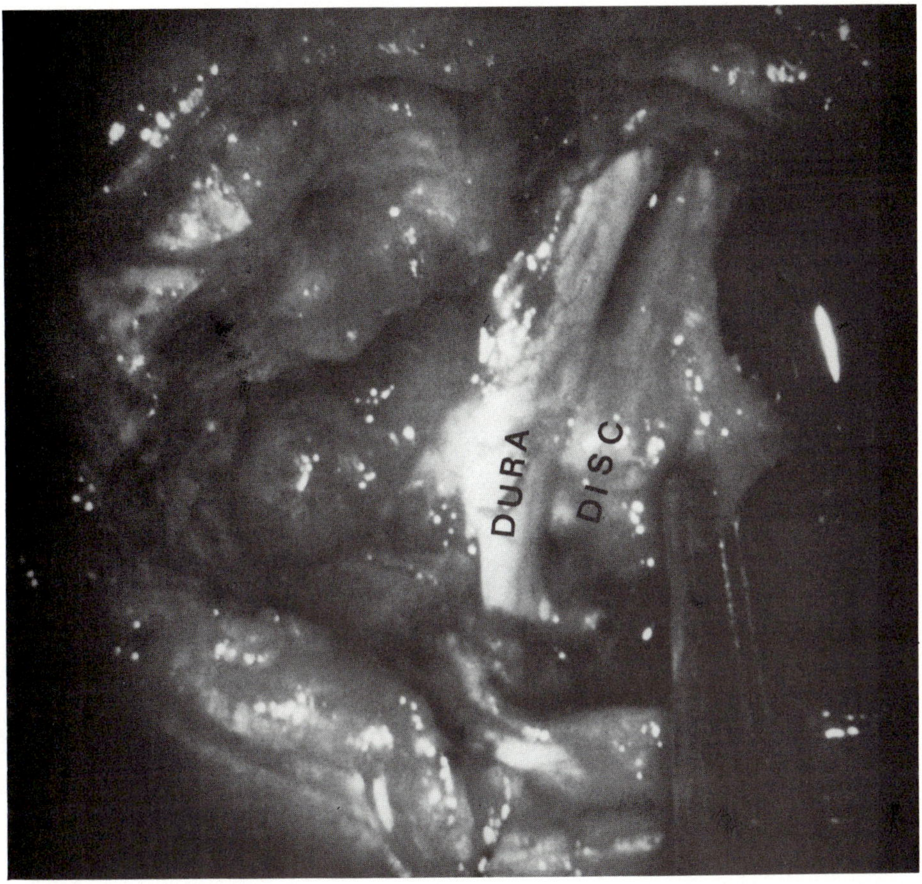

FIG. 30.20. Intraoperative view of removal of the disc complex, showing forceps grasping the lateral margin of the disc (*arrows*).

cases), the dura is sectioned circumferentially and removed with the protrusion. Magnification should be used for this part of the operation, since the arachnoid strands and rootlets may be wrapped around the excrescences of the disc, and they have to be dissected and released before the lesion is removed. The dural opening does not have to be repaired, but if one takes the time it can be patched with a pleural graft.

SPINAL FUSION

Spinal flusion is advisable in the majority of patients, particularly in those who have had previous laminectomies, or if a large portion of the

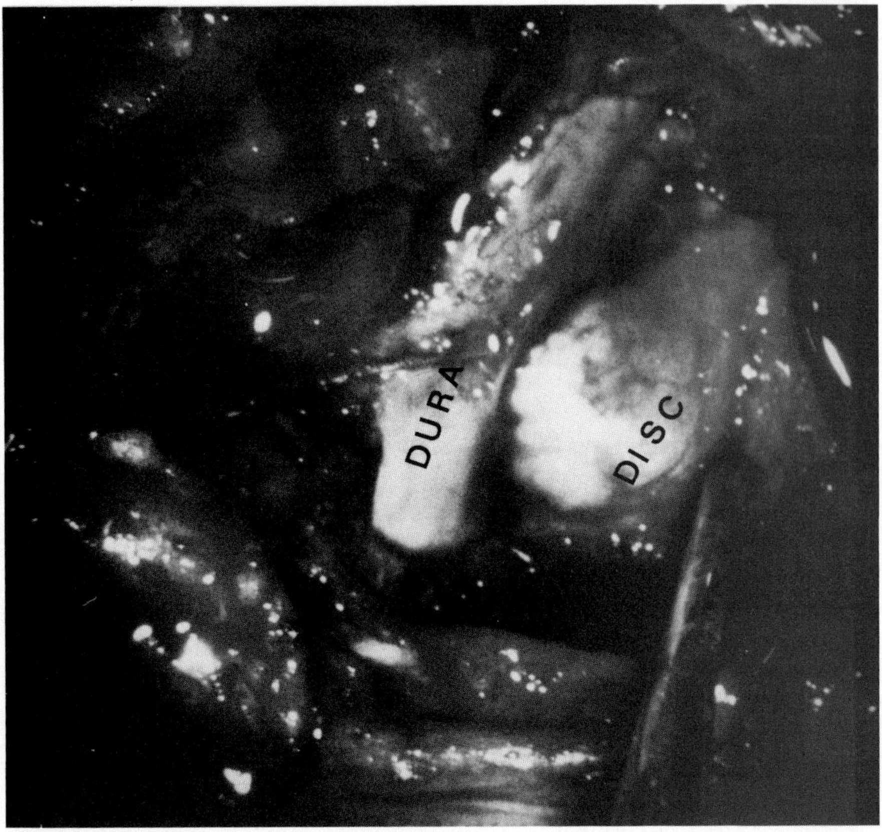

FIG. 30.21. Further extraction of the disc complex showing the ventral aspect of the dura returning to a normal position.

vertebra has been removed. This procedure is simple and can easily be done by utilizing a portion of rib, without the necessity for a separate incision.

SUMMARY

In the last decade there has been a decided improvement in the diagnosis and surgical treatment of thoracic disc protrusions. This has been made possible through the development of water-soluble myelography, CT scan, high speed drills, bipolar coagulation, intraoperative magnification, and the direct frontal approaches to these lesions. Results of surgery have been rather spectacular. These results parallel, if not surpass, the improvements made in the treatment of aneurysms and benign tumors by neurological surgeons. The morbidity rate of 33% has been reduced to less than 1% due to these advances (Table 30.5) (3).

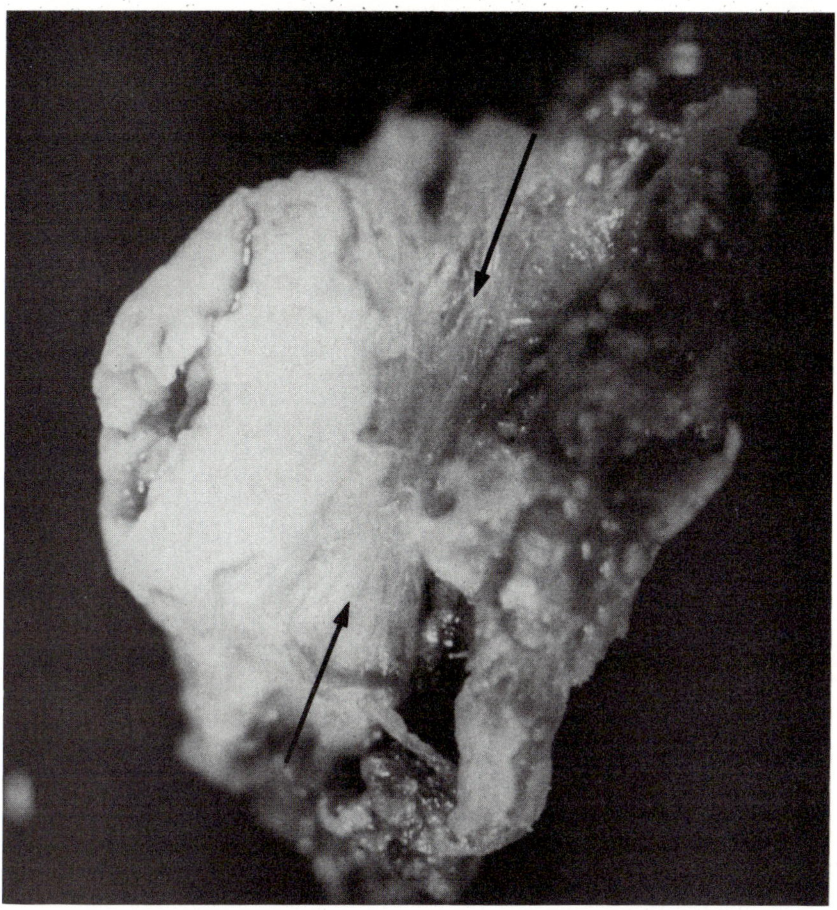

FIG. 30.22. Operative specimen of the same disc as in Figures 30.20 and 30.21, removed *in toto*. To the *left* of the *arrows* is the area of protrusion into the spinal canal.

TABLE 30.5
Complications[a]

Neurological Deterioration	Infection	Death
0	1	0

[a] Data from total of 30 patients.

REFERENCES

1. Albrand, O. W., and Corkill, G. Thoracic disc herniation. Spine. *4:* 41–46, 1979.
2. Arseni, C., and Nash, F. Thoracic intervertebral disc protrusions. A clinical study. J. Neurosurg., *17:* 418–430, 1960.

3. Benjamin, V. Surgical intervention for thoracic disc protrusions and cord compression. The author's experience with 29 patients. Presented at The American Association of Neurological Surgeons, 1982 Annual Meeting, April 25–29, 1982, Honolulu, Hawaii.
4. Benjamin, V. Anterior removal of thoracic disc protrusions. In: *Modern Techniques in Surgery-Neurosurgery*, Chap. 18. edited by J. Ransohoff, pp. 1–11. Futura, Mt. Kisco, N.Y., 1979.
5. Benjamin, V., and Ransohoff, J. Thoracic disc disease. Spine, *1:* 500–507, 1975.
6. Benson, M. K., and Byrnes, D. P. The clinical syndromes and surgical treatment of thoracic intervertebral disc prolapse. J. Bone Joint Surg. *57*(4): 471–477, 1975.
7. Borchi, G. Le ernie discali dorsali. Minerva Neurochir., *7* and *8:* 123–128, 1960.
8. Caron, J. P., Djindjian, R., Julian, H., *et al.* Les hernies discales dorsales. Ann. Med. Intern., *122:* 675–688, 1971.
9. Chesterman, P. J. Spastic paraplegia caused by sequestrated thoracic intervertebral disc. Proc. R. Soc. Med., *57:* 87–88, 1964.
10. Crafoord, C., Hiertonn, T., Lindblom, K., and Olsson, S. E. Spinal cord compression caused by a protruded thoracic disc. Report of a case treated with antero-lateral fenestration of the disc. Acta Orthop. Scand., *28:* 103–107, 1958.
11. Hawk, W. A. Spinal compression caused by ecchondrosis of the intervertebral fibrocartilage: With a review of the recent literature. Brain, *59:* 204–224, 1936.
12. Hulme, A. The surgical approach to thoracic intervertebral disc protrusions. J. Neurol. Neurosurg. Psychiatry, *23:* 133–137, 1960.
13. Jefferson, A. The treatment of thoracic intervertebral disc protrusion. Clin. Neurol. Neurosurg., *78:* 1–9, 1975.
14. Kodama, T., Okubo, K., and Matsukado, Y. Myelopathy due to ossified ligamenta flava in lower thoracic region. No Shinkei Geka, *7:* 867–873, 1979.
15. Logue, V. Thoracic intervertebral disc prolapse with spinal cord compression. J. Neurol. Neurosurg. Psychiatry, *15:* 227–241, 1952.
16. Love, J. G., and Kiefer, E. J. Root pain and paraplegia due to protrusions of thoracic intervertebral discs. J. Neurosurg., *7:* 62–69, 1950.
17. Love, J. G., and Walsh, M. N. Protruded intervertebral disc. Report of one hundred cases in which operation was performed. J.A.M.A., *111:* 396–400, 1938.
18. Marzluff, J. M., Hungerford, D. G., Kempe, L. G., Rawe, S. E., Trevor, R., and Perot, P. L., Jr. Thoracic myelopathy caused by osteophytes of the articular process. Thoracic spondylosis. J. Neurosurg. *50:* 779–783, 1979.
19. Middleton, G. S., and Teacher, J. H. Injury of the spinal cord due to rupture of an intervertebral disc during muscular effort. Glasgow Med. J., *76:* 1–6, 1911.
20. Mixter, W. J., and Barr, J. S. Rupture of the intervertebral disc with involvement of the spinal canal. N. Engl. J. Med., *211:* 210–215, 1934.
21. Müller, R. Protrusion of thoracic intervertebral discs with compression of the spinal cord. Acta Med. Scand., *139:* 99–104, 1951.
22. Omojola, M. F., Cardoso, E. R., Fox, A. J., Drake, C. G., and Durward, Q. J. Thoracic myelopathy secondary to ossified ligamentum flavum. Case report. J. Neurosurg., *56:* 448–450, 1982.
23. Otani, K., Manzoku, S., Shibasaki, K., and Nomachi, S. The surgical treatment of thoracic and thoracolumbar disc lesions using the anterior approach. Report of six cases. Spine *2*(4): 266–275, 1977.
24. Paini, G. P., Baldi, P. G., Di Giovanni, T., Passoni, M., and Barra, N. Ernie discali dorsali. Osservazioni e considerazioni diagnostiche e terapeutiche. Ateneo Parmense [Acta Bio-Med.], *49:* 25–36, 1978.
25. Patterson, R. H., Jr., and Arbit, E. A surgical approach through the pedicle to protruded thoracic discs. J. Neurosurg., *48:* 768–772, 1978.

26. Perrot, P., and Munro, D. D. Transthoracic removal of midline thoracic disc protrusions causing spinal cord compression. J. Neurosurg., *31:* 452–458, 1969.
27. Ransohoff, J., Spencer, F., Wiew, F., and Gage, L. Transthoracic disc protrusions causing spinal cord compression. J. Neurosurg., *31:* 459–461, 1969.
28. Simeone, F. A. The modern treatment of thoracic disc disease. Orthop. Clin. North Am., *2*(2): 453–462, 1971.

CHAPTER

31

Anterior Approaches to the Cervical Spine

JULIAN HOFF, M.D., and DAVID WATERS, M.D.

HISTORY OF THE ANTERIOR APPROACH

Surgeons began to approach lesions of the anterior cervical spine in the early 1950s (4). The procedures usually involved resection of spondylotic osteophytes or removal of herniated disc fragments, followed by autogenous bone grafting to promote intervertebral fusion. Improved instrument design in the late 1950s allowed the anterior procedure for cervical disc disease to be done safely and effectively (5). The Cloward procedure, as it was described in 1958, gained popularity steadily thereafter. Anterior cervical discectomy without bone grafting of the intervertebral space was reported for the first time in 1960 (14). Since then discectomy without fusion has been refined by many surgeons (10, 12, 13, 15, 17, 21, 23, 26). Today, cervical disc disease and spondylosis is approached surgically from a variety of anterior and posterior routes. Some current anterior approaches will be described in this chapter.

In addition to disc disease, other disorders of the cervical spine and spinal cord have been treated by anterior approaches, including tumors, trauma, infections, and intractable pain (6, 7, 15, 16, 27). Consequently, the anterior approach to the cervical spine is an essential technique in the armamentarium of practicing neurosurgeons. A description of pertinent surgical anatomy precedes a description of the various procedures and their application.

ANATOMY

The size and shape of the cervical spine varies considerably in the adult, not only from person to person but also from vertebra to vertebra. The minimum height of the normal canal is 14 mm at C_5, as measured on standard lateral view roentgenographs (19). The width of the canal has little clinical significance and is relevant only if a laterally placed mass within it occupies enough space to compress and displace the spinal cord.

The spinal cord is slightly fusiform in the neck, with maximal girth at C_5. At that level the average height of the cord is 8 mm; its width is 13 mm. Maximum normal height is 10 mm. The remainder of the canal space is occupied by spinal fluid, dura, epidural fat, and epidural veins.

Normal cervical discs are anatomically similar to lumbar discs; both consist of annular and nuclear portions. Clinical syndromes may appear when the nucleus is deformed, either by trauma or degeneration. The degree to which the nucleus can be deformed depends upon the integrity of the surrounding annulus and the investing ligaments. The average height of cervical discs is roughly 45% of the height of the adjacent vertebrae.

The 8 pairs of dorsal and ventral roots of the cervical cord descend slightly to exit from the canal through the intervertebral foramina. The cord moves during flexion and extension of the neck, as much as 3 mm at the C_7 level. The surrounding dura moves slightly more. Cervical roots move within the spinal canal and within the neural foramina, becoming taut with flexion and lax with extension. Angulation of a normal root at the foraminal entrance increases with extension. Dentate ligaments anchor the spinal cord to the dura laterally at intervals, limiting rostrocaudal and side to side movement during neck motion. Stress on the lateral columns of the cord during motion is reduced by the fan-like attachment of the ligaments to the cord.

Radicular arteries, originating from the vertebral, thyrocervical, and deep cervical arteries, pass through the neural foramina within the dural root sleeves to reach the anterior and posterior aspects of the spinal cord in company with the dorsal and ventral roots. A confluence of arteries forms ventral to the cord to become the anterior spinal artery. This artery is usually continuous, passing vertically within the ventral sulcus of the cord. Its branches supply the central and anterolateral regions of the cord, including most of the central grey matter. Paired smaller dorsal arteries supply the posterolateral regions of the cord. Spinal cord veins accompany the arteries, forming radicular veins which pass intradurally through the root foramina to join extravertebral venous plexuses (15).

Anatomical Landmarks

It is often difficult to count the cervical vertebrae by palpating the neck. Some bony prominences are helpful, however, when the neck is in the neutral position. The angle of the mandible corresponds to C_2–C_3, the hyoid bone overlies C_3, and the cricoid cartilage is anterior to C_6–C_7. The carotid tubercle of the C_6 transverse process protrudes anteriorly and can be felt adjacent to the carotid artery (15).

OPERATIVE TECHNIQUE

Anterior Discectomy without Fusion (Fig. 31.1)

The patient is anesthetized in the supine position and ventilated through a nonkinking endotracheal tube. Normal cervical lordosis is maintained by a sandbag or rolled towel placed beneath the neck. The

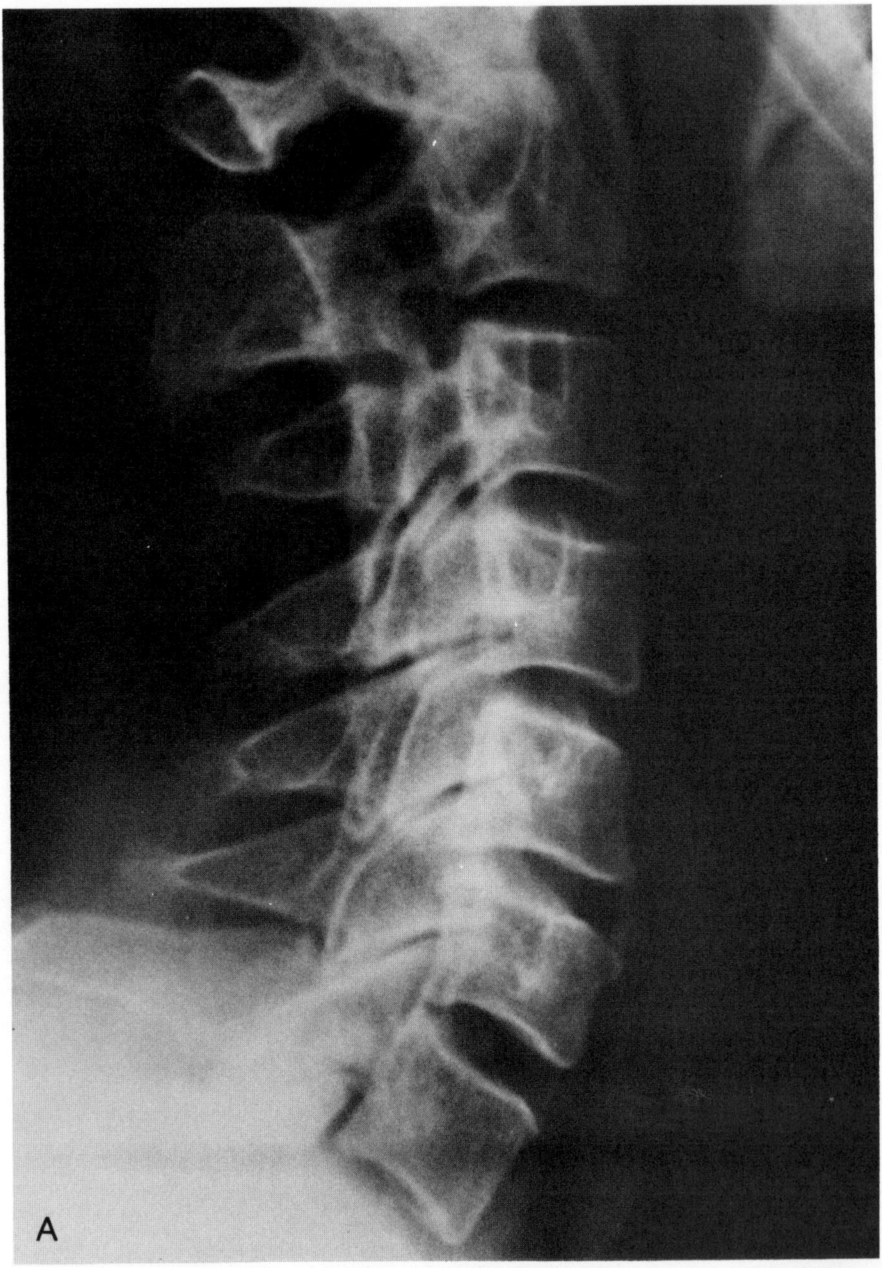

FIG. 31.1. Anterior cervical discectomy without fusion. A 38-year-old man with C_6 radiculopathy. (*A*) Preoperative plain radiograph (lateral view).

head is rotated slightly to the side, opposite that planned for the skin incision.

An approach from the patient's right side is preferred. To expose only one or two or the vertebrae from C_3 through C_7, a collar incision is made from the midline across the anterior border of the sternocleidomastoid muscle. When more than two vertebra must be exposed, a vertical incision along the anterior border of the sternocleidomastoid muscle is usually better.

After transsection of the platysma fibers, that muscle is dissected rostrally and caudally to facilitate deep retraction. The anterior border of the sternocleidomastoid can be readily identified, and the veins within the adjacent fascia are divided.

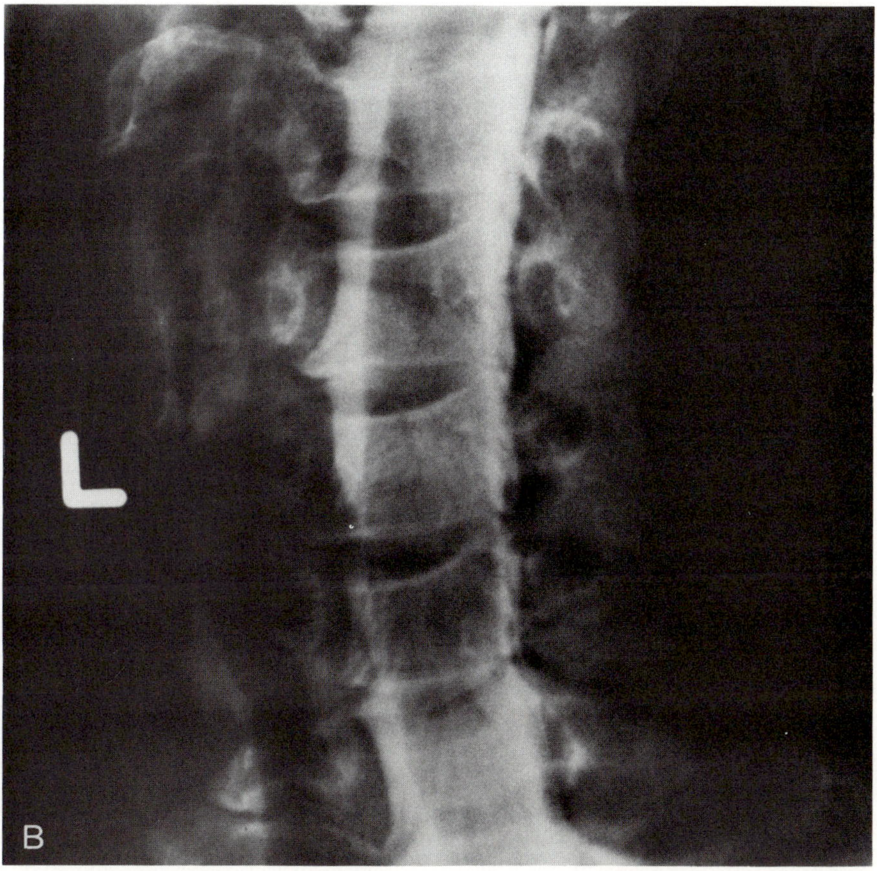

FIG. 31.1. (*B*) Preoperative myelogram (AP view).

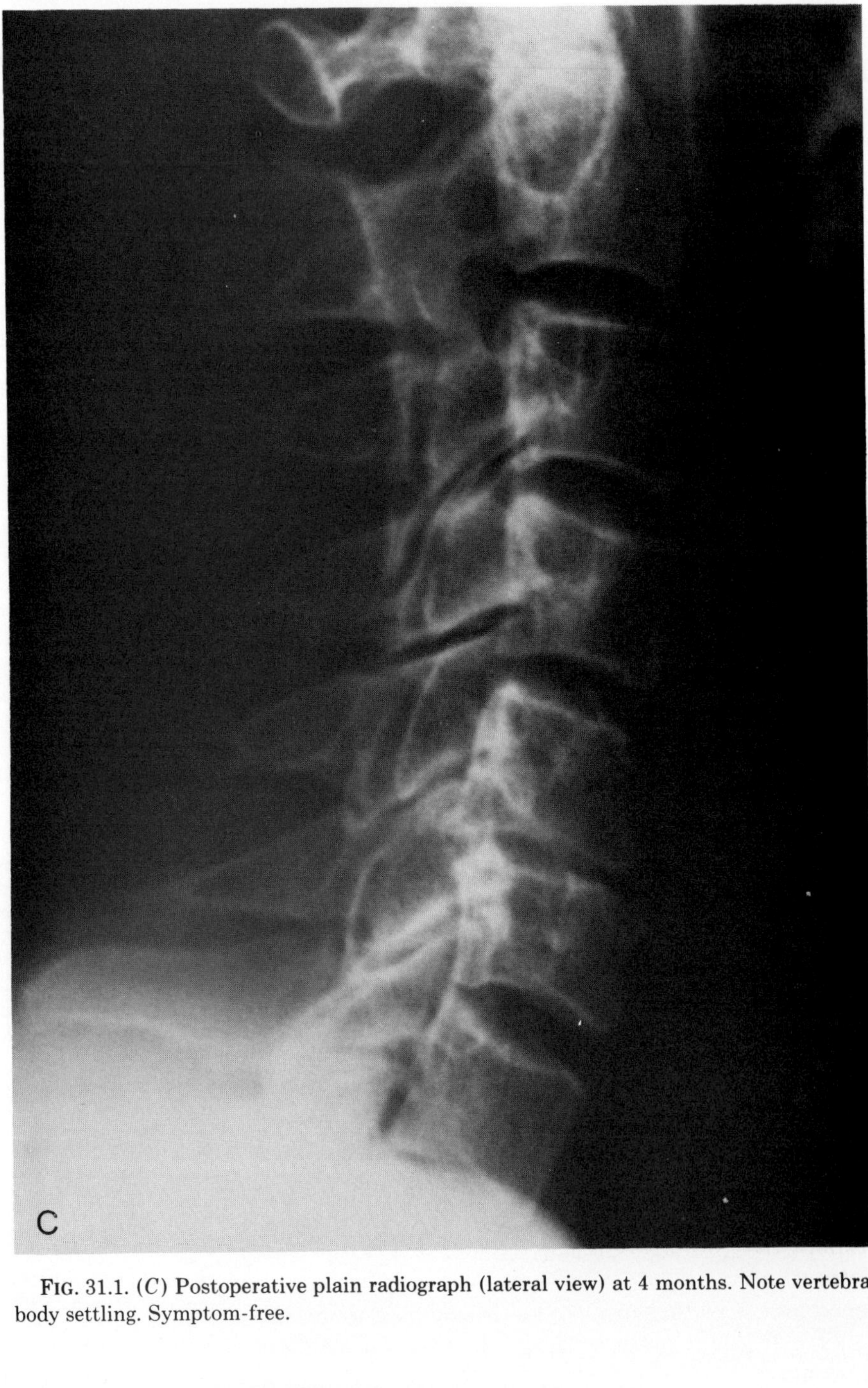

FIG. 31.1. (*C*) Postoperative plain radiograph (lateral view) at 4 months. Note vertebral body settling. Symptom-free.

The middle layer of cervical fascia bridges from the sternocleidomastoid to the strap muscles of the larynx; it is incised, and the exposure is widened and deepened by blunt and sharp dissection. The omohyoid muscle, whose fibers course perpendicularly to those of the sternocleidomastoid, is often encountered; it may be divided.

The carotid sheath and its contents are retracted laterally by finger dissection and, at the same time, the trachea and esophagus are mobilized medially. The deep cervical fascia overlying the longus colli muscles and the anterior longitudinal ligament of the cervical spine is then visible. Rostral and caudal mobilization of the carotid sheath and the tracheoesophageal bundle by blunt and sharp dissection improves exposure.

The prevertebral fascia is incised in the midline, exposing the anterior longitudinal ligament and the longus colli muscles that overlay the anterolateral surface of the vertebral bodies and discs. A lateral radiograph should establish which cervical vertebra is exposed. A spinal needle inserted into one of the exposed discs is a useful radiopaque marker.

When the proper level has been verified radiographically, the longus colli muscles are sharply dissected from the vertebral bodies anteriorly and from the adherent annulus of the disc. A Cloward retractor, its toothed blades carefully placed beneath the dissected margins of the longus colli muscles, then exposes the anterior cervical spine. A second retractor with smooth blades may be used to maximize rostrocaudal exposure.

The surgical microscope is positioned with the pedestal on the patient's left side, and the assistant's observer-attachment is placed on the pedestal side. The light beam is directed into the wound and is angled rostrally in the direction of the intervertebral disc. Suction-irrigation, bipolar cautery, microsurgical instruments, and a high-speed drill with a long handled angled adapter and a small burr are set in place.

The annulus is incised and the nucleus removed with small, straight, and angled curets. When the posterior aspect of the disc space is reached, exposure of the bone may be expanded by drilling away the remaining cartilaginous end plates, above and below, and some of the cortical bone beneath them. The exposure should not exceed 10 mm in width and 5 mm in height. It may be widened a few millimeters posteriorly to gain easy access to the bone adjacent to the neural foramina. Bone wax is not used.

The posterior margin of the annulus is contiguous with the posterior longitudinal ligament. The ligament may be excised by curettage to expose the dura and the proximal 1 to 2 mm of the cervical root sleeves laterally, if a free disc fragment is suspected. If the ligament is intact, it need not be removed.

Free fragments of soft disc material are removed easily. The neural foramina, while not directly visible, are readily palpable with a nerve hook or small, angled curet. Fragments within the foramina can be removed with an angled curet.

If a spondylotic bar projects posteriorly in the midline, it is best removed by curettage proceeding from the midline laterally to the neural foramina. Head traction may be applied at this stage by the anesthetist, or the Cloward disc spreader may be positioned to enlarge the disc space and reveal the narrow gap between osteophytes of the adjacent vertebrae. Spurs of the uncovertebral joints may project into the neural foramina, where they can be palpated and removed by curettage until the foramina are decompressed. It is important to enlarge the neural foramina generously if fusion is not performed. If intervertebral fusion by bone graft is planned, then the neural foramina need not be enlarged as much, but the graft must distract the vertebral bodies to widen the neural foramina.

During this procedure the anterior exposure achieved has disturbed neither the lateral margins of the annulus nor the lateral aspects of the vertebral bodies. Most of the nucleus pulposus has been removed, as well as cartilage from two vertebral end plates and some cortical bone from the articular surfaces. The anterior and sometimes the posterior longitudinal ligaments have been transected, but the uncovertebral joints are undisturbed.

Hemostasis is imperative before closure of the wound. Gelfoam in the intervertebral space usually suffices. When the retractors are removed, the longus colli muscles are not reapproximated. The middle layer of cervical fascia is sutured loosely to approximate the sternocleidomastoid and the laryngeal strap muscles over the carotid sheath. A good platysma closure will ensure a narrow scar, and the skin closure with a fine nylon or paper tapes completes the procedure.

Some settling of the vertebrae occurs, more anteriorly than posteriorly, after operation without fusion. The neural foramina may become slightly narrower after operation than they were before, unless a proper foraminotomy has been done. However, since posterior settling of the vertebral body is slight, the foramina are not narrowed significantly. Spontaneous fusion of adjacent vertebrae can be expected to occur 3 months after operation (13, 15, 24).

Anterior Discectomy with Fusion (Fig. 31.2)

CLOWARD TECHNIQUE

Both the Cloward and the Smith-Robinson techniques involve placement of autogenous bone graft, usually from the ilium, into the evacuated disc space. Osteophytes or disc fragments are removed from the spinal canal and foramina by curettage before fashioning the disc space for the bone graft. The operating microscope provides good light and some magnification for this stage of the procedure.

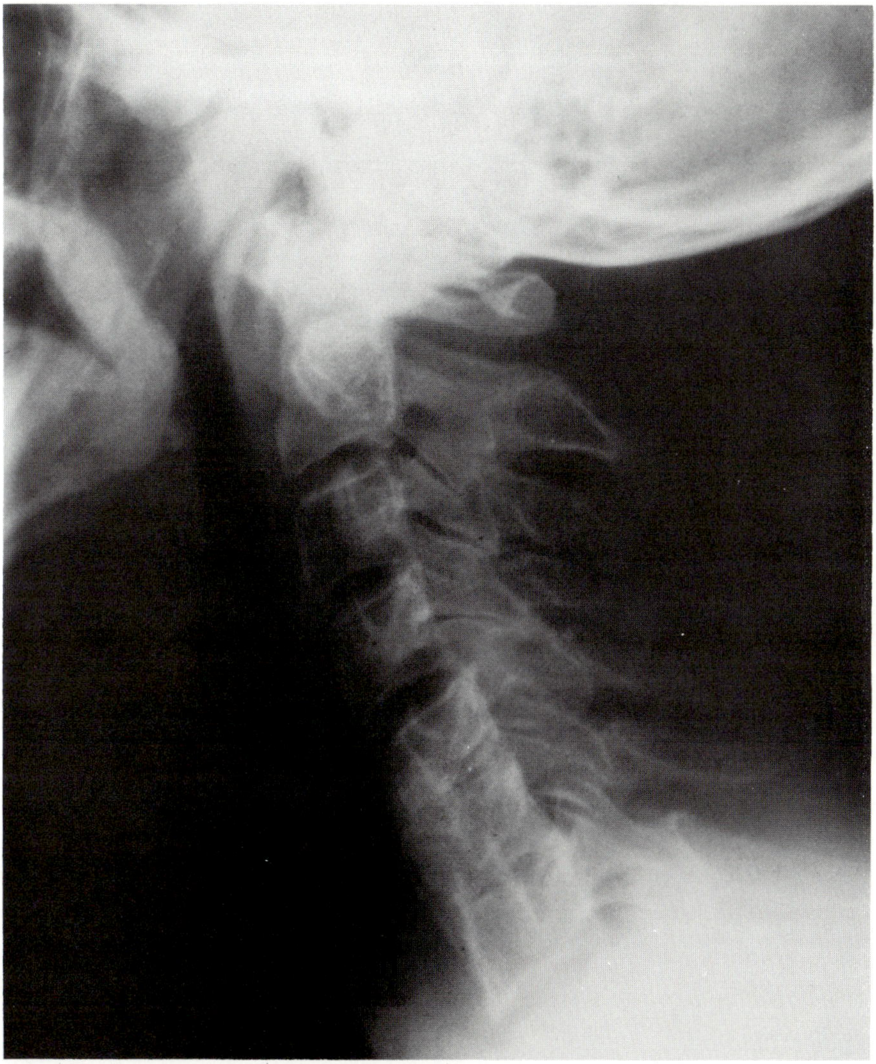

FIG. 31.2. Anterior cervical discectomy with and without bone graft in a 50-year-old man. A Cloward procedure was done at C_6–C_7 3 years earlier; an anterior discectomy without bone graft was done 1 year earlier. Note solid fusion at both levels.

The depth of the interspace is measured after disc removal. The drill guide, seated over the disc space, is set to the measured depth. The drill is then fitted into the drill guide, and a hole is made overlaying the empty disc space, taking care to preserve the posterior cortical rim of the two adjacent vertebral bodies. If more than one disc is resected, the smallest drill and corresponding bone dowel should be used. The dowel is inserted into the hole prepared for it and gently impacted there so that the two

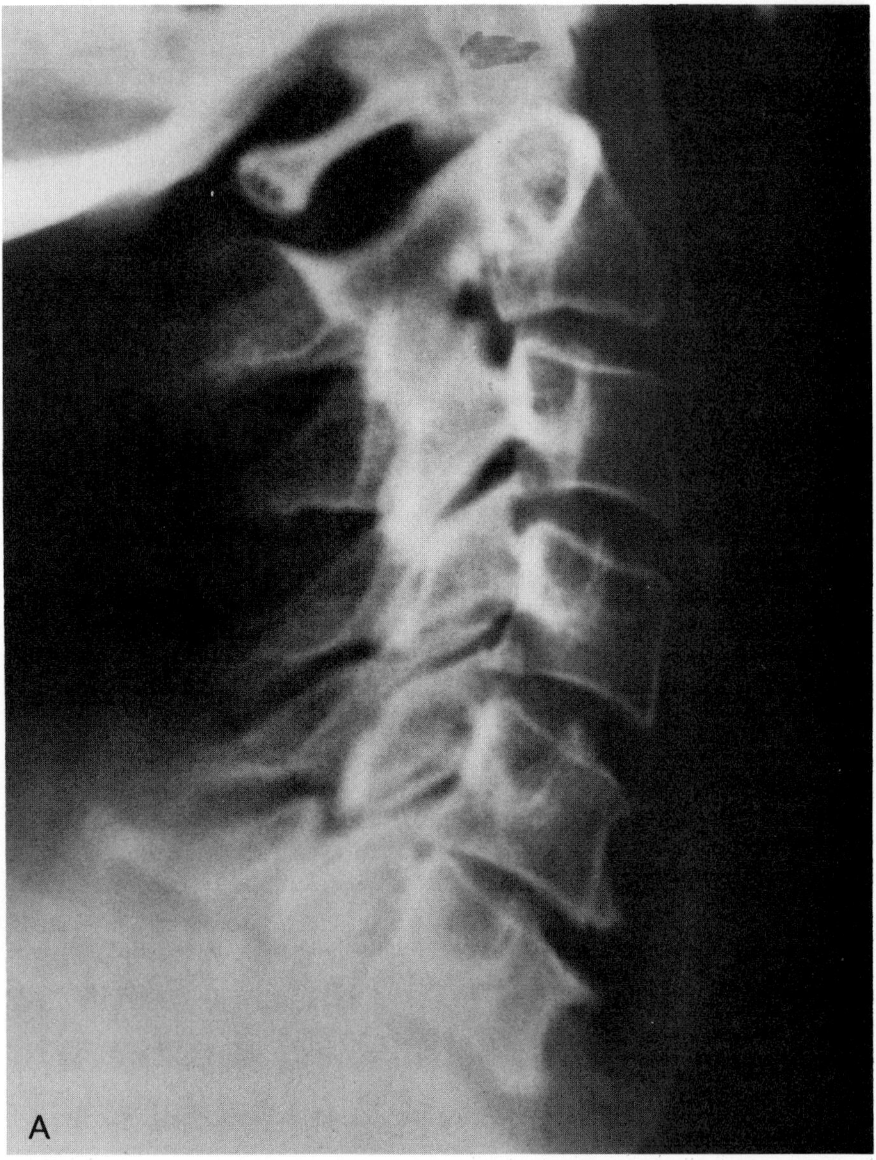

FIG. 31.3. Anterior cervical discectomy with fusion: Smith-Robinson technique. A 45-year-old woman with C_6 radiculopathy. (*A*) Preoperative plain radiograph (lateral view).

cortical surfaces of the dowel are anterior and posterior. Axial traction or use of the disc space spreader allows easy insertion of the graft.

The graft is obtained from the ilium. An incision is made just below the iliac crest. The crest is exposed, and the muscles on its anterior surface and posterior surface are carefully stripped free. The Cloward

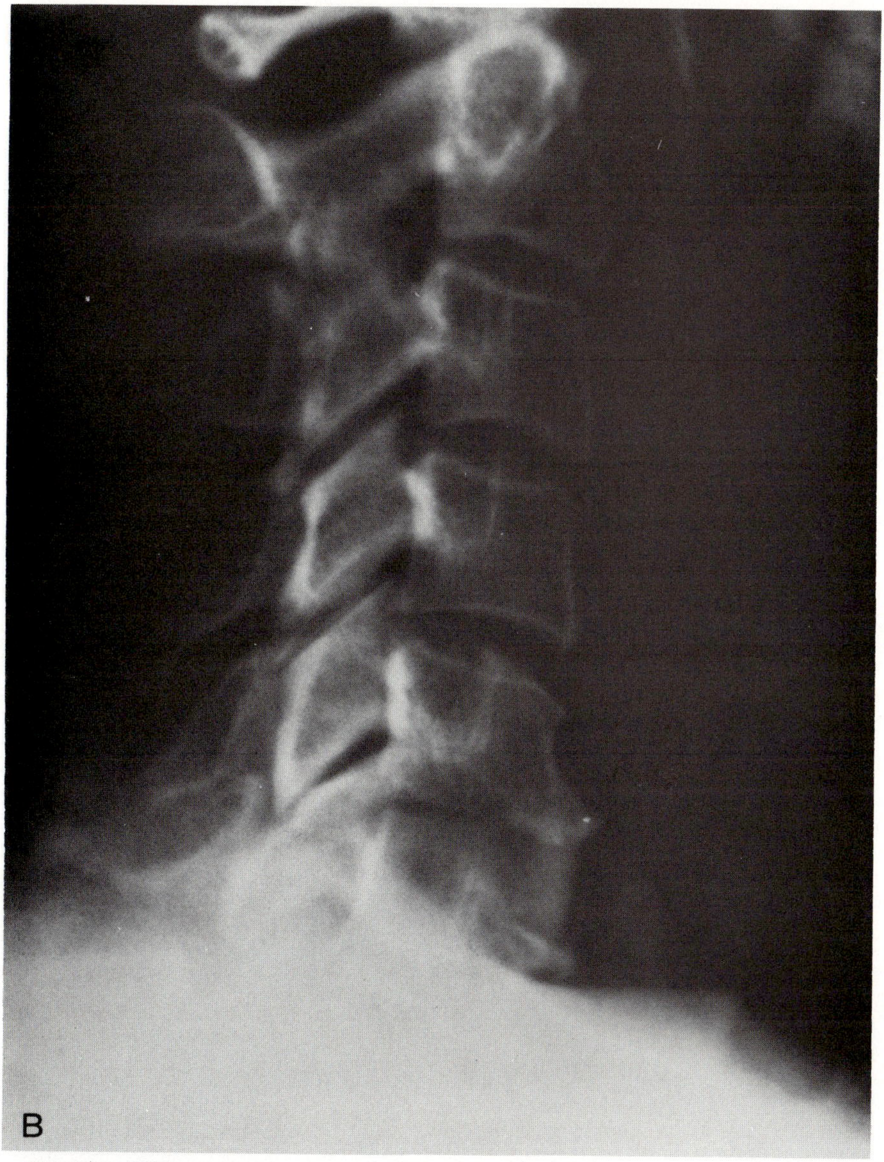

FIG. 31.3. (*B*) Postoperative 4 months. Note intervertebral distraction by graft and inset positioning to prevent extrusion.

bone dowel cutter is passed transversely through the ilium, leaving the crest intact. Several dowels may be obtained if necessary (5, 7, 18).

SMITH-ROBINSON TECHNIQUE (FIG. 31.3)

This procedure is similar to the Cloward method, except that iliac crest bone, with cortical surface on 3 sides, is fashioned to fit the intervertebral space. Thus, it is possible to position the graft so that it rests on the posterior lip of cortical bone of the adjacent vertebral bodies and may be countersunk beneath the anterior edges of cortical bone. Axial traction on the neck by the anesthetist allows maximal spreading of the disc space

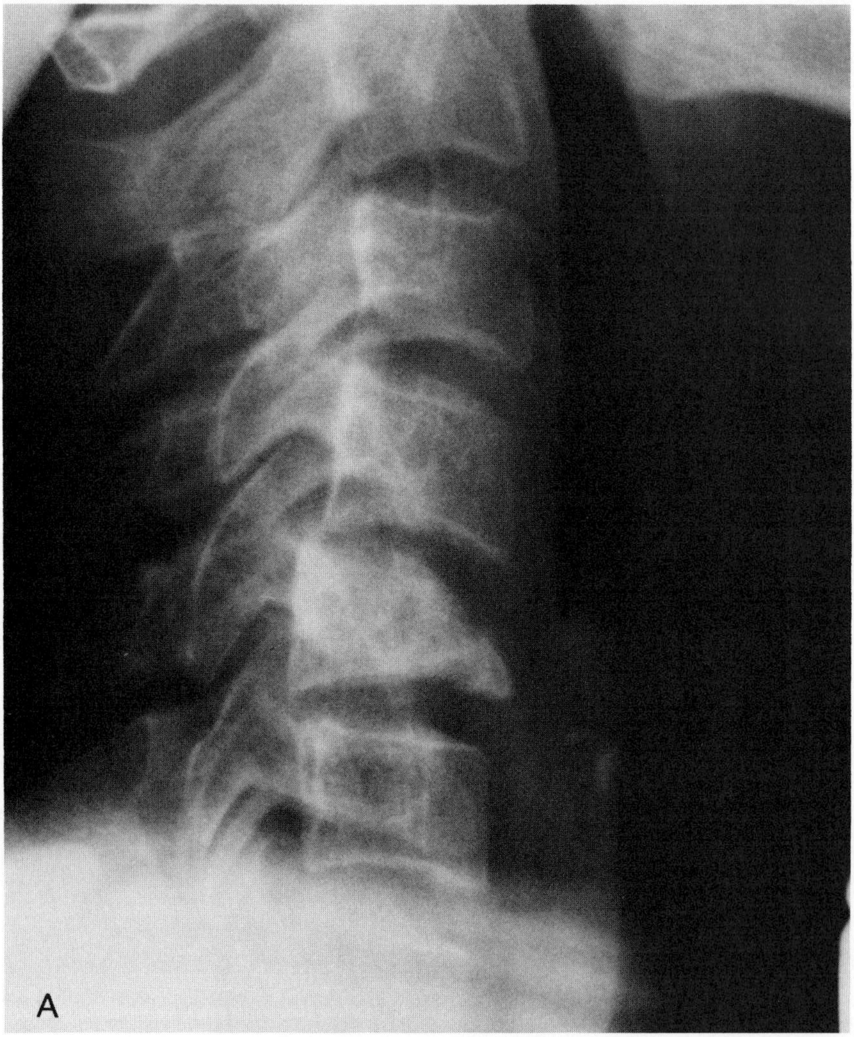

FIG. 31.4. Cervical vertebral body replacement with bone graft. A 29-year-old man suffering from neck pain after motor vehicle accident. Renal recipient 15 years before. (*A*) Preoperative plain radiograph (lateral view). Patient spent 4 months in halo-jacket after injury. Still unstable.

at the time of insertion and gentle impaction of the bone graft (3, 22, 25, 28). The bone graft itself is obtained with an osteotome from the exposed iliac crest. Little or no muscle dissection is necessary.

Postoperative radiographs are made after anterior discectomy with or without bone graft fusion to ensure proper alignment. Patients usually prefer a semirigid cervical collar for comfort for 2 or 3 weeks. If a bone graft has been inserted, we prefer use of a collar for 12 weeks.

VERTEBRAL BODY REPLACEMENT WITH BONE GRAFT (FIG. 31.4)

Replacement of the body of a cervical vertebra may be required because of its destruction by tumor or trauma. The technique is similar to the Smith-Robinson procedure, except that the central two-thirds of the involved vertebral body is resected with a drill, rongeurs, and curets. The bone removal is best carried lateral enough to ensure decompression of the spinal canal but not lateral enough to disrupt the pedicles of the vertebra. An iliac crest tibial or fibular bone strut is then countersunk, as in the standard Smith-Robinson technique, into slots made with the air drill in the vertebral end plates at the rostral and caudal extremes of the resection site. Because of inherent instability at the grafted site, rigid fixation in a halo-jacket apparatus for 12–16 weeks is advisable.

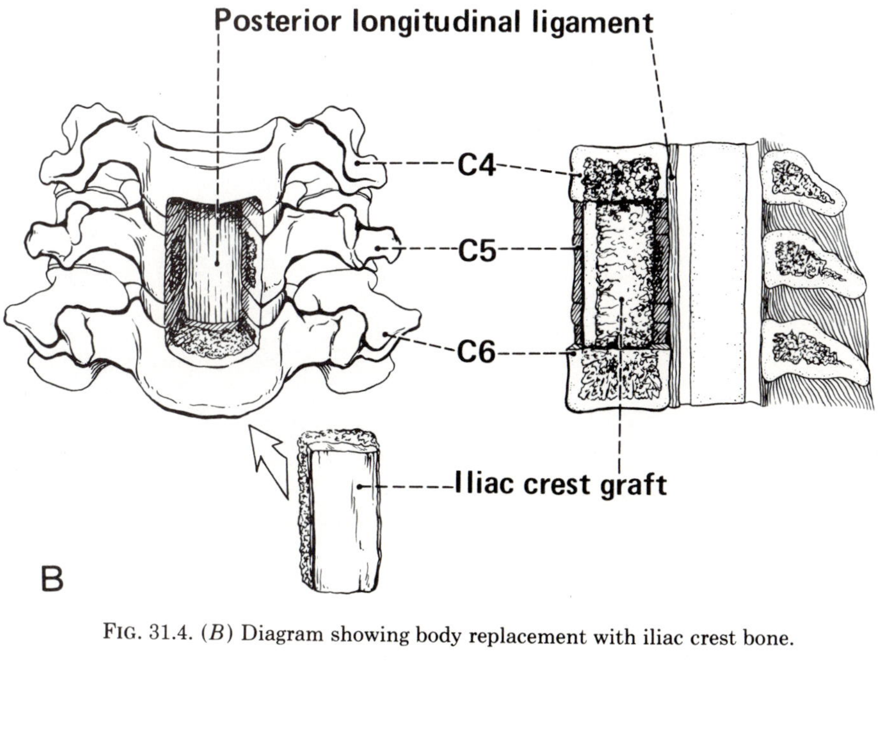

FIG. 31.4. (*B*) Diagram showing body replacement with iliac crest bone.

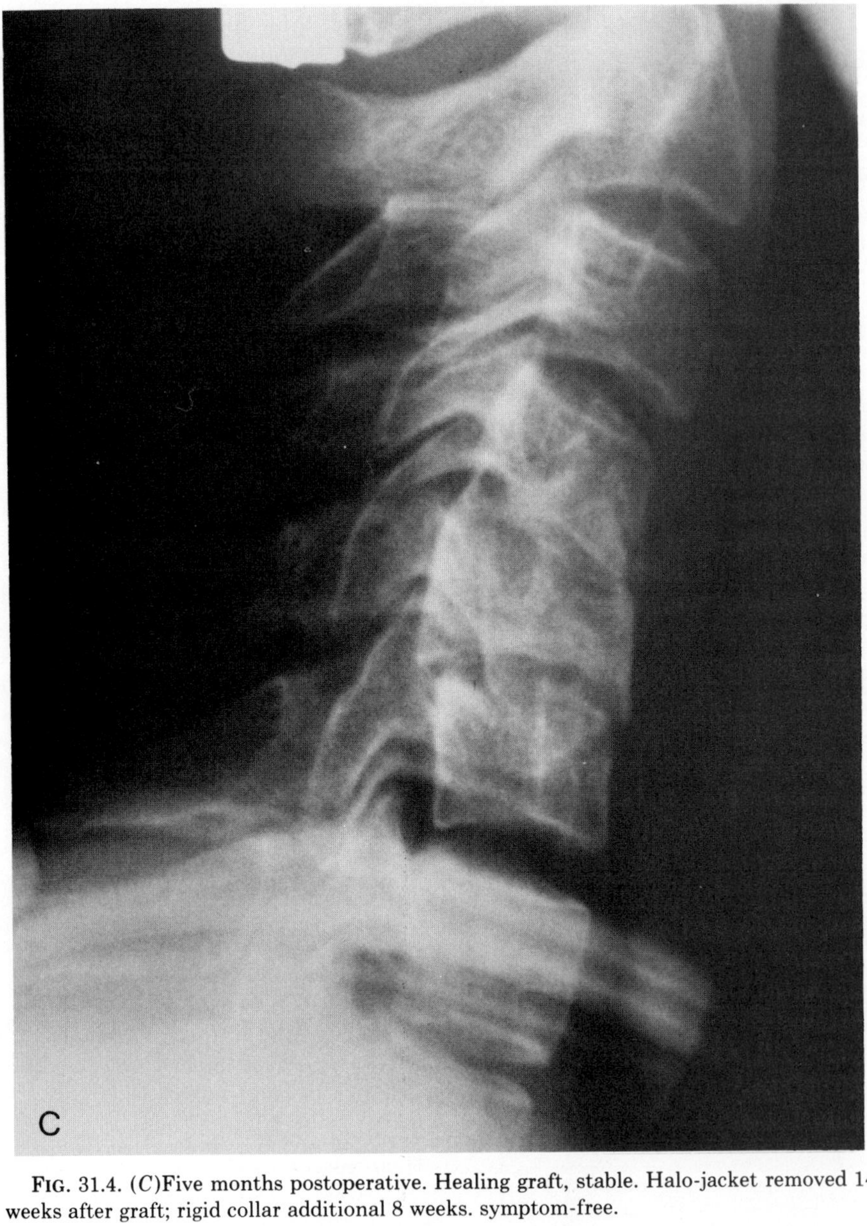

FIG. 31.4. (*C*)Five months postoperative. Healing graft, stable. Halo-jacket removed 14 weeks after graft; rigid collar additional 8 weeks. symptom-free.

VERTEBRAL BODY REPLACEMENT WITH REINFORCED ACRYLIC (FIG. 31.5)

Patients with a tumor in the anterior cervical spine who have cord compression may benefit substantially from anterior decompression and fusion with either bone graft or stabilization with an acrylic vertebral prosthesis. An acrylic prosthesis can be molded precisely to fit the defect. It provides good mechanical stability after operation, allowing early mobilization of patients who face terminal illness (27).

Before operating on patients who have metastatic disease, we establish the exact length of the block by myelography. If the block is more than two segments long, we do not attempt anterior decompression of the cord by resection of the vertebral body, preferring the posterior approach. If the cervical spine is unstable either before or after operation, then external fixation is advisable, initially with skeletal traction, then with a halo-jacket apparatus.

The procedure has 3 stages. First, tumor is resected rostrally and caudally until healthy vertebral bone is exposed, taking care to decompress the spinal canal. Gelfoam is placed in the resection site to cover the dura. Second, 18-gauge Kirschner wires are embedded into the exposed healthy vertebral bodies in a longitudinal direction so that a wire matrix bridges the resection site without impinging on the spinal canal. Third, semisoft methyl methacrylate is poured into the resection site to encase the Kirschner wire matrix. Copious saline irrigation is then carried out until the reinforced acrylic body replacement has hardened and cooled. Postoperative immobilization is accomplished by a rigid collar (15).

Anterior Approach for Cervical Spine Infection

Pyogenic infection of the anterior cervical spine requires drainage and debridement. The use of bone graft to stabilize the spine is contraindicated. Furthermore, bone fusion often occurs spontaneously, provided the infection is controlled and the neck is immobilized adequately. Spontaneous fusion often follows an effectively treated spinal infection, Drainage, debridement, immobilization, and administration of the appropriate antibiotics are fundamentals of treatment. Often, the vertebral body involved nearly reconstitutes itself, and neurological deficits may improve (15).

Anterior Approaches to C_1 and C_2

Because exposure of the anterior surfaces of C_1 and C_2 is difficult by the standard prevertebral route, Fang, Arbit, Mullan, and others (1, 2, 8, 9, 11, 20) have developed retropharyngeal approaches to the upper cervical spine. These techniques are useful for ventrally placed tumors, for fusion or unstable interspaces at C_1–C_2 and C_2–C_3, and for resection of bone compressing the cord, including anomalies and fracture fragments of the odontoid process. The procedures are done in concert with a head and neck surgeon (32).

Complications of Anterior Approaches

Complications of the various procedures can be predicted. Root and cord signs may be increased, regardless of the approach, if the operation is done carelessly. Anterior approaches to the cord and roots may be

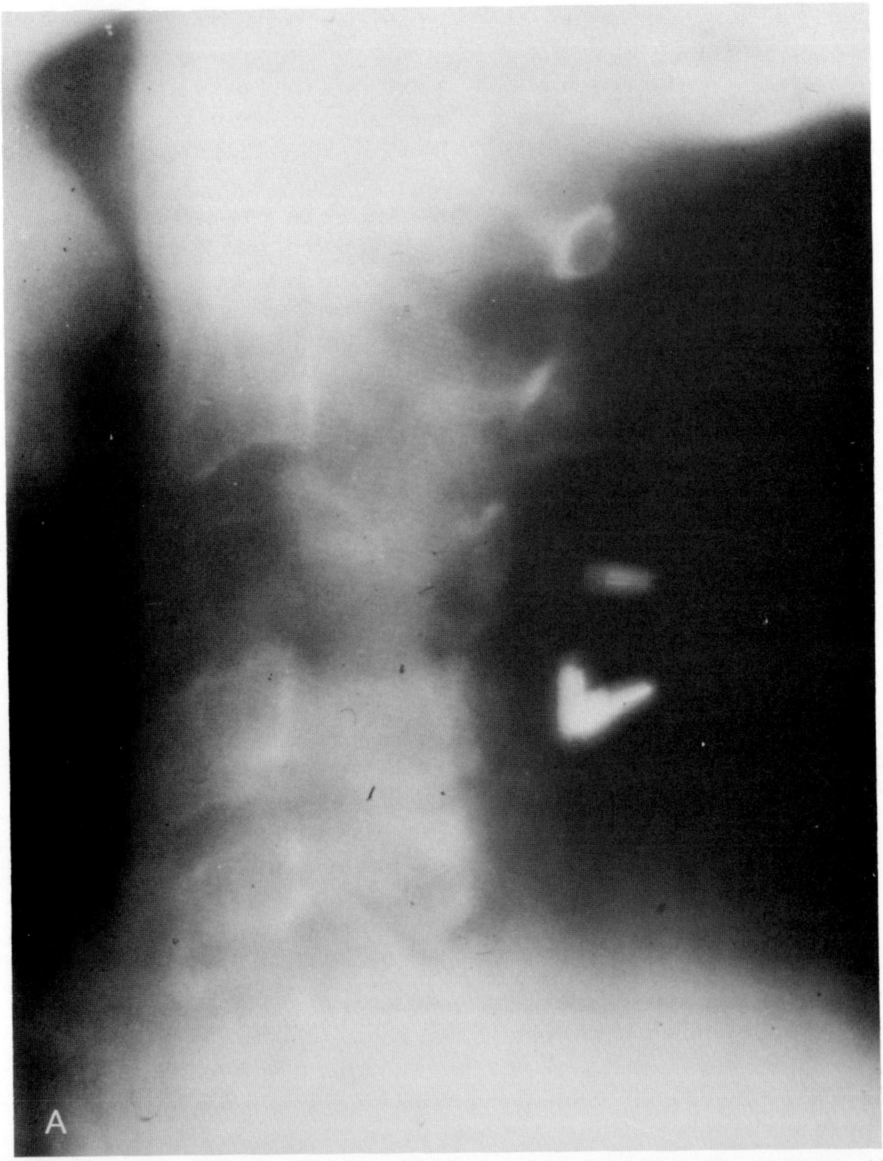

FIG. 31.5. Cervical vertebral body replacement with reinforced acrylic. A 67-year-old woman with metastatic lung carcinoma, neck pain, and no neurological deficit. (*A*) Preoperative tomograph, lateral view.

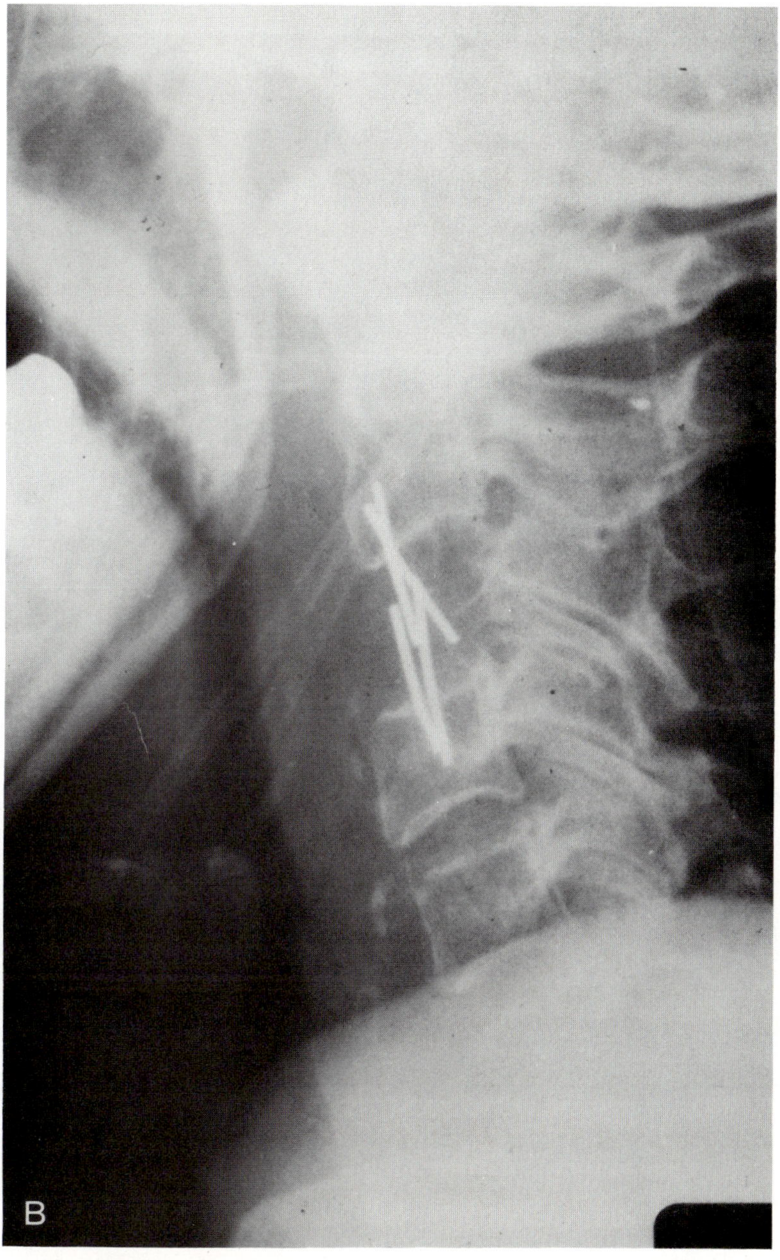

FIG. 31.5. (*B*) Postoperative plain radiograph (lateral view).

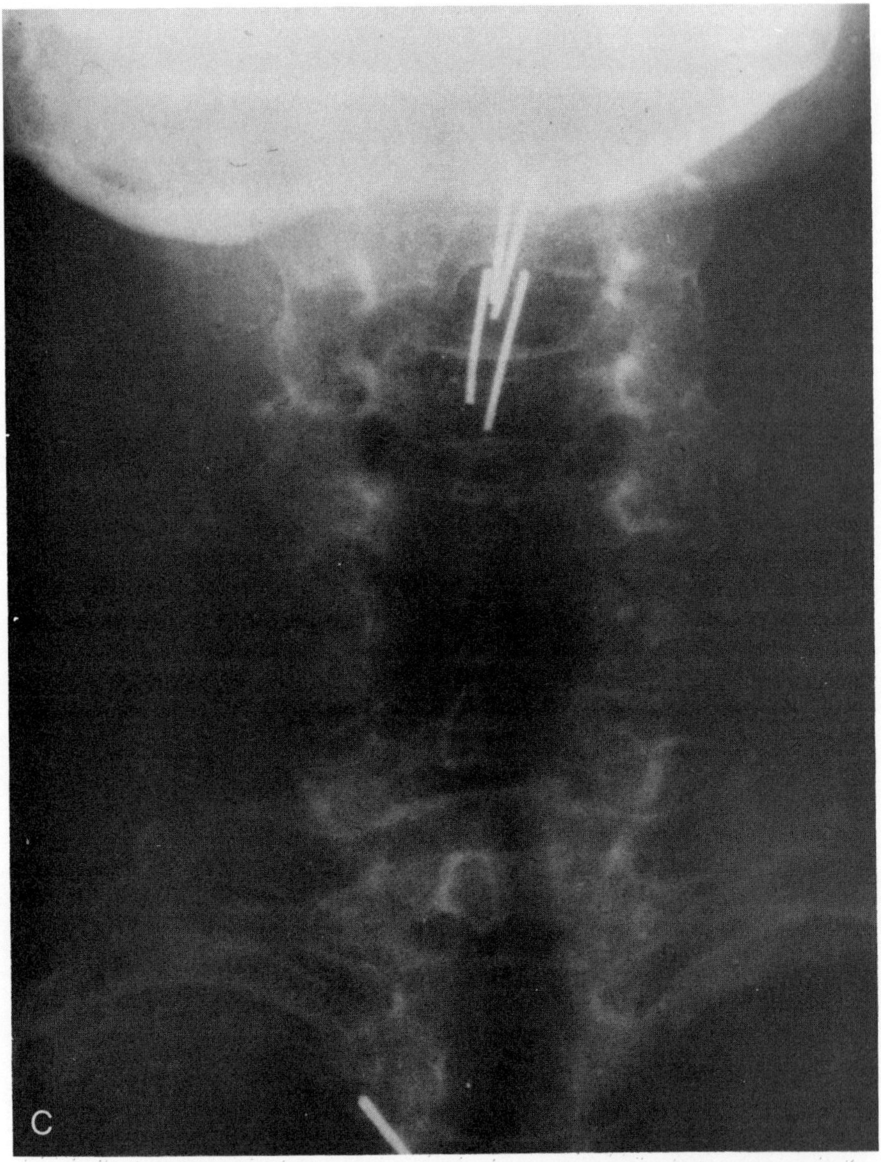

FIG. 31.5. (*C*) Postoperative plain radiograph (AP view).

accompanied by carotid or vertebral artery injury, recurrent laryngeal nerve palsy, hypoglossal palsy, esophageal perforation, and airway obstruction. A postoperative infection or hemorrhage may result. If a bone graft is employed, it may migrate anteriorly or posteriorly. Posterior displacement may result in cord compression. Bone graft harvesting from the ilium may result in a painful wound, bowel perforation, and infection. Instability at the operative site is a threat, particularly when bone removal is extensive and external bracing is insufficient. Nonunion at the site of the resected disc occurs in about 10% of procedures, done with or without intervertebral bone graft. Spinal alignment is superior with either the Cloward or Smith-Robinson technique early after operation, but the ventral angulation that occurs after anterior discectomy without fusion does improve with time (18). Two to 3% of patients develop disc disease at a different level, regardless of the anterior procedure employed (15, 29, 30, 31).

Choice of Approach

Anterior approaches to the cervical spine have evolved because many surgically correctable lesions are situated anteriorly. Whether a discectomy without bone graft, a Cloward, or a Smith-Robinson procedure is used makes little difference in outcome overall, provided the chosen procedure is done carefully and the preoperative diagnosis is correct.

The anterior approach to the cervical spine is easy and safe from the levels of C_3 through C_7, the vertebral segments most often affected by disc disease. The anterior intervertebral route exposes the vertebral bodies, the discs, and the ventral spinal canal and, consequently, osteophytes or disc fragments that impinge on the root foramina and spinal canal can be removed directly. The anterior approach has 2 advantages: osteophytes or disc fragments can be removed safely, and fusion of the affected disc space provides permanent immobility of that joint. The disadvantages of the anterior approach are that it may cause increased stress upon nonfused disc spaces above and below the operated level, and it affords no access to posterior elements that may compress neural structures.

If the anterior spine is affected by trauma or tumor requiring extensive bone removal, then a strut graft is highly effective when combined with halo-jacket immobilization. If life expectancy is short, then we prefer a reinforced acrylic prosthesis and a rigid collar to allow maximum comfort and mobility, free of external bracing.

REFERENCES

1. Apuzzo, M. L. J., Weiss, M. H., and Heiden, J. S. Transoral exposure of the atlantoaxial region. Neurosurgery, *3:* 201–207, 1978.
2. Arbit, E., and Patterson, R. H., Jr. Combined transoral and median labiomandibular glossotomy approach to the upper cervical spine. Neurosurgery, *8:* 672–674, 1981.
3. Aronson, N. I., Filtzer, D. L., and Bagan, M. Anterior cervical fusion by the Smith-Robinson approach. J. Neurosurg., *29:* 397–404, 1968.
4. Bailey, R. W., and Badgley, C. E. Stabilization of the cervical spine by anterior fusion. J. Bone Jt. Surg., *42A:* 565–594, 1960.

5. Cloward, R. B. The anterior approach for the removal of ruptured cervical discs. J. Neurosurg., *15:* 602–617, 1958.
6. Cloward, R. B. Cervical cordotomy by the anterior approach: Techniques and advantages. J. Neurosurg., *21:* 19–25, 1964.
7. Cloward, R. B. Treatment of acute fractures and fracture-dislocations of the cervical spine by vertebral body fusion. A report of 11 cases. J. Neurosurg., *18:* 201–209, 1961.
8. Fang, H. S. Y., and Ong, G. B. Direct anterior approach to the upper cervical spine. J. Bone Jt. Surg., *44A:* 1588–1604, 1962.
9. Fang, H. S. Y., Ong, G. B., and Hodgson, A. R. Anterior spinal fusion: The operative approaches. Clin. Orthop., *35:* 16–33, 1964.
10. Galera, R. G., and Tovi, D. Anterior disc excision with interbody fusion in cervical spondylotic myelopathy and rhizopathy. J. Neurosurg., *15:* 305–310, 1968.
11. Greenberg, A. D., Scoville, W. B., and Davey, L. M. Transoral decompression of atlantoaxial dislocation due to odontoid hypoplasia. Report of two cases. J. Neurosurg., *28:* 266–269, 1968.
12. Gregorius, F. K., Estrin, T., and Crandall, P. H. Cervical spondylotic radiculopathy and myelopathy. Arch. Neurol., *33:* 618–625, 1976.
13. Hankinson, H. L., and Wilson, C. B. Use of the operating microscope in anterior cervical discectomy without fusion. J. Neurosurg., *43:* 452–456, 1975.
14. Hirsch, C. Cervical disc rupture. Acta Orthop. Scand., *30:* 172–180, 1960.
15. Hoff, J. T., and Wilson, C. B. Microsurgical approach to the anterior cervical spine and spinal cord. Clin. Neurosurg., *26:* 523–528, 1979.
16. Lesoin, F., Bouasakao, N., Krivosic, I., DuPont, A., and Jomin, M. Use of acrylic prosthesis for a giant-cell tumor of the cervical spine. Surg. Neurol., *17:* 358–362, 1981.
17. Lunsford, L. D., Bissonette, D. J., Janetta, P. J., Septak, P. E., and Zorub, D. S. Anterior surgery for cervical disc disease. J. Neurosurg., *53:* 1–19, 1980.
18. Martins, A. N. Anterior cervical discectomy with and without interbody bone graft. J. Neurosurg., *44:* 290–295, 1976.
19. McRae, D. L. The significance of abnormalities of the cervical spine. Am. J. Roentgenol., *84:* 3–25, 1960.
20. Mullan, S., Naunton, R., Hekmatpanah, J., and Vailati, G. The use of an anterior approach to ventrally placed tumors in the foramen magnum and vertebral column. J. Neurosurg., *24:* 536–543, 1966.
21. Murphy, M. G., and Gado, M. Anterior cervical discectomy without interbody bone graft. J. Neurosurg., *37:* 71–74, 1972.
22. Riley, L. H., Jr., Robinson, R. A., Johnson, K. A., and Walker, A. E. The results of anterior interbody fusion of the cervical spine. J. Neurosurg., *30:* 127–133, 1969.
23. Robertson, J. T. Anterior removal of cervical disc without fusion. Clin. Neurosurg. *20:* 259–261, 1972.
24. Robertson, J. T. Anterior operations for herniated cervical disc and for myelopathy. Clin. Neurosurg., *25:* 245–250, 1978.
25. Robinson, R. A., Walker, A. E., Ferlic, D. C., and Wiecking, D. K. The results of anterior interbody fusion of the cervical spine. J. Bone Joint Surg., *44:* 1569–1587, 1962.
26. Schmidek, H. H. The anterolateral approach to the cervical spine in the management of cervical spondylosis and its complications. In: *Current Techniques in Operative Neurosurgery*, edited by H. Schmidek and W. Sweet, pp. 303–322. Grune & Stratton, New York, 1977.
27. Scoville, W. B., Palmer, A. H., Samra, A., and Chong, G. The use of acrylic plastic for

vertebral replacement or fixation in metastatic disease of the spine. Technical note. J. Neurosurg., *17:* 274–279, 1967.

28. Smith, G. W., and Robinson, R. A. The treatment of certain cervical spine disorders by anterior removal of the intervertebral disc and interbody fusion. J. Bone Joint Surg., *40A:* 607–624, 1958.
29. Sugar, O. Spinal cord malfunction after anterior cervical discectomy. Surg. Neurol., *15:* 4–8, 1980.
30. Tew, J. M., Jr., and Mayfield, F. H. Complications of surgery of the anterior cervical spine. Clin. Neurosurg., *23:* 424–434,1976.
31. U, H. S., and Wilson, C. B. Postoperative epidural hematoma as a complication of anterior cervical discectomy. J. Neurosurg., *49:* 288–291, 1978.
32. Wood, B. G., Sadar, E. S., Levine, H. L., Dohn, D. F., and Tucker, H. M. Surgical problems of the base of the skull: An interdisciplinary approach. Arch Otolaryngol., *160:* 1–5, 1980.

CHAPTER

32

Thoracolumbar Injuries

EDWARD L. SELJESKOG, M.D., PH.D.

Over the last decade, the management of thoracolumbar injuries has rather dramatically changed. Previous treatment programs have focused, on the one extreme, from nonoperative and noninterventional, in which minimal regard has been given to the neural elements and in which therapy primarily was directed toward a closed reduction of the fracture or subluxation by positioning and closed manipulation. In contrast, there were those proponents, primarily in the neurosurgical community, who advocated radical decompression, usually through a wide and extensive laminectomy, often compounding an already precarious problem of spinal stability. Gradually, however, a number of factors began to alter these concepts.

First was the realization that thoracolumbar injuries are neurologically unique. Many cases, in contrast to those of the cervical and thoracic regions, offer the potential for recovery, in that one is dealing with a combination of spinal cord (conus) injury and an injury to the roots of the cauda equina. In this situation, neurologic recovery can eventually develop in many seemingly complete injuries once decompression or entrapment of nerve roots has been accomplished. Enumerable instances of significant improvement have been reported, even with late decompression. As a result, many patients, although initially impaired rather seriously from the neurologic standpoint, are eventually able to achieve an ambulatory status. Recovery of conus function, however, is another matter, and permanent loss of neurologic function in those areas innervated by the sacral roots, including innervation of bladder and bowel, are common, and certainly the degree of recovery does not parallel that of the cauda equina.

The second factor operant in this changing philosophy of thoracolumbar fracture management has been the development of a better understanding of the injury and its mechanisms of development. This has been particularly aided by the use of polytomography and, more recently, by the use of high resolution CT scanning, best visualized with metrizamide CSF enhancement. Following the introduction of spinal CT scanning has been an appreciation of significant persisting spinal canal compromise by bony elements, despite what was initially thought to be an adequate decompression. As a consequence, CT scanning and tomography can aid immeasurably in the initial assessment of the injury, including its mechanism of production, its stability, its severity and, more importantly, the dimensions of spinal canal. Most importantly, however, this initial complete radiographic evaluation permits one to more appropriately plan therapy and, if necessary, to decide on the most beneficial operative approach.

The third factor in this evolution of management has been the development of various orthopedic techniques and devices for achieving immediate spinal stability until such time as solid bony union has developed across the fracture. Most notable has been the use of Harrington rods (1–3, 6, 9). More recently, anterior bony fusion has been hastened through the use of a vascularized rib graft. The end result has been the achievement in most operative cases of early stability with a minimum of late pseudarthrosis or progressive spinal deformity.

CLASSIFICATION OF THORACOLUMBAR INJURIES

As in analyzing any complex injury, numerous schema of classification have been developed. The studies of Holdsworth (4, 5) are most noteworthy in the thoracolumbar region. He reviewed a large series of cases from the coal mining region around Sheffield, and his classification includes the following:

I. Flexion-compression injuries (including simple wedge fractures).
II. Axial loading or compression injuries (including burst fractures).
III. Lateral rotation fractures (including slice fractures).
IV. Lap belt injuries or tension-stress injuries (including chance fractures).

Flexion-Compression Injuries

In general, most simple compression or wedge fractures at the thoracolumbar junction represent stable injuries. Neurologic impairment is infrequent unless the fracture is significant and accompanied by retropulsion of fracture fragments or disc material. In the event of conus or cauda equina neurologic symptoms, which must include careful testing of the sacral dermatomes, reflexes, and bladder function, tomography and high resolution contrast-enhanced CT scanning then become necessary, chiefly to exclude compromise of the spinal canal by retropulsed fracture fragments or disc material. A similar management philosophy also would seem to be prudent in those cases in which there is *major* compression of the vertebral body, generally over 50% of its anterior height. It is surprising how often significant abnormalities will be identified with this more complete radiographic evaluation, in what initially are thought to be simple injuries. There is a common tendency to grossly underestimate the severity of thoracolumbar fractures, particularly when viewed only in the context of standard x-ray studies.

In considering treatment, minimal compression fractures, without neurologic involvement, can usually be managed quite satisfactorily with a few days bedrest and then progressive ambulation, as recommended by Norrell (8). More significant compression fractures, however, will require bracing or external immobilization with a polypropylene body jacket to prevent fracture collapse and late kyphosis.

In contrast, major compression injuries, involving more than 50% of the anterior body height, should be considered as potentially unstable (Fig. 32.1). If tomography does not reveal involvement of the posterior elements and CT scanning of the canal is unremarkable, we would tend to manage these more significant injuries nonoperatively, with a hyperextension cast or jacket until healing occurs. Involvement of the posterior elements, however, is usually an indication for posterior Harrington rod fusion. Obviously, the development of a progressive kyphosis is another indication for operative intervention.

Axial Loading-Compression Injuries

Axial compression injuries in their severe form produce the so-called burst fracture (Fig. 32.2). Often there is a coexisting element of flexion or lateral rotation, making precise classification in some cases difficult. Nevertheless, with major fractures involving the entire vertebral body, irrespective of the patient's neurologic status, tomography and enhanced CT scanning are nearly always to be recommended. Again, unsuspected significant narrowing of the spinal canal is frequent, along with unsuspected major comminution and disruption of the involved vertebral body.

Since these fractures are usually unstable, some type of immobilization is required. The more simple injuries without spinal canal alteration could be treated with a body jacket and external immobilization, but most injuries are best managed with operative intervention and fusion, preferably with the Harrington rod technique.

In the event that the dimensions of the spinal canal are reduced by bone fragments or disc material and regardless of the patient's neurologic status, we would advocate removal of the offending intraspinal mass. The more significant the degree of constriction, the more strongly we would propose decompression, as prophylaxis against late neurologic symptoms from kyphosis and post-traumatic arthritic change. Late decompressive surgery following bony healing is considerably more difficult

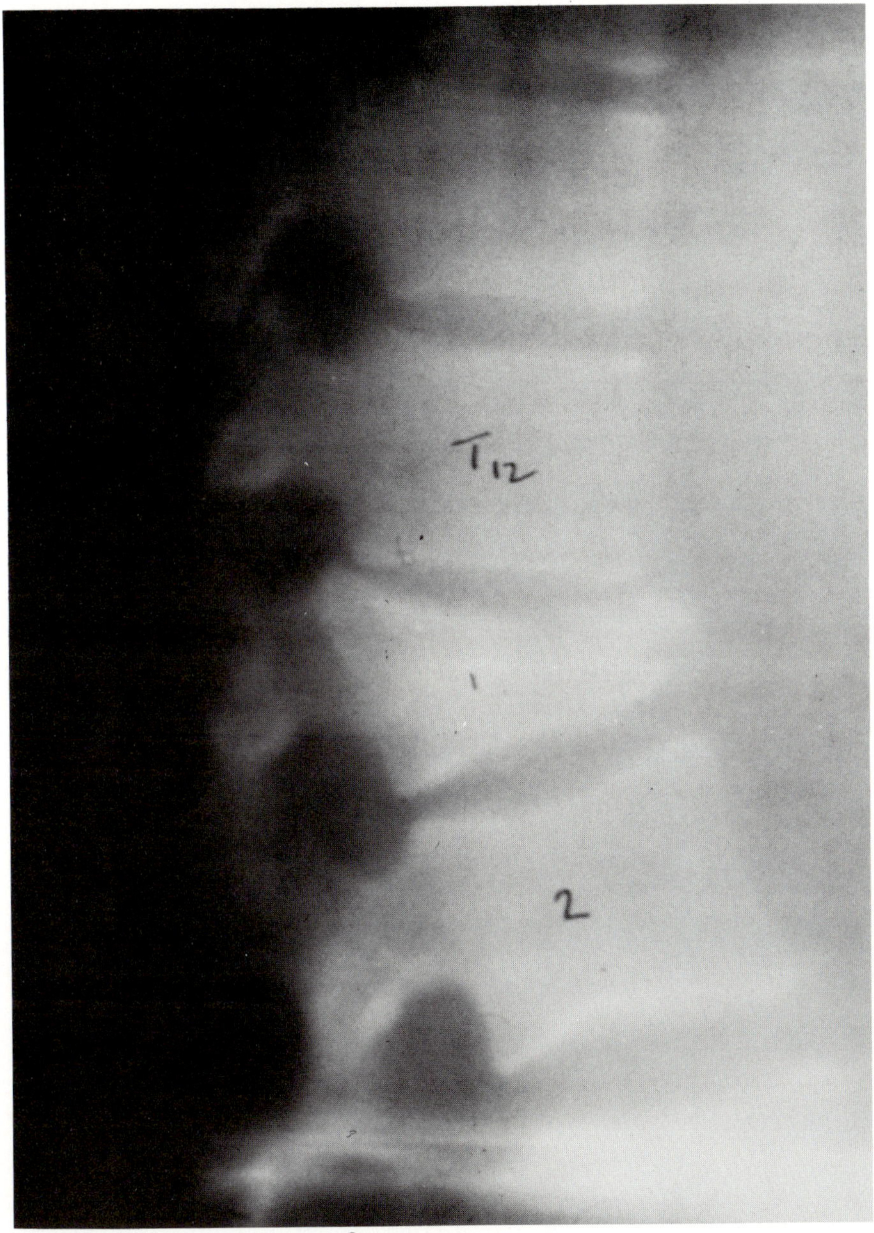

FIG. 32.1. Lateral view of 1st lumbar vertebra, demonstrating a major flexion-compression or wedge fracture.

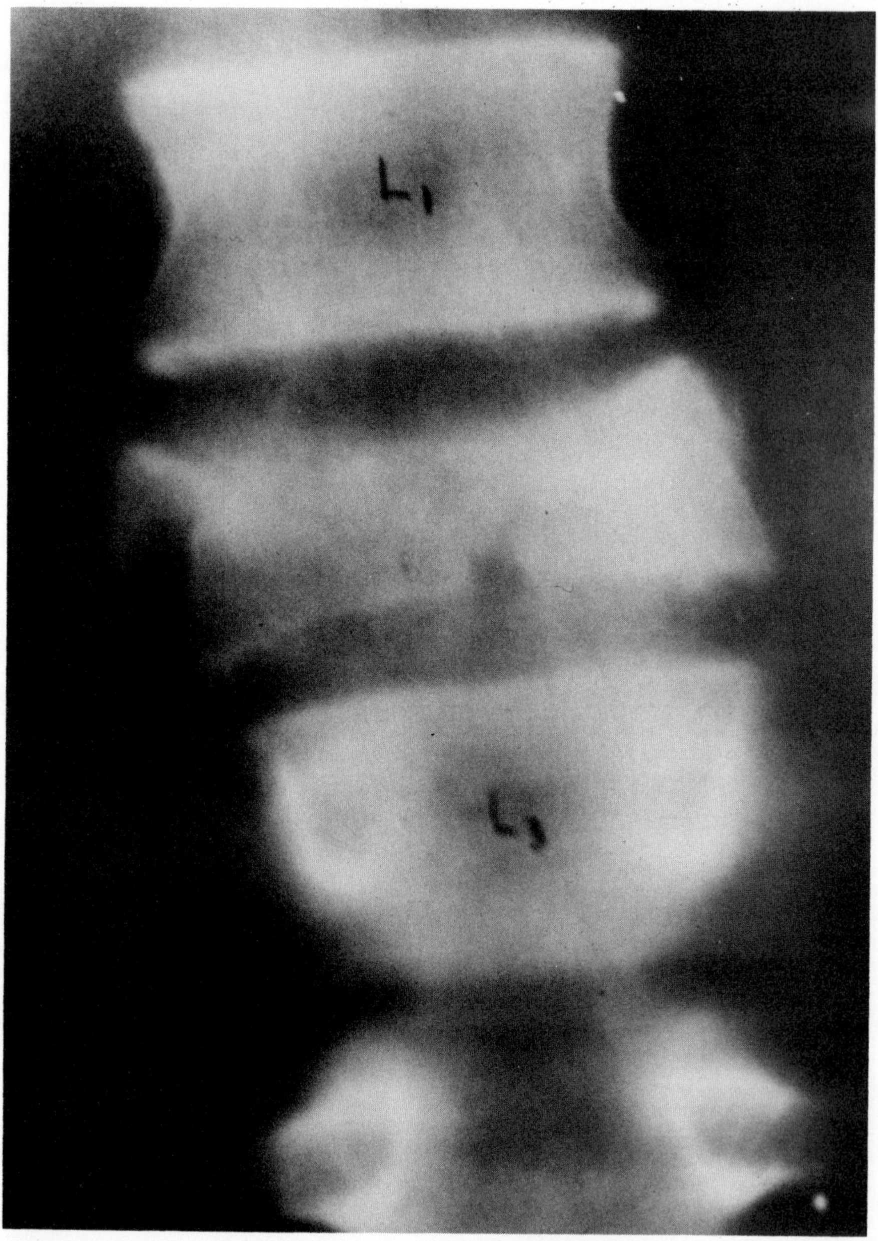

FIG. 32.2. AP view of 2nd lumbar vertebra, demonstrating a major axial loading (burst) fracture.

and may, in itself, recreate spinal instability. It seems reasonable then to advocate this type of early aggressive approach, since most patients will be undergoing operative stabilization and fusion for their initial instability.

Lateral Rotation Injuries

This fracture, in which a rotatory force fractures the posterior elements, along with a fracture of the vertebral body, is generally limited to the thoracolumbar region (Figs. 32.3*A* and *B*). If this fracture passes obliquely through the vertebral body, it produces a so-called slice fracture. In light of the significant forces involved, there is often comminution, dislocation, or retropulsion of fracture fragments. X-ray and CT evaluation are necessary in this injury to determine the need for decompression. Utilizing the principles previously enumerated, operative stabilization is nearly always required, in light of the propensity to develop early and late spinal deformity.

Lap Belt Injuries

Neurologic involvement is less frequent in this group of injuries, which primarily affects the first and second lumbar level (Fig. 32.4). Again, tomography and CT evaluation are in order, as well as principles of management identical to those in the foregoing sections. Posterior Harrington rod fusion is usually necessary in light of the frequent instability and the usual major involvement of the posterior elements. Posterolateral decompression is sometimes necessary in those cases that have intraspinal bone fragments.

SURGICAL CONSIDERATIONS

Since the site of spinal canal compromise in most thoracolumbar injuries is anterior or anterolateral, decompressive laminectomy plays a limited role in the management of these injuries. In the case of encountering a floating fractured lamina, laminectomy, obviously, is prudent, since postoperative intraspinal displacement of fracture fragments is a definite risk. Similarly, removal of a fractured facet or pedicle should be considered, if it will improve visualization or exposure of the ventral fracture site. The need to be assured of an adequate decompression is paramount, and the sacrifice of minor factors of stability is worthwhile, since operative instrumentation and fusion are to be part of the procedure. There seems to be little place for "peek-a'boo" surgery, when compromise of the spinal canal and neural elements are at stake.

In this context, some orthopedic surgeons have advocated a blind fracture reduction utilizing the Harrington rod technique, without de-

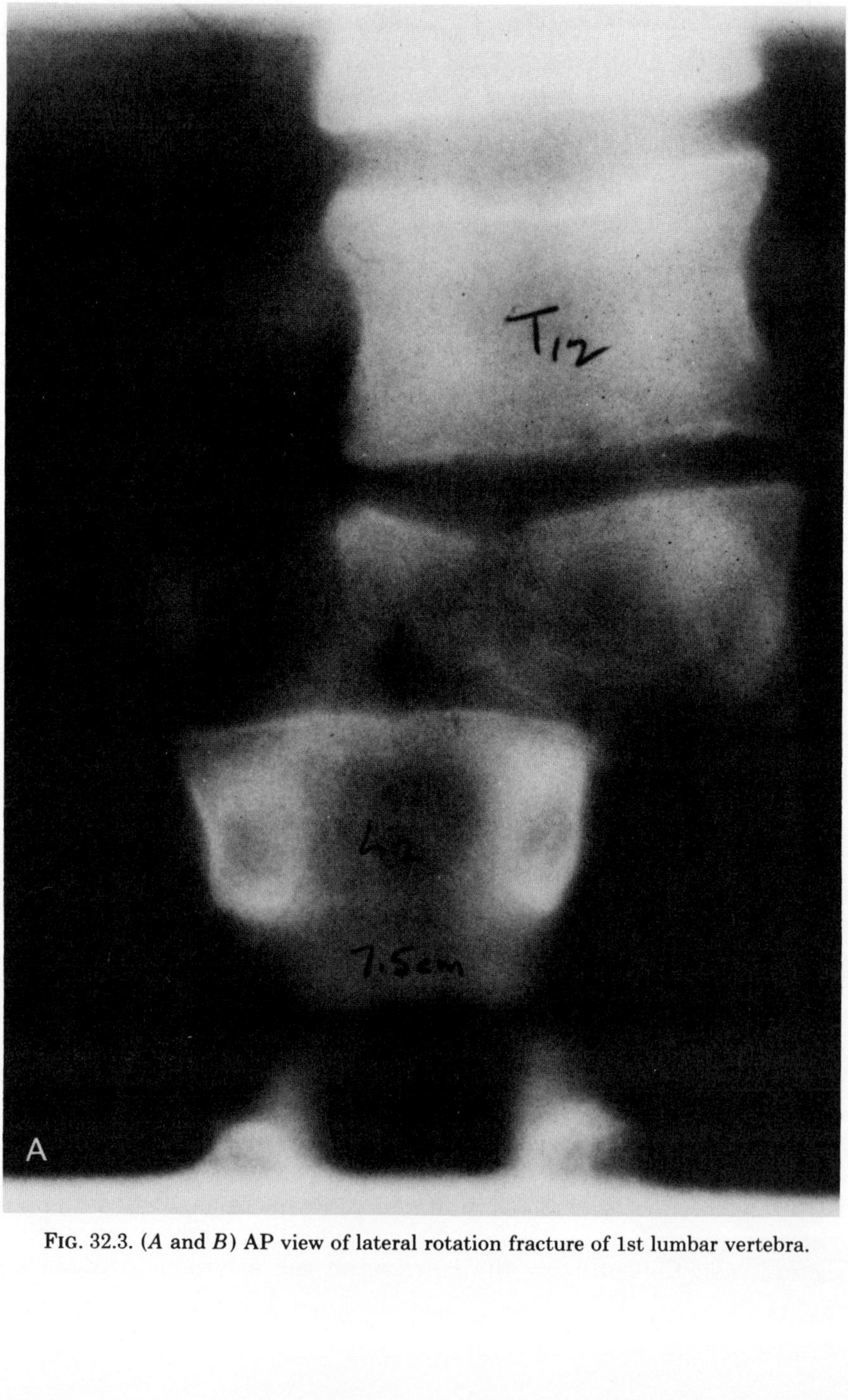

FIG. 32.3. (*A* and *B*) AP view of lateral rotation fracture of 1st lumbar vertebra.

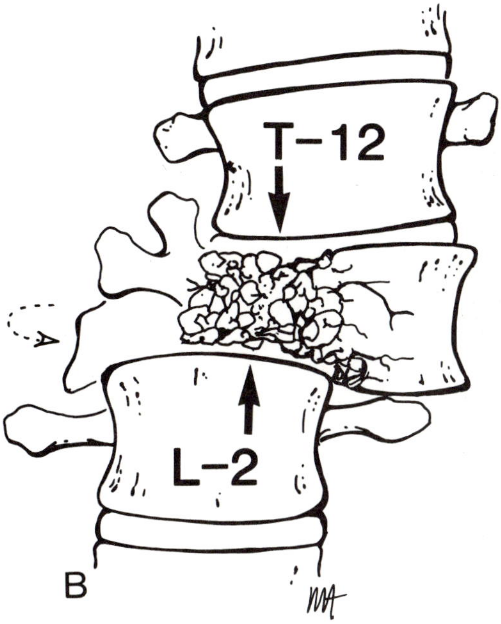

FIG. 32.3*B*

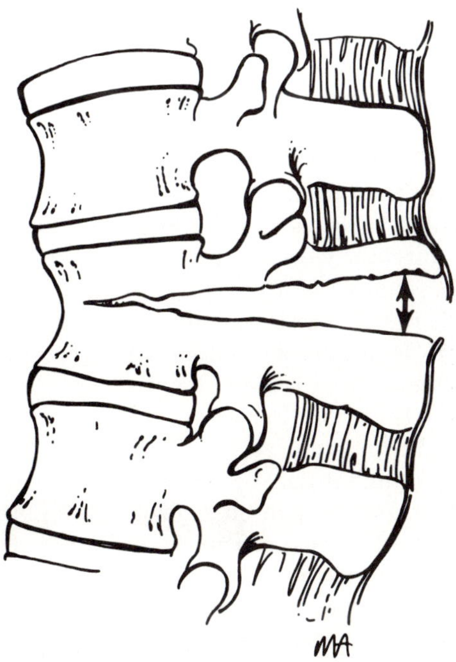

FIG. 32.4. Lateral diagram thoracolumbar lap belt injury illustrating a Chance fracture.

compression or fracture visualization. We have been impressed with the inadequacy of this technique, except in the most minor of fractures and, of course, with significant bony constriction of the spinal canal, it is fraught with the risk of iatrogenic neurologic loss. Despite reduction and realignment of the fracture, fragments and disc material can easily be left behind. In light of this, we always carry out a lateral laminotomy to ensure complete decompression of the canal. At times, this will require bilateral visualization. At the same time, the dura can be inspected for laceration and prolapsed nerve roots can be reduced. Repair of the dura at this time is a comparatively easy matter.

A decision for an anterior, as opposed to a posterolateral decompression, rests with the x-ray studies and CT findings. Unilateral encroachment of the spinal canal and fractured unstable posterior elements are two indicators for considering a posterolateral approach, obviously coupled with a Harrington rod fusion. In contrast, a broad anterior compression and intact posterior elements are indicators for a transthoracic, anterior approach, which can be utilized for lesions as low as the first or second lumbar vertebra (7).

A more significant dilemma is created in thoracolumbar injuries, when confronted with an immediate and complete paraplegia. Generally, these are associated with severe bony injuries of such magnitude as to require decompression and fusion. In these special severe cases, we would tend to favor an approach, especially for those cases at the L_1 or L_2 level, from a posterolateral route utilizing Harrington rod instrumentation for stabilization. The question is always raised as to whether the dura should be opened for inspection for intradural hematoma or bone and disc fragments. Also to be considered is the question of suturing of lacerated nerve roots, since the potential for recovery is present. Often, the decision is easy, since in these severe cases the dura has already been lacerated, and one proceeds directly with a limited laminectomy for dural repair. On inspection, the conus is often softened and hemorrhagic. Usually most of the roots are contused, but intact. If there are lacerated roots and if the patient is otherwise stable, one certainly could consider microneurorraphy but, again, it is to be noted that the value of this latter technique has never been solidly proven.

Finally, there is the question of late operative intervention. Certainly, a very reasonable argument can be made for follow-up reassessment of the patient who continues to exhibit neurologic impairment. Most often this relates to bowel and bladder dysfunction. In these cases, myelography and CT scanning are reasonable, to exclude persisting or recurrent neural compression at the injury site. At the present, a very logical argument can be made for late decompression as advocated by Ransohoff (10). Under some circumstances one could consider intradural exploration and neurolysis. We have had several instances wherein there appeared to be further nerve root recovery following this additional late surgery.

OPERATIVE TECHNIQUE

Posterolateral Approach

In this technique the patient is positioned prone on a Hall 4-poster type of laminectomy frame (Fig. 32.5). This technique allows the abdomen to be free, but most importantly places the thoracolumbar spine in a position of slight hyperextension, aiding the realignment and reduction of the fracture. An alternative, but in our view less satisfactory, approach is the use of the standard laminectomy rolls.

After suitable wide preparation, including both posterior iliac crests and cephalad to the upper thoracic region, a midline skin incision is made down to the spinous processes. This permits a posterolateral exposure from either side or, if necessary bilaterally. The spinous processes are exposed a minimum of 2 to 3 levels above and below the injury, which aids in the posterolateral exposure of the ventral spinal canal, but also is a necessity for the later Harrington rod insertion.

In light of the usual fracture of posterior elements, we use sharp

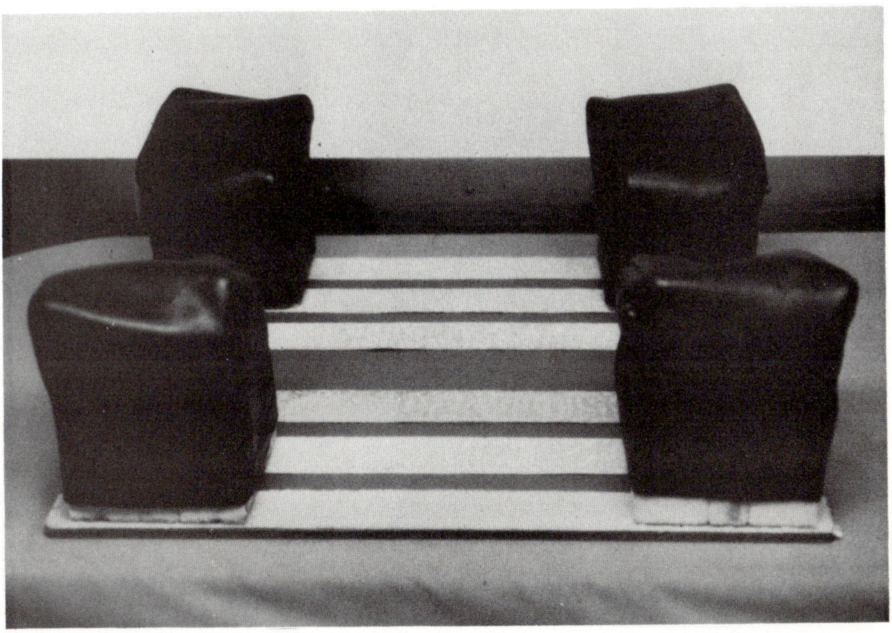

FIG. 32.5. Hall 4-poster-padded laminectomy frame. Note that the abdomen is free and that the net effect is to produce slight thoracolumbar extension, aiding fracture reduction and realignment.

dissection to take down the paravertebral muscles at the level of the injury. At this point, one frequently encounters soft tissue hematoma, especially in the rotatory and lap belt types of injuries. The involved lamina are frequently fractured. If they are found to be free and floating, they are removed to avoid the later risks of inward displacement into the spinal canal.

In order to achieve decompression, a lateral laminotomy is then carried out, utilizing small punches or a burr, along with removal of a portion of the medial aspect of the facet and pedicle (Figs. 32.6*A* and *B*). This procedure allows access to the ventral portion of the canal. One usually approaches the injury from the most severely involved side, as judged by the preoperative CT scan and tomography. At times, with major retropulsion of bone and disc material, exposure is difficult, necessitating removal of the entire facet and pedicle, usually in circumstances in which an anterior decompression might have been preferred. Often, in this type of case, bilateral exposure is necessary and, of course, any removal of the entire facet and pedicle compounds instability. This, however, is a small sacrifice in order to achieve adequate decompression, especially since the area is already unstable, and the patient will be undergoing stabilization and fusion.

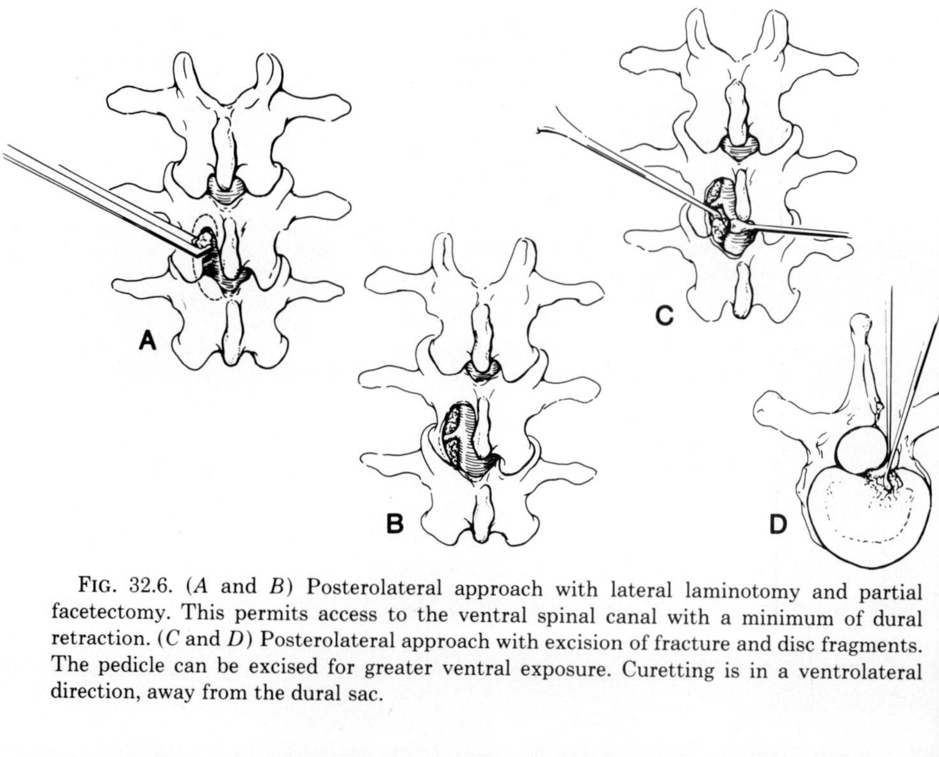

FIG. 32.6. (*A* and *B*) Posterolateral approach with lateral laminotomy and partial facetectomy. This permits access to the ventral spinal canal with a minimum of dural retraction. (*C* and *D*) Posterolateral approach with excision of fracture and disc fragments. The pedicle can be excised for greater ventral exposure. Curetting is in a ventrolateral direction, away from the dural sac.

Once the ventrolateral portion of the canal is exposed through a combination of lateral laminectomy, facetectomy, and gentle dural retraction, the fracture fragments and disc tissue are removed in a piecemeal fashion utilizing long, straight, and angled curettes and small rongeurs. Especially useful is the Dawson-Yue rongeur, which has significant strength despite a relatively small jaw size. Curetting should be directed away from the dural sac, after having undermined and excised some of the vertebral body beneath the fracture fragments (Figs. 32.6*C* and *D*). Once complete decompression has been achieved, as judged by a return of dural pulsations but more particularly as visualized directly or by instrument palpation, hemostasis is achieved in the fracture bed by packing with thrombin-soaked Gelfoam pledgets or Avitene.

In the event that CT scanning and tomography have revealed fracture retropulsion or subluxation to be minimal, we sometimes will consider attempting the minimal reduction solely with operative positioning and Harrington rod instrumentation. The latter should always be under direct visualization through a limited lateral hemilaminotomy. In our view, and as previously noted, there is little place for blind reduction where one hopes for success, but there is always a risk for retained bone and disc fragments.

Dealing with the dura poses another set of problems. In the case of a floating lamina, the dura is readily exposed for inspection following laminectomy. If a laceration is evident, intradural exploration is pursued, along with a reduction of any prolapsed nerve roots. We do not, however, routinely open the dura for exploration, since the majority of cases are incomplete from the neurologic standpoint and, under usual circumstances, one usually does not encounter a dural laceration. In the case of the less frequent, immediate, and complete neurologic injury, a more extensive intradural exploration is advisable, with consideration for microneurorrhaphy.

At this point, attention is then directed to the stabilization phase of the operation, with bilateral placement of Harrington rods, preferably 3 levels above and 3 levels below the fracture. Bone shavings and small fragments from an iliac wing donor site are then placed lateral to the canal over the remaining portions of the facets. In light of the usual and persisting oozing from the fracture fragments, hemovac drainage for 24 hours is usually advisable. In severe injuries which are significantly unstable, postoperative immobilization is usually necessary, utilizing a polypropolene body jacket.

Anterior Transthoracic Approach

In this procedure, carried out with the patient in the lateral decubitus-thoracotomy position, often flexing the table a bit to enhance exposure, we generally utilize the right chest. This approach avoids the need to displace and retract the aorta. On occasion, exposure through the left hemithorax may be indicated to facilitate the anterior decompression. For injuries at the thoracolumbar junction, we generally would utilize the bed of the 9th rib, taking care to preserve its neurovascular bundle and its rib attachment. The lung is then packed away, and the vertebral insertions of the diaphragm are taken down, followed by additional reflection of the pleura, exposing the entire lateral vertebral body. Several intercostal vessels cross the area and are doubly ligated and divided (Fig. 32.7). To date, we have not identified any problems of cord ischemia.

At this point, one can begin the anterior decompression, first by incising and removing the adjacent discs and their associated cartilaginous plates. The posterior portion of the vertebral body is then removed in a piecemeal fashion. This is relatively easy since it is under direct visualization and particularly since the vertebral body is usually comminuted (Fig. 32.8). As cortical bone ventral to the spinal canal is reached, fragments are then excised with long angled curettes as designed by Chou, in combination with the Dawson-Yue rongeur. The decompression

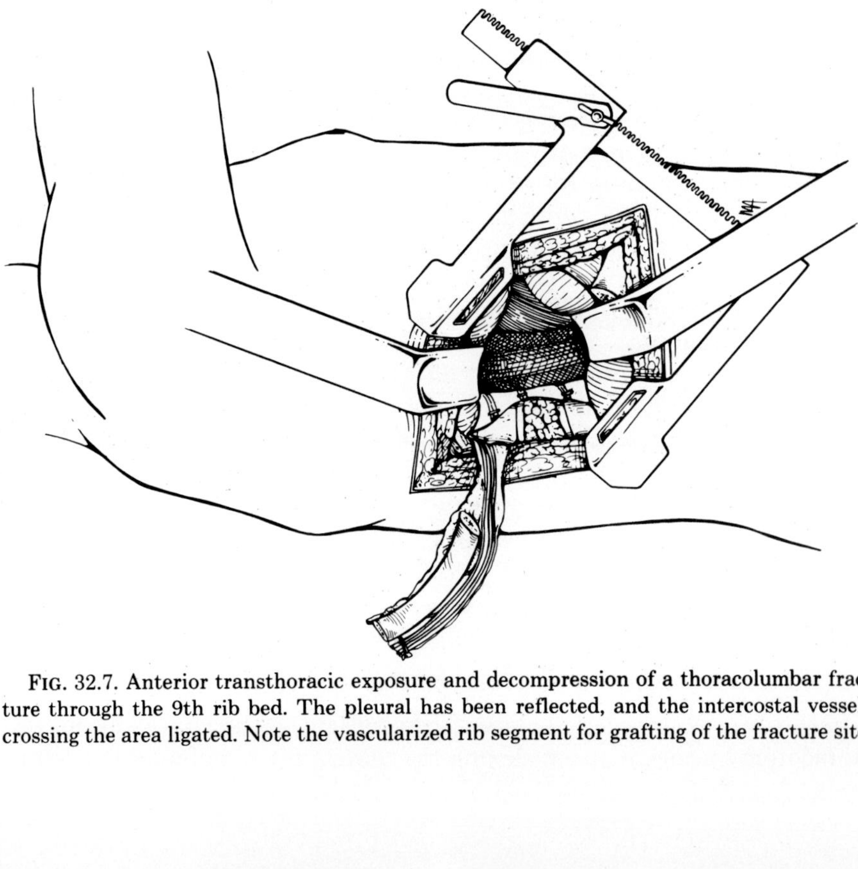

FIG. 32.7. Anterior transthoracic exposure and decompression of a thoracolumbar fracture through the 9th rib bed. The pleural has been reflected, and the intercostal vessels crossing the area ligated. Note the vascularized rib segment for grafting of the fracture site.

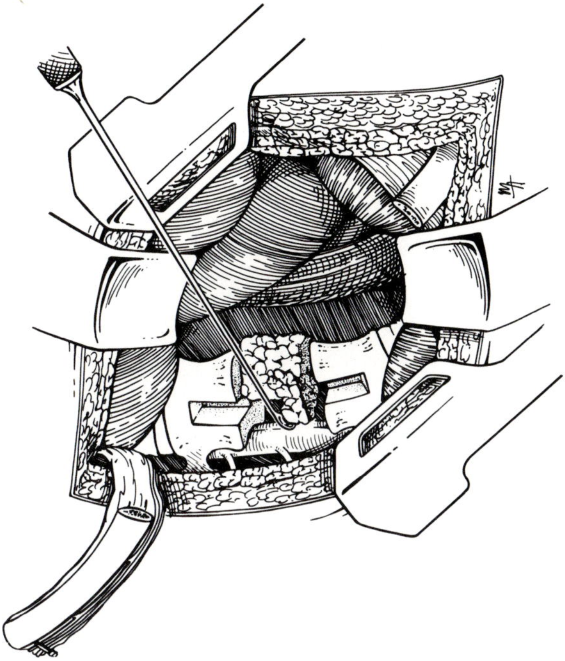

FIG. 32.8. Anterior transthoracic decompression following excision of adjacent intervertebral discs. Note the curetting of fracture fragments away from the dural sac and the troughs fashioned into the adjacent lateral vertebral bodies.

is then carried ventrally across the canal, as far contralaterally as is necessary, to achieve a complete decompression. Care is again exercised to curette fragments away from the canal and into the undermined and excised central vertebral body. With assurance of complete decompression, hemostasis is achieved, as previously described.

Attention is now directed to the lateral aspect of the adjacent vertebral bodies, where in a cephalad and caudad direction, troughs are created for insertion of the vascularized rib graft (Fig. 32.9). The latter has been cleared of periosteum and soft tissue and fashioned to an appropriate length. Prior to its insertion, however, the cavity created within the vertebral body is loosely packed with bone chips preserved from the excised fracture fragments. Recently, our orthopedic colleagues have utilized a large femoral neck ("Bone Bank") graft, fashioned into a central hollowed out area of the adjacent vertebral bodies. Excess rib fragments are then applied adjacent to the vascularized rib graft, along with any extra bone chips. Hemostasis is again achieved. The diaphragm is resutured to its attachment, and the pleura and chest are then closed.

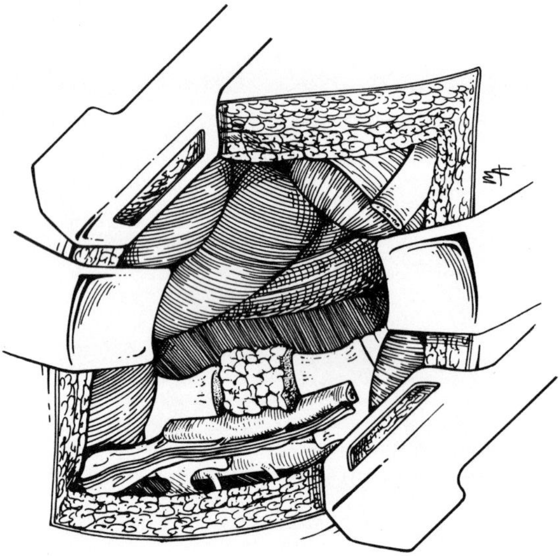

FIG. 32.9. Anterior transthoracic approach following decompression. Note the vascularized rib graft wedged into the previously created channels.

RESULTS

Several years ago, Flesch *et al.* (1) reported our results at the University of Minnesota involving 40 thoracic and lumbar fracture patients who had undergone Harrington rod instrumentation (1). In this particular series, no anterior decompression cases were included. Among these 40 patients there were 25 thoracolumbar injuries, which included 21 significant rotatory injuries, 2 axial loading burst fractures, and 2 simple wedge fractures. Nine of the 25 patients exhibited complete conus injuries. In none of these was there evidence of neurologic recovery, much as one would have predicted, since this is the usual course of recovery from a complete traumatic cord lesion. Injury of the cauda equina roots, however, was another matter. In all patients with incomplete cord or cauda equina injury, there was major postoperative improvement, and all of these patients are now walking. Whether or not this would have occurred as a natural course of events, is open to debate, since there is a tendency for these injuries to improve irrespective of therapy. Judging, however, by the degree of initial nerve root involvement and the significant degree of compression encountered at surgery, we cannot come to any other conclusion than that many of these patients were materially benefited by aggressive decompression.

From the standpoint of spinal stability and postoperative deformity, we have an even brighter picture. All 40 patients in the series had no external evidence of spinal deformity, and 39 had excellent or normal spinal alignment when examined in follow-up over the following years. A similar type of follow-up picture seems to be developing from both the neurological and spinal stability standpoints regarding those patients who have undergone the alternative anterior thoracic decompression.

SUMMARY

Thoracolumbar injuries represent an unique neurologic injury. In light of the potential for recovery in the roots of the cauda equina, an aggressive plan of management should be undertaken, to absolutely ensure an adequate decompression of the spinal canal and neural elements, but in addition to accomplish a simultaneous bony reduction and fusion of the injury site. Traditional laminectomy alone has minimal benefit in most of these cases, since compression is usually anterior and decompression is best achieved through a posterolateral or anterior transthoracic approach. The best avenue of decompression is dictated by a careful and complete preoperative radiographic evaluation, including polytomography and CT scanning. Utilization of this aggressive plan of management can then offer an optimum milieu for neurologic recovery and at the same time produce solid, pain-free bony healing with a minimum of spinal deformity.

REFERENCES

1. Flesch, J. R., *et al.* Harrington rod instrumentation and spine fusion for unstable fractures and fracture dislocations. J. Bone Joint Surg., *59A:* 143–153, 1977.
2. Harrington, P. R. Instrumentation in spine instability other than scoliosis. S. Afr. J. Surg., *5:* 7–12, 1967.
3. Harrington, P. R. Technical details in relation to the successful use of instrumentation. *Orthop. Clin. North Am., 3:* 49–67, 1972.
4. Holdsworth, F. W. Fractures, dislocations and fracture dislocations of the spine. J. Bone Joint Surg., *45B:* 6–20, 1963.
5. Holdsworth, F. W. Fractures, dislocations and fracture-dislocations of the spine. J. Bone Joint Surg., *52A:* 1434–1551, 1970.
6. Jacobs, R. R., *et al.* Thoracolumbar spinal injuries. Spine, *5:* 463–477, 1980.
7. Kelly, R. P., and Whitesides, T. E. Treatment of lumbodorsal fracture-dislocations. Ann. Surg., *167:* 705–717, 1968.
8. Norrell, H. A. Fractures and dislocations of the spine. Spine: 557–562, 1975.
9. Osebold, W. R., *et al.* Thoracolumbar spine fractures. Spine, *6:* 13–34, 1981.
10. Ransohoff, J. Lesions of the cauda equina. Clin. Neurosurg., *17:* 331–344, 1970.

CHAPTER

33

Mechanism of Action of Chymopapain in Ruptured Lumbar Disc Disease

CLARK WATTS, M.D.

INTRODUCTION

Few debates in the neurosurgery-orthopaedic literature have been waged with the intensity and emotion that has been seen in the evaluation of the injection of chymopapain into the lumbar intervertebral disc as a treatment for disc disease (39). Proponents of the treatment cite biochemical evidence for a direct effect of chymopapain upon the lumbar disc. They advocate its use as either a treatment to be interposed between conservative therapy and surgical excision, or as a treatment to replace surgery. Opponents cite the poorly controlled clinical studies as failing to provide evidence of efficacy. Between 1963, when Lyman Smith introduced the drug into clinical use, and 1975, when the Food and Drug Administration and the sponsoring company, Travenol Laboratories (Deerfield, Ill.), closed down a phase III trial of the drug, the debate had become so polarized that objective evaluation of a subsequent double-blind study was not possible.

Throughout the years investigators have reported successful treatment with chymopapain in 50–90% of patients (41, 43). The double-blind study, to which the investigators at Walter Reed Army Medical Center were the major contributors, reported no significant difference in efficacy between chymopapain and a "placebo" (21, 33). The results of this study have been supported primarily by those who have argued that chymopapain has no efficacy in the treatment of lumbar disc disease. Conversely, the study has been criticized by those who have maintained that the efficacy of chymopapain has been shown by previous noncontrolled studies.

Obscured by the debate are known facts concerning degenerative disc disease and the effects of chymopapain upon the lumbar intervertebral disc which, when closely examined suggest a mechanism of action for chymopapain in lumbar disc disease. It is the purpose of this paper to present a hypothesis based upon this data. To accept this hypothesis will require an alteration in the traditional view of symptomatic lumbar disc disease. It will suggest that chymopapain, or similar agents, may be useful in further investigation into the nature of symptomatic degenerative disc disease. I will review pertinent facts known about the anatomy of the lumbar disc and the degenerative process, and the effects of chymopapain upon the various components of the lumbar disc. Following a presentation of the results of conservative therapy, chymopapain injection, and surgery, I will conclude with the hypothesis.

THE DEGENERATIVE DISC

The basic anatomy of the normal lumbar disc is well known (19). The center of the disc, the nucleus pulposus, is a gel-like substance sparse of cellular material and containing an abundant amorphous ground substance (25). This substance is composed largely of mucopolysaccharides which, because of their electrical charges, readily bind water. The normal nucleus of a young person bulges noticeably if the disc is transected, making a sharp distinction between the nucleus pulposus and the more lateral portions of the disc, the annulus fibrosis. With age the mucopolysaccharides are broken down, and water content is lost (5). Increased amounts of a collagen protein, β protein, are found in the region of the nucleus (25). This collagen is different, biochemically, from the normal collagen of the annulus fibrosis, with reduced tensile strength. The combination of a decrease in mucopolysaccharides and water and an increase in nuclear collagenous, as well as noncollagenous, proteins decreases the flexibility and shock-absorbing properties of the disc (26).

The annulus fibrosis is composed of well-oriented fibrils of collagen which give a high tensile strength to the annulus (25). The alternating sheets of collagen are set at an angle to each other, permitting absorption of compression forces applied to the disc. This collagen, α-collagen, is 40% type I, characteristic of cartilaginous collagen, and 60% type II characteristic of tendon cartilage (34). With age there is a slight decrease in the normal or "mature" collagen in the annulus, accompanied by an increase in "immature" collagen and noncollagenous proteins (similar to that found in scar). This is especially noticeable in the portion of the annulus immediately adjacent to the nucleus pulposus such that in the 6th decade it is difficult, grossly, to separate the region of the nucleus pulposus from the more inner aspects of the annulus (5). While the changes described in both the nucleus pulposus and the annulus fibrosis are progressive with age, they appear more rapid in those individuals whose spines have been subjected to more than the average stress and minor trauma of life. The more rapid the change, the more immature is the recently formed collagen, β-protein. This allows for the annulus to be more easily fractured during minor trauma, although some believe the fissuring which occurs with aging in the annulus may be spontaneous (15). This same tendency for the immature collagen and the noncollagenous protein to tear with minor trauma is also found in the degenerating nucleus pulposus (5). It is the expulsion of a fragment of degenerative nuclear material through an annular tear that is the process of disc rupture. The annulus is supported anteriorly and in its most anterolateral portions by a thick anterior longitudinal ligament. A combination of the less substantial posterior longitudinal ligament, the lumbar lordosis, and the biomechanics of the upright spine results in more frequent rupture of the disc through the posterior or posterolateral annulus (1).

Less well known is the nerve supply to the disc. Described is the presence of poorly myelinated nerve fibers in the posterior longitudinal ligament and the more superficial layers of the annulus fibrosis, especially in its posterior and posterolateral extent (14, 31, 45) (Fig. 33.1). Although the function of these nerve fibers is not known, Hirsch *et al.* (14) reminded us that free nerve fiber endings are usually associated with pain perception. The possible role the nerve fibers of the annulus may play in disc syndromes has been virtually ignored. Murphy (23) has demonstrated, during operations on patients for lumbar disc rupture under local anesthesia, that stimulation of the midline posterior longitudinal ligament will produce back pain but stimulation of the lateral aspects of the

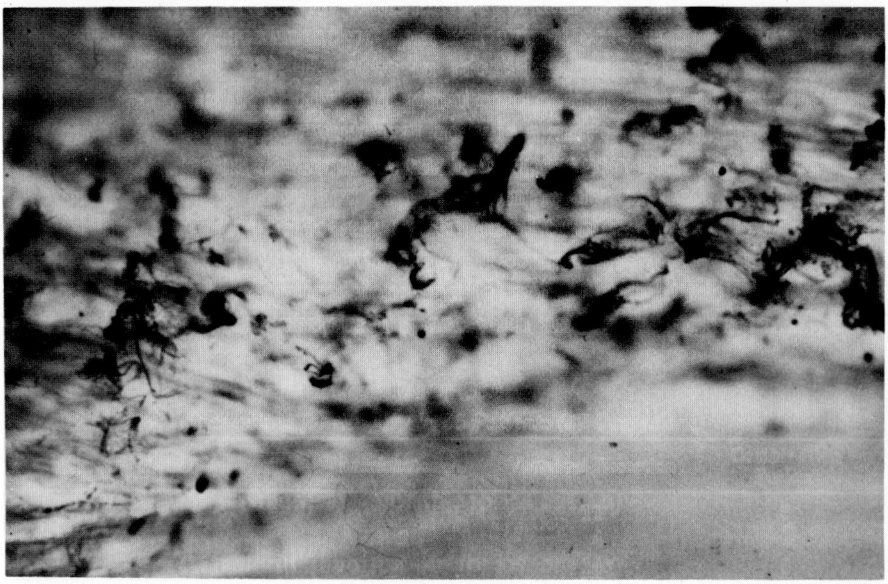

FIG. 33.1. Silver stain (Bielschowsky) demonstrating tangles and clusters of nerve endings in outer annulus. X420. (Reproduced with permission from Yoshizawa *et al.* (45).)

posterior longitudinal ligament or the posterolateral aspect of the annulus will result in not only back pain but also pain which radiates into the appropriate leg. He has also described a patient with "fairly typical back and leg pain, muscle spasm, and limitation of anterior bending, but no neurological deficit" who died from meningitis prior to surgical treatment of his ruptured disc. At autopsy, a small fragment of degenerative nucleus was found approximately halfway through the posterolateral aspect of the annulus, not breaching the outer limits of that structure, with no evidence of nerve root pressure (23). It is crucial to the understanding of the hypothesis to be offered that the importance of Murphy's observations be recognized.

CHYMOPAPAIN

I will not dwell on how chymopapain came to be selected for use in lumbar disc disease, as its choice is well described in the literature (41, 43), and knowledge of the process is not necessary to the understanding of the hypothesis.

Chymopapain is a proteolytic enzyme first isolated in 1941 (18). It catalyzes, both *in vivo* and *in vitro*, a rapid reduction in the viscosity and, hence, the molecular weight of the water insoluble portion of the nucleus pulposus (13, 36). *In vitro*, the digestive activity is terminated within a few hours. The intradiscal injection of chymopapain, both in rabbits and in man, results in transient increased urinary excretion of mucopolysaccharides. Within 4–8 days the rabbit nucleus pulposus is almost completely removed. The human disc following chymopapain injection has not been examined, except on two occasions. Both patients died within 24 hours of injection from acute anaphylactic reactions. The discs injected appeared normal at autopsy (40). Occasionally noted by x-ray is the loss of disc height following injection in man (21, 33, 43).

No effect of chymopapain upon the annulus has been demonstrated in either experimental animals or in man. In human cadaver studies, chymopapain did digest nuclear material from unruptured human lumbar discs, but it had no effect upon the annulus (6). Stern and Smith (37) compared the effects of chymopapain upon normal nuclear material obtained from human cadavers and prolapsed material removed at surgery. They noted first that unruptured degenerative nucleus contained a greater proportion of protein-polysaccharide than did the prolapsed degenerative nuclear material. Conversely, they noted a greater proportion of hydroxyprolene-containing protein (collagen) in the prolapsed material than in the unprolapsed material. They further found that chymopapain more readily dissolved the material containing the higher ratio of protein-polysaccharide and had little effect upon the hydroxyprolene-containing material. They concluded that the "greater soluablization of nucleus pulposus from normal as compared with prolapsed disc material probably reflects the greater proportion of collagen in the latter substrate." Chymopapain has no effect upon collagen (36).

Conflicting data are available concerning the effects of chymopapain upon nervous tissue. Garvin *et al.* (12), studying guinea pigs, applied chymopapain to the cornea and injected it subcutaneously in doses up to 5%. They concluded that chymopapain had no effect upon peripheral nerve endings when they were unable to demonstrate any alteration in the effects of tactile stimulation after 48 hours, even though corneal opacity and tissue necrosis occurred. Additionally, they and MacNab *et al.* (20) reported no acute change in the conduction time or threshold voltage of motor nerves. Brånemark and coworkers (3, 32) demonstrated, pathologically, a direct irreversible effect of chymopapain upon the rabbit tibial nerve. They showed, 4 weeks after the application of 1 ml of 0.4% chymopapain (the approximate dose used for human intradiscal injection), that there was a marked degeneration of nerve fibers as well as fibrosis in both the epineural and endoneural segments of the nerve. While attributing these findings to an alteration in the microvasculature and circulation of the nerve, they could not exclude a direct neurolytic effect (2). Shealy (35) found, in cats, necrosis in peripheral nerves following the extrathecal injection of a 1–2% solution of chymopapain.

TREATMENT OF DISC DISEASE

It is extremely difficult from a review of the literature to evaluate the results of treatment for lumbar disc disease. This is because the end results, usually expressed as "degree of comfort," "return to work with minimal if any difficulty," and other similar descriptions, are subjective ones that may be dramatically influenced by the physician-patient relationship. Equally subjective are the effects of litigation and other sociologic factors (44). The traditional forms of treatment, bed rest, physical therapy, exercise, and surgery, do not lend themselves well to matched-pair study techniques and, of course, double-blind studies are impossible.

Nevertheless, some useful data may be gleaned from the literature. In one of the most respected studies of the value of conservative treatment, defined as up to 4 weeks in bed, followed by slow and progressive increase in activity, 60–70% of the patients had a reduction in pain, loss of abnormal physical findings, and return to work (30). More loosely constructed, yet interpretable studies of the value of surgery in lumbar disc disease are available for analysis. Most of these report a success rate of 80–90% (4, 10, 42), with few exceptions (Nordsby reported a totally unexplainable 49% success rate with laminectomy) (27).

Similar complaints can be registered with regard to the quality of the studies utilizing chymopapain for the treatment of lumbar intervertebral disc disease. With the exception of one double-blind study (21, 33), chymopapain has been studied in uncontrolled protocols, with three groups comparing, in unrandomized series, chymopapain with surgery (9, 27, 42). While the chymopapain success rate varies in the literature from 49 to 90%, most of the investigators report a success rate of 60–70% (41). In the single published double-blind study involving 66 patients, chymopapain had a success rate of 58% on short-term evaluation (33) and 55% on long-term evaluation (21), a response which was determined to be statistically insignificant from that of a placebo.

Study of both the surgical and the chymopapain literature does not permit an objective evaluation of the quality of "conservative therapy" that was given to the patients prior to their surgical or chymopapain treatment. A review of chymopapain treatment protocols (38), and analysis of discussions at medical meetings on the surgical treatment of lumbar disc disease, permit me to conclude that the "conservative therapy" employed in no way approached the strictness of that reported in the study on conservative treatment previously cited (30). The usual explanation given is that "the public will not permit it."

For the purpose of this hypothesis, I am assuming that the success rate of following a strict conservative regimen for the treatment of lumbar disc disease presenting with back and leg pain and an assortment of neurological deficits, both "soft" and "hard", is 60–70%. This is also the result to be expected with treatment by chymopapain. Surgery has a somewhat better result, 80–90%. I'm also assuming that both the chymopapain-treated and surgical patients have been selected following a less than satisfactory trial of conservative therapy.

The hypothesis will be considered in two parts. This is because one can visualize, following the injection of chymopapain into the intervertebral disc, a direct biochemical effect on residual protein-polysaccharide containing nuclear material and a direct neurolytic effect upon the nerve fibers found within the annulus.

This hypothesis is based upon the assumption that fragments of degenerative nucleus pulposus can herniate into tears in the annulus to the superficial levels of the annulus, thus distorting pain fibers and causing pain. The capsule of the annulus need not be disrupted for this to occur. The pain the patient experiences is similar to that of frank rupture with chronic nerve root compression. This pain may also be accompanied by "soft signs" typically associated with signs of disc rupture and thought to be due to nerve root compression. From a study of Granit (11) we learn of suppression of ipsilateral extensor deep tendon reflexes by pain. Peripheral sensory phenomenon may be altered at the spinal level as the result of varied sensory input. The Melzack and Wall (22) gate theory of pain, although not totally accepted today, and the theories behind the use of transcutaneous and peripheral nerve stimulation, support this statement (7). Every experienced examiner has learned the importance of accepting with caution minimal evidence of weakness in the presence of pain.

Since chymopapain is known to reduce the volume of protein-polysaccharide-containing material which, to some extent may be found even in herniating disc fragments, one can postulate that a reduction in the size of a disc fragment by chymopapain might be sufficient to produce an "internal decompression" and effect relief of pain, especially when combined with bedrest that results in reduced intradiscal pressure (16, 24).

It is not unreasonable to believe that chymopapain injected into the intervertebral disc can flow through annular fractures, follow the course of a herniating disc fragment to the region of the nerve fibers in the annulus, and produce a chemical "neurectomy." Discograms reveal the flow of contrast material throughout these fractures and through annular defects into the epidural space (Fig. 33.2). Similar flow of methylene blue has been demonstrated in cadaver and surgical specimens (Fig. 33.3). Chymopapain is bound rapidly and tightly to the protein-polysaccharide component of nuclear material (37); therefore, it is unlikely that it enters the epidural space in a concentration sufficient to alter the function of extradural nervous tissue. In an evaluation of over 400 complications of

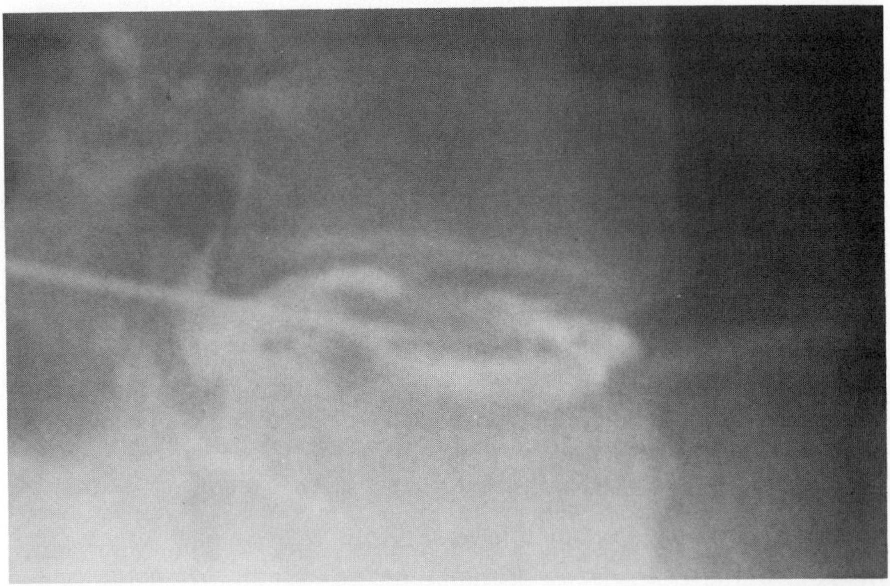

FIG. 33.2. A discogram showing a degenerative lumbar disc with contrast extruding through a defect in the annulus into the epidural space.

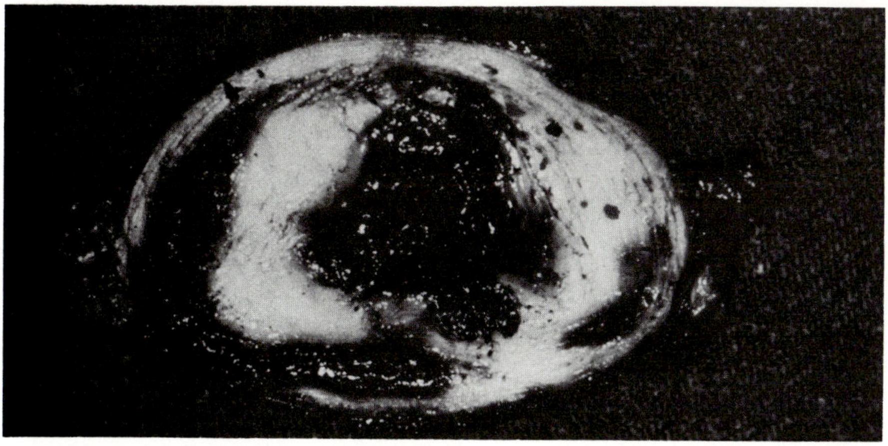

FIG. 33.3. Methylene blue has been injected into the center of this human cadaver disc, prior to section. It can be seen dissecting to the superficial layers of the annulus, especially posterior and posterolateral. (Courtesy of Doctor J. W. Simmons, San Antonio, Texas).

chymopapain treatment in 13,000 patients, not a single case was found which suggested that chymopapain had an adverse effect upon extradural nervous tissue (40).

Some proponents of discography insist that the injection of contrast material into the diseased disc under local anesthesia can reproduce the patient's pain, and they use this as a test of disc disease (8, 29). This pain might be interpreted as a result of transient impaction of the herniated but not extruded disc fragment further into the superficial layers of the annulus, intensifying the stimulation of the annular nerve fibers. MacNab (20) has shown with repeat myelography that chymopapain does not alter the size of the epidural defect; this suggests that chymopapain may have a greater effect upon pain than upon the size of the fragment. Attesting to this possibility are the unpublished observations of myself and others that some patients experience a marked reduction of pain, especially that radiating (referred ?) to the leg, within 1–2 hours of chymopapain injection, suggesting a direct effect upon pain receptors and nerve fibers. On the other hand, a significant number of patients will complain for 2–3 days of an increase in pain, more in the back (with spasms) than the leg, following injection. This could represent an incomplete "neurectomy," leaving the nerve fibers "irritated."

If the mechanism of action of chymopapain is to denervate the annulus in the region of the herniation, reduce the size of the fragment, or both, one would expect the results to be similar to that of surgery where herniation is suspected preoperatively, but no nerve root compression is documented at surgery. This, indeed, appears to be the case. In a nonrandomized comparison of surgery *vs.* chymopapain, my colleagues and I found an 89% surgical success rate in those patients where nerve root compression was established to be present at surgery, compared to a 60% success rate where nerve root compression could not be clearly documented by the presence of either an extruded fragment or a large bulging defect which distorted the position of the nerve root (42). Our success with chymopapain was also 60%. Hudgins (17), in his surgical experience, also found a success rate of approximately 60% in those patients not documented at surgery to have nerve root compression.

It is unlikely that chymopapain directly effects the large protruding or extruded disc fragment. These fragments, containing a high content of collagen, are unaffected by chymopapain *in vitro*. Additionally, in many patients with significant neurological deficits who fail to respond to chymopapain injection, extruded disc fragments with nerve root compression have been found at surgery (20, 28, 42).

Any hypothesis of chymopapain effect must consider the commonality of results obtained with all forms of treatment. Chymopapain is 60–70% effective in all patients thought to have herniated lumbar disc disease. Similar surgical results are obtained when no nerve root compression is identified. Strict adherence to a conservative treatment regimen for up to 4 weeks results in success in 60–70% of patients. Because most patients following chymopapain injection or surgery are advised to continue sedentary activity for several weeks, followed by a progressively increased level of activity culminating in a return to normal levels at approximately 3 months, it is tempting to speculate that the common element is the reduced activity more effectively enforced in patients subjected to a therapeutic protocol as dramatic as chymopapain injection or surgery in a hospital setting rather than at home. This logically leads to the question as to whether chymopapain and, for that matter, surgery in cases when no nerve root compression is identified have a placebo effect.

While it is not possible in an evaluation of the data available to state that chymopapain does have a direct placebo effect, there is indirect evidence that would support this conclusion. One well-analyzed study in the literature reveals chymopapain to have produced no better results than an inactive placebo (21, 33). In addition, the most commonly reported success rate for chymopapain (60–70%) is no better than that accepted for good conservative treatment. While some would argue that the chymopapain was given *after* conservative therapy had failed, a detailed analysis of the study protocols would suggest that in most instances conservative therapy was incomplete and poorly monitored. Emphasizing this was one protocol which stipulated that entry into the study would occur only after "3 weeks of adequate conservative therapy" without outlining what that therapy was to be. On the other hand, the instructions for the posttreatment management consisted of 3 pages of very detailed instructions on a week by week basis for 3 months.

Perhaps this dichotomy is related to pressures, obvious and not so obvious which surround the management of ill health in our country, especially that of low back disability (44) Any physician who sees many patients with low back disorders can identify these factors once a patient is placed at bedrest for a low back disability. Various influences begin to converge on the treatment process that manipulate that process. The patient becomes anxious because "nothing is being done." The physician becomes anxious because he is doing "nothing" positive. The employer and the insurance company wish to know "when" the patient will improve. Friends and family place pressure on the patient to "have something done" and the physician to "do something." If the patient should have sciatica, the pressure becomes greater. It thus becomes quite difficult, in our society, to adequately treat, conservatively, a patient with low back pain and sciatica.

On the other hand, after the patient has been placed in the hospital and "has something done," whether it be chymopapain injection or surgery, the patient and physician are relieved that something has been done and that one now only has to wait for healing to occur. In addition, the patient has invested money and, perhaps more importantly, taken "risks," in order to get well. The employer and insurance company know that within a finite period of time, the patient will either be back to work, or a decision about future disability will be made. Family and friends now tell the patient to "take it easy until you are well."

Thus, it is tempting to ascribe the majority of the effects of chymopapain to the convalescence it forces. However, one cannot ignore the biological effects of chymopapain upon disc and nerve tissue. I am suggesting these effects are twofold. Chymopapain will reduce the size of a fragment of nuclear material impacted in the annulus to the extent that the nuclear fragment contains protein-polysaccharides which may be hydrolyzed. Additionally, it has a direct effect upon pain fibers located within the superficial layers of the annulus, to which it has access along the tract of the herniating disc fragment that is producing the symptoms.

Under this hypothesis, chymopapain would be expected to be as effective as surgery in those patients with herniated discs that do not have nerve root compression and whose symptoms are due to impacted degenerative nuclear fragments within the annulus. Our challenge is to search for clinical clues which will permit us to separate those patients who, following failure of conservative therapy, have herniating disc fragments without nerve root compression. This search should lead to a better understanding of lumbar intervertebral disc disease and its management.

REFERENCES

1. Batts, M., Jr. Rupture of the nucleus pulposus. An anatomical study. J. Bone and Joint Surg., *21:* 121–126, 1939.
2. Brånemark, P. M. Tissue effects of chymopapain (letter to the editor). J. Neurosurg., *42:* 488, 1975.
3. Brånemark, P. I., Ekholm, R., and Lundskog, M. L. Tissue response to chymopapain in different concentrations. Clin. Orthop., *67:* 52–67, 1969.
4. Brown, H. A., and Brown, B. A. Lumbar intervertebral disk disease. Postgrad. Med., *37:* 446–451, 1965.
5. Brown, M. D. The pathophysiology of disc disease. Orthop. Clin. North Am., *2:* 359–370, 1971.
6. Brown, M. D., and Caroff, R. B. The double-blind study comparing disease to placebo: An editorial comment. Spine, *2:* 233–236, 1977.
7. Cauthen, J. C. Transcutaneous and peripheral nerve stimulation for chronic pain states. Surg. Neurol., *4:* 102–104, 1975.
8. Collins, H. R. An evaluation of cervical and lumbar discography. Clin. Orthop., *107:* 133–138, 1975.
9. Fleming, J. F. R. Personal communication. Reported with H. Schutz, G. Vanderlinder, and M. Hogan of Toronto, at the XIII Canadian Congress of Neurological Sciences, 1980.
10. Finneson, B. F. *Low Back Pain*, p. 205. J. B. Lippincott, Philadelphia, 1973.
11. Granit, R. *Receptors and Sensory Perception.* Yale University Press, New Haven, 1955.
12. Garvin, P. J., Jennings, R. B., Smith, L., and Gesler, R. M. Chymopapain: A pharmacologic and toxicologic evaluation in experimental animals. Clin. Orthop., *41:* 204–223, 1965.
13. Gesler, R. M. Pharmacologic properties of chymopapain. Clin. Orthop., *67:* 47–51, 1969.
14. Hirsch, C., Ingelmark, B.-E., and Miller, M. The anatomical basis for low back pain. Studies on the presence of sensory nerve endings in ligamentous, capsular, and intervertebral disc structures in the human lumbar spine. Acta Orthop. Scand., *33:* 1–17, 1963.
15. Hirsch, C., and Schajowicz, F. Studies on structural changes in the lumbar annulus fibrosus. Acta Orthop. Scand., *22:* 184–231, 1952.
16. Hirschberg, G. G. Treating lumbar disc lesion by prolonged continuous reduction of intradiscal pressure. Texas Med., *70:* 48–68, 1974.
17. Hudgins, W. R. Should degenerated disc be removed? Surg. Forum, *25:* 442–445, 1974.
18. Jansen, E. F., and Balls, A. K. Chymopapain: A new crystalline proteinase from papaya latex. J. Biol. Chem., *137:* 459–460, 1941.
19. Joplin, R. J. The intervertebral disc: Embryology, anatomy, physiology and pathology. Surg. Gynecol., Obstet., *61:* 591–599, 1935.
20. MacNab, I., McCullock, J. A., Weiner, D. S., Hugo, E. P., Galway, R. D., and Dall, D. Chemonucleolysis. Can. J. Surg., *14:* 280–289, 1971.
21. Martins, A. N., Ramirez, A., Johnston, J., and Schwetschenau, P. R. Double-blind evaluation of chemonucleolysis for herniated lumbar discs: Late results. J. Neurosurg., *49:* 816–827, 1978.
22. Melzack, R., and Wall, P. D. Pain mechanisms: A new theory. Science, *150:* 971–979, 1965.
23. Murphy, F. Sources and patterns of pain in disc disease. Clin. Neurosurg., *15:* 343–351, 1968.

24. Nachemson, A., and Morris, J. M. *In vivo* measurements of intradiscal pressure J. Bone Joint Surg., *46A:* 1077–1092, 1964.
25. Naylor, A. The biochemical changes in the human intervertebral disc in degeneration and nuclear prolapse. Orthop. Clin. North Am., *2:* 343–358, 1971.
26. Naylor, A. Intervertebral disc prolapse and degeneration: The biochemical and biophysical approach. Spine, *1:* 108–114, 1976.
27. Nordby, E. J., and Lucas, G. L. A comparative analysis of lumbar disk disease treated by laminectomy or chemonucleolysis. Clin. Orthop., *90:* 110–129, 1973.
28. Parkinson, D., and Shields, C. Treatment of protruded lumbar intervertebral discs with chymopapain (disease). J. Neurosurg., *39:* 203–208, 1973.
29. Patrick, B. S. Lumbar discography: A five year study. Surg. Neurol., *1:* 267–273, 1973.
30. Pearce, J., and Moll, J. M. H. Conservative treatment and natural history of acute lumbar disc lesions. J. Neurol. Neurosurg. Psychiatry, *30:* 13–17, 1967.
31. Roofe, P. G. Innervation of annulus fibrosis and posterior longitudinal ligament. Arch. Neurol. Psychiatry, *44:* 100–103, 1940.
32. Rydevik, B., Branemark, P. I., Nordborg, C., McLean, W. G., Sjostrand, J., and Fogelberg, M. Effects of chymopapain on nerve tissue. Spine, *1:* 137–148, 1976.
33. Schwetschenau, P. R., Ramirez, A., Johnston, J., Barnes, E., Wiggs, C., and Martins A. N. Double-blind evaluation of intradiscal chymopapain for herniated lumbar discs: Early results. J. Neurosurg., *45:* 622–627, 1976.
34. Sedowofia, K. A., Tomlinson, I. W., Weiss, J. B., Hilton, R. C., and Jayson, M. I. V. Collagenolytic enzyme systems in human intervertebral disc. Their control, mechanism, and their possible role in the initiation of biomechanical failure. Spine, *7:* 213–222, 1982.
35. Shealy, C. N. Tissue reaction to chymopapain in cats. J. Neurosurg., *26:* 327–330, 1967.
36. Stern, I. J. Biochemistry of chymopapain. Clin. Orthop., *67:* 42–46, 1969.
37. Stern, I. J., and Smith, L. Dissolution by chymopapain *in vitro* of tissue from normal or prolapsed intervertebral disks. Clin. Orthop., *50:* 269–277, 1977.
38. Travenol Laboratories: New Drug Application (chymopapain) to the U.S. Food and Drug Administration, 1981.
39. Watts, C. Chemonucleolysis: An appeal for objectivity. J. Neurosurg., *42:* 488–489, 1975.
40. Watts, C. Complications of chemonucleolysis for lumbar disc disease. Neurosurgery, *1:* 2–5, 1977.
41. Watts, C. Current status of chymopapain. In: *Lumbar Disc Disease*, edited by R. Hardy, pp. 157–164. New York, Raven Press, 1983.
42. Watts, C., Hutchinson, G., Stern, J., and Clark, K. Comparison of intervertebral disc disease treatment by chymopapain injection and open surgery. J. Neurosurg. *42:* 397–400, 1975.
43. Watts, C., Knighton, R., and Roulhac, G. Chymopapain treatment of intervertebral disc disease. J. Neurosurg., *42:* 374–383, 1975.
44. White, A. V. M. The compensation back. Appl. Therap., *8:* 971–974, 1968.
45. Yoshizawa, H., O'Brien, J. P., Smith, W. T., and Trumper, M. The neuropathology of intervertebral discs removed for low back pain. J. Pathol., *132:* 95–104, 1980.

CHAPTER

34

High Resolution CT of the Spine in Lumbar Disc Disease

MOKHTAR GADO, M.D., JASH PATEL, M.D., and FRED J. HODGES, III, M.D.

TECHNIQUE AND ANATOMY

Imaging of the lumbar intervertebral disc depends on the ability of the scanner to provide high spatial resolution with preservation of contrast discrimination. The development of scanning equipment in the past few years has demonstrated this capability. The increase in spatial resolution is obtained by reducing the field of reconstruction of the image such that each picture element represents a smaller part of the object, while at the same time the thickness of the slice is reduced in order to further decrease the volume of tissue represented by each picture element. Customarily, a field of reconstruction of 5 inches × 5 inches and a slice thickness of 4 or 5 mm is adequate for a standard examination of the lumbar spine.

The examination of a single disc space requires the inclusion of the region from the pedicle of the vertebra above to the pedicle of the vertebra below the intervertebral disc. The orientation of the slices in the plane of the intervertebral disc in question has obvious advantages. Therefore, the examination is started by obtaining a digital image (scout view) of the lumbar region by sliding the patient into the gantry aperture while the x-ray tube and detectors are stationary (8). On the lateral scout view, the level and orientation of the slices can be predetermined. A set of 10 images is often required to cover the region of one intervertebral disc. In most cases, when the disc is suspected of being at the level $L_{4\text{-}5}$ or L_5–S_1, it is advisable to examine the last 3 intervertebral disc spaces, *i.e.*, $L_{3\text{-}4}$ as well. The orientation of the set of slices for each intervertebral space is determined by the degree of lordosis of the patient (Fig. 34.1).

The normal anatomy of a single intervertebral disc space may be described at 4 levels. At the level of the pedicle above the intervertebral disc, the complete bony ring of the vertebra is shown (Fig. 34.2). At the next level below, the intervertebral foramen is demonstrated as a gap separating the vertebral body anteriorly from the lamina and root of the inferior articular process posteriorly. Within the intervertebral foramen, the space is occupied by the ganglion of the nerve root that exits at this foramen. The ganglion is surrounded with fat, and the space is not shared by any soft tissue or osseous structure other than those described. This level represents the upper part of the intervertebral foramen. The next level below is the lower part of the foramen. Here, the intervertebral disc is seen occupying the region that was occupied by the vertebral body in the 2 levels just described. The space between the posterior border of the intervertebral disc and the neural arch of the vertebra is reduced by the interposition of the superior articular process of the vertebral below. This narrowing of the foramen at this level should not be interpreted as foraminal stenosis. The latter condition occurs when the superior articular process of the vertebra below is elongated by osteophyte formation and therefore extends into the superior part of the foramen, *i.e.*, in the

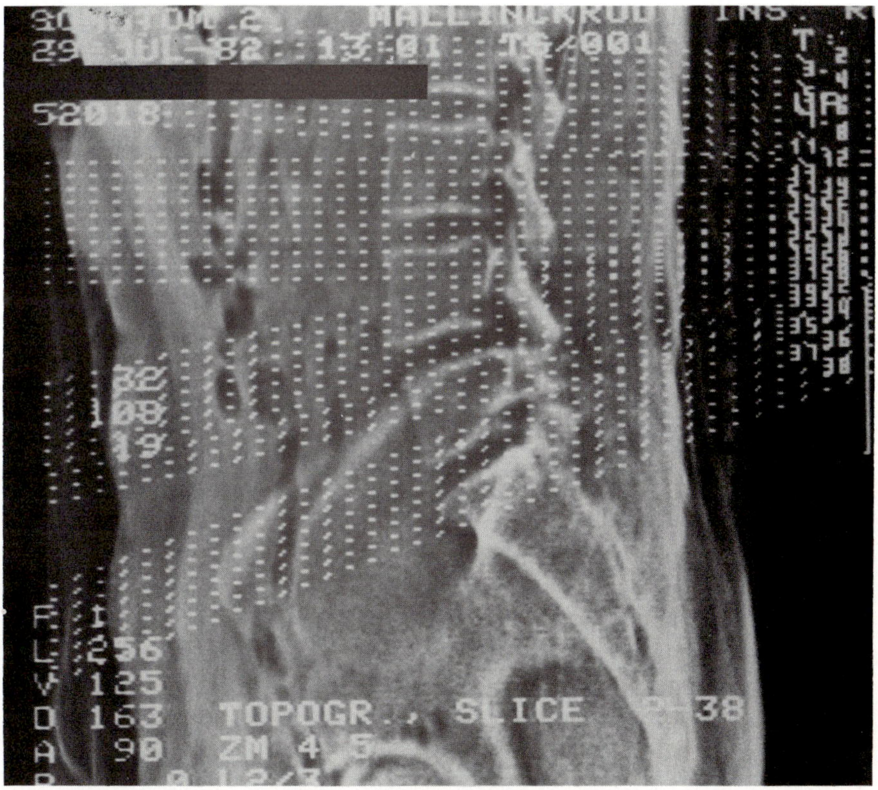

FIG. 34.1. A scout lateral view of the lumbosacral spine. The dotted lines are entered on the digital radiograph determining the level and plane of orientation of the individual slices. The slices are oriented in the plane of the intervertebral discs.

second anatomical level described above. The next level below, the fourth and last level of this series, depicts the complete bony ring of the vertebra below. The neural arch of the vertebra above is replaced in this level by the neural arch of the vertebra below. The pedicle on each side connects the neural arch to the upper part of the vertebral body. As discussed above, it usually takes 10 slices to cover these 4 distinct anatomical levels.

The posterior border of the intervertebral disc is demonstrated in the slice at the anatomical level of the lower part of the foramen. At that level, the greater part of the posterior border of the intervertebral disc abuts on the dural sac. The interface between the disc and the dural sac is shown by the density difference between these 2 structures. This difference is crucial for determining the normality or abnormality of configuration of the posterior border of the disc. The posterior border of the normal intervertebral disc follows that of the posterior border of the bony disc plate. On both sides, the lateral ends of the posterior border of the disc abut on the fat in the intervertebral foramen and the ganglion of the nerve root within the foramen. The low density of fat allows the delineation of this part of the disc border with ease.

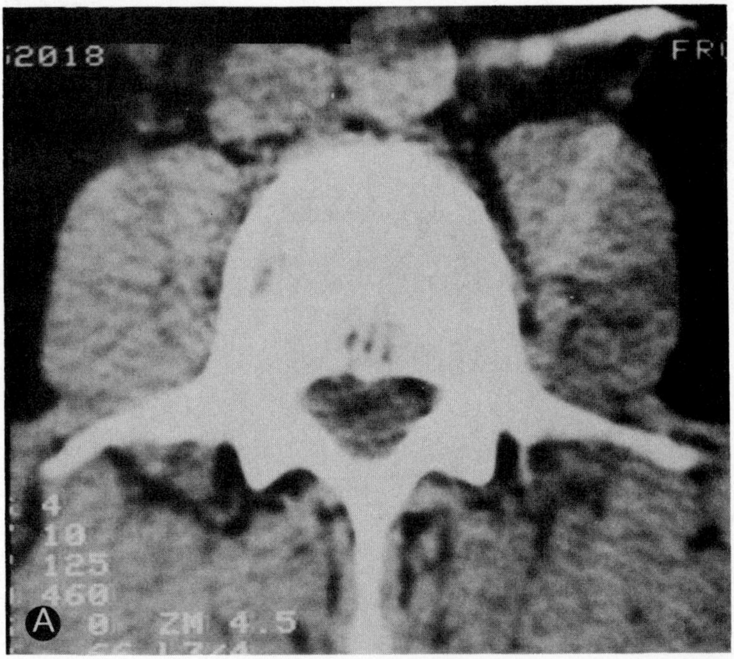

FIG. 34.2. Normal anatomy at 4 anatomical levels covering an intervertebral disc. (*A*) The level of the pedicle of the vertebra above the disc.

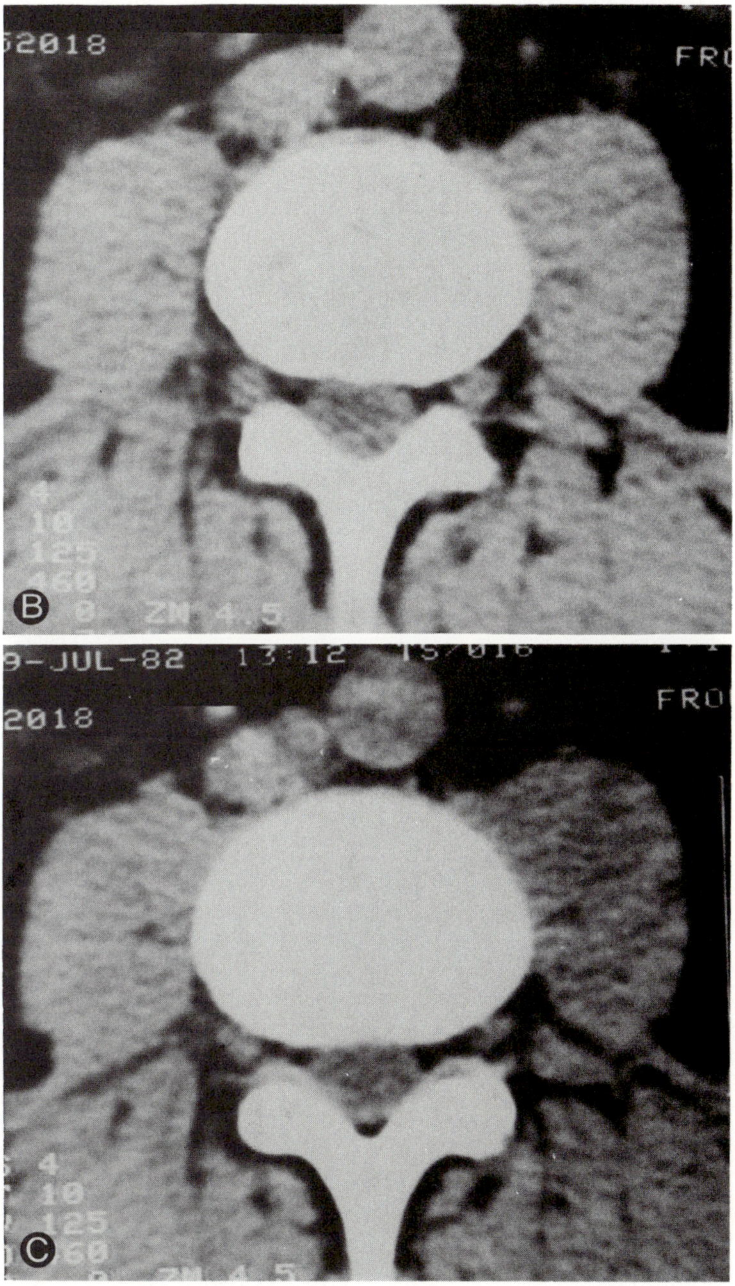

FIG. 34.2. (*B* and *C*) The level of the upper part of the intervertebral foramen.

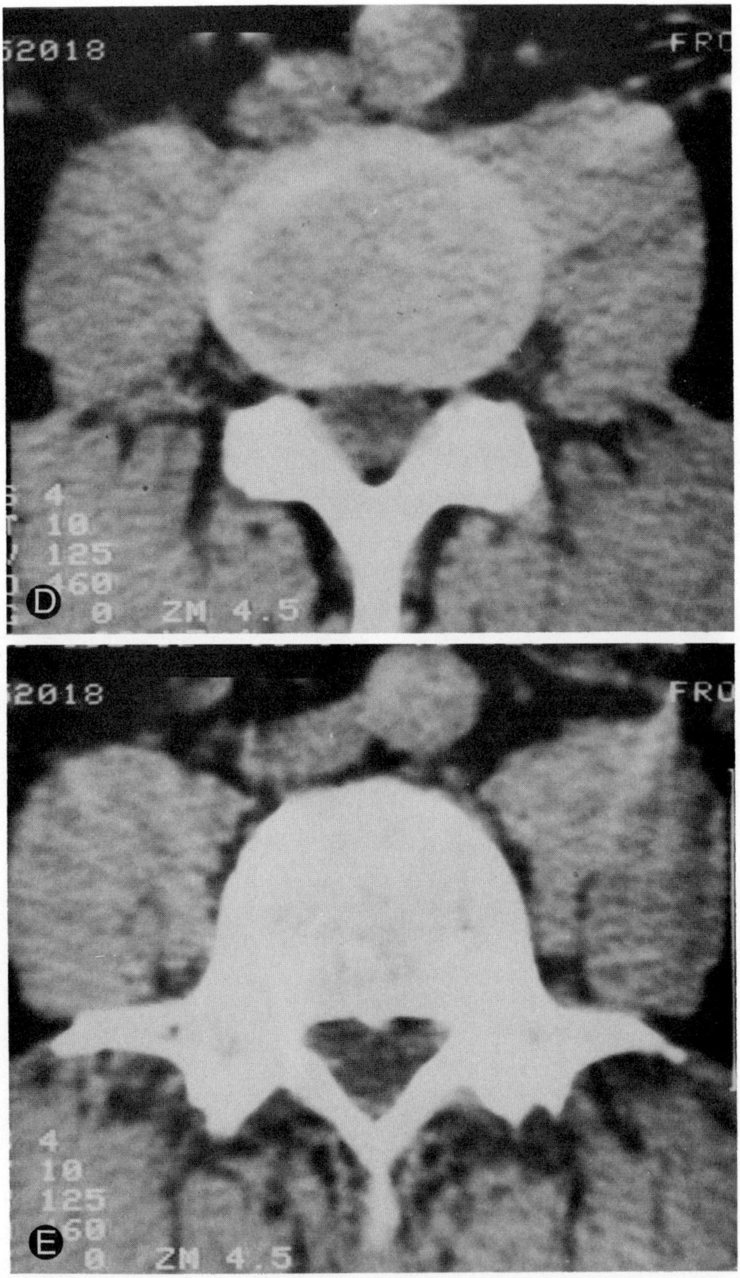

FIG. 34.2. (*D*) The level of the intervertebral disc and the lower part of the intervertebral foramen. (*E*) The level of the pedicle of the vertebra below the intervertebral disc.

The amount of epidural fat within the bony spinal canal is scanty in the upper lumbar region. In contrast, epidural fat is abundant at the lumbosacral junction where the dural sac is significantly smaller in size, in comparison to the bony spinal canal (Fig. 34.3).

CT SIGNS OF RUPTURE OF THE INTERVERTEBRAL DISC (3, 6 8)

Rupture of the intervertebral disc and herniation of the nucleus pulposus results in a focal deformity of the posterior border of the disc and, in turn, the dural sac with which it lies in contact. At the site of deformity, the posterior border of the disc does not follow the contour of the bony disc plate (Fig. 34.4). As a result of the focal deformity, the epidural fat appears asymmetric. In herniation of the nucleus pulposus at the lumbosacral junction, the herniated material may appear as a distinct soft tissue mass within the abundant epidural fat, with little or no deformity of the dural sac (Fig. 34.5). This situation is identical to the well-known case of herniated disc with a normal myelogram encountered at that level.

The presence of calcium or gas within the intervertebral disc space on

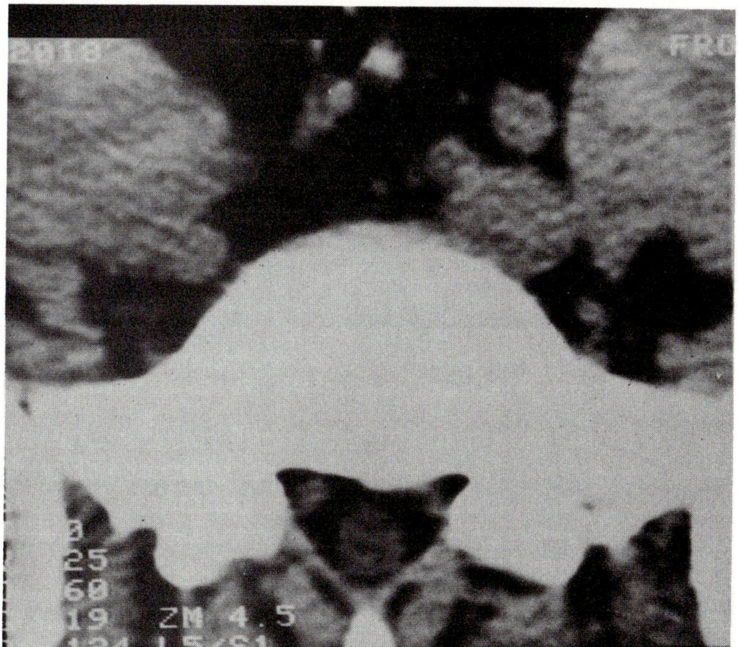

FIG. 34.3. Normal anatomy. At the level of the first sacral segment, the dural sac is small, and the surrounding fat is abundant.

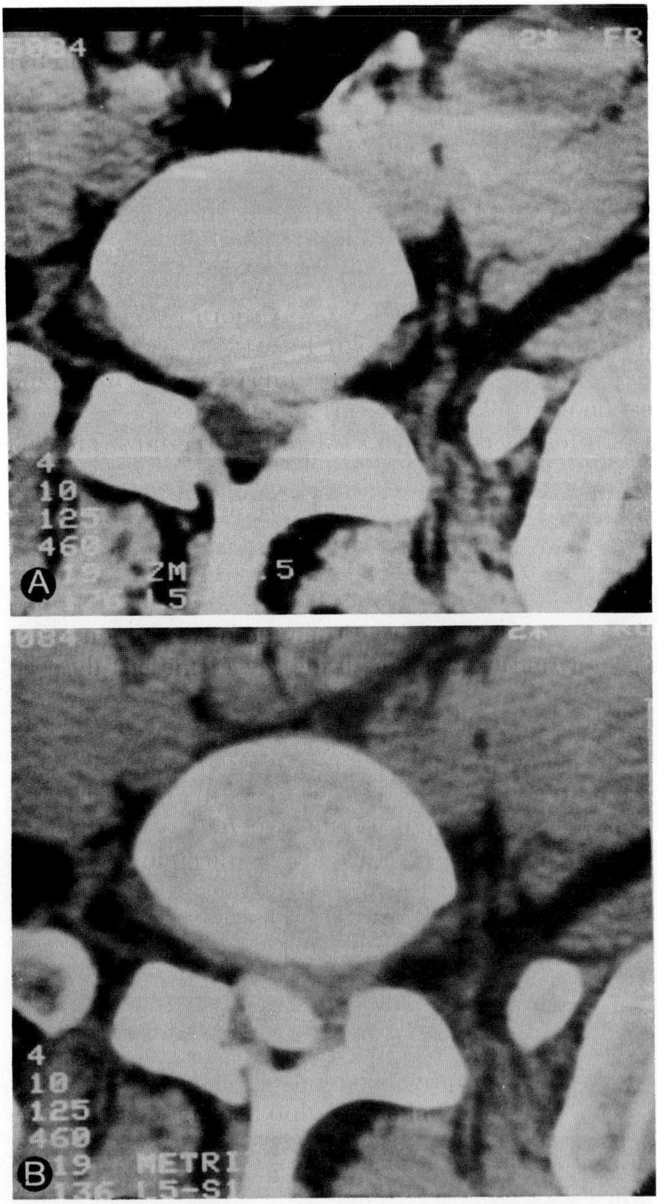

FIG. 34.4. Herniated disc at the L_5–S_1 level. (*A*) Plain CT shows unilateral bulging of the posterior border of the intervertebral disc on the left side, impinging upon the dural sac. (*B*) Repeat scan after a metrizamide myelogram demonstrates the distorted dural sac.

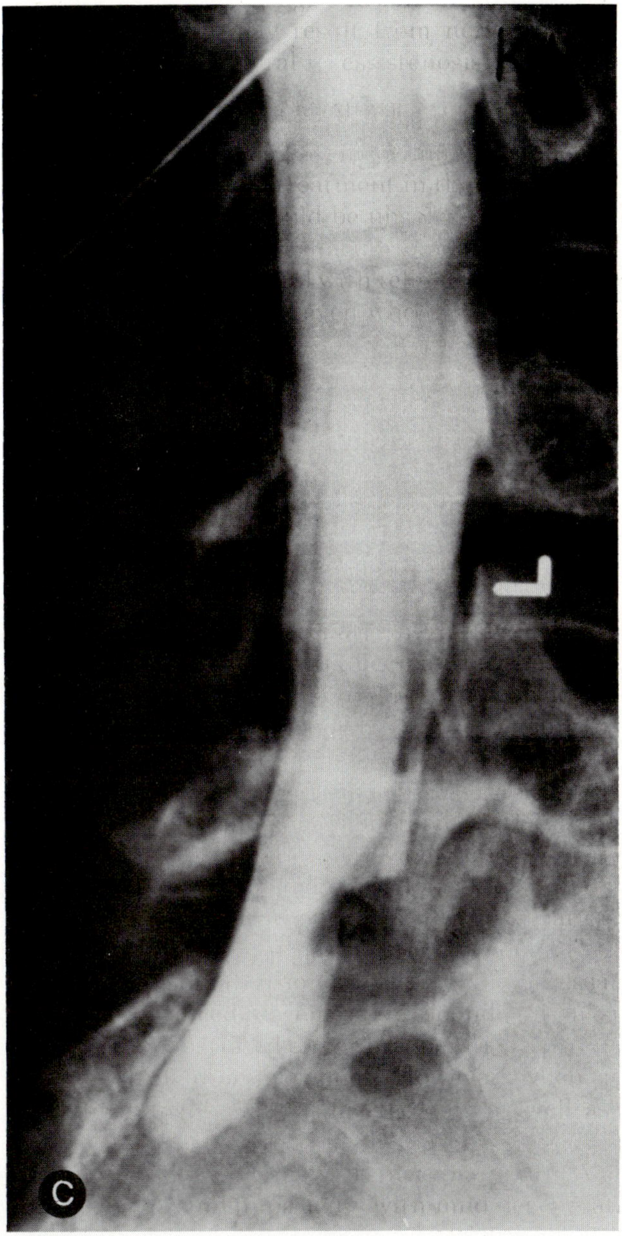

FIG. 34.4. (*C*) Metrizamide myelogram confirms the CT findings in *A* but offers no additional information. (Reproduced with permission from M. H. Gado *et al.* (2).)

the CT image represents disc degeneration (1). When calcium and/or gas appears behind the plane of the bony disc plate, one should consider the possibility of disc herniation (Fig. 34.8).

Depending on the site of the rupture in the annulus, the herniated disc fragment may appear in the midline, *i.e.*, central (Fig. 34.6) or to one side of the midline, *i.e.*, posterolateral (Fig. 34.4) or even in the intervertebral foramen itself, *i.e.*, laterally (Fig. 34.7). In those cases in which the herniated fragment pierces through the posterior longitudinal ligament and lies free in the epidural space, the fragment might migrate away from the level of rupture and lie posterior to the body of the vertebra away from the level of the disc itself (Fig. 34.5). Less commonly, the fragment might migrate cephalad and lie behind the body of the vertebra above the disc. Cephalad migration was seen in our experience more often with lateral disc herniation than with central or posterolateral rupture.

CT AND MYELOGRAPHY

Earlier in our experience, we performed CT scans of the lumbar spine from the level of L_3 to the level of S_1 on 37 consecutive patients who

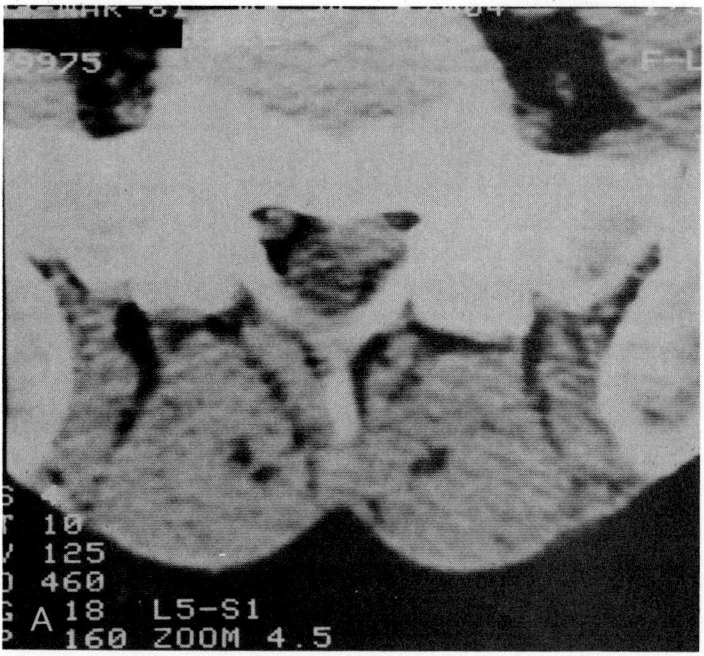

FIG. 34.5. (*A*) Herniated disc at L_5–S_1 on the left side. There is a large fragment with little deformity of the dural sac.

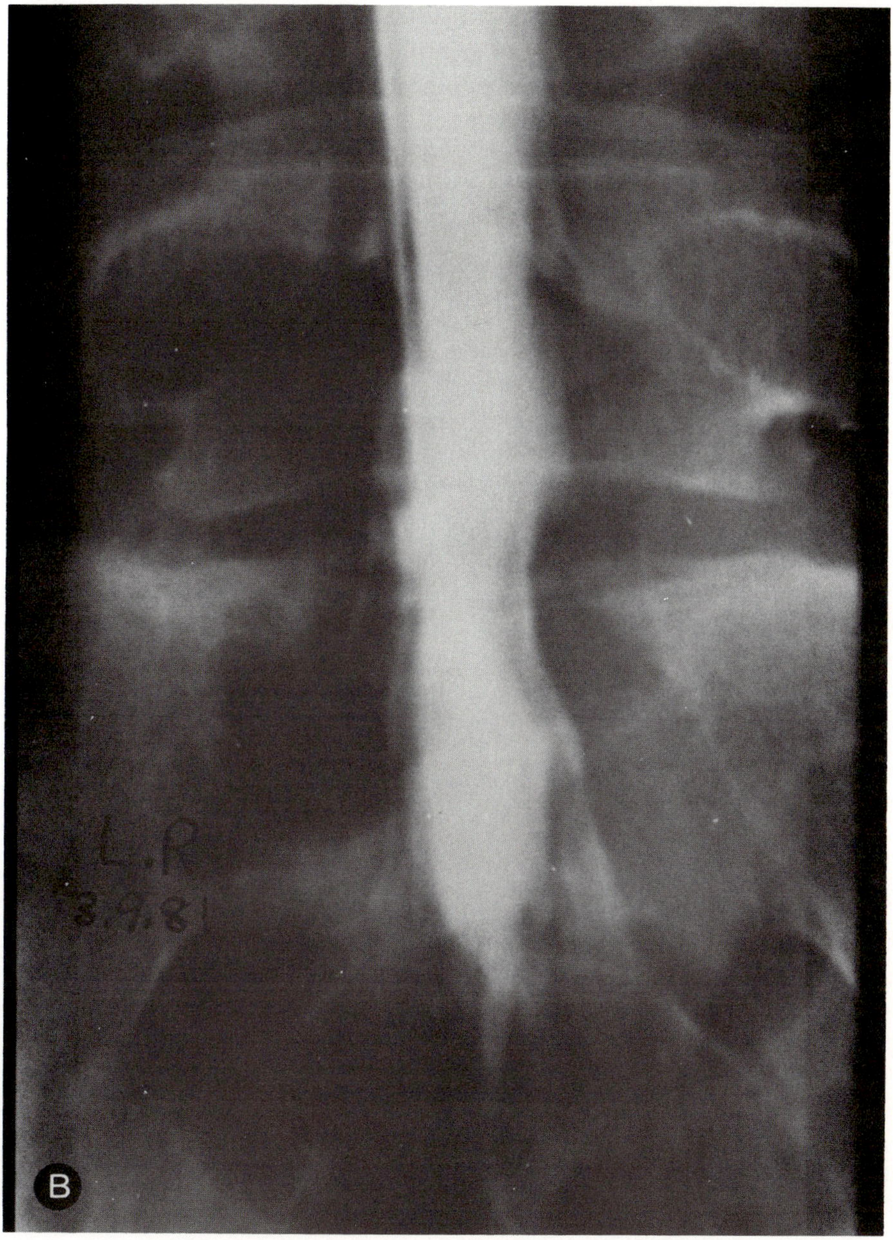

FIG. 34.5. (*B*) Myelogram of the same patients as in *A*.

consented to participate in the study with the clinical diagnosis of suspected rupture of a lumbar intervertebral disc. The cases were reviewed at a later date using the criteria of diagnosis of herniated disc described above. Twenty-five patients had the final diagnosis of herniated disc. Of these, 18 were operated on, and the diagnosis was confirmed. Two underwent enzyme disc injection, and 5 opted for conservative treatment. The results of CT and myelography in the 18 cases confirmed by surgery are shown in Table 34.1. In this small series, there were 9 cases in which both studies were equally helpful and showed similar results (Fig. 34.4). In 3 cases, CT was superior to myelography. These were cases in which the lesion was at the lumbosacral junction (Fig. 34.5). The size of the herniated fragment was sufficient to displace the epidural fat on the image but not sufficient to deform the dural sac at myelography. In 2 more cases, the myelogram was judged as yielding a negative result by 2 experienced radiologists. Therefore, in 14 of 18 cases, the myelogram was equal or inferior to CT.

The 4 cases in which myelography was superior to CT are interesting and should be discussed. In 1 case, the level of the disc rupture was L_{2-3}. That level was not included in the CT. In the remaining 3 cases, there were associated degenerative changes in the posterior articular joints and increased thickness of the soft tissue elements, resulting in obliteration of the epidural fat on both sides. It was not possible therefore to elicit the sign of asymmetry of epidural fat. The disc fragment was rather laterally located, but the diagnosis could not be made on the CT alone, even in retrospect.

One has to consider also, although it was not represented in this small series, the case of an intradural lesion, such as a neoplasm, or arachnoiditis, neither of which is demonstrable by plain CT.

We therefore believe, on the basis of this small series, of reports of other investigators (4, 7), as well as our further experience, that the correct approach to the radiologic diagnosis of suspected intervertebral disc should be a plain CT to start with. If the quality of the scan is optimal, if the diagnosis of a herniated disc is obvious from the criteria

TABLE 34.1

Comparison of CT and Myelography in 18 cases of Disc Rupture (Surgically Proven)

False-negative CT	1
Myelography superior	3
Both studies equal	9
CT superior	3
False-negative myelo	2
	18

discussed above, and if the radiologic diagnosis and clinical signs correlate, myelography need not be performed. Our experience continues to confirm that 70% of the patients with ruptured intervertebral disc should be diagnosed with CT with no need for myelography.

The indications for myelography therefore include a normal CT scan in the face of highly suggestive clinical findings and a positive CT abnormality that does not explain the clinical picture or inability to make a firm diagnosis, either due to poor performance of the scanner or to the presence of degenerative changes obliterating the epidural fat as discussed above.

If myelography is required, it is preferable to perform the study with metrizamide, unless contraindicated. The use of metrizamide gives the opportunity to repeat the CT scan with the contrast material in the subarachnoid space. In certain instances, this postmyelogram CT offers information that clarifies anatomical uncertainties in the relationship of the lesion to the dural sac (Fig. 34.6). The cross-sectional display gives a unique delineation of the entire circumference of the dural sac at a given level.

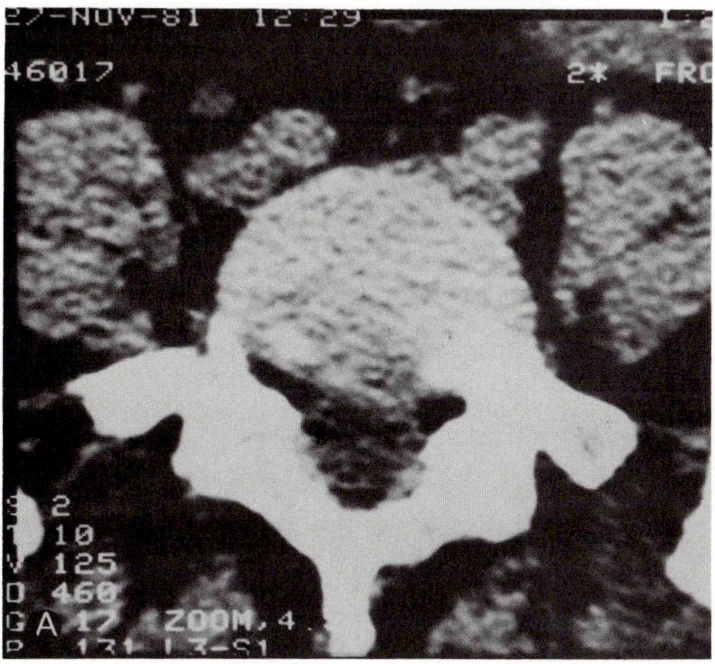

FIG. 34.6. Central disc rupture. (*A*) Plain CT.

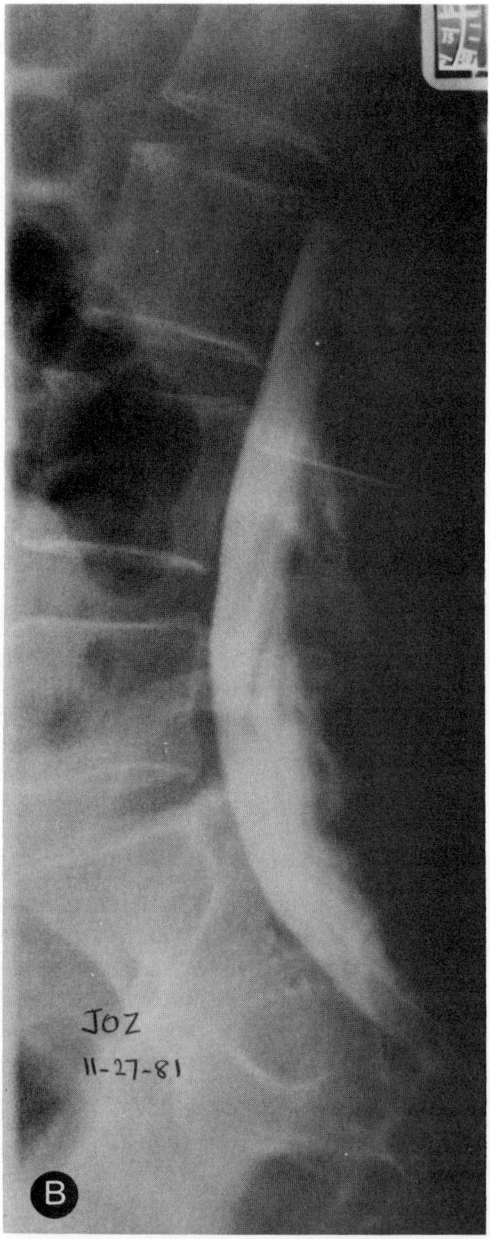

FIG. 34.6. (*B*) Negative myelogram.

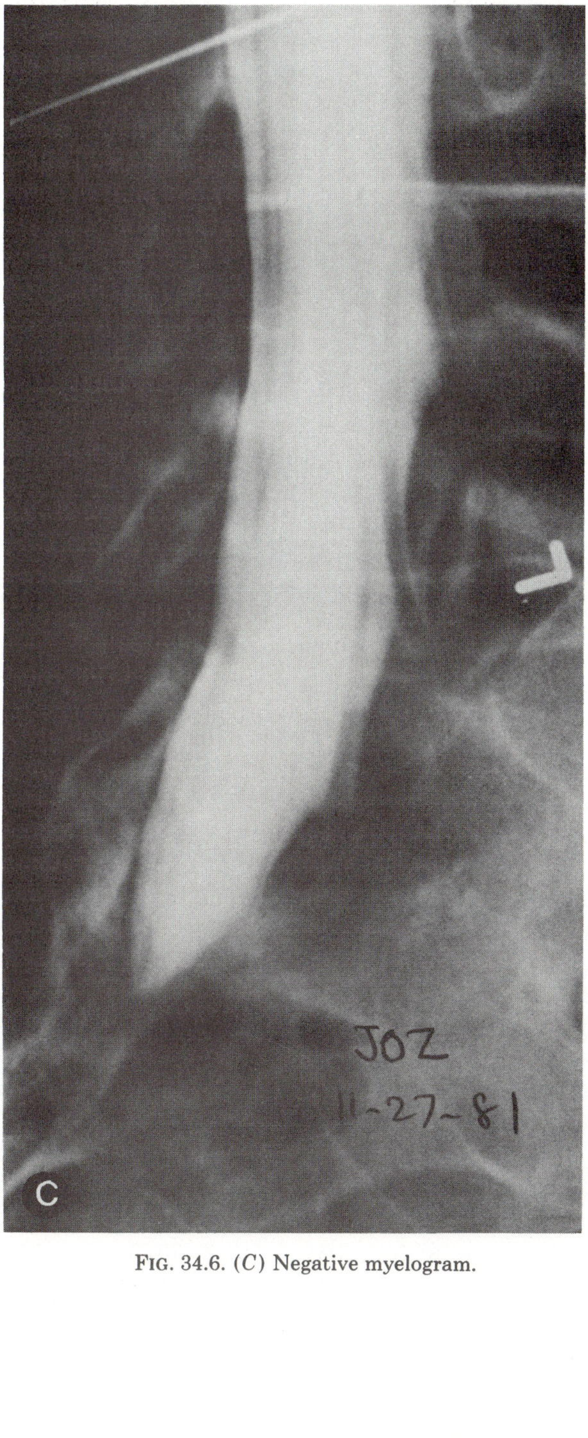

FIG. 34.6. (*C*) Negative myelogram.

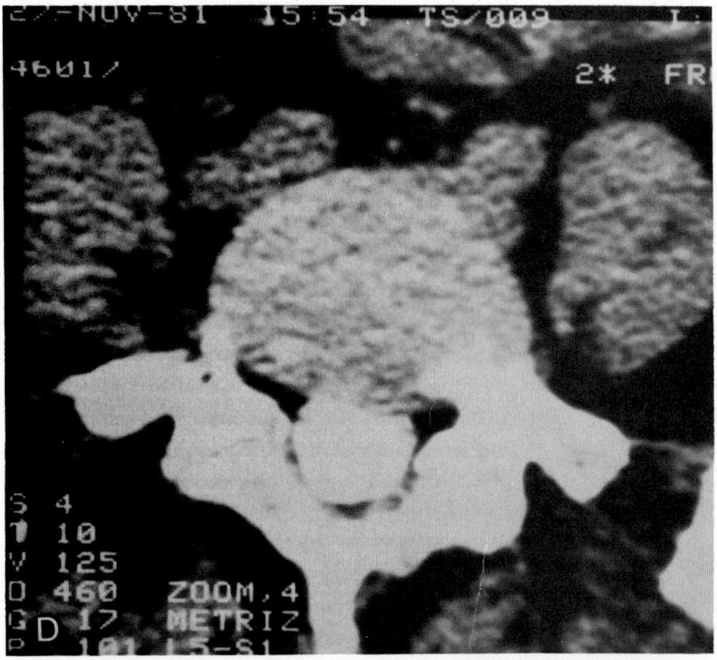

FIG. 34.6. (*D*) Postmyelogram CT. Confirms the deformity of the anterior border of the dural sac.

LATERAL DISC HERNIATION

We are reporting in this section the results of CT scans of 8 patients with lateral disc herniation in the intervertebral foramen encountered during the past 8 months. In addition, we are reporting one more case that was encountered 1 year earlier. Each of these 9 patients had a high resolution CT scan of the spine with the technique described above, and each case was confirmed surgically with removal of the herniated disc material. There were 2 females, age 47 and 65, as well as 7 males ranging in age from 29 to 79 years. Each patient presented with symptoms and/or signs of unilateral lumbar radiculopathy for a period of less than 3 months' duration. In 2 patients, there was, in addition, a long history (8 years in 1 and 20 years in the other) of backache. CT scans were done in all cases, and myelograms were done in 8 of 9 cases.

All patients were operated on by a partial or complete hemilaminectomy. In each case, a lateral herniated disc fragment was encountered in the foramen, causing compression of the nerve root at that location. In addition, in 2 cases there was also a large fragment within the bony spinal canal continuous with the lesion in the foramen. All these findings were demonstrated by CT. The location of the disc herniation in the

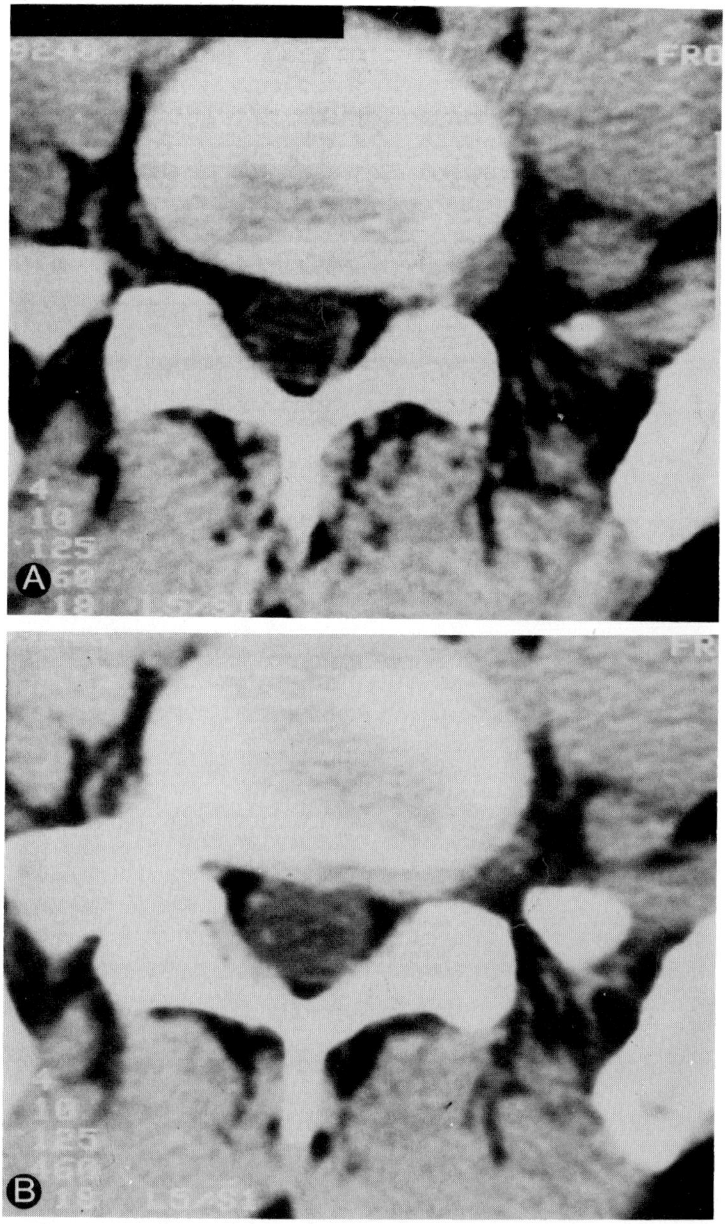

FIG. 34.7. Lateral disc herniation in the intervertebral foramen at L_5–S_1 on the left side. (*A*) Soft tissue mass in the foramen. (*B*) Protrusion of the posteior border of the L_5–S_1 disc encroaching upon the lower part of the foramen on the left side.

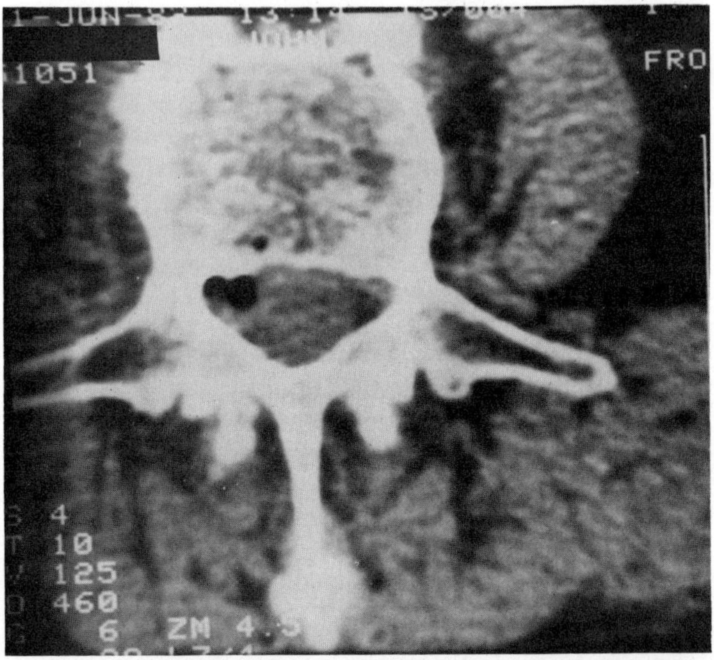

FIG. 34.8. Gas in a herniated disc fragment behind the lower part of the body of L_3.

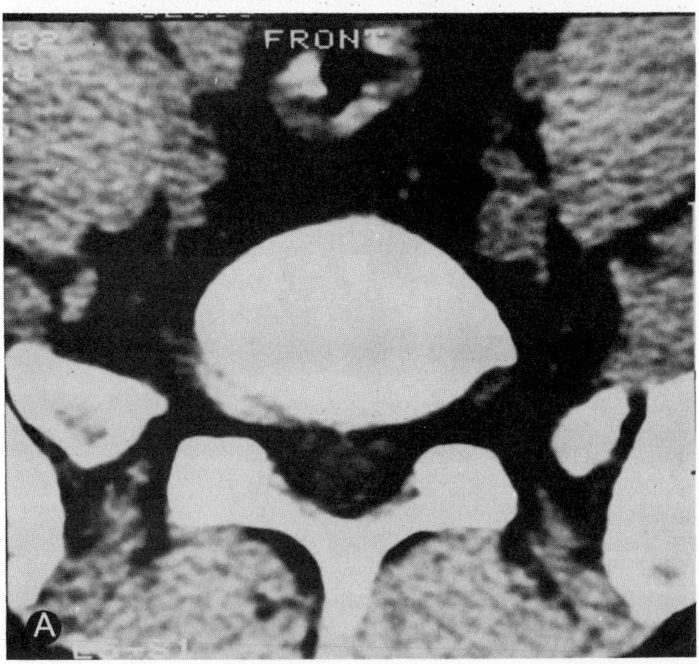

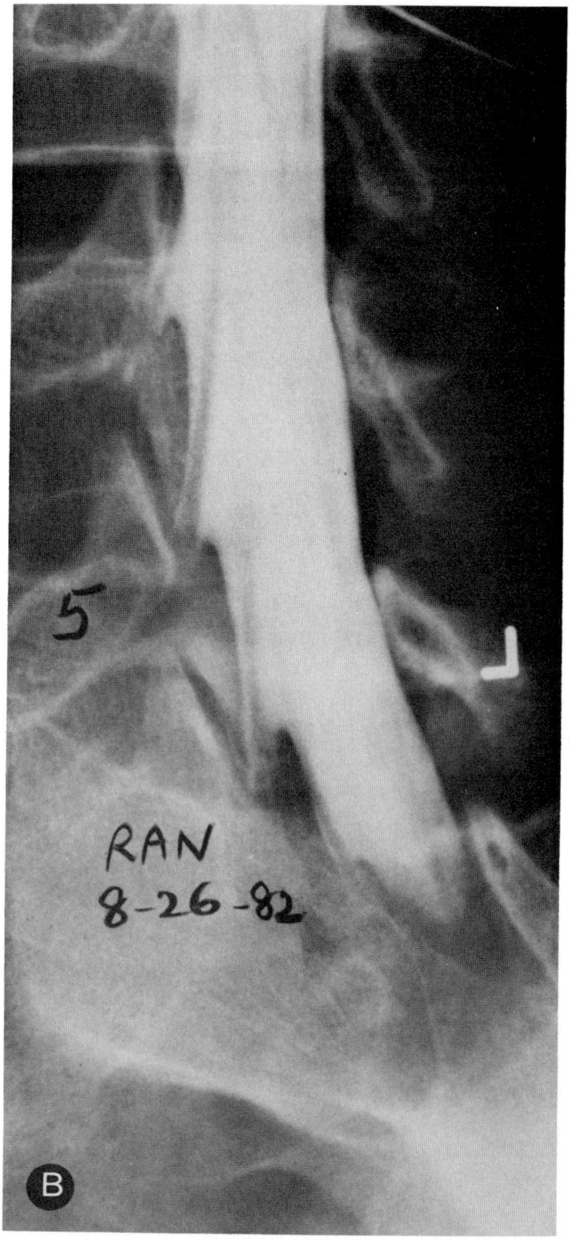

FIG. 34.9. (*B*) Myelogram on the same patient shows no abnormality at the level on that side.

FIG. 34.9. Lateral disc herniation at the level L_5–S_1 on the right side. (*A*) Plain CT. The herniated fragment encroaches upon the intervertebral foramen.

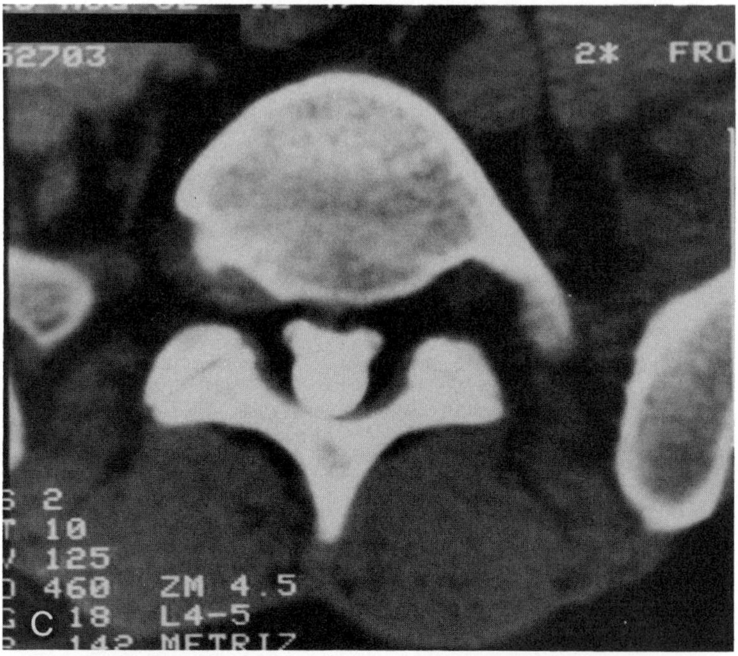

FIG. 34.9. (*C*) Postmyelogram CT shows no deformity of the contrast column. Note the calcification within the disc fragment, which responsible for its higher density.

foramen was as follows: L_{3-4} in 4 cases, L_{4-5} in 2 cases, and L_5–S_1 in 3 cases.

The CT findings of lateral disc herniation may be summarized as follows. In all 9 cases, CT demonstrated a soft tissue mass displacing the fat in the intervertebral foramen. This finding was demonstrated in the slice at the level of the upper part of the foramen just below the pedicle of the vertebra above the disc (Fig. 34.7*A*). In 3 cases, there was in addition a focal protrusion of the posterior border of the disc encroaching upon the intervertebral foramen. This finding was demonstrated in the slice at the level of the lower part of the intervertebral foramen (Fig. 34.7*B*). Furthermore, in 2 cases as described above, there was, in addition, a large component of herniated disc material within the bony spinal canal (Fig. 34.8). On the CT image, the density of the herniated disc fragment was distinctly higher than that of the dural sac in 8 of the 9 cases. In the remaining case, the herniated fragment contained a significant amount of gas, and the density was lower than that of the epidural fat (Fig. 34.8). In 2 patients, the density of the herniated fragment was higher than the denisty of the nucleus pulposus within the intervertebral disc space. In these 2 cases, calcium was demonstrated within the herniated fragment (Fig. 34.9). In the remaining 6 cases, the herniated

TABLE 34.2
CT and Myelographic Findings in Lateral Disc Herniation in the Intervertebral Foramen

No.	Sex	Age	Level of Foramen	Density Measurements by CT[a]			Location of Lesion by CT		Myelographic Findings	
				Dural sac	Lesion	Nucleus Pulposus	Intervertebral Foramen	Bony Spinal Canal	Nonfilling of Root Sheath	Extradural Defect
1	F	47	3/4	23	62	73	+	+	+	+
2	M	60	3/4	12	55	70	+	0	?+[b]	+[b]
3	M	56	3/4	13	76	54	+	0	+	+
4	M	57	4/5	18	46	75	+	0	+	−
5	F	65	5/1	14	74	97	+	0	0	0
6	M	34	5/1	8	73	75	+	0	Not done	
7	M	79	3/4[c]	3	−800	−760	+	+	+	+
8	M	63	4/5	13	78	85	+	0	0	0
9	M	29	5/1	16	90	62	+	0	0	0

[a] In Hounsfield units.
[b] Bilateral nonfilling of the root sheath and a very small extradural defect.
[c] Originated from L2/3 disc.

fragment, although denser than the dural sac, was lower in density than the nucleus pulposus. This is almost certainly the result of the partial volume effect caused by the surrounding epidural fat and also by the degenerative process that precedes or accompanies disc herniation. The apparent density of the herniated fragment, in comparison with that of the dural sac or the nucleus pulposus, was confirmed by actually measuring the density on the display monitor of the scanner using the interactive computer program. The results of these measurements are shown in Table 34.2.

In 8 patients, a myelogram was performed following the CT scan. The results of myelography are also shown in Table 34.2. In 3 of 8 patients, there was no asymmetry in root sheath filling nor was there a defect in the contrast column at the level of the lateral disc herniation. The myelogram therefore appeared normal. In one case, the myelogram was considered unhelpful. The root sheath was not filled on either side at the level of the disc herniation (L_{3-4}). There was a questionable indentation of the lateral border of the contrast column on the side of the disc herniation. In the remaining 4 cases, the myelogram was positive. Two of these had a large component in the bony spinal canal, and the

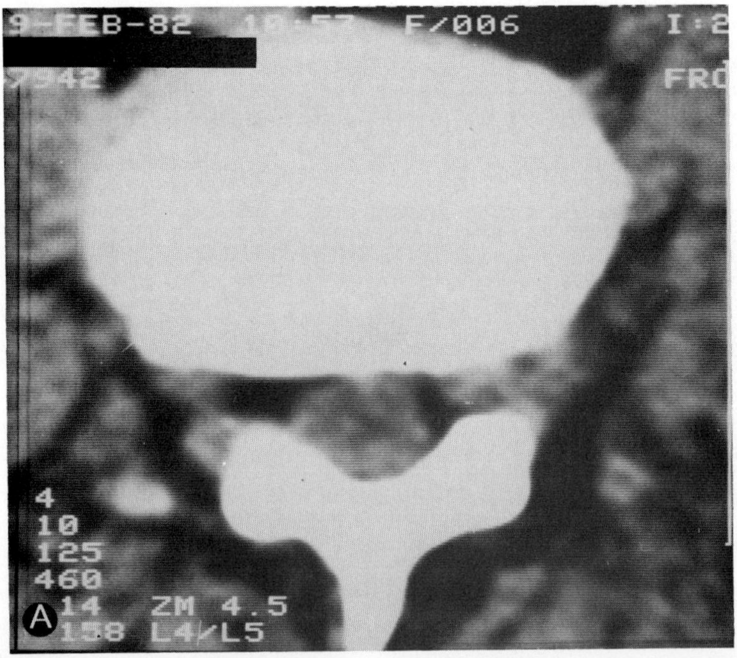

FIG. 34.10. Lateral disc herniation in the left intervertebral foramen. (*A*) CT showing the mass in the foramen.

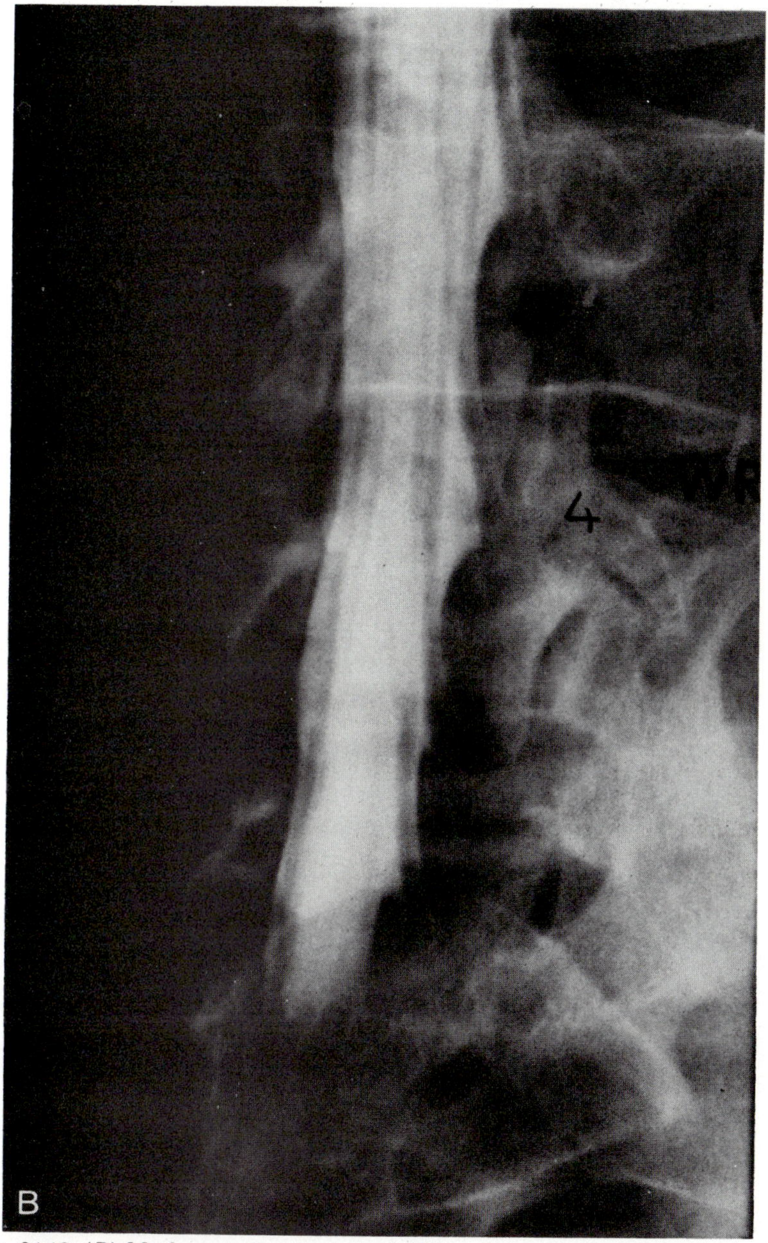

FIG. 34.10. (*B*) Myelogram showing lack of filling of the root sheath and flattening of the root itelf.

remaining 2 showed asymmetry of root sheath filling with apparent widening of the root, presumably due to flattening by compression (Fig. 34.10).

Therefore, in half of the cases, CT was the informative diagnostic procedure, while myelography was noncontributory.

The high incidence of negative myelographic examination in the face of a positive CT in cases of surgically confirmed disc herniations is not surprising. In the past, positive explorations were made after a negative myelogram when the clinical findings were overwhelming. Furthermore, in two of our cases, the main bulk of the lesion was virtually lateral to the intervertebral foramen. The recognition of the lesion on CT helped in planning surgery with lateral exploration in mind. The presence of disc herniation lateral to the foramen explains the previously reported negative explorations of patients who later on were found to have lateral disc herniations at reexploration (5).

REFERENCES

1. Ford, L. T., Gilula, L. A., Murphy, W. A., and Gado, M. Analysis of gas in vacuum lumbar disc. A.J.R., *128:* 1056–1057, 1977.
2. Gado, M. H., Patel, J., Chandra-Sekar, B., Kapila, A., and Hodges, F. J. An integrative approach to the diagnosis of lumbar disc disease by CT and myelography. Presented at the 67th Scientific Assembly and Annual Meeting of the Radiological Society of North America, Chicago, Ill. November 15–20, 1981.
3. Gulati, A. N., and Weinstein, Z. R. Gas in the spinal canal in association with the lumbosacral vacuum phenomenon: CT findings. Neuroradiology, *20:* 191–192, 1980.
4. Haughton, V. M., Eldevik, O. P., Magnaes, B., and Amundsen, P. A prospective comparison of computed tomography and myelography in the diagnosis of herniated lumbar disks. Radiology, *142:* 103–110, 1982.
5. MacNab, I. Negative disc exploration—An analysis of the cause of nerve root involvement in 68 patients. J Bone Joint Surg., *53A*(5): 891–903, 1971.
6. Meyer, G. A., Haughton, V. M., and Williams A. L. Diagnosis of herniated lumbar disk with computed tomography. N. Engl. J. Med., *301:* 1166–1167, 1979.
7. Sachsenheimer, W., Hamer, J., and Muller, H. A. The value of spinal computed tomography in diagnosis of herniated lumbar discs. Acta Neurochir (Wien), 60: 107–114, 1982.
8. Williams, A. L., Haughton, V. M., and Syvertsen, A. Computed tomography in the diagnosis of herniated nucleus pulposus. Radiology, *135:* 95–99, 1980.
9. Williams, A. L., Haughton, V. M., Daniels, D. L., and Thorton, R. S. CT recognition of lateral lumbar disc herniation. A.J.R., *139:* 345–347, 1982.

CHAPTER

35

Diagnosis and Management of Lumbar Spinal Stenosis

PHILIP R. WEINSTEIN, M.D.

INTRODUCTION

The problem of lumbar spinal stenosis has received considerable attention in the medical and surgical literature during the past 10 years. Clinical features of the syndrome as well as principles of diagnosis and management have been described in detail and should now be familiar to neurologists, neurosurgeons, and orthopedists (14, 26, 27). The normal and pathological anatomy of the lumbar spine and its contents has been described, and the pathophysiology of lumbosacral radiculopathy due to spinal stenosis has been reviewed (24, 25). Since the advent and refinement of CT lumbar spine scanning, stenosis has been diagnosed more frequently and more accurately even when the condition is relatively asymptomatic. As our experience with this disorder increases, it becomes clear that a number of special problems remain in understanding the pathogenesis of lumbar stenosis, as well as in confirming the diagnosis and planning of appropriate and successful surgical management. In an attempt to elucidate some of these issues the results of our own more recent experience and that published in the current literature will be reviewed.

The importance of continuing to expand our understanding of the more elusive features of this disorder is emphasized by its prevalence. In a series of 383 cases of lumbosacral radiculopathy reviewed by Paine and Huang (19) in 1972, only 30% were due to disc herniation alone, and 70% were caused by various combinations of stenosis, spondylosis, and superimposed disc displacement. With the advancing average age of the population it is reasonable to expect that narrowing of the lumbar spinal canal will require treatment even more frequently.

PATHOGENESIS

Since the pioneering work of Verbiest (22) and later Epstein *et al.* (5) defined developmental variations in dimensions of the lumbar spinal canal with intraoperative and cadaver spine measurements, dysplastic reduction of the anteroposterior and transverse canal diameters has been clearly defined. At that time one could hardly have imagined that radiographic CT technology would develop the capacity to image the configuration of the neural canal and foramina in axial sections with the exquisite detail which is now available. On the other hand, the embryological basis for failure of the pedicles to attain normal height and orientation in association with inadequate width of the laminar arch remains unexplained (16). Although occasional cases of both cervical and lumbar spinal stenosis are encountered, no other skeletal or systemic disorders have been associated with developmental lumbar stenosis. As regards pedicle and laminar enlargement, it is not possible to determine whether or not degenerative hypertrophy due to ordinary or excessive wear and tear plays a role in the development of the acquired features of lumbar stenosis. Careful histological examination of surgical specimens obtained in our series reveals no evidence of inflammatory or degenerative abnormalities in the bone. Sclerosis and hypertrophy are observed in some cases. Thus, one is tempted to conclude that the presence of excessively thick dorsal elements in spinal stenosis patients represents a feature of the developmental error.

Additional experience in a large number of cases reported recently by Verbiest (23) indicates that significant variations in the morphology of lumbar spinal stenosis must be suspected and anticipated. In some cases stenosis may be unilateral with the side varying from level to level. Skipped levels have been observed with a normal segment situated between stenotic vertebra above and below. Midline stenosis at one level may be associated with a normal midline diameter at other levels, but with narrowing laterally. CT spine scanning is helpful in delineating these variations on the theme of lumbar stenosis.

In our experience, it has not been possible to correlate patient habitus or life and work style with the occurrence of either developmental or spondylotic lumbar stenosis. Despite the observation that lumbar stenosis is more prevalent in males, we have treated 8 female patients in the past 2 years for extensive stenosis and spondylosis associated with complete or partial myelographic block. These patients were all within the 50- to 70-year age range and of average height and weight. In only one case was the patient unusually short and heavy set, as might be expected if lumbar stenosis were associated with a typical body growth pattern. None of these women had a history of having sustained serious spinal trauma or of having engaged in strenuous physical labor. Moreover, 8 of our more severe male age-matched cases presenting over the same 2-year period were also of average height and build.

On the other hand, facet hypertrophy does appear to be associated with the proliferative responses of lumbar spondylosis. Surgical specimens reveal degenerative and hypertrophic changes, with chondroid and osseous metaplasia in the articular capsule. Osteophyte formation may involve the articular processes, and cartilaginous degeneration of the apophyseal surfaces results in reactive changes in the underlying bone. In addition, the well-known hypertrophic changes of spondylosis affect the disc and vertebral body margins as well as the posterior longitudinal ligament to add additional sources of encroachment within the developmentally narrowed lumbar spinal canal. Again, the history in patients with the most severe degenerative and hypertrophic changes does not consistently include an unusual amount of repetitive stress upon the lumbar spine structures.

The ligamentum flavum is a special case insofar as it is often the structure contributing most significantly to constriction of the dural sac in the midline and the nerve roots in the lateral recesses or foramina. Using special histological staining techniques, scanning electron microscopy, and biochemical analysis for elastin, collagen, lipid, and DNA content, we have examined surgical specimens in 16 patients for comparison with normal tissue obtained at autopsy. Despite a 4-fold increase in thickness of the ligamentum, there was no statistically significant evidence of disproportionate increase in any of its components. Although focal areas of granulation or collagen scar deposition and disruption of the normal elastin fiber pattern were commonly observed, there was no significant alteration in the elastin to collagen ratios comparing surgical spondylosis specimens with autopsy controls. Although focal inflammation was occasionally seen in association with microscopic areas of hemorrhage within the ligament, the overall ratio of cells to ground substance was also not altered in the pathological material. In 3 cases amyloid-like deposits were seen without evidence of any systemic disorder. Islands of cartilaginous and osseous metaplasia were also occasionally identified. Thus, it would appear that pathological enlargement of the ligamentum flavum in lumbar stenosis and spondylosis patients reflects excessive growth of this strategically located interlaminar ligament without occurrence of fibroblast hyperplasia or selective increase of any of its components.

Again, the issue of the role of stress and strain must be raised, but here with perhaps a different conclusion. We have now collected 3 cases of males in their fifth or sixth decade in whom hypertrophy of the ligamentum flavum at L_{4-5} was the predominant cause of focal spinal stenosis associated with complete myelographic block in 2 and partial block in 1. The former 2 patients had severe neurogenic claudication with aggravation of symptoms upon assuming erect posture, and the latter had bilateral sciatic radiculopathy. In all 3 cases there was a previous history of major lumbar injury in a position of flexion that can be expected to cause stretching or tearing of the ligamentum flavum. In addition, one patient had an old compression fracture of L_4.

Another important aspect of the development of acquired features of lumbar stenosis is the presence of an unstable joint. The occurrence of degenerative or pseudospondylolisthesis as a cause of lumbar stenosis has been described in detail (6, 8, 18). Radiographic and operative observations indicate that the facet joint is oriented more toward the sagittal plane in these cases, and that it may actually present a 90° angle to the horizontal. Excessive movement or lack of restraint in the facet joint may promote or be associated with laxity of the joint capsule, as well as the interspinous and longitudinal ligaments. Progressive slip either as an anterolisthesis or retrolisthesis can be clearly visualized on the plain spine radiographs in the lateral projection. However, it is also important to obtain lateral flexion-extension views even when, as is usually the case, the disc appears chronically collapsed, and bridging osteophytes suggest stability of the joint. In 6 of 10 cases treated during the past 2 years, significant alteration of the subluxation was demonstrated on the motion films. Interestingly, these patients were females aged 50 to 75. Posterolateral or posterior interbody fusion was peformed to supplement decompression in 3 of these cases (Fig. 35.1).

Also of considerable interest was the observation that massive facet and ligamentous hypertrophy was responsible for spinal stenosis at the level of spondylolisthesis in each case. These patients may be examples of intraspinal ligamentous and articular hypertrophy due to the abnormal forces applied to soft tissues attached to an unstable joint. Additional evidence in favor of this hypothesis is provided by recent experimental work which indicates that ligamentous hypertrophy and epidural scar formation was significantly increased after wide laminectomy in dogs when stability of the spinal column was disrupted by discectomy and anterior longitudinal ligament section (10).

Finally, the importance of biomechanical and postural factors in determining the neural canal and foramen diameters cannot be overemphasized. Radiographic measurements during myelography and metrizamide CT scanning have now been obtained documenting substantial alteration of space available for nerve roots within the stenotic lumbar spine during flexion and extension (29). As in the cervical area, anterior displacement and infolding of the ligamentum flavum in association with posterior protrusion of the disc is aggravated by spinal extension and relieved by flexion. Accordingly, the pincer effect may be demonstrated with standing flexion-extension views obtained during myelography. Even in patients with a relatively normal midline AP diameter who show no evidence of dural sac constriction, narrowing of the lateral recess and foramen may

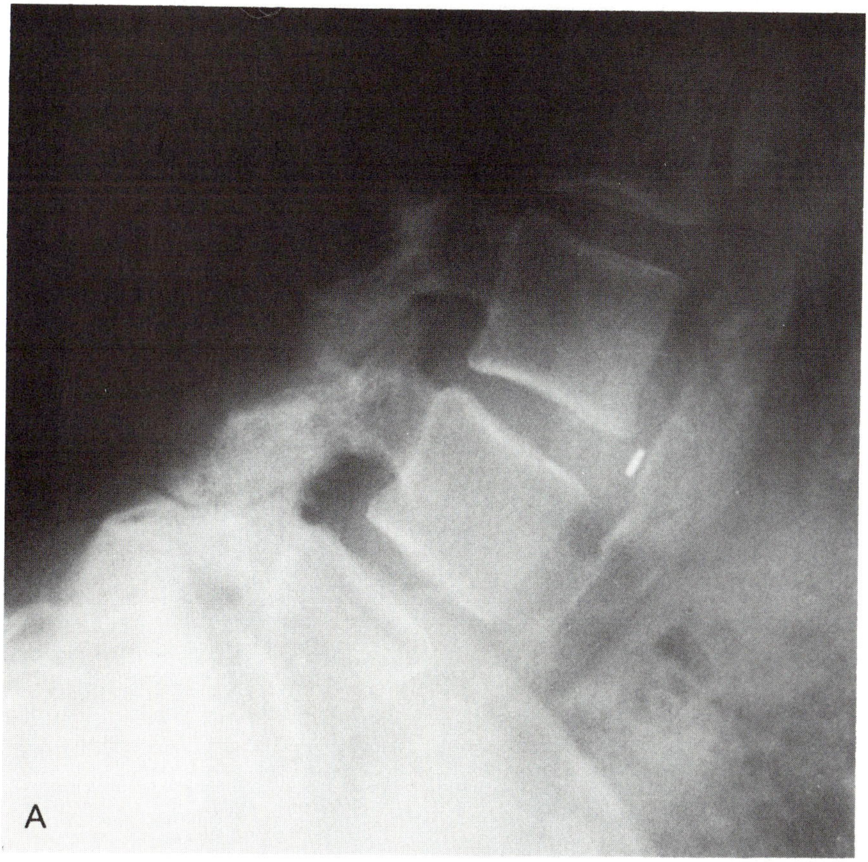

FIG. 35.1. (*A*) Lateral radiograph in a 57-year-old female with disabling leg pain and paresthesias in the L_5 distribution, especially on the left. Slight anterior subluxation due to degenerative spondylolisthesis at L_{4-5} increased to 6 mm in flexion as shown here.

occur in extension due to "shingling" of the overlying lateral third of the lamina and the articular processes. The superior facet migrates superiorly into the roof of the foramen during extension, causing further encroachment within the foramen. These dynamic factors, which cannot be routinely demonstrated by CT scanning, must be considered during the evaluation of patients with postural aggravation of caudal radiculopathy or symptoms of neurogenic claudication.

DIAGNOSIS

Problems in diagnosis of lumbar stenosis appear to arise in the young patients and in older individuals with chronic illness. Patients in the

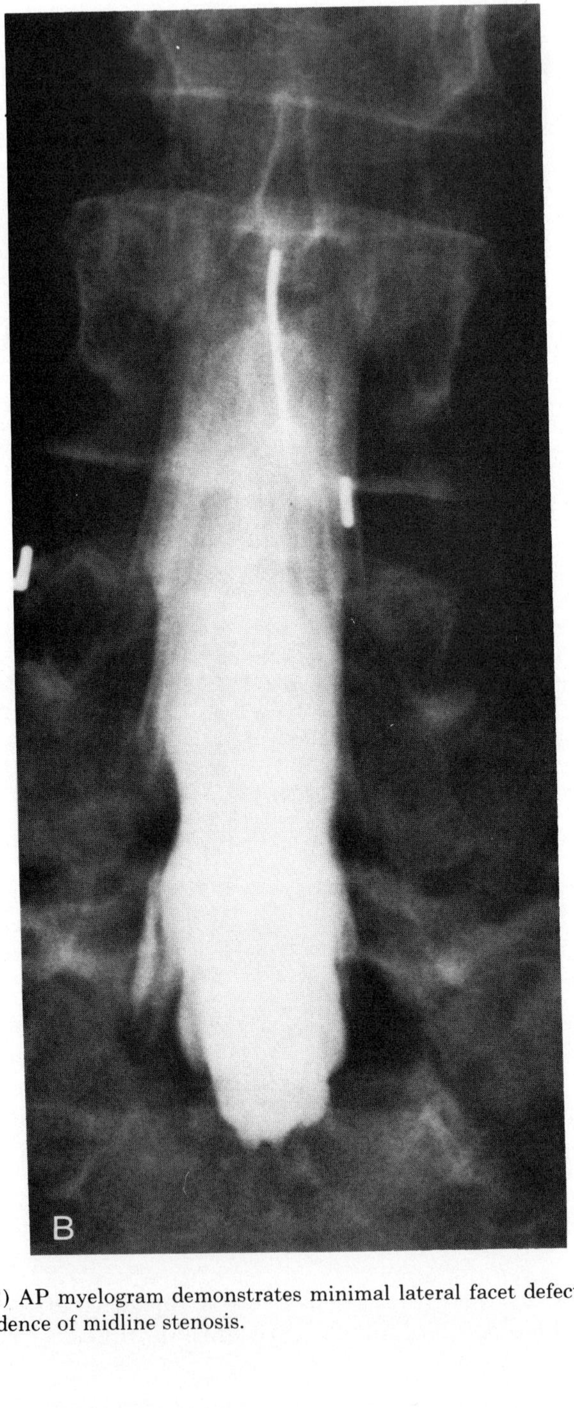

FIG. 35.1. (*B*) AP myelogram demonstrates minimal lateral facet defect at L_{4-5} on the left with no evidence of midline stenosis.

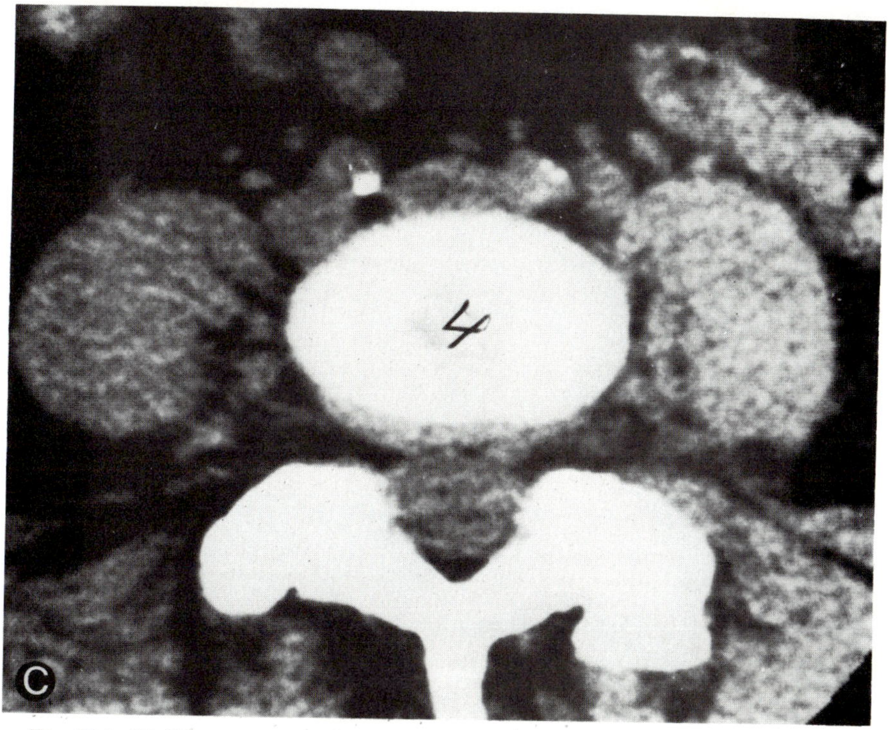

FIG. 35.1. (*C*) CT scan at L_4 is normal except for thickening of the posterior longitudinal ligament.

second or third decade presenting with bilateral lumbosacral radiculopathy should always have the diagnosis of lumbar stenosis considered. Even if there is a history of trauma or acute onset of symptoms, and disc rupture is the most likely diagnosis, the presence of spinal stenosis should be suspected, since primary disc rupture is less common in this age group. Similarly, in the few cases of pure spinal stenosis we have treated where there was no evidence of disc protrusion or spondylosis, the patients were in the younger age group. Accurate anatomical diagnosis is essential in planning the appropriate surgical procedure which should include decompressive foraminotomy or laminectomy in addition to discectomy, especially if a partial or complete myelographic block is present. Information obtained from CT scanning can be helpful in this regard.

Diagnostic difficulties presented by older patients are characterized by the puzzling nature of chronic poorly localized pain syndromes and progressive disability which may also be due to other unrelated diseases. The diagnosis of lumbar stenosis has been missed for years in some of

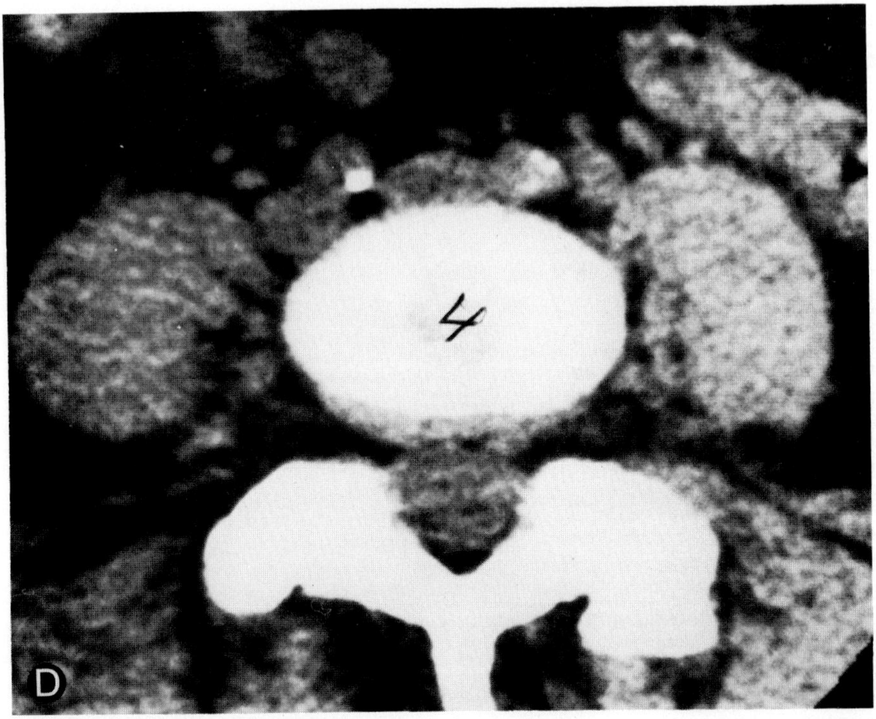

FIG. 35.1. (*D*) CT scan at the L_4 disc level shows facet hypertrophy without significant foramen or lateral recess narrowing. At surgery (interlaminar foraminotomy and posterolateral fusion) severe entrapment of both L_5 roots was encountered due to ligamentum flavum and facet capsule hypertrophy.

our elderly patients treated for degenerative hip joint disease, aortofemoral occlusive vascular disease, and diabetic peripheral neuropathies. Degenerative spinal joint disease or osteoarthritis is commonly invoked as a diagnosis in the older patient who is becoming progressively incapacitated by inability to stand and walk. A careful neurological, spinal and extremity joint examination as well as an effort to palpate the peripheral pulses is essential for evaluation of such patients. Missed diagnosis may lead to prolonged immobilization and unnecessary suffering. We have recently treated a 67-year-old woman who had been confined to bed in her mobile home under the care of neighbors and a visiting nurse for more than a year due to the occurrence of excruciating pain and neurogenic claudication associated with attempts to stand and ambulate. In 2 recently treated males aged 67 and 74, progression of the cauda equina syndrome to advanced radiculopathy associated with muscle atrophy and chronic neurogenic bladder, resulted in only partial recovery after extensive decompressive surgery. In the older gentleman, pain and neurogenic claudication were relieved and bladder function eventually recovered within 6 months after surgery, but bilateral foot drop persisted and required the use of braces. On the other hand, after extensive surgical decompression from L_3 to L_5, a 64-year-old woman experienced unexpected partial resolution of a foot drop which had been present for 12 years since a previous laminotomy for discectomy. In general, somewhat disapppointing results must be expected in older patients with advanced caudal radiculopathy which has been present or progressive for over 1 to 5 years.

Perhaps one of the most difficult diagnostic problems is presented by patients with progressive and disabling back and upper leg pain who were found to have degenerative joint disease on their lumbar spine radiographs. Often they have had previous disc surgery with only partial or temporary relief as long as 10 or 20 years previously. As is the case with many back pain patients, their symptoms are aggravated by standing and walking and relieved by sitting, resting, or lying down. These cases often are referred for neurosurgical consultation from orthopedic or medical clinics by colleagues who have learned about neurogenic claudication and lumbar stenosis. The diagnosis is suggested by the occurrence of segmental radiation of the pain into the upper legs, which is rarely associated with lancinating pain in a radicular distribution or a significant focal neurological deficit. The pain may be aggravated by straight leg raising, although it is often produced as well by hip flexion with the knee flexed. If a lumbar spine CT scan is obtained, facet hypertrophy with borderline foraminal narrowing may be demonstrated. It has been our policy to treat such patients conservatively, avoiding myelography and even CT spine scanning whenever possible. The absence of a clear-cut pattern of radicular pain and neurological deficit, even if the pain described is intermittent and brought on only by activity, has been useful in ruling out the diagnosis of clinically significant lumbar stenosis. This is often a somewhat subjective determination, however, since findings of a positive straight leg raising sign and progressive neurological deficit may be absent in some of the most severe cases of surgically documented stenosis. Another useful point is the observation that lumbar flexion is often quite painful in degenerative joint disease, whereas it should relieve symptoms of nerve root compression in spinal stenosis.

A difficult diagnostic problem is presented by patients who demonstrate unusual patterns of claudication pain (3, 12, 28). Pain which begins distally in the calf and migrates proximally during ambulation, even though it is associated with leg weakness and back pain, should be considered as possibly being due to vascular insufficiency. On the other hand, further aggravation of claudication pain by bending backward and pain that is quickly relieved by sitting, although not by standing after ambulation, is more consistent with neurogenic claudication. The bicycling test is helpful in distinguishing vascular from neurogenic forms of claudication. Since elderly patients with spinal stenosis may also have abnormal pedal pulses or femoral bruits, we refer many of these cases for Doppler flow studies of the lower extremity circulation. When significant abnormalities are detected, digital subtraction intravenous angiography has been a useful screening test for definitive vascular evaluation.

Equivocal cases may also be evaluated with somatosensory evoked potentials obtained before and after ambulation or before and after assuming a hyperlordotic posture in patients suspected of having neurogenic claudication with postural aggravation of caudal radiculopathy. Although consistent changes in latency have not always been demonstrated in our patients, a significant reduction in amplitude of the potentials evoked by stimulation of the posterior tibial and peroneal nerves has occurred following ambulation productive of paresthesias and weakness in the legs. This response to ambulation has been abolished following surgical decompression in our cases as well as those reported by Larson *et al.* (15).

Differential diagnosis in patients with caudal radiculopathy and neurogenic claudication should also include both benign and metastatic tumors. We have a patient with schwannoma of the L_3 root who presented in this manner, as did a patient reported in the literature with lumbar epidural metastasis (17). Claudication may also occur in patients with massive midline disc herniation without spinal stenosis. Occasionally a lateral disc extrusion has been associated with unilateral leg claudication (7). Cervical spinal stenosis has also been associated with intermittent leg numbness and weakness aggravated by ambulation but not by neck extension. Although the symptoms have been characterized by paresthesias and incoordination rather than by leg pain and weakness in both of our cases, a diagnosis of primary or associated cervical stenosis should be considered, especially when long tract signs or cervical radiculopathy are also present.

Plain radiographs of the lumbar spine may be useful for purposes other than to demonstrate the presence of degenerative osteoarthritis. Measurement of the distance between the floor of the spinal canal at the vertebral body margin to the midline roof of the spinal canal as represented by the spinolaminar line may provide a helpful estimate of the midline anteroposterior diameter of the lumbar canal. However, this measurement should be taken at the rostral edge of the lamina which is the narrowest portion of the canal, since the lamina slants anteriorly to lie in front of the caudal edge of the lamina above. In evaluating patients with back pain and equivocal leg symptoms, plain film measurements of 14 to 16 mm midline AP diameter can be interpreted as suggesting that adequate space should be available for the nerve roots. The AP diameter of the foramen can also be measured on the lateral radiograph. On oblique views it is possible to estimate canal diameter by measuring the length of the lamina as represented by the distance between the pedicle or pars interarticularis and the base of the spinous process (1). However, the presence of thickened soft tissue, such as disc and ligamentum flavum, cannot be estimated from the bony configuration seen on the plain films. In addition, comparison of plain x-rays with CT scan in a number of our recent cases suggests that the spinolaminar line may be situated well above the actual roof of the neural canal, especially when the laminar arch is thickened and triangular in shape in association with vertical orientation of the lamina.

At the present time, CT spine scanning has not entirely replaced myelography in our experience for the diagnosis of lumbar stenosis. We rely upon physiological as well as anatomical information derived from myelography to indicate the severity of dural sac and nerve root compression as reflected by the flow and distribution of subarachnoid contrast material. We find myelography especially useful to supplement upper lumbar CT scan images. Since nerve roots at L_{2-3} and above leave the dural sac more caudally and have a shorter extradural course, CT demonstration of facet hypertrophy and lateral recess narrowing may not be clinically significant. On the other hand, CT scanning has been invaluable for visualization of levels below a partial or complete myelographic block (Fig. 35.2). At levels of severe midline stenosis causing an hour glass-shaped partial myelographic block, CT may also demonstrate the configuration of lateral recesses and foramina that do not fill with contrast.

The relative contribution of midline or subarticular hypertrophy to stenosis at individual levels can often be clearly documented by CT scanning. Furthermore, it may be possible to determine preoperatively whether or not a ventral myelographic bulge or nonosseous mass on the floor of the spinal canal consists of disc or osteophyte. Careful review of sequential axial sections or sagittal and coronal reconstructions may determine whether lateral recess encroachment is due to enlargement of the inferior facet of the vertebra above, the superior facet and pedicle of the vertebra below, or both. Scan images may also distinguish the relative contributions to dorsolateral impingement due to thickening of the lamina or ligamentum flavum.

True foraminal stenosis can, of course, only be demonstrated by CT

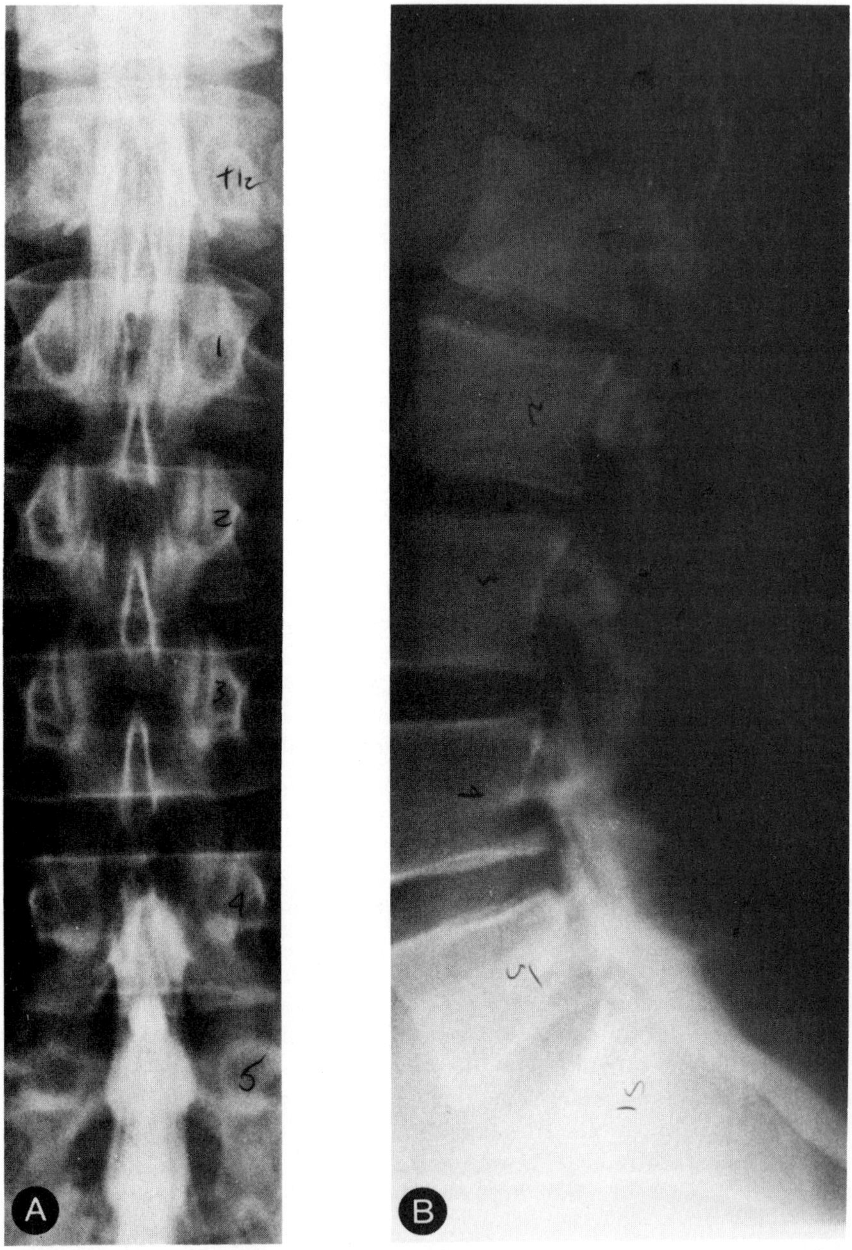

FIG. 35.2. (*A* and *B*) AP and supine lateral myelogram in a patient with back and leg pain aggravated by standing and walking. There was no focal radicular deficit. A partial myelographic block was present at L_{1-2} above and L_{3-4} below. The subarachnoid space in between could not be visualized.

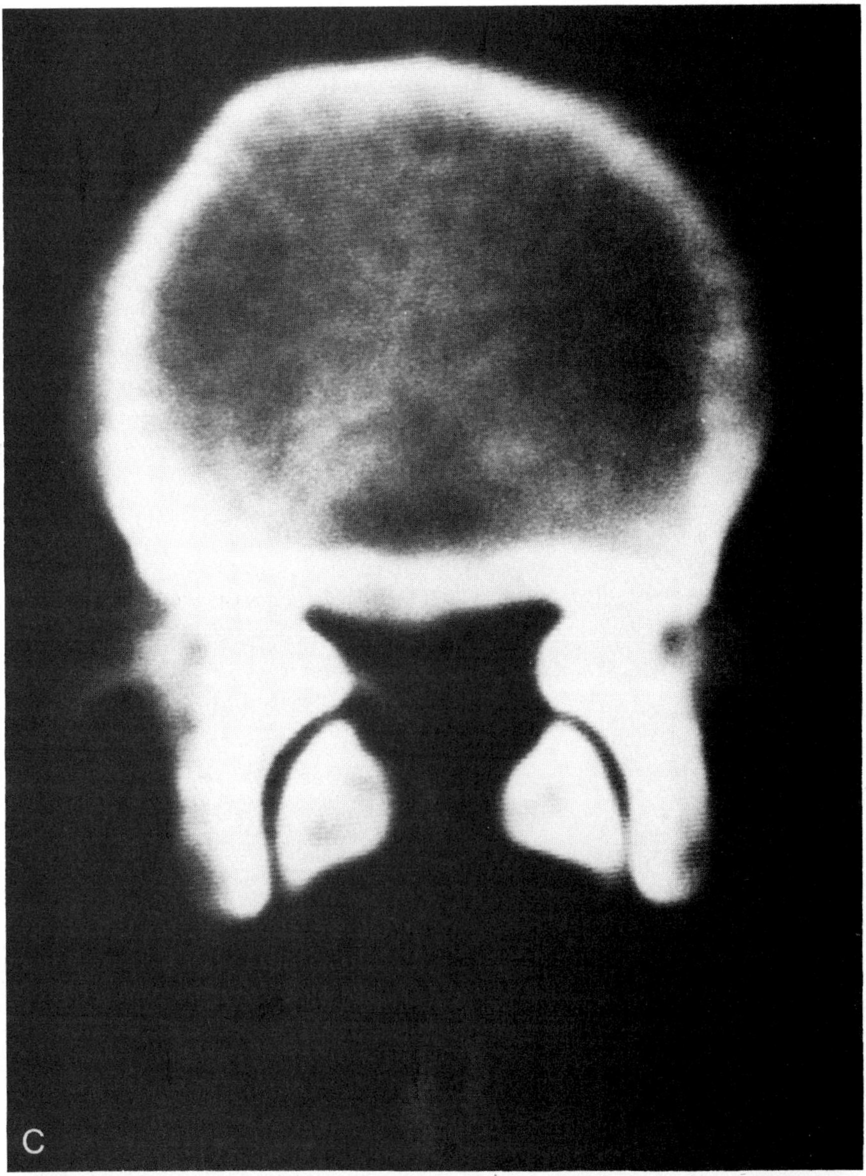

FIG. 35.2. (*C*) CT scan at L_{2-3} shows midline and lateral recess stenosis due to shortened pedicles and large facets. A faint shadow of dorsolateral contrast is seen on the *right*.

scanning, since even water-soluble contrast agents rarely diffuse that far laterally. However, it is important to recall that the normal lumbar neural foramen measures 7–10 mm in the anteroposterior plane and that the interpedicular distance normally measures 18–20 mm in the su-

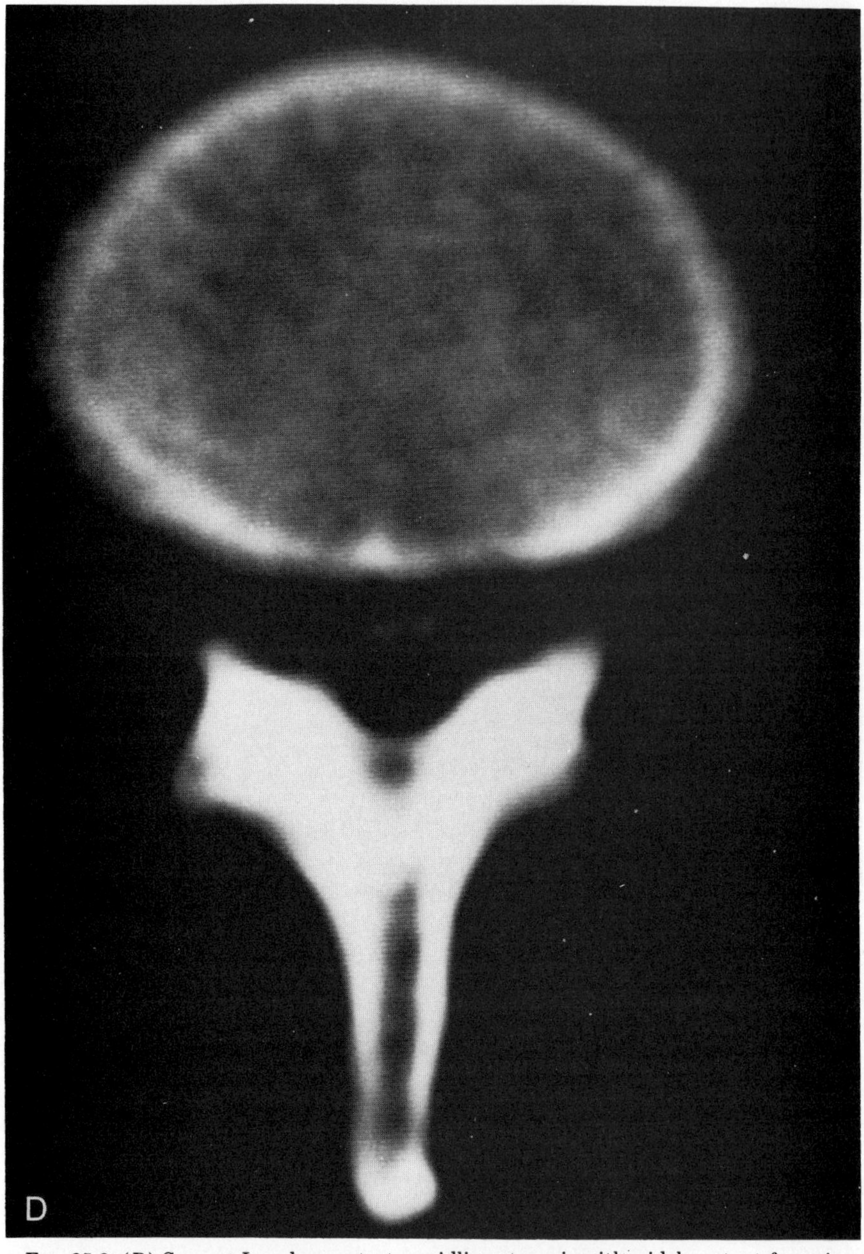

FIG. 35.2. (*D*) Scan at L_{3-4} demonstrates midline stenosis with widely patent foramina.

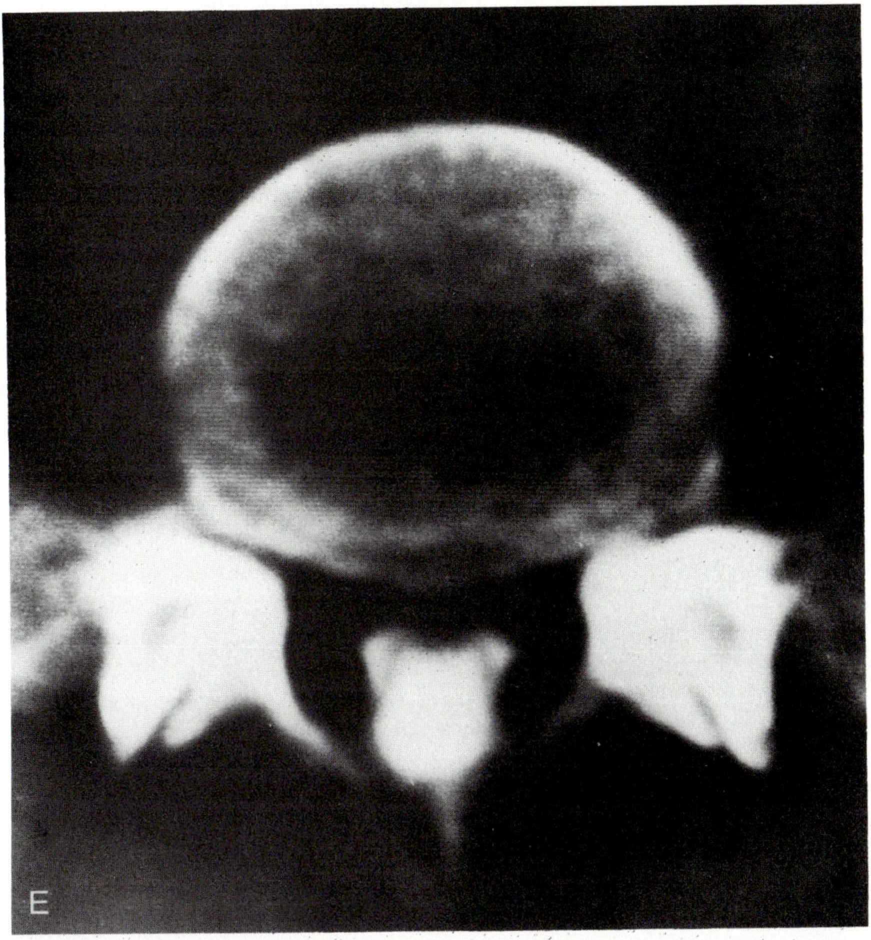

FIG. 35.2. (*E*) Scan at L_5–S_1 reveals constrast filling a narrow dural sac surrounded by a widely patent and normal neural canal which did not require surgical decompression. Note that facet joints touch the disc at a site far lateral to the nerve roots.

peroinferior dimension. The actual location of a given nerve root and ganglion which normally measures 4–7 mm in diameter depends upon a highly variable anatomical configuration determining its site and angle of exit from the dural sac as well as the obliquity of the course that it assumes. Therefore, a CT image showing decrease in the AP diameter of the foramen must be correlated with the position of the nerve root as demonstrated with soft tissue window settings as well as with exact level of each CT section as identified on the localizer scout view.

With this problem in mind we have undertaken extensive foraminal exploration by inspection or palpation in our recent lumbar stenosis cases in order to obtain correlation with CT images. We have regularly observed inferior facets touching the floor of the canal at the level of nonherniated discs and at a point well lateral to the nerve root where it just begins to exit from the dural sac. In addition, we have confirmed contact between the disc and the anterior surface of superior facets, especially at the L_5–S_1 level at a point which is also situated lateral to the S_1 root within the canal and inferior to the L_5 root exiting through its foramen. Therefore, interpretation of CT evidence of foraminal stenosis must be cautious, especially when associated lateral recess or midline stenosis is not also present to provide a more convincing indication for surgical exploration.

Other potential pitfalls in the CT diaganosis of lumbar stenosis relate to variations in scanning technique. False-positive or false-negative results may occur when the angle of the scanner gantry is not set parallel with the plane of the intervertebral discs. Although the soft tissue window setting is useful for imaging neural and ligamentous structures, it can provide an exaggerated impression of the degree of bone thickness and encroachment. Thin or overlapping section techniques are often needed at 3–5 mm intervals in order to avoid missing a site of nerve root compression due to a small osteophyte or disc fragment. Similarly, scan sections should not be taken only at the disc levels but rather at regular intervals through the entire vertebral segment. Otherwise, sites of significant focal subarticular or sublaminar stenosis may be missed.

A final diagnostic problem in lumbar stenosis relates to the evaluation of patients with unilateral monoradiculopathy consistent neurologically and by history with acute disc syndrome. In these patients the myelogram may be negative or there may be multilevel disc bulges making it difficult if not impossible to determine which root is involved. CT scan results may again be equivocal or suggestive of facet hypertrophy without clear-cut demonstration of subarticular nerve root compression; it is difficult to determine the exact site of compression unless the involved root can be identified by the neurological examination or EMG. In a series of 22 cases recently reviewed at our institution there were 6 normal myelograms, 7 with posterolateral defects, 6 with anterolateral defects, 1 with a lateral defect, and 2 with complete myelographic blocks (20). Although lumbar stenosis was diagnosed only in the latter 2 cases and disc herniation was considered to be the diagnosis by the neuroradiologist in 14 patients, the operative diagnosis was stenosis due to facet syndrome in all 22 cases. Root compression was due to the inferior facet in 8 cases and the superior facet in 14. Relief of back pain resulted in 12 of 15, and leg pain resolved postoperatively in 19 of 21. Certainly, standard laminotomy and discectomy would have been inadequate for most if not all of these patients. Furthermore, aggravation of radiculopathy and permanent nerve root damage may result from nerve root retraction for discectomy in patients with lateral recess stenosis.

MANAGEMENT

Special problems in the management of lumbar stenosis include the difficulty of defining appropriate treatment in the small group of patients in whom surgery is refused or would be unsafe because of advanced age or severe medical illness. In cases of acute caudal radiculitis, bed rest in a position of flexion has been helpful with relief of both pain and radicular deficit occuring within a few days even when a cauda equina syndrome has developed after spinal anesthetic or general anesthesia for surgery in the lithotomy position (4). Relief of nerve root compression by flexing the lumbar spine may provide temporary relief and it eliminates mechanical trauma so that radiculitis can resolve. However, in many cases symptoms will recur when erect posture and ambulation is resumed. Occasionally, flexion exercises help to correct a hyperlordotic posture that is aggravating lumbar stenosis. Weight reduction also may be beneficial in this regard. Epidural anesthetic block or steroid administration should be avoided if severe spinal stenosis is suspected on radiographic or CT examination. Especially in the postoperative patient, where adhesions or epidural scar tissue may be present, the risk of attempting to needle the epidural space may be considerable. On the other hand, in patients who have not had previous surgery, the L_5–S_1 interspace may be utilized, since it is often normal or far less narrow than the midlumbar segments. The caudal route can also be utilized in patients who have not been previously operated. Although implantation of epidural electrodes for pain relief may be effective in certain selected patients, even the multiply operated chronic back patient should not be referred for neurostimulation without a complete evaluation to rule out a diagnosis of spinal stenosis that has not been adequately treated.

As mentioned above, spinal fusion should only be necessary following decompression for advanced degenerative spondylolisthesis or when spinal instability is demonstrated either preoperatively or during surgery following completion of foraminotomies. However, when adequate decompression requires total bilateral facetectomy as well as removal of disc or marginal osteophytes, destablization of the intervertebral joint can be anticipated, and fusion may be necessary (9). A more subtle management problem occurs in patients with mild degenerative spondylolisthesis and a stable 3–4 mm subluxation who present with severe back pain in addition to their radiculopathy. It has been our policy to defer fusion in these cases in the hope that surgical decompression alone may relieve pain in the back as well as the legs. In 5 of our 8 such cases operated in the last 2 years by decompression without fusion, persistent back pain has been a significant problem. However, none of these patients is willing to consider additional surgery, even if it has been recommended by the orthopedic consultant. This experience raises the question as to whether the presence of severe back pain in cases of degenerative spondylolisthesis should be considered as an indication for surgical fusion at the time of initial operation. Such management decisions must be individualized and based upon consideration of all available clinical information, such as response to preoperative lumbar immobilization.

Other causes of surgical failure or recurrence of radiculopathy include inadequate initial decompression, bone and osteophyte regeneration, epidural fibrosis in marginally decompressed areas, and iatrogenic stenosis due to additional laminar hypertrophy or bony ingrowth after posterior fusion over an underlying unrecognized spinal stenosis. In our experience the most frequent cause of surgical failure is found in patients referred because of persistent symptoms after discectomy alone or "keyhole" midline laminectomy. CT scan in these cases dramatically demonstrates the cause of residual nerve root entrapment. Thus, decompression must be carried out far enough laterally to include the medial 30–60% of the facet joints to the level of their junction with the pedicles before nerve root compression has been satisfactorily relieved. In some cases the longitudinal extent of laminectomy and foraminotomies has been inadequate. For example, patients with stenosis at L_{2-3} as well as at L_{3-4} and L_{4-5} may not be adequately decompressed unless at least the caudal half of the lamina and facets of L_2 are removed as well. Similarly, a need for L_5–S_1 decompression may be overlooked in patients with a complete or partial myelographic block at L_{4-5}. If bony removal has been adequate, occurrence of epidural fibrosis should not be clinically significant. Attempts to prevent bone regeneration have not been necessary in our experience, since we have observed clinically significant ossification of epidural scar only in patients who had been fused posteriorly or who have had an inadequate initial decompression. Intraneural hemorrhage or ischemia as well as stretch or compressive nerve root injury may result in permanent damage, intraneural fibrosis, or arachnoiditis. Under these circumstances, additional surgical decompression will be of little or no value.

An important issue regarding surgical technique as well as outcome is raised by the question, "How wide is a wide laminectomy?" Although total facetectomy can be accomplished bilaterally in patients over 50 without development of spinal instability, it has rarely been necessary for adequate decompression in our experience. Satisfactory decompression can usually be obtained by undercutting the facet and by achieving total removal of the lateral attachments of the ligamentum flavum. However, after completion of the decompression, it should be possible to easily palpate both the roof and floor of the foramen as well as the pedicle above and below with an angled dissector in order to be sure that the nerve root is fully decompressed. Foraminal palpation should be executed with great caution and should not be attempted until the nerve root has been well visualized within the lateral recess. Otherwise, blind instrumentation of the foramen may result in additional nerve root injury or profuse venous bleeding.

Use of the high speed air drill, initially with a cutting burr and later with a diamond burr, has been invaluable for facilitating atraumatic decompression of lumbar stenosis patients. The medial third of the facets is removed prior to laminectomy, leaving only a paper-thin layer of bone overlying the ligamentum flavum and epidural fat. Sharp osteotomes are also useful in order to accomplish removal of thickened bone posteriorly without inserting large angled rongeurs into the neural canal or foramina. Angled sharp curettes may be useful for undercutting subarticular osteophytes and for removal of the lateral attachment of the ligamentum flavum. Insertion of an interlaminar spreader may dramatically facilitate exposure by enlarging the interlaminar space and separating the articular processes. The ligamentum flavum is placed on a stretch as is the posterior longitudinal ligament which may also be bulging into the canal. This method is especially useful for accomplishing bilateral foraminotomies and interlaminar decompression without laminectomy for decompression of focal stenosis at 1 or 2 levels.

Although decompression for extensive lumbar stenosis is a lengthy and tedious operation, the final stages of nerve root exposure and decompression are most delicate and require utmost attention and care. We routinely use the operating microscope or magnification loupes with a headlight. Magnification of vision and intense illumination greatly facilitate dissection, decompression, and hemostasis in the lateral recesses and foramina. Magnification has not been helpful during the initial midline decompression unless repair of a dural laceration is required.

Hemostasis is essential following completion of the decompression. Bleeding from the cut bone edges as well as from epidural veins and paravertebral muscles must be controlled, since formation of a blood clot in the epidural space may contribute significantly to development of epidural fibrosis. Recent studies indicate that placement of an autogenous graft of the patient's subcutaneous fat in the epidural space may reduce the amount of scarring (11). We recently had the occasion to reexplore 3 patients, 1 year after epidural fat grafts had been placed at surgery for disc herniation. Although a reconstituted epidural fat layer was not present, adhesions were not dense, and a clear epidural plane of dissection was easily established at the site of previous surgery.

Perhaps the most significant factor in determining satisfactory operative results is the surgeon's ability to follow the anatomical road map of the stenotic lumbar canal provided by the CT scan and myelogram. With knowledge of the nature and severity of various compressive elements at every level, the appropriate surgical approach and technique may be selected in order to provide adequate space for passage of the nerve roots. For example, a limited unilateral foraminotomy or bilateral interlaminar decompression can be performed in patients who demonstrate acquired thickening of the ligamentum flavum and facet joints without developmental shortening and thickening of the pedicles and lamina; the latter condition would require complete laminectomy for adequate decompression. Recently proposed modifications in standard decompressive surgical techniques include interlaminar decompression with or without posterior interbody fusion or interlaminar decompression with posterior wiring (2), internal decompression after removal of the laminar arch followed by its replacement with metal screws, and osteoplastic laminotomy (13, 21). Whether or not these modifications will result in significant improvement in results will have to be determined on the basis of future experience.

REFERENCES

1. Babin, E. Radiology of the narrow lumbar canal. In: *The Narrow Lumbar Canal*, edited by A. Wackenheim, and E. Babin, pp. 1–10. Springer-Verlag, New York, 1980.
2. Cloward, R. B. Operations for spinal stenosis. Presented at the PLIF Workshop II, Honolulu, April 23, 1982.
3. Dyck, P., Pheasant, H. C., Doyle, J. B., and Rieder, J. J. Intermittent cauda equina compression syndrome: Its recognition and treatment. Spine, *2:* 75–81, 1977.
4. Ehni, G. Significance of small lumbar spinal canal: Cauda equina compression syndromes due to spondylosis. Part 4. Acute compression artificially induced during operation. J. Neurosurg., *31:* 507–512, 1969.
5. Epstein, B. S., Epstein, J. A., and Lavine L. The effect of anatomic variations in the lumbar vertebrae and spinal canal on cauda equina nerve root syndromes. Am. J. Roentgenol. Radium Ther. Nucl. Med., *91:* 1055–1063, 1964.
6. Epstein, J. A., Epstein, B. S., Lavine, L., Carras, R., and Rosenthal, A. D. Degenerative lumbar spondylolisthesis with an intact neural arch (pseudospondylolisthesis). J. Neurosurg., *44:* 139–147, 1976.
7. Evans, J. G. Neurogenic intermittent claudication. Br. Med. J., *2:* 985–987, 1964.
8. Farfan, H. F. The pathological anatomy of degenerative spondylolisthesis: A cadaver study. Spine, *5:* 412–418, 1980.
9. Hazlett, J. W., and Kinnard, P. Lumbar apophyseal process excision and spinal instability. Spine, *7:* 171–176, 1982.
10. Honma, S. Influence of unstable spine on the post-laminectomy scar tissue formation. Jpn. (Nippon) Orthop. Assoc., *54:* 553–562, 1980.

11. Jacobs, R. R., McClain, O., and Neff, J. Control of postlaminectomy scar formation: An experimental and clinical study. Spine, *5:* 223–229, 1980.
12. Johansson, J. E., Barrington, T. W., and Ameli, M. Combined vascular and neurogenic claudication. Spine, *7:* 150–158, 1982.
13. Kawai, S., Hattori, S., Oda, H., Yamaguchi, Y., and Yoshida, Y. Enlargement of the lumbar vertebral canal in lumbar canal stenosis. Spine, *6:* 381–387, 1981.
14. Kirkaldy-Willis, W. H. Pathology and pathogenesis of lumbar spondylosis and stenosis. Spine, *3:* 319–328, 1978.
15. Larson, S. J., Sances, A., Jr., Walsh, P. R., Bressler, B. C., and Hemmy, D. C. Evoked potentials in neurogenic claudication. Presented at the 47th Annual Meeting of the American Association of Neurological Surgeons in Los Angeles, 1979.
16. Lee, C. K., Hansen, H. T., and Weiss, A. B. Developmental lumbar spinal stenosis. Spine, *3:* 246–259, 1978.
17. Martin, N. A., Gutin, P. H., Newman, A. B., and Pickett, J. B. Neurogenic claudication due to narrowing of the lumbar canal by extradural metastatic tumor. Neurosurgery, *9:* 436–439, 1981.
18. McIvor, G. W. D., and Kirkaldy-Willis, W. H. Pathological and myelographic changes in the major types of lumbar spinal stenosis. Clin. Orthop., *115:* 72–76, 1976.
19. Paine, K., and Haung, P. Lumbar disc syndrome. J. Neurosurg., *37:* 75–82, 1972.
20. Reynolds, A. R., Weinstein, P. W., and Wachter, R. D. Lumbar monoradiculopathy due to unilateral facet hypertrophy. Neurosurgery, *10:* 480–486, 1982.
21. Tsuji, H. Laminoplasty for patients with compressive myelopathy due to so-called spinal canal stenosis in cervical and thoracic regions. Spine, *7:* 28–34, 1982.
22. Verbiest, H. A radicular syndrome from developmental narrowing of the lumbar vertebral canal. J. Bone Joint Surg., *36B:* 230–237, 1954.
23. Verbiest, H. Fallacies of the present definition, nomenclature, and classification of the stenoses of the lumbar vertebral canal. Spine, *1:* 217–225, 1976.
24. Weinstein, P. R. The application of anatomy and pathophysiology in the management of lumbar spine disease. Clin. Neurosurg., *27:* 517–540, 1980.
25. Weinstein, P. R. Anatomy of the lumbar spine. In: *Lumbar Disc Disease*, edited by R. W. Hardy, pp. 5–15. Raven Press, New York, 1982.
26. Weinstein, P. R. Lumbar stenosis. In: *Lumbar Disc Disease*, edited by R. W. Hardy, pp. 257–276. Raven Press, New York, 1982.
27. Weinstein, P. R., Ehni, G., and Wilson, C. B. Clinical features of lumbar spondylosis and stenosis. In: *Lumbar Spondylosis. Diagnosis, Management and Treatment*, edited by P. R. Weinstein, G. Ehni, and C. B. Wilson, pp. 115–133. Year Book Medical Publishers, Chicago, 1977.
28. Wilson, C. B. Significance of the small lumbar spinal canal: Cauda equina compression syndromes due to spondylosis. Part 3. Intermittent claudication. J. Neurosurg., *31:* 499–506, 1969.
29. Yamada, H., Ohya, M., Okada, T., and Shiozawa, Z. Intermittent cauda equina compression due to narrow spinal canal. J. Neurosurg., *37:* 83, 1972.

CHAPTER

36

Management of Spinal Epidural Metastases

NEAL E. SLATKIN, M.D., and JEROME B. POSNER, M.D.

INTRODUCTION

Compression of the spinal cord and/or its roots by metastatic epidural tumor is a common and often devastating neurological complication of cancer. At Memorial Sloan-Kettering Cancer Center (MSKCC) we treat approximately 60–80 patients with this problem each year, and estimates projected from autopsy series place the clinical occurrence of symptomatic epidural metastases in the United States at 18,000 new patients annually (4, 17). Although the disorder usually affects patients with advanced disease, spinal cord compression may complicate any stage of a patient's illness, and in 8% of patients the complication announces the underlying malignancy (4). If the disorder is unrecognized and untreated, patients experience progressive pain followed by weakness and ultimately paralysis, all of which diminish the quality and at times the length of survival. Early clinical diagnosis and vigorous treatment with the nonsurgical modalities of radiation therapy and chemotherapy often relieve symptoms and prevent progression (4, 16, 32). However, a significant number of patients either fail to respond or relapse within months of the initial treatment, leaving the physician facing a patient with advanced cancer (and therefore often not a good surgical risk) but suffering intractable pain and/or progressive paralysis. This report reviews the evidence for efficacy of the therapeutic modalities currently available and recommends an approach to treatment based on our own experience and that culled from the literature. The reader is cautioned to recognize that many of the conclusions in this report represent personal bias, since, with the exception of the report of Young *et al.* (40), a small, randomized study comparing decompressive laminectomy with radiation therapy, there are no controlled trials in the literature on which to base judgments.

THERAPEUTIC MODALITIES

Table 36.1 lists the therapeutic modalities currently available to the physician treating patients with epidural spinal cord compression. *Chemotherapy* may be either specific, *i.e.*, directed at the epidural tumor itself, or nonspecific, *i.e.*, directed either at complications of the tumor

TABLE 36.1
Spinal Epidural Metastases: Therapeutic Modalities

Chemotherapy
Specific
Nonspecific
Radiation therapy
External
Internal
Surgical decompression
Laminectomy
Vertebral body resection

(*e.g.*, spinal cord edema) or at symptoms produced by the tumor (*e.g.*, pain). *Radiation therapy* is usually delivered from an external source, but sometimes surgical decompression can be combined with internal radiation therapy using radioactive seeds (brachytherapy). *Surgical approaches* for decompressing the spinal cord or cauda equina include decompressive laminectomy with or without extrinsic stabilization and anterior vertebral resection with replacement by acrylic polymer. Because patients with spinal cord compression caused by epidural metastases have, by definition, tumors that have spread from a primary site and thus are no longer curable by local measures, surgical procedures are, like radiation therapy, palliative and not curative.

CHEMOTHERAPY

Specific Chemotherapy

If the primary tumor is known or believed to be sensitive to chemotherapeutic agents, those agents should be used in patients suffering from cord compression. The blood-brain barrier, which is often a consideration in the treatment of other central nervous system metastases, is not a factor in the treatment of spinal cord compression by epidural disease. Epidural metastasis arising from primary tumors showing good chemotherapeutic response are likely (but not certain (14)) to respond to chemotherapy, particularly early in the course of a patient's disease. An example is the response shown by certain spinal lymphomas to corticosteroid treatment (29). Unfortunately, this area has drawn little in the way of investigative interest, although in one animal model cyclophosphamide was more effective than either radiation therapy or laminectomy (37). In the human, the extent to which the results of trials comparing radiation and surgical treatments have been confounded by therapeutic benefit derived from concomitantly administered chemotherapy is uncertain. Hormonal therapy for the treatment of spinal metastasis arising from breast and prostatic tumors is often useful in relieving pain, but its value in ameliorating neurological dysfunction is not established. Because of the uncertainty of its response and the irreversibility of severe spinal cord dysfunction, it is our policy never to use specific chemotherapy alone as the primary treatment of patients with spinal cord compression, but, whenever possible, to combine it with other therapeutic modalities.

Corticosteroids are a specific chemotherapy for lymphomas and certain other tumors. The use of corticosteroids in these tumors may lead to rapid resolution of the symptoms caused by epidural metastasis and sometimes even disappearance of the tumor. Figure 36.1, for example, illustrates a patient whose tumor disappeared each time it was treated with corticosteroids, only to recur when the corticosteroids were tapered (29). Because corticosteroids are also used in almost all patients as nonspecific chemotherapy (see below), their occasional specific effect often surprises and confuses the treating physician.

Nonspecific Chemotherapy

ADRENOCORTICOSTEROIDS

The role of glucocorticoids in the therapy of epidural spinal cord compression is less well-established than their role in metastatic brain tumors. Certainly glucocorticoids rarely, if ever, produce the dramatic relief of neurological disability in patients with spinal cord compression that they do in patients with brain metastases (32). Experimental evidence indicates that there is substantial vasogenic edema in spinal cord compressed by tumor and that both the edema and clinical symptoms can be improved by the use of high dose corticosteroids (37). Anecdotal

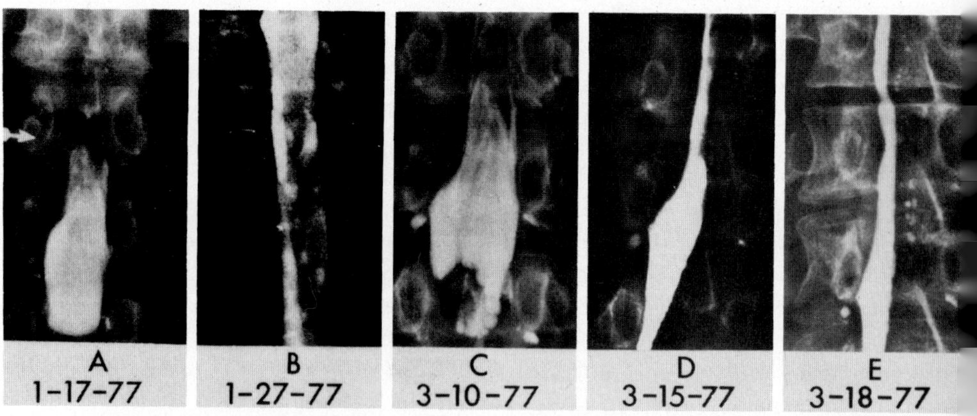

FIG. 36.1. X-rays of case wherein each time corticosteroids were used to treat the tumor, the tumor disappeared, only to recur when the corticosteroids were tapered.

evidence in humans also supports this conclusion. When high doses of corticosteroids are used in the treatment of cord compression, most patients experience dramatic relief of pain (5, 17). Some experience an arrest of progressively deteriorating neurological function, and a few actually improve from the use of corticosteroids alone. Therefore, it has been our policy over the past several years to treat patients suspected of epidural spinal cord compression with 100 mg of dexamethasone intravenously, preferably before a myelogram is performed but if not, immediately after the diagnosis is established by myelography. We then begin patients on a tapering course of dexamethasone while other therapy is being instituted. After the initial 100 mg bolus, we begin oral treatment at 96 mg a day, halving the dose each 2–3 days if the patient stabilizes or improves, but raising the dose again if the patient experiences neurological deterioration.

High dose steroid treatment is not without its problems (1), although there is evidence that when used for short periods of time high doses are no more deleterious than conventional doses of steroids (6, 26). The serious side effects of high dose, short-term steroids include *hyperglycemia* in some patients, at times severe enough to lead to hyperosmolar *seizures* or *encephalopathy*, *gastrointestinal bleeding*, and *intestinal perforation.* The last complication can be difficult diagnostically. We have encountered several patients on high dose corticosteroids who have developed abdominal pain without rigidity or loss of bowel sounds. The apparently benign findings on abdominal examination have at times led to a delay in diagnosis, the true cause of the abdominal pain being established only by the presence of free air under the diaphragm on appropriate x-rays. Even the abdominal pain may be muted in patients on high dose steroids, particularly if the cord compression has damaged pain pathways. Thus, the physician must always be alert to the possibility of intestinal perforation in patients on corticosteroids.

A true *steroid psychosis* is rare in patients treated with dexamethasone, but as many as 40% of patients on high dose steroids experience hallucinations during the first several days of treatment. The hallucinations are usually mild and nonthreatening and do not bother patients if they are reassured that these are a potential side effect of the drug.

Dexamethasone given by intravenous bolus frequently causes a severe *burning* sensation in the genitalia (10). The sensation lasts several minutes and is very unpleasant, but easily tolerated by patients if they are warned of its possibility in advance. More diffuse burning occasionally occurs as well.

Another annoying side effect of high dose steroids is *hiccups.* Many of our patients have suffered intractable hiccups which respond only to tapering the steroid dose.

Steroid therapy can sometimes confuse the clinical picture of epidural spinal cord compression. In addition to causing rarely the disappearance of tumor, as noted above, the drug can produce proximal weakness of the extremities (*steroid myopathy*), which can at times be confused with progressive neurological dysfunction resulting from cord compression. Rapid taper of the drug sometimes causes severe pain in muscles and joints (steroid *pseudorheumatism*) which at times is mistaken for the radicular pain of spinal cord compression. Rapid relief of pain caused by epidural metastases when high dose steroids are given is not a useful diagnostic test, since other kinds of pain, particularly pain caused by metastatic brachial or lumbar plexopathy, also at times responds dramatically to steroids (5). As well, one cannot always equate pain relief with arrest of clinical progression since neurological deterioration can continue despite effective analgesia.

OSMOLAR AGENTS

One author reports temporary reduction of epidural compression after hyperosmolar agents have been infused intravenously (18). There are, however, no data on which to base a judgment about the general efficacy of such agents in treating spinal cord compression. Since we have little experience with hyperosmolar agents, we cannot even hazard an opinion as to their usefulness.

ANALGESIA

Since pain is the common problem in patients with epidural metastasis, it is essential that the principles of good analgesic management be applied (15). On occasion, neurosurgical procedures directed at pain control (*e.g.*, cordotomy) may be useful treatment adjuncts for patients with intractable pain. Although the benefit conferred by these procedures is often of short duration (27), they may spare the patient with limited life expectancy from the risks of more extensive interventions. One of the problems in assessing the outcome of various treatment modalities with respect to pain is that few studies address the question of whether analgesic agents are continued after more definitive treatments and, if so, in what dose. At MSKCC the adjustment of analgesic agents often occurs *peri passu* with more definitive treatment, making it sometimes difficult to determine which modality had improved the patient's pain.

BLADDER AND BOWEL DYSFUNCTION

Bladder and bowel dysfunction are common accompaniments of spinal cord compression. Proper attention to the management of such problems may avert needless patient discomfort and medical complications. Urinary tract infection represents the major complication of neurogenic bladder. In the population suffering metastatic cord compression, compromised immune function may significantly increase the risks of urosepsis (22). Morbidity is decreased by strict adherence to antiseptic technique in the handling of urinary appliances and prompt diagnosis and treatment of infection. Certain patients, particularly those anticipated to have a prolonged survival, should receive urological consultation to address such questions as urinary diversion, pharmacologic manipulation of urodynamics, and chronic urinary antisepsis (24, 39). Problems of neurogenic bowel may be additionally exacerbated by narcotic analgesics and radiation therapy. In equigesic doses, all narcotics are equally as likely to arrest bowel motility. Adjustment of analgesic dose and combination with nonnarcotic pain relievers may be of benefit in allowing for more normal bowel activity. Since neurological worsening may attend the performance of valsalva maneuvers in patients straining at stool, coordination of a bowel regimen including the use of stool softeners is an important management goal.

RADIATION THERAPY

External Beam Irradiation

Several series (Table 36.2) report the results of radiation therapy in ameliorating the signs of epidural spinal cord compression in patients suffering from a variety of metastatic tumors. In general, between 35 and 50% of patients so treated either regain or maintain ambulation at the end of therapy, and of those who show such improvement or stabilization, 50% or more who survive a year maintain that improvement (16). Studies that have addressed the question of pain relief indicate that more than half of the patients with pain are relieved by radiation therapy alone (9, 17). The efficacy of radiation therapy depends in part on the radiosen-

TABLE 36.2
Radiation Therapy of Epidural Metastases (16, 17)

Series	Year	No. of Patients	No. Improved (%)	No. Worse (%)
Mones	1966	41	14 (34%)	
Kahn	1967	82	34 (42%)	
Posner	1971	75	35 (47%)	
Brady	1976	19	9 (47%)	
Gilbert	1977	170	84 (49%)	
Marshall	1977	29	12 (41%)	
Cobb	1977	18	9 (50%)	4 (22)
Greenberg	1980	83	47 (57%)	6 (7)
Stark (36)	1982	31	11 (35%)	

sitivity of the tumor and in part on the patient's clinical condition at the time radiation therapy is undertaken. Table 36.3, from a study of 170 patients with epidural metastases treated by radiation therapy (16), demonstrates that patients with highly radiosensitive tumors are far more likely to regain or maintain ambulation than those with less radiosensitive tumors (64 *vs.* 45%) and that patients who are ambulatory when treatment is undertaken are far more likely to maintain ambulation than those who are paraparetic or paraplegic when treatment begins. Other studies have yielded similar results.

There are no controlled studies comparing various dose and fractionation schedules of radiation therapy, but if one compares the several studies reported in the literature, neither the dose nor the fractionation schedule appears to have a major effect on outcome. In experimental animals, a high dose protracted course (500 rad 3 times every other day) is more effective for a longer time than either a protracted low dose course (200 rad 8 times) or a single dose of 1000 rad (37). We are currently treating most patients with newly diagnosed epidural spinal cord compression with a dose of 500 rad daily for 3 days, followed by 400 rad daily for 3 days. The rationale is to give as high a dose as possible early in an attempt to prevent progression and to complete the course as rapidly as possible to allow these patients with advanced disease an opportunity to spend more time at home.

Because most patients are treated to spinal cord tolerance when they first develop spinal cord compression, patients who respond and then relapse are usually not candidates for reirradiation, especially if the lesion extends over several spinal segments or is located in thoracic or thoracolumbar watershed areas (12). An exception should be made in terminal patients who have previously responded and subsequently developed progressive pain or weakness. Such patients can be retreated with radiation therapy for relief of symptoms when the physician recognizes that their disseminated disease will cause their demise before spinal cord necrosis becomes a problem (28). Lesions compressing the cauda

TABLE 36.3

Radiation Therapy of Epidural Spinal Cord Compression: MSKCC Series (16)

Pretreatment Condition	Total Series (170 Cases)	More Radiosensitive Tumors (39 Cases)	Less Radiosensitive Tumors (131 Cases)
	No. Ambulatory *vs.* No. Treated (%)	No. Ambulatory *vs.* No. Treated (%)	No. Ambulatory *vs.* No. Treated (%)
Grade 1 (ambulatory)	46/58 (79%)	10/12 (83%)	37/47 (79%)
Grade 2 (paraparetic)	37/83 (45%)	14/19 (74%)	22/64 (34%)
Grade 3 (paraplegic)	1/29 (3%)	2/8 (13%)	0/20 (0%)
Totals	84/170 (49%)	25/39 (64%)	59/131 (45%)

equina pose less of a problem. They may be irradiated with greater impunity than those overlying the cord proper.

Brachytherapy

Brachytherapy has theoretical advantages and disadvantages when compared with external beam irradiation. The major disadvantage is that a surgical operation is required to place the radioactive seeds or the afterloading catheters for internal radiation. The major theoretical advantage is that one can deliver high doses of radiation to the tumor without endangering normal structures that are more than 1 mm or so away. Brachytherapy appears to have its most practical advantage in the treatment of paravertebral tumors that cannot totally be removed by surgical resection. We have combined internal radiation with spinal decompression in 14 patients treated here between 1977 and 1982. All of these patients had previously received external radiation therapy and relapsed after an initial response. Surgical procedures performed included anterior decompression (see below) in 12, decompressive laminectomy in 1, and a combined procedure in 1. ^{125}I-labeled seeds were implanted at the time of surgery; 71% improved. Although the numbers are small, the results appear comparable with, but no better than, the results in those patients treated by surgical decompression alone.

SURGERY

Decompressive Laminectomy

The time-honored approach to the treatment of spinal cord compression has been decompressive laminectomy, with or without postoperative radiation therapy. As Table 36.4 indicates, ambulation is maintained or regained in between 35 to 50% of the patients, a result similar to that achieved by radiation therapy (Table 36.2). In the one controlled study comparing radiation therapy with decompressive laminectomy (40), ambulation was regained or maintained in 43% of the patients operated and 54% of those irradiated, not statistically different from each other. The study, however, included only 16 patients in the surgical group and 13 patients in the radiation therapy group, and thus cannot be considered definitive. Our own data of 65 patients treated with decompressive laminectomy indicate a 73% ambulation rate for those with radiosensitive tumors and a 38% ambulation rate for those with less radiosensitive tumors (Table 36.5). Similarly, Brady's study (7) of surgery alone compared with surgery and radiation therapy indicates a 29% improvement rate for the former and 61% improvement rate for the latter. As with radiation therapy, patients who are ambulatory at the time treatment is undertaken do far better than those who are paraparetic or paraplegic

TABLE 36.4

Laminectomy for Epidural Spinal Cord Compression (16, 17)

Series	Year	No. of Patients	No. Improved (%)	No. Worse (%)	Operative Mortality (%)
Mullan	1957	36	8 (22)	12 (33)	
Perese	1958	30	4 (13)		1 (3)
Barron	1959	38	11 (29)	7 (18)	
Wright	1963	86	28 (33)		
Brice	1965	139	44 (32)	10 (7)	(6)
Smith	1965	51	13 (25)	7 (14)	2 (4)
Vieth	1965	34	13 (38)	3 (9)	3 (9)
Auld	1966	41	15 (36)	9 (20)	
Bansal	1967	51	20 (33)		
Chade	1968	162	62 (38)	25 (15)	
Haerer	1968	65	20 (30)	2 (3)	
White	1971	226	78 (36)	23 (10)	(8.7)
Posner	1971	34	17 (50)		
Hall	1973	129	39 (30)		
Brady	1976				
surgery alone		24	7 (29)		
surgery + RT[d]		90	55 (61)		
Gilbert	1977	65	29 (45)		
Merrin	1976	22[a]	18 (22)	0	0
Hattori	1976	9	4 (44)	0	0
Kleinman	1978	20	3 (15)	1 (5)	3 (15)
Marshall	1977	17	5 (29)		
Dahlstrom	1979	19	6 (32)		
Cobb	1977	26	12 (46)	6 (23)	
Gianotta	1978	33	10 (30)	6 (18)	4 (12)
Gorter	1979	31	12 (39)		4 (13)
Livingston	1978	100	58 (58)		0
Baldini (3)	1979	140	42 (30)	27 (19)[c]	0
Dunn (11)	1980	104	34 (33)	24 (23)	(10)
Levy	1982	39[b]	32 (82)	6 (15)	3 (8)
Stark	1982	84	31 (37)		

[a] GU tumors.
[b] All ambulatory preoperatively.
[c] Pain decreased for these patients.
[d] RT, radiotherapy.

(Table 36.3). For example, in Levy's study (25) of 39 patients all ambulatory preoperatively, 32 (or 82%) continued to walk. Several studies that address the question of pain indicate that pain is improved in 50 to 70% of patients after laminectomy, results similar to that with radiation therapy, but these studies were like the radiation therapy results contaminated by concomitant use of analgesics.

Decompressive laminectomy is not without its complications. Operative mortality varies from 3 to 15%, and operative morbidity including worsening of neurological symptoms, vertebral instability, infection, hematomas, etc., varies from 5 to 30% (4). The frequency of laminectomy treatment failures may be ascribed to 2 problems inherent in the performance of this procedure. The first relates to the tendency for most epidural tumors to originate from vertebral body metastasis directly. With the majority of tumor located anterior or anterolateral to the cord, decompression via a posterior approach is both difficult and risky. Tumors localized to the lower lumbar area are often an exception in this regard, the cauda equina proving less of an obstacle to tumor resection than the spinal cord. Since only 15% of cord metastases are present at the lumbar level (4, 16), the surgeon is seldom able to take advantage of this feature of the local anatomy. The second drawback to laminectomy follows from the first. With the anterior vertebral elements weakened by metastatic disease, vertebral stability is more easily compromised following surgical removal of the posterior support elements. If vertebral destruction is advanced, the potential for acute collapse and subluxation with resultant cord compression is apparent. In an effort to offset these limitations, some surgeons have begun to perform "supported" laminectomies using Harrington rods, steel plates, and bony fusion to secure better vertebral stability (20, 23). Aside from occasional complications ensuing from poor graft fusion, osteomyelitis at the donor site and rod slippage, such additional support does not guarantee against angulation arising from the collapse of a vertebral body. It is of interest that even such a recognized authority in the field as Harrington (21) counsels in most instances against decompressive laminectomy in the treatment of vertebral metastases.

We have recently examined the results of decompressive laminectomy with Harrington rods to stabilize the vertebral column, performed by orthopedic and neurological surgeins at MSKCC, in a group of patients who had failed radiation therapy, relapsed after initially successful irradiation, or who could not be radiated because the spinal cord had previously been included in a radiation portal. Of 12 such patients, 10

TABLE 36.5

Laminectomy for Epidural Spinal Cord Compression: MSKCC Series (39)

Pretreatment Condition	Total Series (65 Cases)	More Radiosensitive Tumors (15 Cases)	Less Radiosensitive Tumors (50 Cases)
	No. Ambulatory *vs.* No. Treated (%)	No. Ambulatory *vs.* No. Treated (%)	No. Ambulatory *vs.* No. Treated (%)
Grade 1 (ambulatory)	14/22 (64%)	5/6 (83%)	9/16 (56%)
Grade 2 (paraparetic)	15/33 (45%)	5/8 (63%)	10/25 (40%)
Grade 3 (paraplegic)	1/10 (10%)	1/1 (100%)	0/9 (0%)
Totals	30/65 (46%)	11/15 (73%)	19/50 (38%)

were treated for intractable pain and 6 for progressive weakness (some had both) (Table 36.6); 6 of the 10 patients treated for pain received substantial pain relief such that they were much improved on a stable dose of analgesic agents or were able to decrease or discontinue narcotic drugs (Table 36.7). Of the 6 patients undergoing decompressive laminectomy for progressive weakness, 4 had that procedure alone, and in an additional 2 patients it was combined with a vertebral resection (see below). Of the 4 patients treated with laminectomy alone, 3 were ambulatory in the preoperative period; one patient with carcinoma of the prostate remained ambulatory for 3 months and then died of disseminated disease. Two died without leaving the hospital, one on the 26th hospital day and the other on the 44th hospital day. The fourth patient, with carcinoma of the breast, was not ambulatory before treatment and remained unable to walk after treatment. Two patients with combined vertebral resection and posterior laminectomy were nonambulatory before treatment and did not regain ambulation. One died in the hospital and the other at home. Thus, decompressive laminectomy in patients who have failed radiation therapy appears to be frequently effective for relief of pain and occasionally allows patients to maintain ambulation, but is rarely functionally effective in nonambulatory patients.

Vertebral Body Resection

Several studies in recent years have recommended a different surgical approach to the treatment of epidural spinal cord compression (Table 36.9) (21, 30, 34, 35). Because in most instances the tumor initially involves the vertebral body and spinal cord compression arises ventrally, anterior resection of the vertebral body is a more rational cancer operation than posterior decompression. The operation has 3 objectives: (a) the bony tumor is debulked or even completely excised, lessening the probability of tumor regrowth; (b) epidural tumor excision is facilitated by direct exposure of the anterolateral compartment, thereby allowing for better neural decompression; and (c) spinal stability is improved by reconstruction of the vertebral space with an acrylic polymer. Most of

TABLE 36.6

Indications for Surgery in 45 Patients (47 Operations)

	Laminectomy	Vertebral Resection	Combination Fusion[a]
Pain (20)	6	11	3
Weakness (6)	2	4	
Pain + weakness (21)	4	14	3
	12	29	6

[a] Two patients with fusion stabilized with Harrington rods, 3 with transthoracic resection and laminectomy, and 1 with transcervical resection and laminectomy.

TABLE 36.7
Results of Surgery for Epidural Metastasis (% Improved)

	Laminectomy	Vertebral Resection	Combination Fusion	Total
1. Pain	4/6 (67%)	8/11 (73%)	2/3 (67%)	14/20 (70%)
2. Weakness	1/2 (50%)	3/4 (75%)		4/6 (67%)
3. Pain + weakness	2/4 (50%)	7/14 (50%)	0/3[a] (0%)	9/21 (43%)
4. Pain (1 + 3)	6/10 (60%)	15/25 (60%)	3/6[a] (50%)	24/41 (59%)
5. Weakness (2 + 3)	3/6 (50%)	10/18 (56%)	0/3[a] (0%)	13/27 (48%)
Totals	7/12 (58%)	18/29 (62%)	2/6 (33%)	27/47 (57%)

[a] One patient had relief of pain but not paresis.

these goals can be accomplished without resorting to external support either with rods or rigid bracing. Although some report few postoperative complications, others consider the technique demanding and have warned of potentially serious complications (21). Siegal *et al.* (34) reported successful operations with relief of neurological signs and symptoms in 11 patients suffering from cord compression. Five patients had failed prior radiation; 2 were progressing despite radiation. Radiation therapy was continued postoperatively in the 2 progressive patients and in 4 others who had not received preoperative radiation. In one of these patients, paraplegia resolved. They have subsequently reported the success of second operations after tumor had regrown following the first operation (35). There are other reports of success using this procedure, but no controlled study comparing it with either posterior laminectomy or radiation therapy alone (21, 30). The MSKCC experience with patients who for the most part either progressed during radiation therapy or relapsed after radiation therapy extends to 29 patients (Tables 36.6–36.8). Twenty-three operations were transthoracic resections, 5 transabdominal resections, and 1 transoral resection for cervical cord compression. Twenty-five were performed for pain, with 15 patients having substantial relief of pain; 18 were performed for progressive weakness, and 10 patients improved. Of 7 patients nonambulatory before treatment, 3 regained ambulation and were able to walk for periods of 4 to 7 months, with improvement persisting in 1 patient beyond 6 months. Two patients (7%) died within 30 days of the operation, and 12 (41%) suffered some operative morbidity, including worsening of neurological symptoms in 3, CSF leak in 2, wrong vertebral body removed in 1, pneumothorax in 1, hematoma requiring reexploration in 1, pleural cutaneous fistula in 1, and wound dehiscence in 1.

Several differences exist between our series and those of Harrington and Siegal, which may in part explain why the outcome for our patients appeared less favorable: (a) 43% of our patients had paravertebral tumor which typically was surgically unresectable. Such tumor may have been

TABLE 36.8

Morbidity and Mortality after Surgery for Epidural Metastases (45 Patients)[a]

	Laminectomy	Vertebral Resection	Combination Fusion	Total
Mortality				
30-Day deaths	1	2	0	3
In-hospital deaths after 30 days	2	3	1	6
Morbidity				
Neural	1	5	1	7
Extremity weakness		3		3
Paraparesis	1			1
CSF leak		2	1	3
Other	5	9	1	15
Wrong vertebra removed		1		1
Pneumothorax		1		1
Hematoma, re-explored	1			1
Pleurocutaneous fistula		1		1
Wound dehiscence		1		1
Displaced Harrington rod	2			2
Meningitis	1			1
GI bleed		1[b]		1
Wound infection	1[b]	1[b]	1[b]	3
Chest infection		1[b]		1
Carcinomatous peritonitis	1[b]			1
Leptomeningeal carcinomatosis	1[b]			1

[a] Includes 1 patient with extremity weakness + CSF leak, 1 with paraparesis + displaced Harrington rod, and 1 with hematoma + meningitis.

[b] Patient died.

TABLE 36.9

Results of Vertebral Resection for Epidural Metastasis

Author	Year	No. of Patients	Improved	
			Pain	Weakness
Harrington[a]	1979	14	9/10 (90%)	9/10 (90%)
Siegal[b]	1982	11 (5)	10/10 (100%)	7/8 (88%)
Siegal[c]	1982	9 (32)		6/7 (86%)
MSKCC	1982	29	15/25 (60%)	10/18 (56%)

[a] All patients either pre- or postoperative irradiation, with the temporal correspondence of preoperative irradiation to surgery unclear. Four patients with pain and 3 with weakness received postoperative radiation therapy. Four patients had previous laminectomies. Distribution of patients skewed to more radiosensitive tumors (breast 7, prostate 2).

[b] Six patients with pain received postoperative radiation therapy; 4 with weakness.

[c] Data from an abstract.

responsible for pain and radicular weakness beyond that caused by the spinal lesion. (b) All of our patients had received preoperative radiation therapy and only 3 received postoperative external beam therapy. A much higher percentage of patients in both the Harrington and Siegal series received postoperative radiation therapy, and in Harrington's series many had received preoperative radiation therapy, perhaps immediately before surgery.

All in all, both the literature and the experience at MSKCC indicate that when a single or perhaps 2 contiguous vertebral bodies are involved by tumor and epidural cord compression has failed to respond to radiation therapy, anterior vertebral body resection with acrylic stabilization frequently relieves pain and allows the patient to maintain or regain ambulation. Although a major operation, the morbidity and mortality appear acceptable for this group of often seriously ill patients.

RECOMMENDATIONS FOR MANAGEMENT

Given the above findings, how should the management of a patient suffering from epidural spinal cord compression be approached? The marked variability in such factors as the extent of the cancer, the location of the vertebral and epidural lesion, the type, degree, and rapidity of development of neurological signs and symptoms, and the general condition of the patient all make each patient different and thus each management decision unique. One can, however, construct certain guidelines, recognizing that there will be exceptions in many instances.

In patients with mild or equivocal spinal cord signs, myelography can be deferred for several hours (until the next day), but in patients with deteriorating cord signs, we treat with dexamethasone prior to the myelogram, which is performed as soon as possible. In patients with major epidural masses or deteriorating cord signs, radiation therapy is begun as an emergency. In less urgent patients, radiation can be begun the next day. During and at the end of radiation therapy, the steroids are tapered to tolerance but always raised again if the patient begins to deteriorate. Six to 8 weeks after the end of radiation therapy, the myelogram is repeated (with the lipid-soluble contrast material left in at the time of the original myelogram) to determine if the block has resolved. There is no fixed correlation between change in the block and change in the patient's neurological symptoms. Some patients improve substantially despite a myelographic block remaining present; others deteriorate despite the block opening. For patients with radiosensitive tumors and nonprogressive neurological dysfunction, we advise that an adequate period of observation be allowed for clinical improvement to occur after spinal irradiation before considering surgical intervention. Only if the clinical response remains unsatisfactory at 8 weeks following the completion of treatment can radiation therapy confidently be considered to have failed.

Exceptions to these guidelines include the following.

UNKNOWN PRIMARY TUMOR

Surgery is indicated to obtain tumor tissue for pathologic identification, since the type of tumor may have significant implications for systemic chemotherapy. If other, more accessible, bony lesions are present, these should be given first consideration for biopsy. Surgery may also help to exclude rare cases of epidural lipomatosis (8, 19), protruded intervertebral discs (33), abscesses (2), and hematomas (13) which may simulate tumor, although careful myelography, transaxial CT scanning, and a good history will usually allow these to be distinguished without surgery.

RESECTABLE LESIONS

Tumors shown on myelography to be located posterior to the spinal cord may be surgically resectable by a laminectomy (21). In the presence of plain x-ray or bone scan changes suggestive of vertebral body involvement, no additional advantage over radiation therapy alone is likely to be gained.

VERTEBRAL BODY INSTABILITY AND ANGULATION

Since the anterior vertebral elements are most commonly subject to collapse, neurological symptoms which are thought to arise on this basis should most likely be treated by anterior decompression of the collapsed vertebra with methyl methacrylate replacement. Laminectomy with extrinsic rod stabilization has certain theoretical advantages over simple laminectomy, but thus far it has not been shown to have a clear clinical benefit.

PROGRESSION DURING RADIATION THERAPY

The question of what to do with the patient who appears to progress during the course of radiation therapy or who has rapidly progressive neurological deterioration before beginning radiation therapy is an unanswered one. Our own experience has been that decompressive laminectomy is not helpful in reversing these progressive courses, and others have reported similar findings. The efficacy of anterior decompression is not yet established, although it appears promising.

OTHER POSSIBLE INDICATIONS FOR SURGERY

Marrow suppression may on occasion complicate the administration of radiation therapy, particularly among patients receiving chemotherapy. Depending upon the progression of neurological dysfunction, the schedule of radiation treatments may either be amended or surgery considered. Radioresistant tumors (many sarcomas, and cancers of the thyroid, kidney, and cervix) also pose a therapeutic problem. Again, depending upon the tempo of clinical progression, we advise a trial of radiation therapy prior to electing surgery.

Previously Untreated Patients

Figure 36.2 outlines our approach to the patient known to have cancer who presents with previously untreated signs of epidural spinal cord compression. In patients whose only symptom is pain, spine films are procured and reviewed by the physician together with the radiologist. If there is a vertebral body lesion, the likelihood, even in the absence of neurological findings other than pain, of finding a complete or almost complete block to the passage of myelographic dye is about 20% (31). We perform a lumbar myelogram, injecting only 3 ml of lipid-soluble contrast material to determine if there is a complete block. A lateral cervical myelogram defines the upper end of the port if the lumbar contrast is blocked. The patient is placed on steroids, and radiation therapy is begun. In patients with pain only and a vertebral lesion on plain x-ray that coincides with the pain, it also seems reasonable to give radiation therapy in the absence of a myelogram, recognizing that on rare occasions myelography would have revealed an epidural mass outside the planned radiation port, and therapy may fail for that reason. However, every effort must be made to exclude other diagnoses which may either resemble the clinical presentation of cord compression or complicate its occurrence. These include metastatic plexopathies, pathologic extremity fractures, spinal radionecrosis, steroid-induced weakness, and leptomeningeal metastases. Since the last often carries a poor prognosis even with treatment (38), it is essential that appropriate CSF studies be done to exclude its consideration, particularly if surgery is contemplated. This may be made difficult when a complete myelographic block requires that a limit be placed on the amount of CSF obtained caudal to the lesion. Under these circumstances, fluid obtained from the cervical puncture should be submitted for cytologic study as well.

Previously Treated Patients

Patients who relapse after radiation therapy should be considered for a surgical decompression. The exceptions include the group of patients with cancer so widely disseminated that they are not candidates for surgery. In those patients that have responded to radiation therapy in the past, that treatment modality should be repeated despite exceeding the tolerance of the spinal cord to radiation. Spinal cord necrosis follows excessive radiation therapy by several months to several years, and terminal patients can reap the early benefits of radiation without surviving long enough to suffer its hazards.

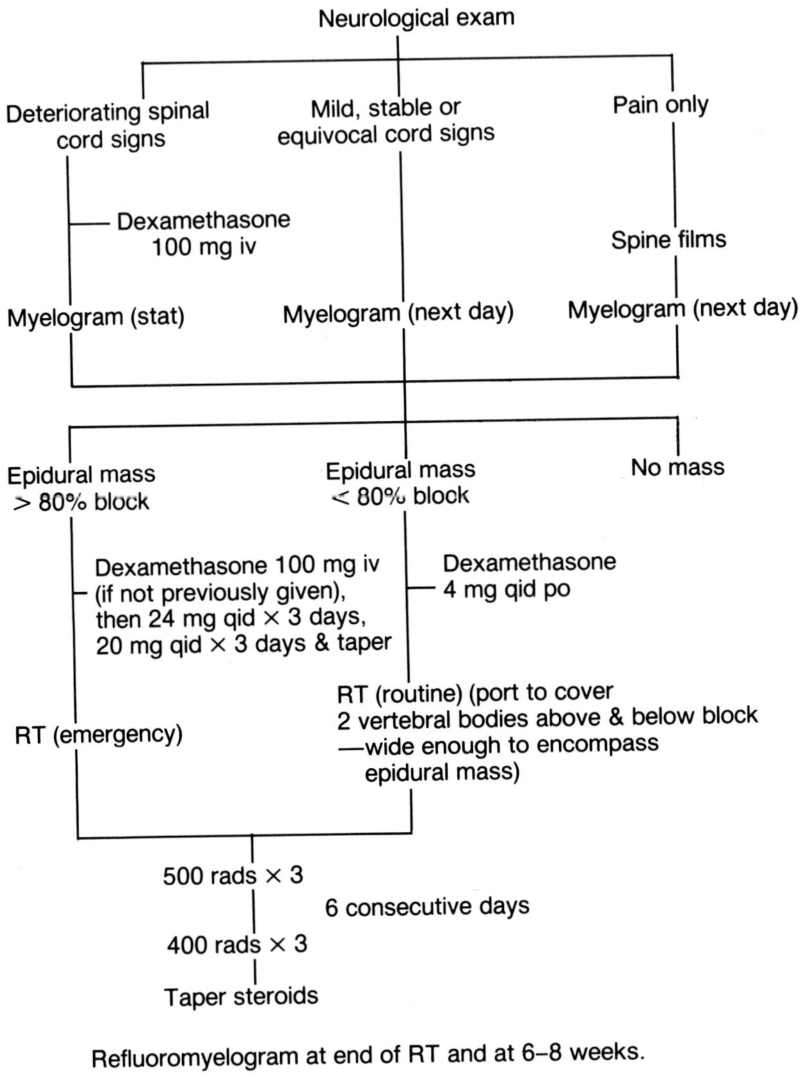

FIG. 36.2 Treatment of previously unknown signs of epidural spinal cord compression.

The choice of operation to be performed in those patients selected for surgery depends on a number of factors, including the number of vertebral bodies involved and the site of vertebral involvement. Evidence is accumulating that in most instances anterior vertebral decompression with fixation by acrylic is the operation of choice when technical factors allow it to be performed.

REFERENCES

1. Axelrod, L. Glucocorticoid therapy. Medicine, *55:* 39–65, 1976.
2. Baker, A. S., Ojemann, R. G., Swartz, M. N., and Richardson, E. P. Spinal epidural abscess. N. Engl. J. Med., *293:* 463–468, 1975.
3. Baldini, M., Tonnarelli, G. P., Princi, L., *et al.* Neurological results in spinal cord metastases. Neurochirurgia, *22:* 159–165, 1979.
4. Black, P. Spinal metastasis: Current status and recommended guidelines for management. Neurosurgery, *5:* 726–746, 1979.
5. Bonica, J. J. Cancer pain. In: *Pain*, Vol. 58, edited by J. J. Bonica, pp. 335–362. ARNMD, Raven Press, New York, 1980.
6. The Boston Collaborative Drug Surveillance Program. Acute adverse reactions to prednisone in relation to dosage. Clin. Pharmacol. Ther., *13:* 694–698, 1972.
7. Brady, L. W., *et al.* The treatment of metastatic disease of the nervous system by radiation therapy. In: *Tumors of the Nervous System*, edited by H. G. Seydel, pp. 177–188. John Wiley & Sons, New York, 1975.
8. Butcher, D. L., and Sahn, S. A. Epidural lipomatosis: A complication of corticosteroid therapy. Ann. Intern. Med., *90:* 60, 1979.
9. Cobb, C. A., Leavens, M. E., and Eckles, N. Indications for nonoperative treatment of spinal cord compression due to breast cancer. J. Neurosurg., *47:* 653–658, 1977.
10. Czerwinski, A. W., Czerwinski, A. B., Whitsett, T. L., and Clark, M. L. Effects of a single, large, intravenous injection of dexamethasone. Clin. Pharmacol. Ther., *13:* 638–642, 1972.
11. Dunn, R. C., Kelly, W. A., Wohns, R. N. W., and Howe, J. F. Spinal epidural neoplasia. A 15-year review of the results of surgical therapy. J. Neurosurg., *52:* 47–51, 1980.
12. Dynes, J. B., and Smedal, M. I. Radiation myelitis. Am. J. Roentgenol., *83:* 78–87, 1960.
13. Edelson, R. N., Chernik, N. L., and Posner, J. B. Spinal subdural hematomas complicating lumbar puncture. Arch. Neurol., *31:* 134–137, 1974.
14. Fidler, I. J., and Hart, I. R. Biological diversity in metastatic neoplasms: Origins and implications. Science, *217:* 998–1003, 1982.
15. Foley, K. M. The management of pain of malignant origin. In: *Current Neurology*, Vol. 2, edited by H. R. Tyler, and I. M. Dawson, Chap. 18, pp. 279–302. Houghton-Mifflin, Boston, 1979.
16. Gilbert, R. W., Kim, J.-H., and Posner, J. B. Epidural spinal cord compression from metastatic tumor: Diagnosis and treatment. Ann. Neurol., *3:* 40–51, 1978.
17. Greenberg, H. S., Kim, J.-H., and Posner, J. B. Epidural spinal cord compression from metastatic tumor: Results with a new treatment protocol. Ann. Neurol., *8:* 361–366, 1980.
18. Greenwood, J., Jr. Spinal cord tumors. In: *Neurological Surgery*, edited by J. R. Youmans, pp. 1514–1534. W. B. Saunders, Philadelphia, 1973.
19. Guegan, Y., Fardoun R., Launois, B., and Pecker, J. Spinal cord compression by extradural fat after prolonged corticosteroid therapy. Case report. J. Neurosurg., *56:* 267–269, 1982.
20. Hansebout, R. R., and Blomquist, G. A., Jr. Acrylic spinal fusion. A 20-year clinical series and technical note. J. Neurosurg., *53:* 606–612, 1980.
21. Harrington, K. D. The use of methylmethacrylate for vertebral-body replacement and anterior stabilization of pathological fracture-dislocations of the spine due to metastatic malignant disease. J. Bone Joint Surg., *63-A:* 36–46, 1981.
22. Jameson, R. M. Prolonged survival in paraplegia due to metastatic spinal tumours. Lancet, *1:* 1209–1211, 1974.

23. Lane, J. M., Boland, P., Sundaresan, N., and Beattie, E. J. Spinal cord decompression treated by laminectomy with spinal stabilization and realignment. Clin. Bull. (Mem. Sloan-Kettering Cancer Cent.), *11:* 83–87, 1981.
24. Lapides, J. Neurogenic bladder. Principles of treatment. Urol. Clin. North Am., *1:* 81–97, 1974.
25. Levy, W. J., Latchaw, J. P., Jr., Hardy, R. W., and Hahn, J. P. Encouraging surgical results in walking patients with epidural metastases. Neurosurgery, *11:* 229–233, 1982.
26. Marshall, L. F., King, J., and Langfitt, T. W. The complications of high-dose corticosteroid therapy in neurosurgical patients: A prospective study. Ann. Neurol., *1:* 201–203, 1977.
27. Pagni, C. A. General comments on ablative neurosurgical procedures. In: *Advances in Pain Research*, Vol. 2, edited by J. J. Bonica, and V. Ventafridda, pp. 405–423. Raven Press, New York, 1979.
28. Pallis, C. A., Louis, S., and Morgan, R. L. Radiation myelopathy. Brain, *84:* 460–479, 1961.
29. Posner, J. B. P., Howieson, J., and Cvitkovic, E. "Disappearing" spinal cord compression: Oncolytic effect of glucocorticoids (and other chemotherapeutic agents) on epidural metastases. Ann. Neurol., *2:* 409–413, 1977.
30. Raycroft, J. F., Hockman, R. P., and Southwick, W. O. Metastatic tumors involving the cervical vertebrae: Surgical palliation. J. Bone Joint Surg., *60-A:* 763–768, 1978.
31. Rodichok, L. D., Harper, G. R., Ruckdeschel, J. C., *et al.* Early diagnosis of spinal epidural metastases. Am. J. Med., *70:* 1181–1188, 1981.
32. Rodriguez, M., and DiNapoli, R. P. Spinal cord compression with special reference to metastatic epidural tumors. Mayo Clin. Proc., *55:* 442–448, 1980.
33. Schramm, J., and Umbach, W. Simultaneous occurrence of spinal tumor and lumbar disk herniation. Neurochirurgia, *20:* 22–28, 1977.
34. Siegal, T., Siegal, T., Robin, G., *et al.* Anterior decompression of spine for metastatic epidural cord compression: Is it a promising avenue of therapy? Ann. Neurol., *11:* 28–34, 1982.
35. Siegal, T., Siegal, T., Robin, G., *et al.* Recurrent metastatic cord compression: Results of repeat anterior spinal decompression. Neurology, *32:* A156, 1982.
36. Stark, R. J., Henson, R. A., and Evans, S. J. W. Spinal metastases. A retrospective survey from a general hospital. Brain, *105:* 189–213, 1982.
37. Ushio, Y., Posner, R., Kim, J.-H., Shapiro, W. R., and Posner, J. B. Treatment of experimental spinal cord compression caused by extradural neoplasms. J. Neurosurg., *47:* 380–390, 1977.
38. Wasserstrom, W. R., Glass, J. P., and Posner, J. B. Diagnosis and treatment of leptomeningeal metastases from solid tumors: Experience with 90 patients. Cancer, *49:* 759–772, 1982.
39. Wein, A. J., Raezer, D. M., and Benson, G. S. Management of neurogenic bladder dysfunction in the adult. Urology, *8:* 432–443, 1976.
40. Young, R. F., Post, E. M., and King, G. A. Treatment of spinal epidural metastases. Randomized prospective comparison of laminectomy and radiotherapy. J. Neurosurg., *53:* 741–748, 1980.

CHAPTER

37

Intramedullary Spinal Cord Tumors

BENNETT M. STEIN, M.D.

Of all spinal cord tumors, intramedullary tumors affect a small but important segment of patients. Controversy has developed over the best treatment for these tumors, which oftentimes afflict patients during their most productive years (8, 12, , 17, 20).

Intramedullary spinal cord tumors comprise approximately 15% of all spinal cord tumors, if metastases are excluded (1, 2, 11, 12). This figure is subject to distortion, depending upon a particular neurosurgeon's interest, referral pattern, and adult-child ratio of patients. Within the category of intramedullary tumors, the two groups which comprise approximately 30% each are the astrocytoma (excluding the malignant variety) and the ependymoma. The remaining 30% of tumors are a miscellaneous group, including the malignant astrocytoma, dermoid, teratoma, and hemangioblastoma (1, 15, 20). In this discussion, intramedullary lipomas are excluded, as their neoplastic nature is questionable.

In my series of 31 intramedullary tumors, I have not selected patients according to age. Therefore, the mixture of pediatric *vs.* adult intramedullary tumors is probably appropriate to the general population. Using age 16 as a division, I have treated 12 children with intramedullary tumors and during the same period 19 adults. Astrocytic tumors predominated in children, and including the malignant variety, this group comprised 7 patients. In adults, there were 6 astrocytomas and 11 ependymomas. There were no ependymomas in children. In the miscellaneous group of tumors, the teratoma and dermoid predominated in children whereas the hemangioblastoma predominated in adults (Table 37.1). In the astrocytoma group, the benign low-grade astrocytoma, regardless of patient age, outnumbered the malignant astrocytoma by a ratio of 3 to 1. None of the ependymomas were malignant. Unfortunately, a number of both major groups of tumors had been previously treated by decompressive laminectomy and radiation, somewhat distorting their gross and microscope appearance.

HISTORICAL PERSPECTIVES

It is interesting to review the history of treatment of intramedullary spinal cord tumors. Before the popularity of radiotherapy for all types of

TABLE 37.1

Types of Intramedullary Spinal Cord Tumors

Astrocytoma	10
Glioblastoma	3
Ependymoma	11
Mixed Tumor	1
Dermoid	2
Teratoma	1
Hemangioblastoma	2
Cavernous Hemangioma	1
Total	31

tumors of the central nervous system, surgery appeared to be the only reasonable treatment for these tumors (2). Considering the lack of sophisticated microsurgical techniques that existed 5 decades ago, the accomplishment of neurosurgeons in attempting and, in some cases, accomplishing removal of these tumors was quite remarkable. In reviewing his broad experience with spinal cord tumors, Elsberg (2) recorded 13 patients with intramedullary tumors. These were operated on by laminectomy and, via a myelotomy, an attempt was made to remove the tumor. In the 13 patients, 3 tumors were totally removed, and the remainder were biopsied or partially removed. He emphasized that certain tumors had well-defined cleavage planes between their margin and that of the normal spinal cord and therefore were appropriate for removal. He also documented that other tumors, although partially encapsulated, had borders that shaded into the normal spinal cord, precluding their removal. Based on his early experience, he suggested that an initial myelotomy with no concerted effort to remove the tumor could be followed in a week or two by a second operation, at which time the tumor then extruding from the myelotomy could be removed. Detailed analysis of his cases would indicate that lacking current microsurgical techniques, Elsberg performed myelotomy over the entire area of spinal cord widening and then removed the exophytic portion of the tumor as it was forced from the interior of the cord by the intrinsic pressure of the cord substance. In the few instances noted, the whole tumor extruded and could be plucked from the dorsal surface of the cord. In most instances only small portions of the tumor were removed, and often second and third operations were performed, removing tumor each time. Many of these patients had gliomas and enjoyed a long useful survival. This ingenious management has been reiterated subsequently, but no single neurosurgeon has utilized it in a significant number of patients to determine its effectiveness (10). My limited experience would indicate that tumors which might extrude through a myelotomy at a second stage can probably be removed at the primary operation with less difficulty. In those tumors which are removable, it is unlikely that they will define themselves in the interim between the two stages of the operative procedure.

Subsequent to Elsberg, despite isolated case reports of satisfactory removal of intramedullary tumors (9, 20), the importance of the surgical treatment of these lesions was lost to the literature for a number of years. The reason for this is not apparent, although it is probably related to unpublished futile attempts at removal of these tumors without sufficient experience or availability of microsurgical techniques. Therefore, during this period, radiotherapy following a decompressive procedure was the recommended treatment for most intramedullary tumors. Reports reached the literature about successful remission or stabilization of intramedullary tumors of all varieties by standard radiotherapeutic techniques (12–14, 18, 19). Unfortunately, these patients were followed only on a clinical basis and not by myelography, and therefore there was no objective evidence of regression of the tumor following radiotherapy. Furthermore, it has been recognized that the symptomatology and clinical course of the benign intramedullary tumors of the common varieties (astrocytomas and ependymomas) without radiation may span many years, if not decades (1, 4, 6, 7, 8, 11, 15, 20). In fact, there have been instances where tumors have been partially removed without additional treatment that have been associated with long-term survival and a static or even improving clinical picture (1, 2, 20). Baker, in discussing Greenwood's work (6), cited 2 cases, one an ependymoma, the other an astrocytoma, who had 25 and 40 years, respectively, of useful life following only myelotomy with no significant tumor removal or radiotherapy. Therefore, any therapy directed at intramedullary spinal cord tumors must stand the scrutiny of a detailed objective follow-up plus the test of a significant time frame in terms of clinical and radiological evaluation.

The committment to surgery as the primary treatment of these tumors was reaffirmed by the reports of Greenwood (6, 7), in which he reported the successful removal of 9 intramedullary ependymomas and 1 teratoma. The tumors were removed without mortality and without significant morbidity. His reports came at a time of burgeoning interest in microsurgery and stressed the use of microinstrumentation and magnified vision in order to accomplish successful removal of these lesions. He also pointed out the difference between the astrocytoma and the ependymoma, with the former not reliably associated with a plane between tumor and spinal cord whereas the latter was invariably associated with an identifiable interface between tumor and spinal cord. Following this, there have been a number of reports emphasizing the appropriateness of surgery and the excellent results obtained by radical surgical removal of these tumors (3–5, 8, 11, 15, 21).

ANALYSIS OF PERSONAL EXPERIENCE

Pathology

In my series of 31 intramedullary tumors, 10 were benign low-grade astrocytomas (Table 37.1). In approximately half of these astrocytomas, regardless of previous radiation, I was able to develop a plane around the tumor and remove it grossly. Anatomically, these resectable tumors were similar in appearance to the cystic cerebellar astrocytomas. They were often associated with cysts of varying volumes, and the lining of the cyst was gliotic, thin-walled, and not tumorous, according to representative biopsies. In many instances, cysts of unequal volume were present at both the rostral and caudal extent of the tumor. The interface between the resectable astrocytoma and the normal but compressed cord was well defined and consisted of a thin gliotic layer traversed by small adhesions representing blood vessels and gliotic tissue (Fig. 37.1). The primary blood supply for these relatively avascular tumors came from the ventral median raphe region. These vessels tended to be small, and in no instance were the tumors highly vascular. The internal consistency of the astro-

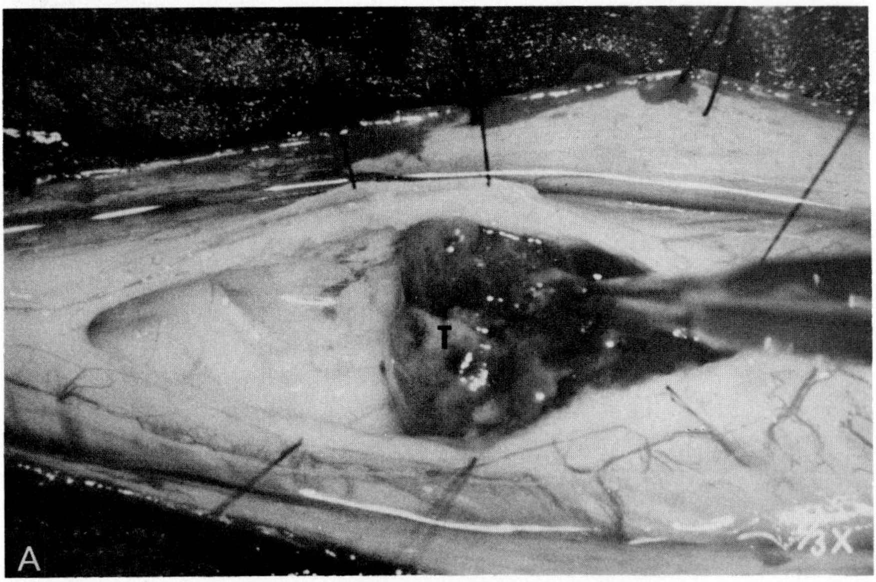

FIG. 37.1. (*A*) Operative photograph showing myelotomy with traction on intramedullary astrocytoma as the tumor is being removed from the dorsal central portion of the cord. *T*, tumor.

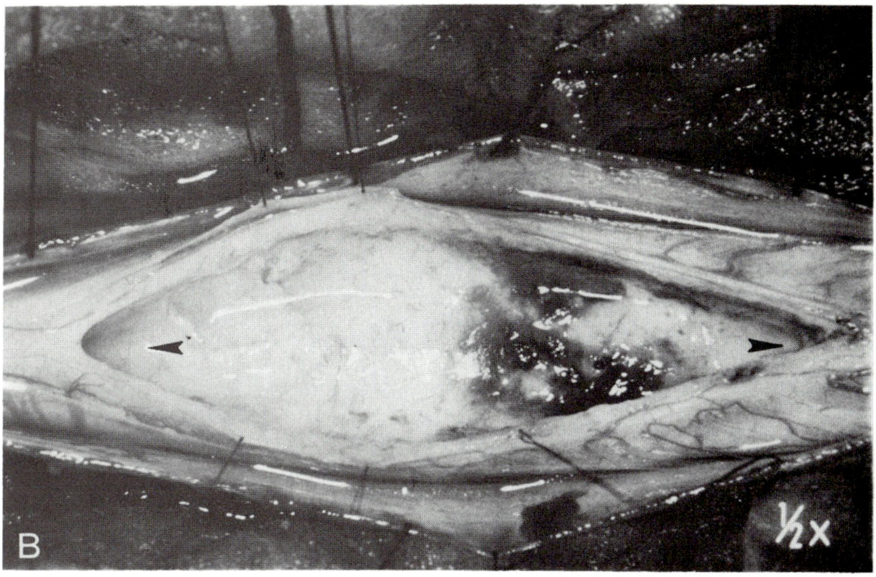

FIG. 37.1. (*B*) Interior of the spinal cord after total resection of astrocytoma associated with cysts at either end of the tumor. *Arrows*, cysts.

cytoma was firm to soft but generally uniform. The color of the tumor was distinguishable from the surrounding normal cord tissue. The astrocytoma, like other well-defined intramedullary tumors, tends to be elliptical in shape, does not have significant "pseudopod" extensions into the surrounding cord tissue, and is located toward the dorsal aspect of the cord. It would appear that the fibrous nature of the central canal near the ventral median raphe prevents the tumor from growing predominantly in this direction and, therefore, its growth tends toward the dorsal aspect of the cord, lying only millimeters under the dorsal pial surface of the spinal cord (Fig. 37.2). Neither do the tumors appear to be eccentric. These tumors, as with other intramedullary tumors, may gain enormous size despite minimal symptoms and signs.

Those astrocytomas which were not totally definable from the spinal cord had varying degrees of resectable portions. In some, the tumor appeared grossly removed while histologic examination of the specimen showed inclusion of anterior horn cells surrounded by tumor (Fig. 37.3). This establishes the infiltrating nature of at least a portion of the tumor. In some instances these tumors were associated with cysts, and it was in this part of the tumor that a plane could best be identified between tumor and spinal cord (Fig. 37.4). Unfortunately, beyond this point, the tumor often shaded imperceptibly into the surrounding spinal cord and was impossible to remove totally. In those areas, planes were ill-defined, and

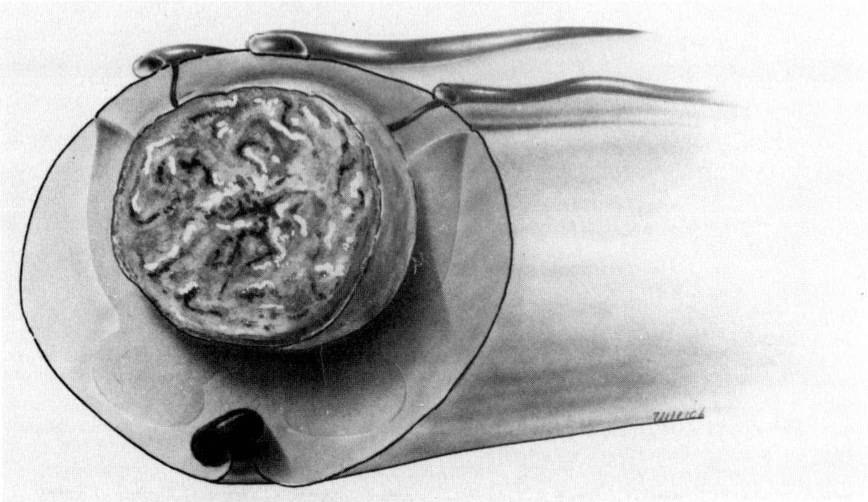

FIG. 37.2. Drawing showing the relationship of most intramedullary tumors which lie more toward the dorsal aspect of the spinal cord.

color changes were gradual between the normal and abnormal so that one could not expect to create a clean division between tumor and spinal cord.

In the more malignant varieties of astrocytoma (glioblastoma), the tumor tended to be more vascular and hemorrhagic without a distinguishable plane between tumor and spinal cord. In many instances the tumor would be exophytic in an eccentric position at the dorsal or lateral surface of the spinal cord (Fig. 37.5). Even though part of the interior of these tumors could be removed, their growth was rapid and unregulated by any form of treatment.

The other large group of intramedullary tumors are the ependymomas, all of which in my series were benign. Unlike the astrocytoma, a number of these tumors occur in the region of the conus medullaris of the spinal cord and in this situation may be both intrinsic and extrinsic (Fig. 37.6). They may also be associated with cysts and invariably with a well-defined anatomical and color differential between tumor and the spinal cord. Their interface with the normal spinal cord is through fine adhesions around their circumference, except for the ventromedian area, where the major blood supply enters the tumor. Although somewhat more vascular as a group than the astrocytoma, they have an easily controlled blood supply. The shape and size relationship to the spinal cord are similar to the astrocytomas. In one instance, we observed the presence of an ependymoma associated with a small rostral component that was a subependymal astrocytoma.

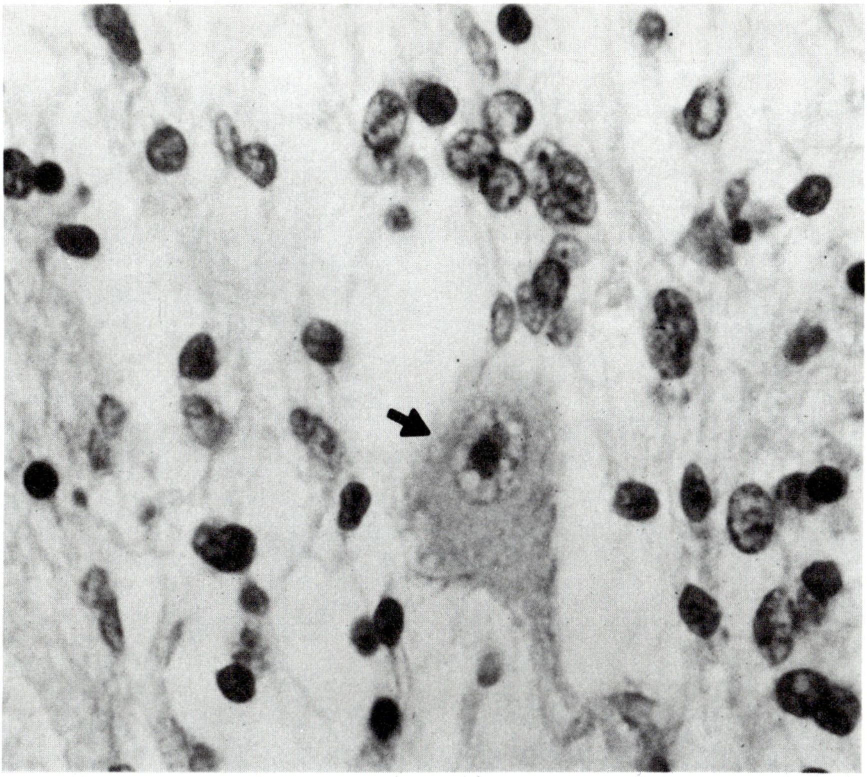

FIG. 37.3. Photomicrograph (×250) from specimen of a grossly removed low grade astrocytoma from the cervical spinal cord of a child. The infiltrating nature of the tumor is characterized by the astrocytic tumor cells surrounding an anterior horn cell (*arrow*).

Two dermoid tumors were primarily intramedullary, but a small portion was visible at the dorsal surface of the spinal cord (Fig. 37.7). In one instance, this portion of the tumor was associated with a fibrous band that penetrated the dura leading to the extraspinal tissue. The interior of the tumor was filled with grumous material containing hairs. The capsule of the tumor was diaphenous and partially adherent to the spinal cord. These tumors, in gaining a large size, were located in the region of the conus medullaris and penetrated the cord from dorsal to ventral.

The single case of a teratoma represents a rare variety of intramedullary tumor. It was encapsulated, located in the conus, and had a markedly irregular configuration within the substance of the spinal cord. It could be removed totally and had a variegated internal consistency. Of similar rarity, was the occurrence of a cavernous angioma which was associated with a 14-year history of spinal cord symptomatology and was both intrinsic and exophitic (Fig. 37.8). It had the appearance of a thrombosed

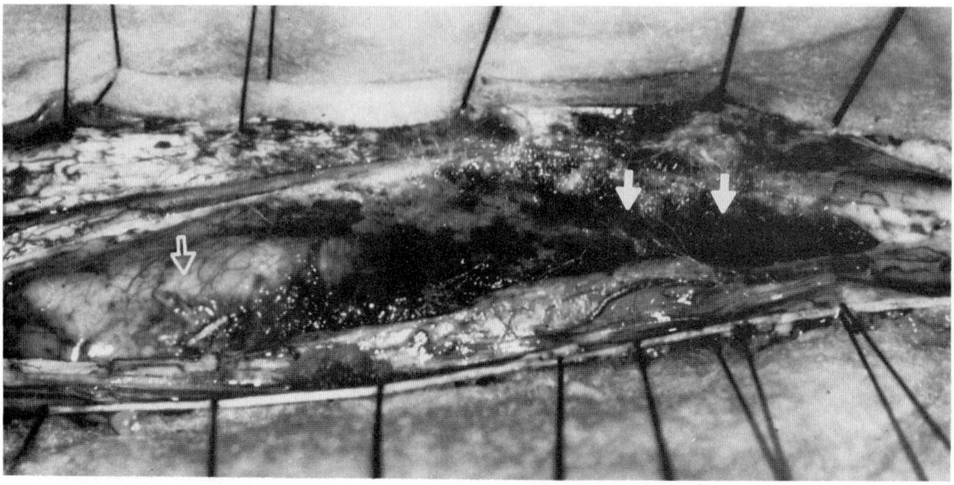

FIG. 37.4. Operative photograph of a portion of an intramedullary low grade astrocytoma which extended throughout the entire spinal cord. At the upper portion one sees the remains of a cyst (*open arrow*) from which a large amount of tumor has been removed from the portion of the spinal cord (*two arrows together* denote the area where the tumor blended with the spinal cord tissue and could not be further removed).

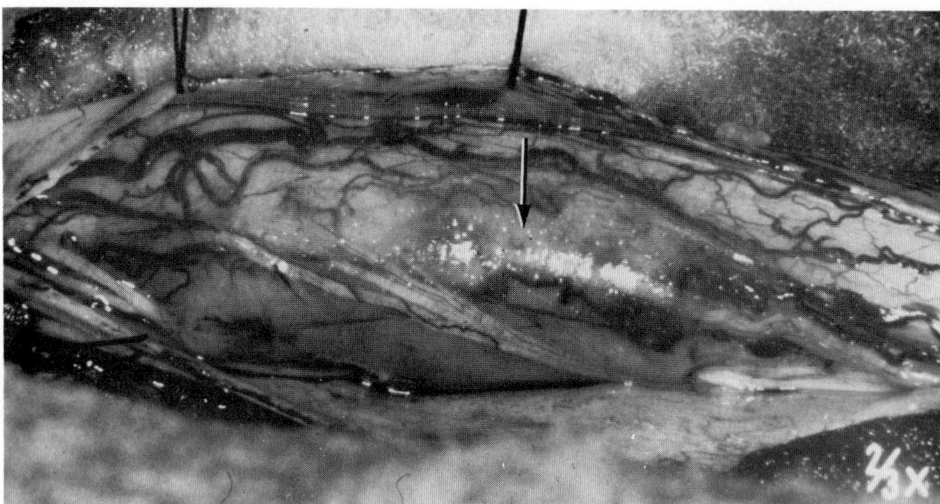

FIG. 37.5. Operative photograph of the dorsal surface of the spinal cord of a thoracic spinal cord infiltrated by a glioblastoma which is distorting the normal surface anatomy of the cord and blends with the cord tissue. *Arrow*, a portion of the glioblastoma.

intramedullary arteriovenous malformation (AVM), with poorly defined planes between it and the interior of the spinal cord, while occupying approximately 90% of the interior of the spinal cord. It could not be resected *in toto*.

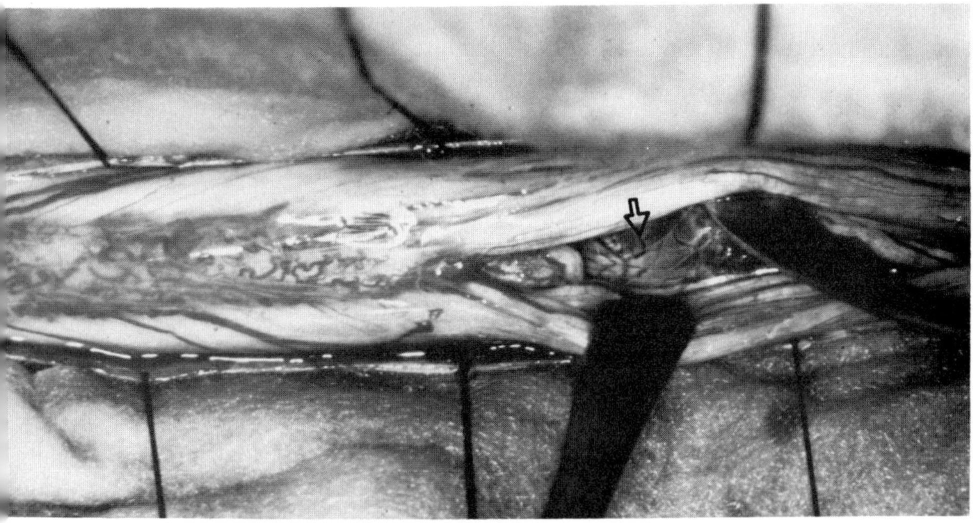

FIG. 37.6. Operative photograph with retraction of the nerve roots of the cauda equina showing an ependymoma (*arrow*) both intrinsic and extrinsic to the region of the conus.

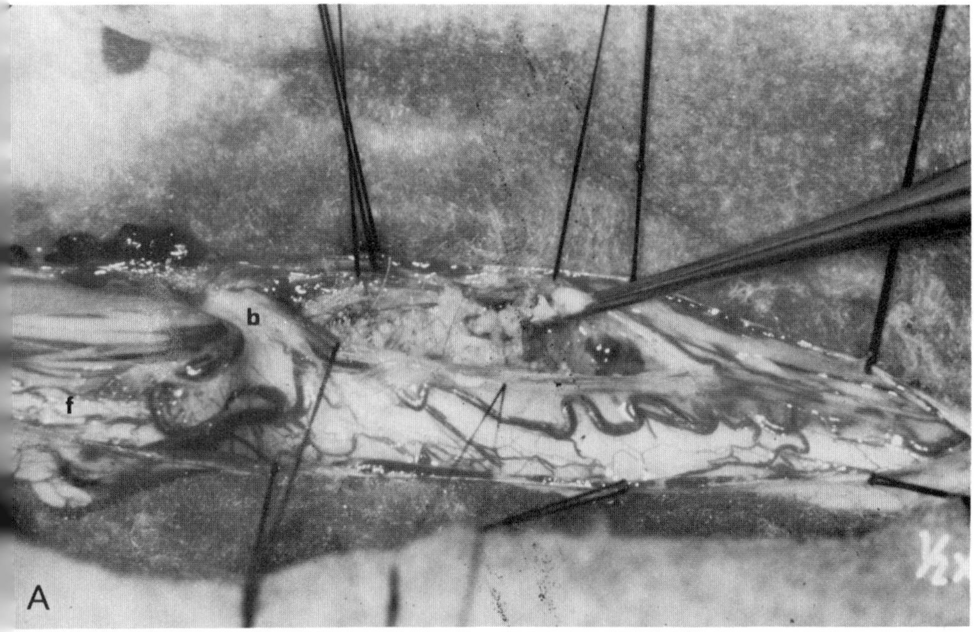

FIG. 37.7. (*A*) Operative photograph of the conus of the spinal cord involved by an intramedullary dermoid. Associated abnormalities of a fibrous band (*b*) to the dura and an enlarged filum terminale (*f*) are noted. A myelotomy exposes the dorsal surface of the tumor.

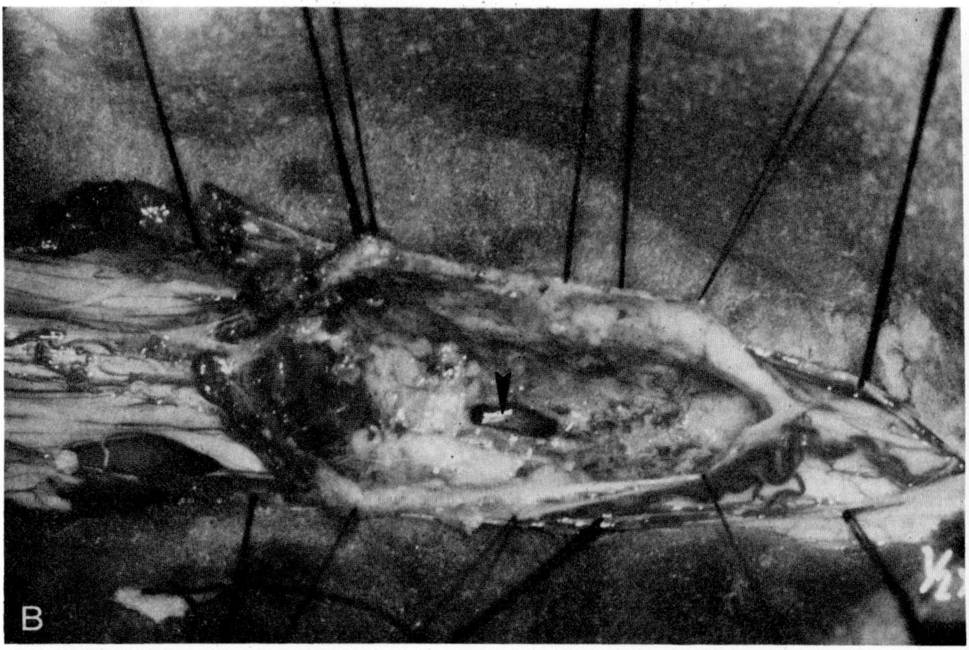

FIG. 37.7. (*B*) Cord held widely open by stay sutures following removal of intramedullary dermoid, which extended from dorsal to ventral, leaving a defect in the anterior margin of the cord (*arrow*).

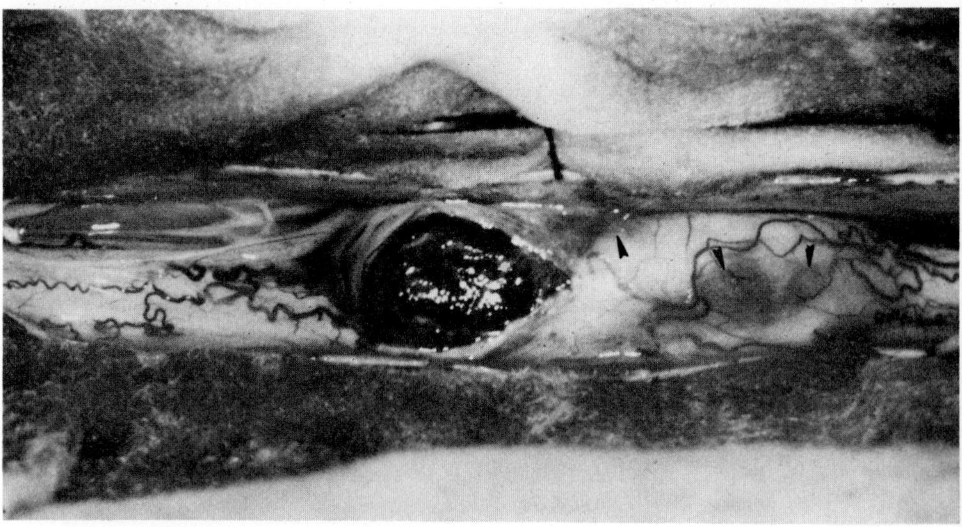

FIG. 37.8. Operative photograph of the conus region of the spinal cord showing a cavernous angioma both intrinsic and extrinsic to the cord. *Arrowheads indicate multiple areas of intrinsic involvement of the spinal cord.*

The two cases of hemangioblastoma were identical in unusual anatomical appearance. Both of these lesions occupied a discrete two segmental area in the upper cervical region, were visible on the dorsal surface of the cord, and resided, for the most part, in an intramedullary position. They were both associated with a uniform enlargement of the spinal cord that extended 5 to 6 segments caudally, as observed on the myelogram and at surgery. In one of these cases, incision into the widened spinal cord below the obvious pathology was negative for tumor or cyst. In both cases, follow-up myelography done months after the resection of the hemangioblastoma showed a return of the spinal cord below the level of the lesion to a normal or atrophic caliber (Fig. 37.9). The explanation of this enlargement, lacking cyst or identifiable tumor within this portion of the spinal cord, was not apparent. We presumed that the hemangioblastoma had created spinal cord edema or venous congestion that extended beyond the tumor due to the vascular shunting within the tumor.

Clinical Features

The clinical syndrome produced by these tumors tends to be stereotyped and related to the location of the tumor and to the age of the patient. In children the presentation is primarily one of a gait disturbance with appendicular or spinal deformities. The latter takes the form of a scoliosis (often under treatment by orthopedic surgeons), the former associated with deformities of the feet or intrinsic muscles of the hands. The gait disturbance is commensurate with the deformity and or weakness produced by the tumor. Pain in the younger child is not a prominent early symptom. In the adult, unlike children, radicular or a girdle type of pain is an early and persistent symptom. The progression of the disorder in children and adults is insidious, often unrelenting. The chain of events is weakness and spasticity involving the extremities, decreased posterior column function with impairment of position sense, and other sensation below the level of the lesion. Involvement of the pain and temperature pathways tends to be late in the course of tumor growth. A typical pattern of dissociated sensory loss in the upper extremities seen with cervical cysts or syringomyelia was not frequently noted with intramedullary tumors of this region. Those lesions both in children and in adults that involve the conus medullaris region of the spinal cord are often associated with early symptomatology related to bladder dysfunction. In children this may take the form of failure of toilet training and enuresis while in the adult this takes the form of stress incontinence. In many cases, because of the insidious and ill-defined progression of symptomatology, these disorders were not recognized for their true nature until many years had passed.

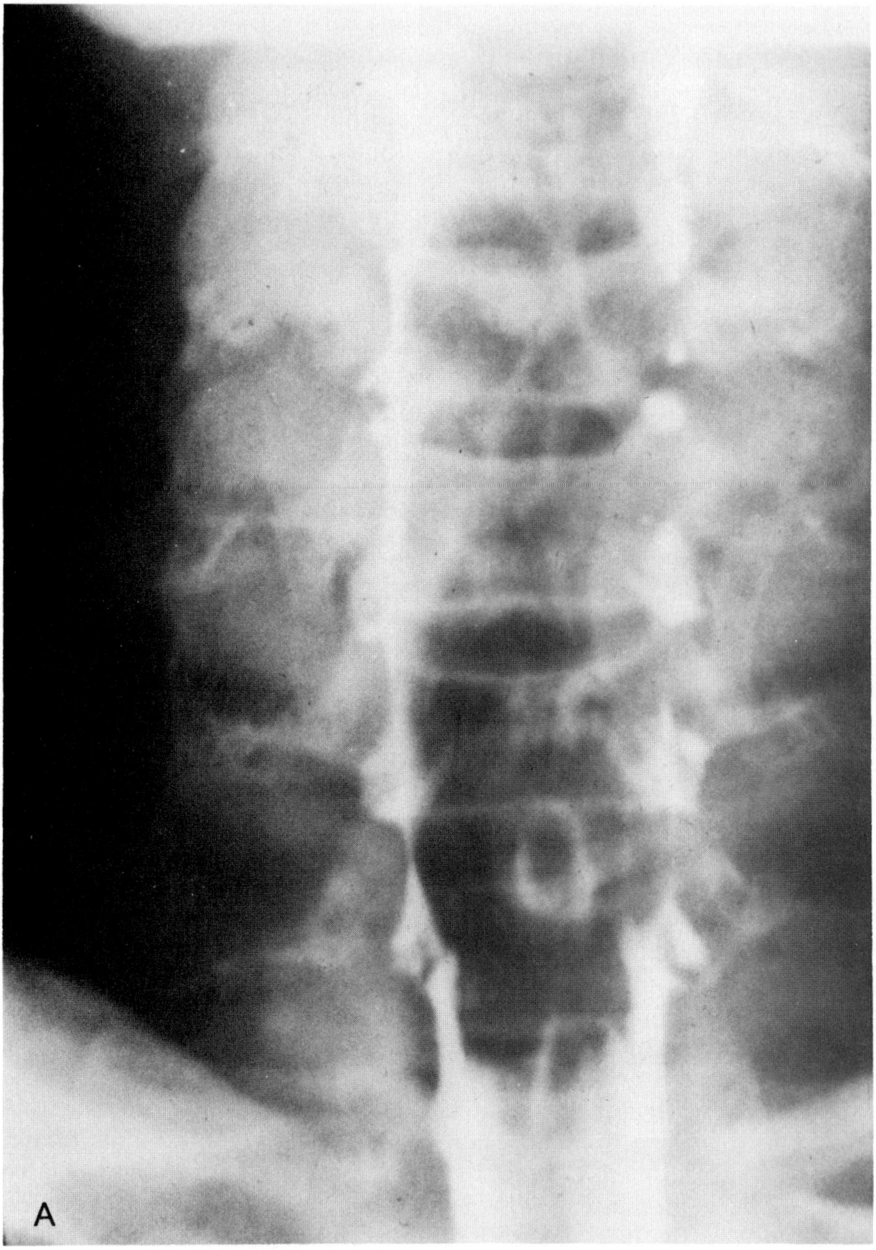

FIG. 37.9. (*A*) Myelogram showing widening of the entire cervical spinal cord by intramedullary process.

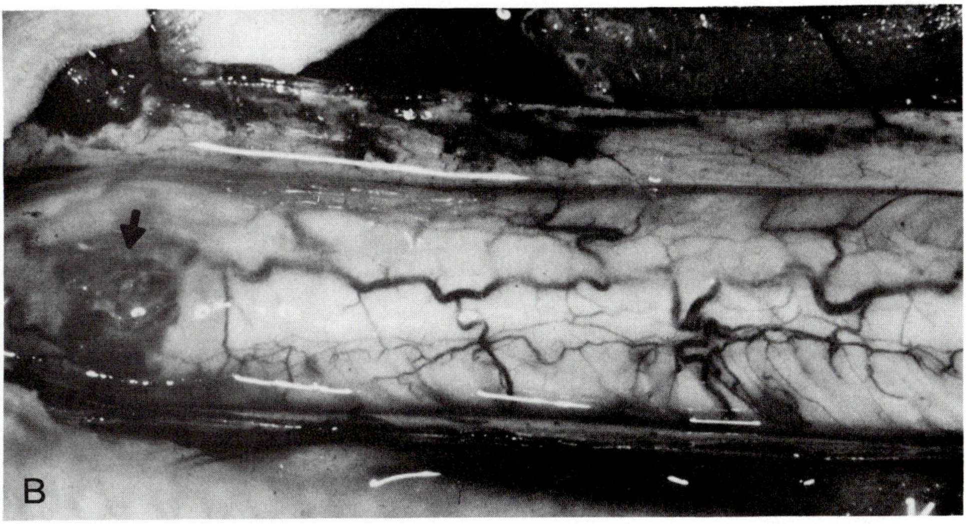

FIG. 37.9. (*B*) Exposure of the spinal cord showing the hemangioblastoma (*arrow*) localized to the upper segments of the cervical spinal cord with unexplained widening of the remainder of the spinal cord extending caudally.

Radiological Findings

Changes seen on the routine x-ray views of the spinal canal depend on the growth characteristics of the tumor more than they do on the nature of the tumor. In approximately 50% of the cases, there will be changes that include widening of the interpedicular distance, widening of the spinal canal in general, and scalloping of the posterior margin of the vertebral bodies.

The presence of an intramedullary tumor is best defined by a standard myelogram. If necessary because of complete block, the dye should be placed above the lesion as well as below in order to define the entire extent of the tumor. Currently, the definition as to the location of the tumor and confirmation that the tumor is within the spinal cord, rather than compressing it from anteriorly, are obtained by the use of metrizamide and computed tomography (CT scan). This will give exquisite detail as to the exact location of the tumor, and in some cases with refined scan technique it may demonstrate the consistency of the intramedullary process showing a cystic as opposed to solid tumor. In rare cases, contrast enhancement of the intramedullary component of the tumor may be observed on the CT scan. Spinal angiography has not been of significant value in the diagnosis or identification of the type of intramedullary tumor, except for the hemangioblastoma. In the latter instance, one may

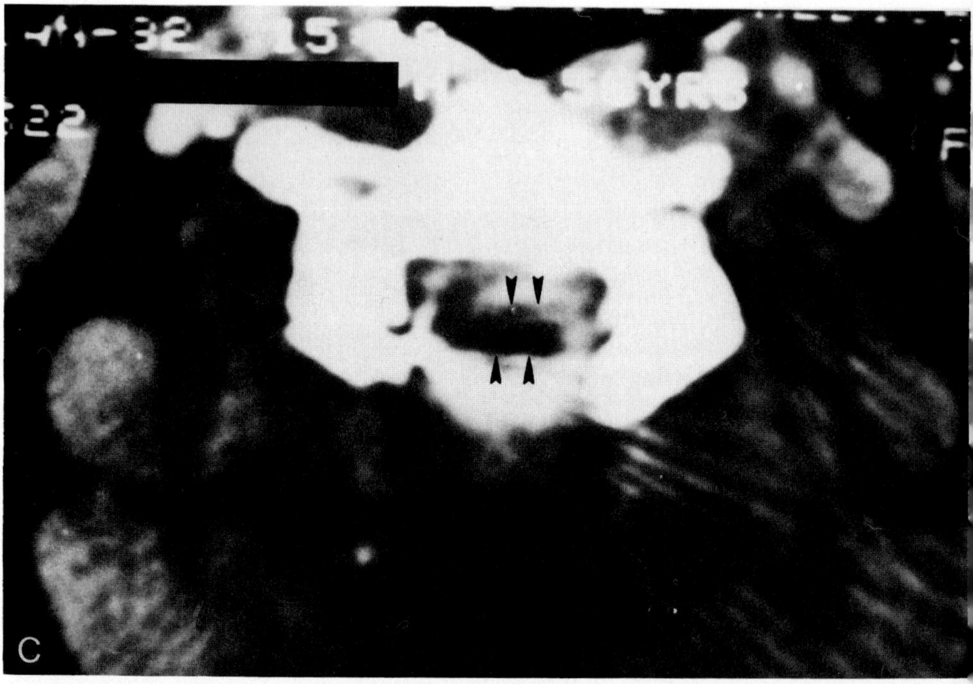

FIG. 37.9. (*C*) **Metrizamide CT study performed on the same patient 9 months after** surgery at the intermediate level of cervical enlargement now showing an atrophic spinal cord (*arrowheads*). This area was well removed from the hemangioblastoma and initially represented an unexplained widening of the spinal cord associated with the hemangioblastoma at a higher level.

suspect this tumor when prominent vascular markings are seen on the myelograms, although many of the intramedullary tumors are associated with distended venous channels below the level of the lesion.

Even in cases of intramedullary tumors which are of a size capable of obstructing the spinal subarachnoid spaces we have not been concerned about shifts of tumor and spinal cord and rapid deterioration of the patient following myelography. Therefore, surgery can be scheduled on an elective basis once the nature and extent of the tumor have been diagnosed from the various x-ray evaluations.

The patient is prepared for surgery by steroid medication and a medical evaluation that is aimed at turning up any coagulation deficiencies or any pulmonary problems, especially in the instance of cervical intramedullary tumor, in which one may be confronted by additional respiratory problems postoperatively. It is amazing how many of these patients who have taken aspirin or other platelet-inhibiting medications to relieve their pain do not make the physician aware of these circumstances prior to operation. Such medications may create difficult problems in terms of hemostasis. The operation is discussed in detail with the patient and family, indicating that these tumors often occupy a high percentage of the intramedullary space severely compressing spinal cord tissue and that their symptomatology and signs may not truly reflect the true extent of the tumor. The implication of this is that any additional injury or compression to the spinal cord may lead to a neurological disaster during and immediately after the operation. In the case of cervical intramedullary tumors, they should be warned that it may be necessary to maintain intubation for 24–48 hours postoperatively to ensure, in the awake patient, an adequate airway and ventilation. It is also well-established that the patient's postoperative deficits are related most closely to the preoperative condition of the patient. Therefore, an individual who has been ravished by the disease process prior to operation and has major neurological deficits such as paraplegia or quadriplegia may not be expected to gain much recovery, even though the tumor may be successfully removed. Those with lesser neurological deficits can expect improvement after successful removal of the tumor.

Surgical Technique

The majority of operations, regardless of the site of the tumor, have been carried out with the patient in the prone position. In those lesions which involve the cervical region, because flexion on the head on the cervical spine is necessary, a test in flexion for 15–20 minutes should be carried out with the patient awake before the operation to see if he/she can tolerate this position. The reason for operating on the patients in the prone position is to maximize the use of the surgical assistant. The operating microscope may be used so that the surgeon and his assistant work vis-à-vis across the operating table. In this fashion the assistant may be able to use both hands in assisting the surgeon in the removal of the tumor. This is important, as will be recorded later, in terms of providing traction and countertraction in order to divide the adhesions between the tumor and the spinal cord tissue. The area of surgery is kept relatively high above the heart in order to maximize venous drainage and prevent any congestion around the area of the surgery. A free abdomen or chest, as well as excellent ventilation, is absolutely essential. The midline incision is utilized, and a relatively wide laminectomy sparing the intervertebral articulations is carried out. In many of these patients, especially in children, because of the tumor there is local atrophy and weakness of the paraspinal muscles and, therefore, the structural integrity and stability of the spine must be preserved whereever possible. It is not only for this reason that the joint spaces are preserved but also for this reason that a laminotomy has been recommended in the case of children, as opposed to laminectomy. The removal of the posterior elements and then replacement after the operative procedure are more effective in preserving spinal stability than anything else that can be done at the time of the operative procedure.

In most instances, the tumor spans a number of segments in an elliptical or fusiform fashion. The dura will be tense due to the underlying compression by tumor and should be opened at either extreme of the tumor. In the caudal region one is more apt to encounter dilated veins, and therefore it may be safer to open the dura from the rostral region. In rare instances the tumor protruding from the spinal cord may be adherent to the dura, especially when the tumor has been previously operated on or treated by radiation. In those instances, we have found dense adhesions between the dura and the spinal cord which may require sharp dissection to liberate under the microscope. Unfortunately, this scar tends to obscure the plane that one wishes to develop between the tumor and the spinal cord.

Once the entire area of spinal cord widening has been exposed, one must select a site for myelotomy. In the minority of instances, the tumor will be visible through the translucent dorsal or dorsolateral portions of the spinal cord. In most instances, the tumor lies well enough beneath the surface so that it is not readily visible (Fig. 37.10). A myelotomy should be carried out as close to the midline as possible. A stringent criteria that must be followed is that the incision be straight and parallel to the longitudinal plane of the spinal cord. With the ladder-like arrangement of arteries and veins that occurs over the dorsal surface of the spinal cord, in performing a myelotomy it will be necessary to interrupt a number of small vascular channels. This is accomplished with the bipolar cautery set at low level under irrigation, and the myelotomy is then made by a very sharp dissection. The myelotomy should be carried over the entire extent of widening of the spinal cord so that any planes between the tumor and the spinal cord will not be missed by a too short myelotomy (Fig. 37.11). Once this has been performed, the pial margins are held back with fine sutures under tension opening the cord as one would open a book (Fig. 37.12). If the myelotomy has been extensive, a plane between tumor and spinal cord will be readily visible. This plane is further developed by gentle use of dissectors, bipolar cautery, and cottonoids so that the tumor at its dorsal, lateral, and rostocaudal extent becomes apparent. If one is fortunate to encounter a cyst at either or both ends of the tumor, it significantly facilitates the removal of the tumor. In many instances, it may not be necessary to debulk the interior of the tumor in order to effect a total removal. If there is any question about undue compression of the spinal cord tissue with the removal of

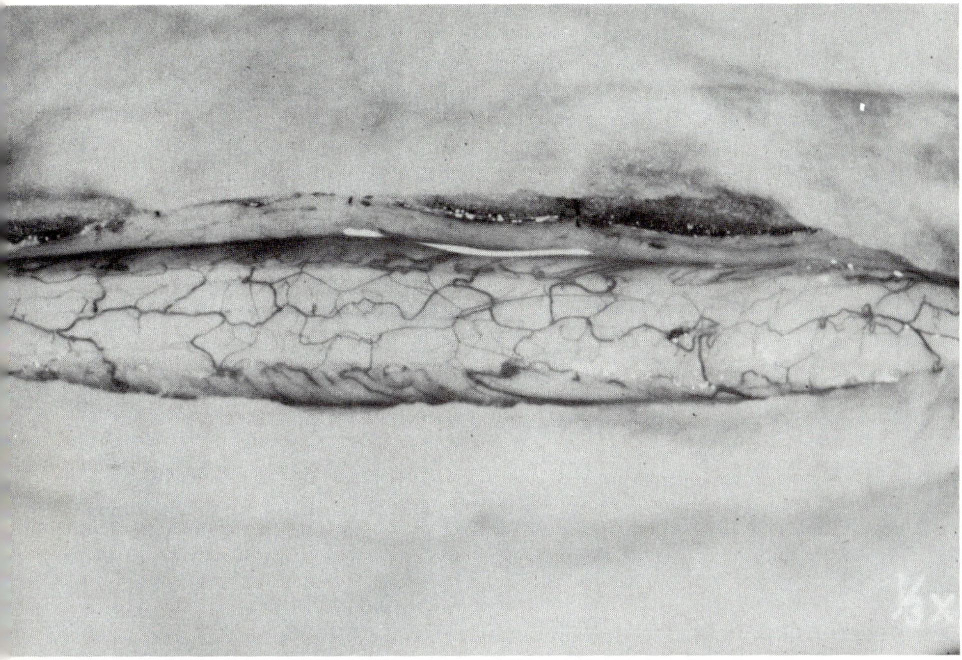

FIG. 37.10. Exposed surface of the cervical spinal cord with an intramedullary tumor. No visible evidence of the tumor is seen on the dorsal surface of the spinal cord.

the tumor, then the interior of the tumor should be resected first. In terms of debulking the interior of the tumor, care must be taken not to allow any bleeding which spills over and obscures the plane between the external surface of the tumor and the spinal cord. It is absolutely essential that this area be kept dry so that the surgeon may carefully follow the contour and coloration provided by the margin of a resectable tumor. It is in these maneuvers that it is important to utilize one's assistant in terms of traction on the tumor, irrigation, and even cutting of the adhesions between tumor and the surrounding spinal cord (Fig. 37.13). Combining these maneuvers allows one to remove the tumor expeditiously (Fig. 37.14). In the case of the astrocytoma there may be a plane which encompasses the majority of the tumor but in some places tends to fade into the surrounding spinal cord. In these instances, judgment must be used in defining where this plane is or should be, and removal should be carried out radically.

Epstein and Epstein (3) have recently reported the use of the CUSA (*C*avitron *U*ltrasonic *S*urgical *A*spirator, Cooper Medical, Stamford, Conn.) in the removal of intramedullary astrocytomas in children. They state that these tumors are probably different from those in adults, are

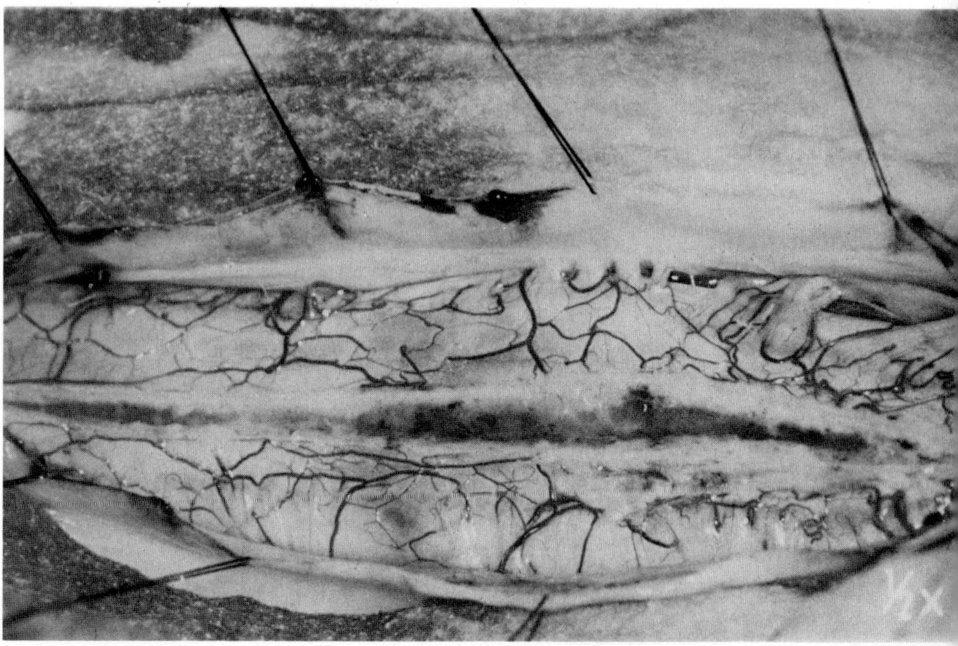

FIG. 37.11. Extensive myelotomy performed over the dorsal surface of the spinal cord in a longitudinal direction exposing the characteristic differentiation of the intramedullary spinal cord tumor. In this case, the tumor is an ependymoma.

of slower and more indolent growth and, for the most part, can be debulked, not removing all fragments, with excellent postoperative results. The use of the CUSA permits one to work very close to the ill-defined margin of these tumors without distorting or otherwise injuring the normal tissue. Utilizing this technique, the spinal cord has been filleted over many segments, and a radical removal of the tumors has been accomplished. Hemostasis should be accurate after maximum resection of the tumor.

Recently, we have utilized sensory evoked potential monitoring during radical tumor removal. The potentials are recorded from the spinal cord above the surgery and from the cortex (Fig. 37.15). The usefulness of this procedure is yet to be determined. It appears to warn when cord function is affected during the removal of tumor. However, if the surgeon is carefully dissecting with the microscope, it may not be necessary to give up at this point since the loss of potentials appears reversible on occasion.

In the case of the dermoid tumors, it may be impossible to remove every filament of the fine tumor capsule, in which case one should attempt

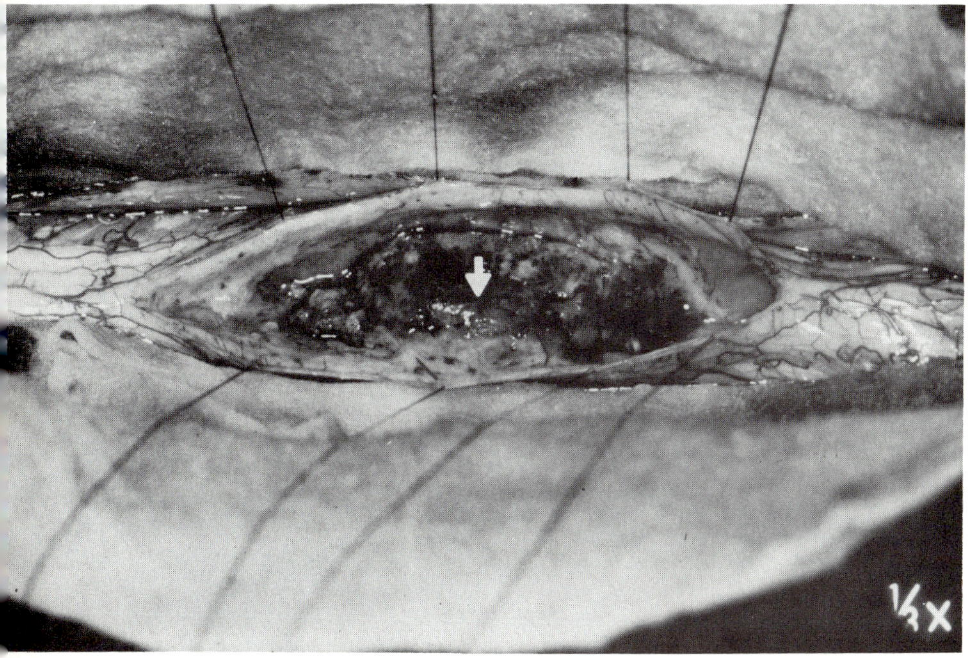

FIG. 37.12. Myelotomy opened by fine traction sutures to the pial margin, revealing the intramedullary tumor (*arrow*), which has been partially dissected from the surrounding spinal cord.

the most radical removal possible without injury to the surrounding spinal cord tissue.

In the instance of the hemangioblastoma, it is treated in similar fashion to hemangioblastomas of the cerebellum or to arteriovenous malformations, in that the arterial supply to the lesion which is obvious is secured first, and the single- and multiple-draining veins are preserved until the end of the resection (21). In certain instances, the hemangioblastoma may be associated with small or large cysts which are drained when the solid component of the tumor is removed.

I have found no need to appose by suture the pial margins of the opened spinal cord. These are released and tend to collapse within the spinal cord (Fig. 37.16). I have not had the development of cysts under tension within the spinal cord following these resections.

The dura is closed or a dural substitute is used, preferably fascia, to close the opening. I prefer not to cover the exposed spinal cord with Gelfoam (Gelfoam; Upjohn Co., Kalamazoo, Mich.) alone, although this procedure has been recommended by others as a satisfactory means of

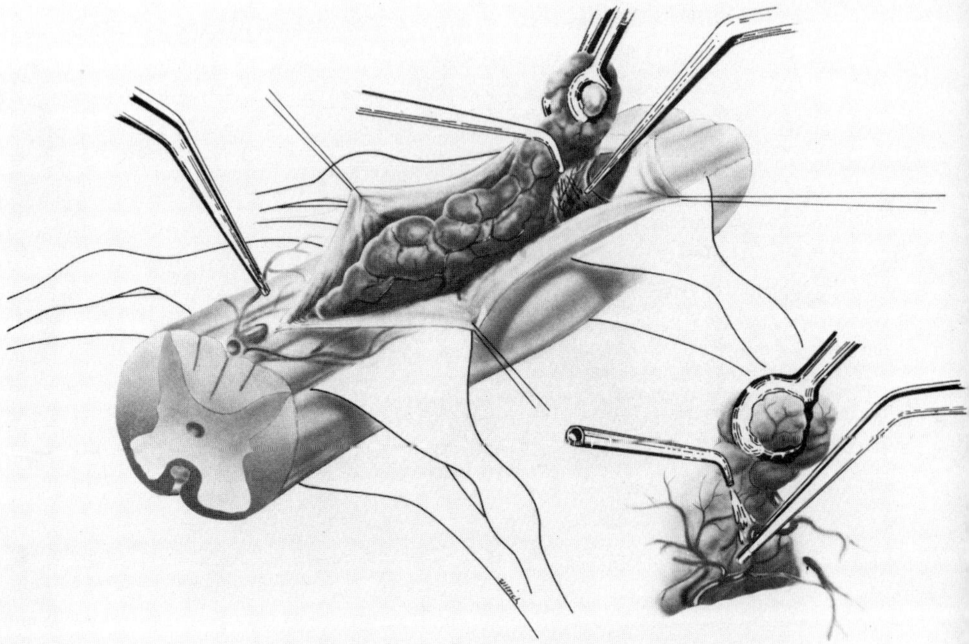

FIG. 37.13. Drawing showing the essential steps in the removal of an intramedullary spinal cord tumor, including the opened myelotomy held by stay sutures, bipolar coagulation of the adhesions, and vessels between the tumor and spinal cord with irrigation and traction upon the tumor. (Courtesy of *Clinical Neurosurgery*, Vol. 26).

closure. One is doubly concerned about those patients that have been previously operated on and radiated in terms of the integrity and water-tightness of the closure. Any leakage from the area of operation may lead to a disastrous infection or, at the very least, to a nagging inflammatory reaction in the surrounding tissues and agony for both the surgeon and the patient in the postoperative period. If a laminotomy has been done, then these fragments are wired or sewn back into position, and the muscles are then closed with the fascia in meticulous fashion. I generally use drains in the epidural space if the integrity of the dura has been reconstituted. These drains are left for a period of 12 hours.

It is most important to ensure adequate airway and pulmonary function postoperatively. In the cervical region the cervical collar is utilized to support the suture line for a week or two, but the patients are generally

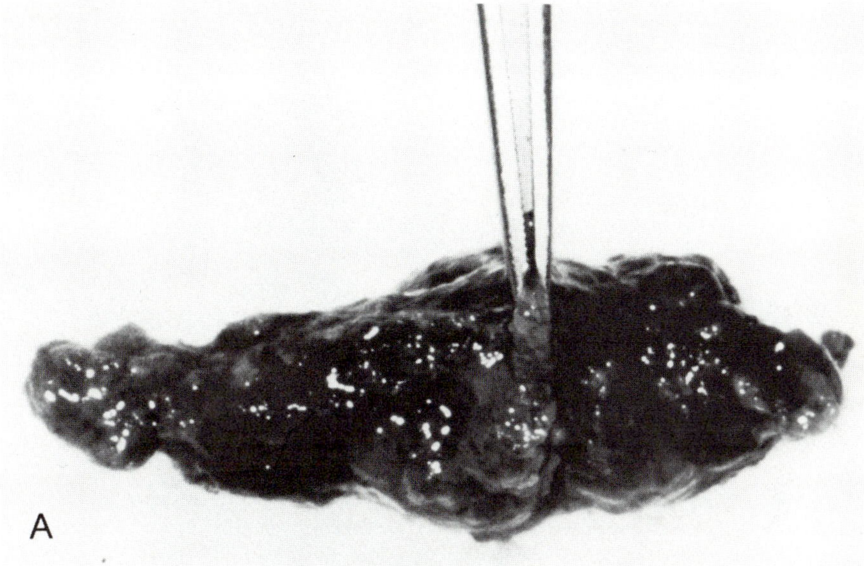

FIG. 37.14. (*A*) Intramedullary ependymoma removed *in toto*.

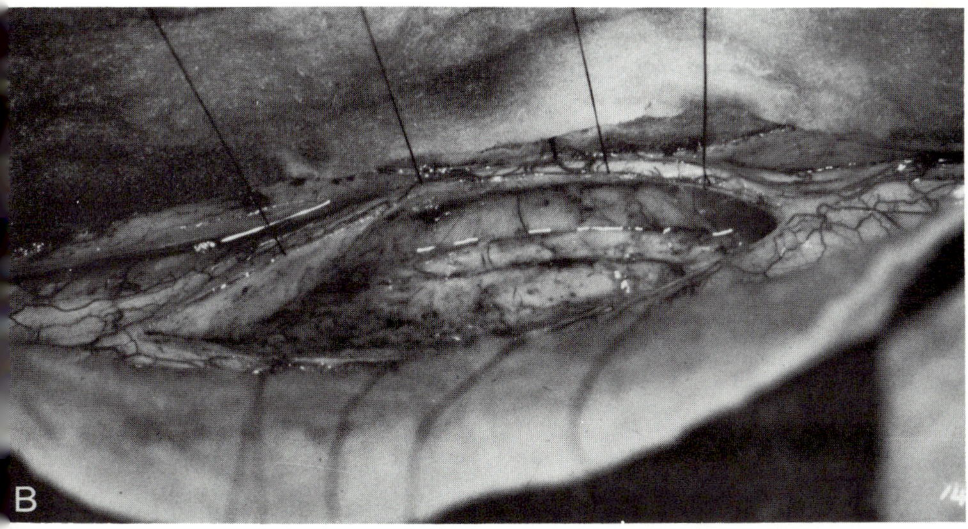

FIG. 37.14. (*B*) Interior of the spinal cord clear of tumor, with margins still being kept open by stay sutures. There was no grossly visible tumor in this clean resection of an ependymoma.

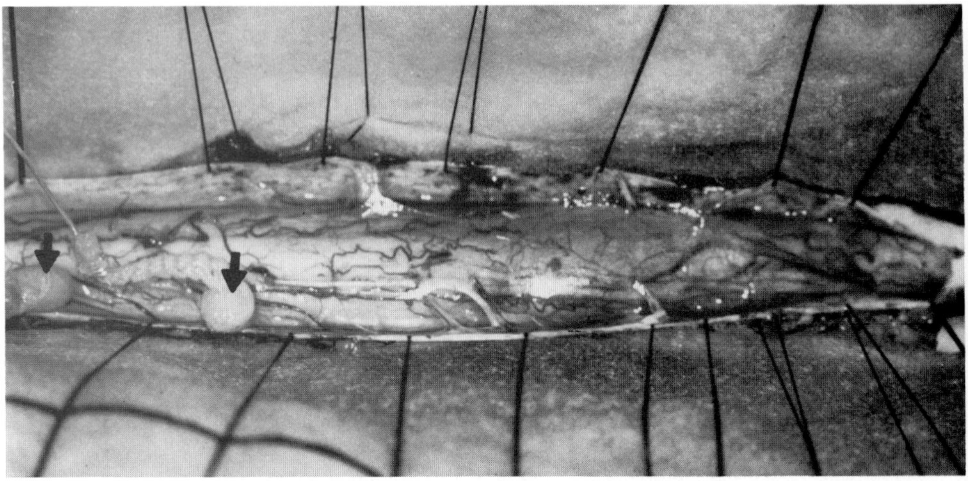

FIG. 37.15. Operative exposure of an infiltrating low grade astrocytoma of the thoracic spinal cord. Note electrodes (*arrows*) used in the sensory evoked potentials study in this case.

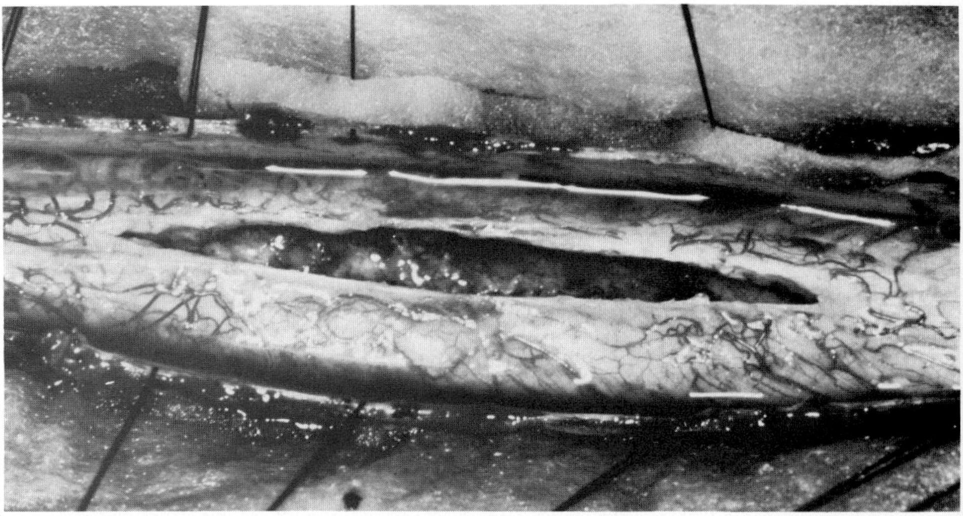

FIG. 37.16. Stay sutures removed from the pial margins and dorsal columns, thinned by the total removal of an intramedullary cord tumor are allowed to fall back into position. No apposition of the pial margins is attempted.

mobilized as quickly as possible following this surgery. Endotracheal tubes, when left in place, are generally removed 12–48 hours postoperatively. Any longer intubation should be replaced by a tracheotomy, if one anticipates long-term respiratory problems.

Radiation Therapy

If the intramedullary tumor has been totally resected, no other treatment is required. In those astrocytomas where a scrap of tumor has been left in place, I have not utilized postoperative radiotherapy. The real dilemma comes in the various grades of astrocytoma when a significant portion of tumor has been left behind following attempts at radical resection. Radiotherapy has not only been recommended in these cases but also has been recommended with the ependymoma as primary therapy (12–14, 18, 19). I feel that there is no substantive information that would indicate radiotherapy has any effect whatsoever on the ependymoma. In fact, it is probably deleterious since we have reason to believe that gliotic changes are produced in the interior of the spinal cord, and no impact is noted on the tumor. In those patients that have received previous radiotherapy in appropriate doses I have found a high incidence of intramedullary gliosis. This has been most apparent in those tumors of ependymal origin where I have found a thickened discoloration either rostral or caudal to the tumor in the central portion of the presumed normal spinal cord. This area has been in the field of radiotherapy, and the tissue which has been biopsied shows intense gliosis, which is quite different in histological nature from the tumor. It is my opinion that this gliosis is a deleterious effect of the radiotherapy. In the case of astrocytoma, both benign and malignant, where there is a significant intramedullary component I have seen no proof of the effect of radiotherapy (1, 11, 15, 20). In children, radiotherapy to the growing spine may result in further spinal deformities or the onset of spinal deformities if these have not existed before (10, 16). Therefore, the removal must be as radical as possible, and I do not now recommend radiotherapy of the low-grade astrocytomas in which portions remain following surgery. Rather these patients should be watched; observed from a clinical viewpoint and appropriate radiographic studies when indicated. In the case of the malignant astrocytoma or glioblastoma we have had very discouraging results from the use of radiotherapy but nevertheless failing any other form of treatment to significantly retard the disastrous effects of the tumor growth, we have been utilizing radiotherapy in these cases. In the other intramedullary cord tumors that I have encountered, we have not utilized radiotherapy.

Results of Treatment

In my series of 31 intramedullary tumors, there has been no mortality (Table 37.2). The result of the surgery is predicated on the preoperative neurological condition of the patient. Those individuals who have maximum neurological deficits prior to the operation have made no significant functional recovery following the successful removal of the tumor. In

TABLE 37.2
Intramedullary Tumors

Operations	32
Operative Mortality	0
Postoperative Deterioration	7

those individuals with mild to modest neurological deficits, when the tumor has been totally removed, excellent functional recovery may be expected. In those instances where only a portion of the tumor has been removed, the subsequent course depends upon the growth pattern of the tumor. If the tumor growth is static or indolent, the neurological deficits may improve or remain static for many years. In the case of malignant tumors, the postoperative course tends to be disastrous with rapid growth and seeding of the tumor. I have not as yet used a second look operation to remove, many years from the primary surgery, more of these incompletely removed tumors. This, however, is a viable option and, in my estimation, is preferable to radiotherapy. If cysts in association with an incompletely removed tumor occur, these may be tapped percutaneously, alleviating symptoms and pressure within the spinal cord.

I have had no incidence of recurrence in those cases of totally removed tumors, which comprise the majority of this series, over a follow-up which varies from 6 months to 10 years. One can draw few conclusions from this statement since these disease processes, as previously mentioned, may span not only years but decades.

One unique problem in intramedullary tumor surgery and also with intramedullary vascular malformations has been the development of a pain syndrome following successful surgery. The physiological mechanism for this phenomenon is poorly understood, and the treatment defies the grasp of most physicians dealing with these problems. The pain is often comprehensive and involves many portions of the body. It is almost impossible to control except by psychological preparation and treatment of the patient pre- and postoperatively. I have seen no ameliorating effect from the use of various drugs or stimulators as used in other pain problems of spinal origin.

REFERENCES

1. DeSousa, A. L., Kalsbeck, J. E., Mealey, J., Campbell, R. L., and Hockey, A. Intraspinal tumors in children: A review of 81 cases. J. Neurosurg., *51:* 437–445, 1979.
2. Elsberg, C. A. *Tumors of the Spinal Cord and the Symptoms of Irritation and Compression of the Spinal Cord and Nerve Roots: Pathology, Symptomatology, Diagnosis, and Treatment.* Paul B. Hoeber, New York, 1925.
3. Epstein, F., and Epstein, N. Surgical management of "holocord" intramedullary spinal cord astrocytomas in children. J. Neurosurg., *54:* 829–832, 1981.
4. Fischer, G., and Mansuy, L. Total removal of intramedullary ependymomas: Follow-up study of 16 cases. Surg. Neurol., *14:* 243–249, 1980.

5. Garrido, E., and Stein, B. M. Microsurgical removal of intramedullary spinal cord tumors. Surg. Neurol., *7:* 215–219, 1977.
6. Greenwood, J., Jr. Intramedullary tumors of spinal cord: A follow-up study after total surgical removal. J. Neurosurg., *20:* 665–668, 1963.
7. Greenwood, J., Jr. Surgical removal of intramedullary tumors. J. Neurosurg., *26:* 276–282, 1967.
8. Guidetti, B. Intramedullary tumours of the spinal cord. Acta Neurochir. (Wien), *17:* 7–23, 1967.
9. Horrax, G., and Henderson, D. G. Encapsulated intramedullary tumor involving whole spinal cord from medulla to conus: Complete enucleation with recovery. Surg. Gynecol. Obstet., *68:* 8–819, 1939.
10. Katzman, H., Waugh, T., and Berdon, W. Skeletal changes following irradiation of childhood tumors. J. Bone Joint Surg., *51A:* 825–843, 1969.
11. Malis, L. I. Intramedullary spinal cord tumors. Clin. Neurosurg., *25:* 512–540, 1978.
12. Rand, R. W., and Rand, C. W. *Intraspinal Tumors of Childhood.* Charles C Thomas, Springfield, IL, 1960.
13. Schwade, J. G., Wara, W. M., Sheline, G. E., Sorgen, S., and Wilson, C. B. Management of primary spinal cord tumors. Int. J. Radiation Oncol. Biol. Phys., *4:* 389–393, 1978.
14. Sloff, J. L., Kernohan, J. W., and MacCarty, C. S. *Primary Intramedullary Tumors of the Spinal Cord and Filum Terminale.* W.B. Saunders, Philadelphia, 1964.
15. Stein, B. M. Surgery of intramedullary spinal cord tumors. Clin. Neurosurg., *26:* 529–542, 1979.
16. Tachdjian, M. O., and Matson, D. D. Orthopedic aspects of intraspinal tumors in infants and children. J. Bone Joint Surg., *47A:* 223–248, 1965.
17. Turnbull, F. Intramedullary tumors of the spinal cord. Clin. Neurosurg., *8:* 237–247, 1962.
18. Woltman, H. W., Kernohan, J. W., Adson, A. W., and Craig, W. M. Intramedullary tumors of spinal cord and gliomas of intradural portion of filum terminale: Fate of these patients who have these tumors. Arch. Neurol. Psychiatry, *65:* 378–395, 1951.
19. Wood, E. H., Berne, A. S., and Taveras, J. M. The value of radiation therapy in the management of intrinsic tumors of the spinal cord. Radiology, *63:* 11–24, 1954.
20. Woods, W. W., and Pimenta, A. M. Intramedullary lesions of the spinal cord: A study of 68 consecutive cases. Arch. Neurol. Psychiatry, *52:* 383–399, 1944.
21. Yasargil, M. G., Antic, J., Laciga, R., dePreux, J., Fideler, R. W., and Boone, S. C. The microsurgical removal of intramedullary spinal hemangioblastomas: Report of twelve cases and a review of the literature. Surg. Neurol., *6:*141–148, 1976.

Index

N

P

Q

R

S

T

Cumulative Index: 1972–1983 (Volumes 20–30)

F

G

H

I

N

O

P

R

T

U

V